...ok of

...cal

...esia

Handbook of **Clinical Anaesthesia**

third edition

Edited by

Brian J Pollard BPHARM MB CHB MD FRCA
Professor of Anaesthesia
University Department of Anaesthesia
Manchester Royal Infirmary
Manchester, UK

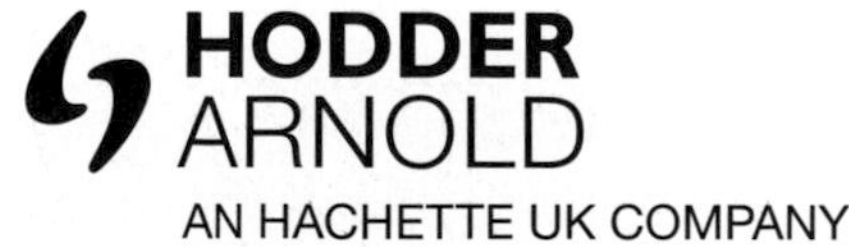

First published in Great Britain in 1996 by Pearson Professional Limited
Second edition 2004, Elsevier Ltd.

This third edition published in 2011 by
Hodder Arnold, an imprint of Hodder Education, an Hachette UK Company,
338 Euston Road, London NW1 3BH
http://www.hodderarnold.com

British Library Cataloguing in Publication Data
A catalogue record for this book is available from the British Library

Library of Congress Cataloging-in-Publication Data
A catalog record for this book is available from the Library of Congress

ISBN-13 978 1 444 108 620

1 2 3 4 5 6 7 8 9 10

Commissioning Editor: Gavin Jamieson
Project Editor: Joanna Silman
Production Controller: Joanna Walker
Cover Designer: Helen Townson

Typeset in 9/11 Rotis Semi Sans by MPS Limited, a Macmillan Company
Printed and bound in India by Replika Press

What do you think about this book? Or any other Hodder Arnold title?
Please visit our website: www.hodderarnold.com

This book is dedicated to my three children, Kathryn, Christine and Alexander. They are my future.

Contents

Contributors

Iurie Acalovschi MD PhD FCARCSI(HON) FRCA(HON)
Consultant and Professor Emeritus, Department of Anesthesia and Intensive Care, Octavian Fodor Emergency Clinical Hospital, Cluj-Napoca, Romania

José A Aguirre MD DESRA FMH(Anesthesiology) SGNOR(Emergency Medicine) SFG-LNA
Consultant Anesthetist, Balgrist University Hospital, Zurich, Switzerland

Baha Al-Shaikh FCARCSI FRCA
Consultant Anaesthetist and Honorary Senior Lecturer, William Harvey Hospital, Ashford, Kent, UK

Ian Appleby FRCA
National Hospital for Neurology and Neurosurgery, University College London Hospitals, London, UK

Dougal Atkinson MBBS MRCP(UK) FRCA
Consultant in Anaesthesia and Critical Care, Manchester Royal Infirmary, Manchester, UK

Craig R Bailey MB BS FRCA
Consultant Anaesthetist, Guys and St Thomas' NHS Foundation Trust, London, UK

Mark C Bellamy BA MBBS MA FRCA
Intensive Care Unit, St James's University Hospital, Leeds, UK

Alain Borgeat
Head of the Department of Anesthesiology, Orthopedic University Hospital Balgrist, Zurich, Switzerland

Carol L Bradbury FRCA
Specialist Registrar in Anaesthesia, University Hospitals Coventry and Warwickshire, Coventry, UK

David Brealey MRCP PhD FRCA
University College London Hospitals, London, UK

Helen Buglass MBChB FRCA
Consultant in Anaesthesia and Critical Care, Pinderfields Hospital, Wakefield, UK

Giorgio Capogna MD
Professor of Obstetric Anesthesia, University La Sapienza, Rome; Head of Department of Anesthesia, Città di Roma Hospital, Rome, Italy

Andrew J Charlton
Department of Paediatric Anaesthesia, Royal Manchester Children's Hospital, Manchester, UK

Thomas Allen Crozier MScBiol PhD MD
Department of Anesthesiology, University Medical Center, University of Göttingen, Germany

Stefan De Hert MD PhD
Professor, Department of Anesthesiology, University Hospital Ghent, Belgium

Susanne Eberl MD DEAA
Department of Anesthesiology, Academic Medical Center, Amsterdam, The Netherlands

Veronika Evers MD MAE
Department of Anesthesiology, Academic Medical Center, Amsterdam, The Netherlands

Jan Fräßdorf DESA MD
Staff Anesthesiologist, Department of Anaesthesiology, Academic Medical Centre (AMC), University of Amsterdam, The Netherlands

Amy Greengrass BM
Core Trainee in Anaesthesia, William Harvey Hospital, Ashford, Kent, UK

Stephen Greenhough BSc MB ChB FRCA
Department of Paediatric Anaesthesia, Royal Manchester Children's Hospital, Oxford Road, Manchester, UK

Tamsin Gregory BSc MBBS MRCP FRCA
National Hospital for Neurology and Neurosurgery, University College London Hospitals, London, UK

Rashan Haniffa FRCA MRCP
Academic Clinical Fellow in Anaesthesia, University College London Hospitals, London, UK

Richard J Harding MBBS BMedSci FRCA
Department of Anaesthesia, St James's University Hospital, Leeds, UK

David Highton MBChB FRCA
National Hospital for Neurology and Neurosurgery, University College London Hospitals, London, UK

Nicholas Hirsch FRCA FRCP
Department of Neuroanaesthesia and Neurocritical Care, The National Hospital for Neurology and Neurosurgery, University College London Hospitals, London, UK

Philip M Hopkins MB BS MD FRCA
Professor of Anaesthesia, University of Leeds; Honorary Consultant Anaesthetist, Leeds Teaching Hospitals NHS Trust, Leeds, UK

Marianne Hösele MD
Division of Anesthesiology for Neurosurgical and Craniofacial Surgery and Intensive Care Medicine, Medical University of Graz, Graz, Austria

Katharine Hunt FRCA
Consultant Neuroanaesthetist, National Hospital for Neurology and Neurosurgery, University College London Hospitals, London, UK

Chandran Jepegnanam FRCA
Consultant in Anaesthesia and Acute Pain Management, Department of Anaesthesia, Manchester Royal Infirmary, Central Manchester University Hospitals NHS Foundation Trust Hospital, Manchester, UK

Rohit Juneja
National Hospital for Neurology and Neurosurgery, University College London Hospitals, London, UK

Payal Kajekar FRCA
Specialty Registrar in Anaesthesia, University Hospitals Coventry and Warwickshire, Coventry, UK

Swati Karmarkar MD FRCA
Consultant Anaesthetist, Manchester Royal Infirmary, Manchester, UK

Rick Keays MD FRCP FRCA
Magill Department of Anaesthetics and Intensive Care, Chelsea & Westminster Hospital, London, UK

Paul Knott RN Dip HE BSc(Hons) PGCE
Resuscitation & Simulation Practitioner, Central Manchester University Hospitals, NHS Foundation Trust, Manchester, UK

Robin Kumar MBBS BSc FRCA
Clinical Fellow in Neuroanaesthesia, National Hospital for Neurology and Neurosurgery, Queen Square, London

Michelle Leemans
Department of Neuroanaesthesia and Neurocritical Care, The National Hospital for Neurology and Neurosurgery, University College London Hospitals, Queen Square, London, UK

William R Macnab BSc MBChB FRCA
Consultant Anaesthetist, Manchester Royal Infirmary, Manchester, UK

Gerlinde Mausser MD
Division of Anesthesiology for Neurosurgical and Craniofacial Surgery and Intensive Care Medicine Medical University of Graz, Graz, Austria

Denise McCarthy MB BCh BAO FCARCSI
Specialist Registrar in Anaesthesia, Department of Anaesthesia and Intensive Care Medicine, Cork University Hospital, Cork, Ireland

George H Meakin ChB MD FRCA
Consultant and Senior Lecturer, Department of Paediatric Anaesthesia, Royal Manchester Children's Hospital, Manchester, UK

Peter Meijer
Department of Anesthesiology, Academic Medical Center, Amsterdam, The Netherlands

Cyprian Mendonca MD FRCA
Consultant Anaesthetist and Honorary Senior Clinical Lecturer, University Hospitals Coventry and Warwickshire, Coventry, UK

Zoka Milan MD MSc PhD
Consultant Anaesthetist and Intensivist, St James's University Hospital, Leeds, UK

Lisa Milligan BSc(Hons) MBChB FRCA FFICM
Consultant in Anaesthetics and Intensive Care Medicine, Sherwood Forest Hospitals NHS Foundation Trust, Nottinghamshire, UK

John A Moore BSc MBChB FRCA MRCP
Consultant in Anaesthesia and Intensive Care, Manchester Royal Infirmary, CMFT, Manchester, UK

Andrew J Mortimer BSc(Hons) MD FRCA FFPMRCA MEWI
Consultant in Anaesthesia and Intensive Care, Department of Anaesthesia, University Hospital of South Manchester, Wythenshawe Hospital, Manchester, UK

Paul Murphy MA(Cantab) MBChB FRCA
Neurosciences Critical Care Unit, The General Infirmary at Leeds, Leeds, UK

Mary Newton MB BS FRCA
National Hospital for Neurology and Neurosurgery, University College London Hospitals, Queen Square, London, UK

Deborah M Nolan MBChB FRCA
Consultant Anaesthetist, University Hospital of South Manchester, Manchester, UK

Niall O'Keeffe BAO BCh FRCA FICM
Consultant in Cardiothoracic Anaesthesia and Intensive Care, Manchester Royal Infirmary, Manchester, UK

Davandra Patel MBChB FRCA
Consultant Paediatric Anaesthetist, Royal Manchester Children's Hospital, Manchester, UK

Mark R Patrick BSc FRCA
Consultant Cardiothoracic Anaesthetist, University Hospital of South Manchester, Wythenshawe Hospital, Manchester, UK

Rajesh Pattanayak FRCA
Consultant Anaesthetist, William Harvey Hospital, Ashford, Kent, UK

Brian J Pollard BPharm MBChB MD FRCA MEWI
Professor of Anaesthesia, Manchester Medical School, Department of Anaesthesia, Manchester Royal Infirmary, Manchester, UK

Dr Chris JD Pomfrett BSc PhD Clinical Scientist,
Lecturer in Neurophysiology applied to Anaesthesia, Department of Anaesthesia, Manchester Royal Infirmary, Manchester, UK

Benedikt Preckel MD MA DEAA
Associate Professor of Anesthesia, Department of Anesthesiology, Academic Medical Center, Amsterdam, The Netherlands

Jeremy Radcliffe FRCA
Department of Neuroanaesthesia and Neurocritical Care, The National Hospital for Neurology and Neurosurgery, University College London Hospitals, Queen Square, London, UK

Shilpa Reddy FRCA MRCP
Perioperative Research fellow in Anaesthesia, University College Hospitals, London, UK

Ugan Reddy BSc MBChB FRCA
Consultant in Neuroanaesthesia, The National Hospital for Neurology and Neurosurgery, University College London Hospitals, London, UK

Andrew Roscoe MBChB FRCA
Assistant Professor, Department of Anaesthesia, Toronto General Hospital, University of Toronto, Canada

Isolde Rötzer MD
Division of Anesthesiology for Neurosurgical and Craniofacial Surgery and Intensive Care Medicine, Medical University of Graz, Graz, Austria

Rajneesh Sachdeva DA FCARCSI
Specialty Trainee in Anaesthesia, University Hospitals Coventry and Warwickshire, Coventry, UK

Charles Marc Samama MD PhD FCCP
Professor and Chairman, Department of Anaesthesiology and Intensive Care, Hotel-Dieu University Hospital, Paris, France

Andreas Schöpfer MD
Division of Anesthesiology for Neurosurgical and Craniofacial Surgery and Intensive Care Medicine, Medical University of Graz, Graz, Austria

Jean-François Schved MD, PhD
Professor and Chairman, Department of Hematology, Hôpital Saint -Eloi, Montpellier University Hospital, Montpellier France

Gerhard Schwarz MD
Professor and Chairman, Division of Anesthesiology for Neurosurgical and Craniofacial Surgery and Intensive Care Medicine, Medical University of Graz, Graz, Austria

Sandeep Sharma BSc MBBS FRCA
National Hospital for Neurology and Neurosurgery, University College London Hospitals, London, UK

George Shorten FFARCSI FRCA MD PhD
Professor of Anaesthesia and Intensive Care Medicine, Department of Anaesthesia and Intensive Care Medicine, Dean of Medicine, Cork University Hospital, University College Cork, Ireland

Suveer Singh BSc MBBS PhD FRC EDIC DICM FFICM
Consultant Intensivist and Respiratory Physician, Honorary Senior Lecturer, Chelsea and Westminster Hospital NHS Foundation Trust, Imperial College London, UK

Roger M Slater MRCP(UK) FRCA
Consultant Anaesthetist, Department of Anaesthesia, Manchester Royal Infirmary, Manchester, UK

Martin Smith MBBS FRCA FFICM
Consultant and Honorary Professor in Neuroanaesthesia and Neurocritical Care, The National Hospital for Neurology and Neurosurgery, University College London Hospitals, London, UK

Mark Snazelle MRCP FRCA
Specialist Registrar, William Harvey Hospital, Ashford, Kent, UK

Neil Soni MBChB FRCA FANZCA FCICM MD
Consultant in Critical Care and Anaesthesia, Chelsea and Westminster Hospital, London, UK

R Kadayam Sreenivasan MD FRCA
ST5, The Royal London Hospital, London, UK

Simon Stacey FRCA
Consultant Anaesthetist, St Bartholomew's Hospital, London, UK

Arabella P Stevens MBChB MRCP FRCA
Locum Consultant Anaesthetist, University Hospital of South Manchester, Manchester, UK

Silvia Stirparo MD
Staff Anesthesiologist, Department of Anesthesiology, Città di Roma Hospital, Rome, Italy

Rachel A Stoeter MBChB DTM&H FRCA
Specialist Trainee, Department of Anaesthesia, University Hospital of South Manchester, Wythenshawe Hospital, Manchester, UK

Chris Taylor BSc MBBS MRCP FRCA
Department of Neuroanaesthesia and Neurocritical Care, National Hospital for Neurology and Neurosurgery, University College London Hospitals, London, UK

Sarath Varghese
Core Trainee, William Harvey Hospital, Ashford, Kent, UK

Simon Varley MB BS FRCA
Consultant in Anaesthesia, Department of Anaesthesia, Manchester Royal Infirmary, Manchester, UK

Akbar Vohra MB ChB DA FRCA FFICM
Department of Anaesthesia, Manchester Royal Infirmary, Manchester, UK

Richard Wadsworth BSc MB BChir FRCA
Consultant Anaesthetist, Manchester Royal Infirmary, Manchester, UK

Robert WM Walker MBChB, FRCA
Department of Paediatric Anaesthesia, Royal Manchester Children's Hospital, Manchester, UK

Stuart White BSc FRCA MA
Consultant in Anaesthesia, Brighton and Sussex University Hospitals NHS Trust, Brighton, UK

Sally Wilmshurst MB ChB MRCP FRCA
Great Ormond Street Hospital for Children NHS Trust, London, UK

Sally Wilson FRCA
Department of Neuroanaesthesia and Neurocritical Care, National Hospital for Neurology and Neurosurgery, University College London Hospitals, London, UK

James DA Wood FRCA
Consultant Anaesthetist, Maidstone Hospital, Kent. UK

Quanhong Zhou MD MSc
Anaesthesia Department, Shanghai No. 6 People's Hospital, Shanghai, China

Preface

A third edition represents a significant step forward in the life of a book. The first edition represents the coming to fruition of an idea. A second edition indicates that the idea was good and that the first edition sold well, was popular and was valued by its readers. To move into a third edition is a huge step forward again and is an indication that the book has an established place in clinical practice and education. It is also an appropriate time to critically evaluate again the contents and to ensure that the book is up-to-date and keeps abreast of changes in practice.

The general structure of this third edition of the *Handbook of Clinical Anaesthesia* is identical to that of the previous two, namely that individual problems are approached and addressed in a concise and readable form, readily assimilated by busy clinicians. Each article tries to maintain a fairly consistent format beginning with the background or pathophysiology of the condition or situation and continuing through anaesthetic management ending with postoperative care and outcome. This sort of structured approach tends to be that favoured by examiners in postgraduate specialty examinations. Some topics do not lend themselves directly to this exact approach and in these cases as logical a structure as possible has been followed.

This third edition differs from the previous two with respect to the authors of the different sections. In the first two editions, the authors were principally UK based. In this third edition, authors are drawn from a much wider international field. The monographs are written as much as possible by experts in their fields, who are practising clinicians with an appreciation of the important issues.

There are some areas of overlap between sections and topics but these are inevitable and have been reduced to a minimum. Like the previous two editions, the book is divided into three principal parts, **Patient Conditions, Surgical Procedures** and **Anaesthetic Factors**. Each of these is sub-divided systematically. An overall index is supplied to guide the reader rapidly to specific places and cross references are supplied at the end of most of the chapters to guide the reader in appropriate onward directions. A short bibliography is included at the end of most of the chapters directing the reader to further reading and recent review articles.

Not every eventuality has been covered of course – that would be impossible in a book of this size. It is not a replacement for major texts or review articles but a supplement to them. In this text the reader will find guidance to cover most everyday problems and also many less common ones. The previous editions were popular with trainees preparing for examinations and it is hoped that the new edition will prove to be just as useful. The editor is a past examiner for the FRCA diploma in the UK and thus has knowledge of the expectations of examiners at this level. There will be many ways to use this book and individuals will develop their own method, probably annotating the margins with additional points relevant to their own particular practice.

I must finally thank each and every contributor who has written for this book. I also want to thank the contributors to the first and second editions. Their original contributions have been taken and updated as necessary for this edition. Those contributors of the first and second editions are too numerous to list but I should like to thank each and every one of them. Finally I must thank you the reader for purchasing this book. It has been written for you. I hope that you find it useful.

BJP

Part 1
Patient Conditions

1 Central nervous system

Martin Smith

Autonomic dysfunction and autonomic dysreflexia

Katharine Hunt and Sandeep Sharma

Autonomic dysfunction occurs as a result of central or peripheral nervous system disease, most commonly in patients with diabetes, Parkinson disease and Guillain-Barré syndrome. The symptomatology and treatment of these conditions are covered elsewhere in this book.

Autonomic dysreflexia is a syndrome of massive reflex sympathetic discharge occurring in patients with spinal cord injury, usually at or above the level of the splanchnic sympathetic outflow tract at T6. It is typified by a sudden increase in blood pressure associated in many cases with headache, sweating and pallor. It poses a significant risk to patients, and is of major importance to the anaesthetist.

Autonomic dysreflexia occurs in 60% of cervical lesions and 20% of thoracic lesions above T6. It is more common in complete spinal cord injury and may occur at any time from 3 weeks to 12 years after injury.

Pathophysiology

Autonomic dysreflexia is caused when a loss of descending inhibition coupled with changes in neuronal pathways within the distal spinal cord lead to abnormal sympathetic responses. This may be potentiated by the increased sensitivity to catecholamines that is often seen in patients with spinal cord injury. Many stimuli are known to trigger autonomic dysreflexia, and bladder distension is well documented. Abdominal pathology, including bowel distension, anal fissures and visceral stimulation, such as uterine contraction in the obstetric patient, are other known triggers.

Clinical features

Hypertension caused by vasoconstriction is the most striking clinical feature of autonomic dysreflexia. The hypertension is paroxysmal and severe, with systolic pressures of greater than 260 mmHg and diastolic pressures of 170–220 mmHg being reported. This can result in headache, intracranial and retinal haemorrhage, pulmonary oedema and myocardial ischaemia. A compensatory vasodilatory response may occur in the segments above the level of spinal cord injury, causing flushing and sweating. Cardiac arrhythmias, in particular reflex bradycardia, are also commonplace.

Autonomic dysreflexia is sometimes associated with a Horner syndrome, nausea and anxiety.

Acute management

Removal of the trigger usually results in the resolution of the hypertension, although prevention of the most common causes of autonomic dysreflexia, such as blocked urinary catheters, urinary tract infection and faecal impaction, is paramount in preventing attacks.

Many short-acting antihypertensive agents have been used during the acute attack and in long-term therapy for prevention of hypertensive crises in autonomic dysreflexia (Box 1.1). Some, such as nifedipine, may also be employed preoperatively, prior to an intervention such as hysteroscopy or cystoscopy, and to prevent attacks, although care must be taken if resting blood pressure is already low because of the spinal cord injury.

Box 1.1 Antihypertensive therapy used in the treatment of autonomic dysreflexia

- Nifedipine (10 mg sublingual)
- Phentolamine
- Glyceryl trinitrate (bolus or infusion)
- Labetalol
- Prazosin
- Guanethidine
- Hydralazine
- Clonidine

Anaesthetic implications

The anaesthetist should remember that spinal cord-injured patients may have many other physiological abnormalities, such as respiratory dysfunction, as well as autonomic dysreflexia. Each patient should be individually assessed with this in mind (see Spinal cord injury, p. 36).

Preoperative assessment

Patients who are vulnerable to autonomic dysreflexia are usually very aware of the problem and its triggers. A careful history and assessment of blood pressure, including the presence of both hypertension and postural hypotension, should be taken. Preoperative antihypertensive therapy should be considered.

Anaesthetic monitoring

In addition to standard monitoring, invasive blood pressure monitoring should be employed in all cases. Urinary catheterization may also be required to prevent bladder distension from triggering autonomic dysreflexia during surgery.

Anaesthetic technique

Spinal anaesthesia obliterates autonomic dysreflexia. Although it can be difficult to detect the level of the block, loss of spasms or a decrease in muscle tone may be helpful indicators. Epidural anaesthesia is not as reliable as spinal anaesthesia in preventing autonomic dysreflexia intraoperatively but may prevent postoperative autonomic dysreflexia after abdominal surgery. Obstetric patients are at particularly high risk, and epidural analgesia is recommended for up to 48 hours after birth.

General anaesthesia offers some protection from autonomic dysreflexia. Fluid preloading is advisable to prevent the dramatic hypotension during induction of anaesthesia in patients with chronic spinal cord injury.

Bibliography

Fox R, Watling G. Anaesthesia for patients with chronic spinal cord injury. *Curr Opin Anaesth Crit Care* 2001; **12**: 154–8.

Cross-references

Diabetes mellitus, 60
Parkinson disease, 26
Spinal cord injury, 36

Brainstem death

Paul Murphy

Death is defined as the irreversible loss of capacity for consciousness combined with the irreversible and complete loss of capacity to breathe. The state of death can be arrived at in various ways, and different circumstances may require different diagnostic criteria to be used. For instance, the criteria that are necessary to confirm death that follows failed cardiopulmonary resuscitation differ from those used in cases of advanced decomposition. Neurological criteria are the most direct examination of the essential components of death and are applicable when patients are suspected to be brain dead.

Pathophysiology of brain death

Multiple physiological changes occur after the onset of brain death.

Cardiovascular

A transient sympathetic storm (increases in heart rate, blood pressure, systemic vascular resistance), followed by more prolonged hypotension, myocardial impairment, pulmonary oedema and arrhythmias, often follows brain death.

Endocrine

- Failure of secretion of antidiuretic hormone (ADH) from the posterior pituitary results in diabetes insipidus, causing excessive diuresis, hypovolaemia, hypernatraemia, hyperosmolality and hypokalaemia.
- Variable loss of function of the anterior pituitary results in low levels of cortisol and thyroid hormones.
- Hyperglycaemia may occur secondary to reduced insulin secretion, treatment of hypernatraemia with 5% dextrose or high levels of circulating catecholamines.

Coagulation

- Tissue thromboplastin release causing disseminated intravascular coagulation.

Temperature regulation

- Loss of hypothalamic temperature control.
- Fall in metabolic rate/muscle activity.
- Peripheral vasodilatation.

Metabolism

- Reduced myocardial energy stores.
- Increased anaerobic metabolism.
- Increased lactate and free fatty acids.
- Metabolic acidosis.

Confirmation of death using neurological criteria

The brainstem controls the ability to breathe independently, is an integrative control centre for the cardiovascular system, provides a conduit for ascending and descending neuronal pathways and, via the reticular activating system, maintains the capacity for consciousness. Diagnostic criteria for brain death were first described by the Harvard Medical School in 1968. Initial UK criteria (1976) have recently been updated by the Academy of the Medical Royal Colleges (2008).

There are two key components of brain death testing in the UK – fulfilment of essential preconditions/exclusion criteria and clinical evaluation of coma, brainstem areflexia and apnoea. While the latter demonstrates the absence of brainstem function, it is the former which determines irreversibility and which requires the greater expertise for confirmation.

Preconditions

- Apnoeic coma: the patient is unresponsive and ventilator dependent.
- Proven irremediable structural brain damage. Major causes of brain death include spontaneous intracranial haemorrhage, hypoxic brain injury, trauma, ischaemic stroke and intracranial infection.

Exclusion criteria

Clinicians must be confident that reversible influences do not significantly contribute to a patient's coma/apnoea. Factors that should be excluded include the following.

Residual sedation

- Allow more than three times half-life of drug before testing.
- Establish that plasma levels of thiopental or benzodiazepine are subtherapeutic.
- Consider the administration of specific antagonists such as flumazenil or naloxone or the possible role for confirmatory investigation.

Physiological/metabolic derangements

- Only consider testing when the temperature is >34°C.
- Ensure mean arterial pressure (MAP) >60 mmHg, P_aCO_2 <6.0 kPa, P_aO_2 >10 kPa, pH 7.35–7.45.
- Confirm normoglycaemia and avoid diabetic ketoacidosis (blood glucose 3–20 mmol L^{-1}).
- Hypernatraemia secondary to brainstem death-related diabetes insipidus can be ignored and does not need correction before testing.

Clinical assessment of brainstem function

In the UK, clinical examination must be carried out by two physicians working together and must be repeated. At least one of the doctors must be a consultant and both must have been fully registered with the GMC for more than 5 years. Neither must be part of any transplant team.

Clinical examination of brainstem reflexes

Demonstration of brainstem areflexia variously reveals loss of hind-brain function at the level of the mesencephalon, pons and medulla oblongata by examination of specific cranial nerves.

- The pupils are fixed and do not respond to sharp changes in the intensity of incident light (mesencephalon, cranial nerves II and III).
- There is no corneal reflex (pons, cranial nerves V and VII).
- The oculovestibular reflexes are absent. No eye movements are seen during or following the slow injection of at least 50 mL of ice-cold water over 1 minute into each external auditory meatus in turn. Clear access to the tympanic membrane must be established by direct inspection (pons, cranial nerves VIII, III, IV, VI).

Access to the above reflexes may be prevented on one or other side by local injury or disease, but this does not invalidate clinical testing. In the case of bilateral injury or disease, ancillary testing should be considered.

- No motor responses within the cranial nerve distribution can be elicited by adequate stimulation of any somatic area, e.g. by supraorbital pressure or pressure applied to the nailbed of a finger (the latter may be contraindicated by a spinal injury). Care must be taken to distinguish central response from primitive spinally mediated reflexes that can be ignored in this context.
- There is no cough reflex response to bronchial stimulation by a suction catheter placed down the trachea to the carina, or gag response to stimulation of the posterior pharynx with a spatula (medulla, cranial nerves IX, X).

Apnoea test

The apnoea test should only be considered once brainstem areflexia has been confirmed. It should be performed as follows:

1. increase F_iO_2 to 1.0
2. check arterial blood gases to confirm that the measured P_aCO_2 and S_aO_2 correlate with the monitored values
3. with oxygen saturation greater than 95%, reduce minute volume ventilation by lowering the respiratory rate to allow a slow rise in end-tidal CO_2 ($ETCO_2$)
4. once $ETCO_2$ rises above 6.0 kPa, check arterial blood gases to confirm that P_aCO_2 is at least 6.0 kPa and that the pH is less than 7.40
5. if cardiovascular stability is maintained, disconnect the patient from the ventilator and oxygen should be delivered by bulk flow, preferably using a Mapleson C-type rebreathing circuit rather than an intratracheal catheter. If the maintenance of adequate oxygenation proves difficult, then continuous positive airway pressure (and possibly a prior recruitment manoeuvre) may be used
6. after 5 minutes of apnoea, repeat arterial blood gas, confirm a minimum of a further 0.5 kPa rise in P_aCO_2 above 6.0 kPa. Loss of respiratory drive is confirmed at this point and mechanical ventilation resumed.

The legal time of death is that at completion of the first set of tests. However, this must be confirmed by the second set of tests. All brain-dead patients should be considered as potential organ donors and referred to the local specialist nurse for organ donation for assessment. The possibility of donation as part of end-of-life care should only be introduced to the family of the patient when they have accepted the inevitability of their loss.

Confirmatory tests

Many parts of the world have a legal requirement (e.g. Sweden) or allow professional discretion (e.g. USA, UK) for the use of a confirmatory investigation to support the clinical diagnosis of brain death. Potential confirmatory tests involve either:

- measures of cerebral blood flow
  - four-vessel cerebral angiography
  - CT angiography
  - MR angiography
  - transcranial Doppler ultrasonography
  - radioisotope perfusion scanning
- measures of cerebral electrical activity
  - electroencephalography
  - brainstem-evoked potentials.

EEG is the most popular and best validated ancillary test, but is little value in cases of drug intoxication since sedative drugs suppress neuronal, and therefore EEG, activity.

The absence of cerebral blood flow at angiography establishes the irreversibility of coma in such circumstances, but may be more difficult to organize. CT angiography may be more readily available but has yet to be properly validated in this context.

Bibliography

Academy of the Medical Royal Colleges. *A Code of Practice for the Diagnosis and Confirmation of Death*. London: AoMRC, 2008. See www.aomrc.org.uk/reports.aspx.

Murphy PG. Death and donation in critical care: the diagnosis of brainstem death. In: Adams JP, Bell MDD, McKinlay J (eds) *Neurocritical Care*. London: Springer, 2010.

Wijdicks Eelco FM. The diagnosis of brain death. *N Engl J Med* 2001; **344**: 1215–21.

Cross-references

Heart transplantation, 520
Kidney transplantation, 522
Liver transplantation, 527
Lung and heart–lung transplantation, 530
Pancreas transplantation, 533

Diseases of the neuromuscular junction

David Brealey and Nicholas Hirsch

The neuromuscular junction (NMJ) can be affected by a number of rare but diverse disease processes (Box 1.2), leading to severe weakness and bulbar and respiratory failure. A sound knowledge of the NMJ in health and the impact of disease are vital to enable the appropriate anaesthetic management of these complex patients.

Box 1.2 Disease affecting the neuromuscular junction

- Myasthenia gravis
- Lambert–Eaton myasthenic syndrome
- Autoimmune neuromyotonia
- Toxins and drugs
  - Botulism
  - Tetanus
  - Organophosphates

Myasthenia gravis

Aetiology and pathology

Myasthenia gravis (MG) is the commonest disease of the neuromuscular junction, affecting two in 100 000 of the population. It arises from an autoimmune-mediated destruction of the postsynaptic acetylcholine (ACh) receptor. There is a strong link between MG and disorders of the thymus gland, which is thought to be responsible for production of the antibodies.

Clinical presentation and diagnosis

Initially, patients may complain of double vision and have evidence of ptosis. This can progress to bulbar and proximal limb weakness and fatigue. The weakness is often fluctuant. Approximately 20% of patients have respiratory muscle involvement and, if severe, this will require intubation and ventilation. Diagnosis can be difficult and a high index of suspicion is required. The Tensilon test consists of the intravenous administration of the short-acting anticholinesterase drug edrophonium. Patients with MG show a rapid improvement in muscle strength lasting about 5 minutes after injection of the drug. Unfortunately, the Tensilon test has low sensitivity and specificity. Electromyography (EMG) shows a diminishing response of the muscle action potential on repeated stimulation, but again has low specificity. However, the presence of anti-acetylcholine receptor antibodies is diagnostic.

Rarer forms of MG include a seronegative variant with antibodies directed against muscle-specific kinase (anti-MuSK) or drug induced (e.g. penicillamine). MG is associated with other autoimmune diseases.

Management

The management of MG involves:

- enhancing neuromuscular transmission with the use of long-acting anticholinesterases
- immunosuppression with steroids and, if required, azathioprine or cyclophosphamide
- thymectomy for those with evidence of an enlarged thymus on CT scan
- intravenous immunoglobulin or plasma exchange is usually reserved for those with a myasthenic crisis or resistance to standard therapy (e.g. anti-MuSK myasthenia)
- withdrawal of precipitating drugs.

Anaesthetic implications

Preoperative

Patients with MG may present for incidental surgery or for thymectomy. A preoperative history of symptoms and functional ability, with particular reference to respiratory and bulbar function, is important to predict the postoperative course. Evidence of respiratory failure and consistently low forced vital capacity (FVC) may indicate the need for postoperative ventilation. A soft voice and a history of dysphagia and choking indicates bulbar dysfunction. Close cooperation with a neurologist is vital to optimize patients prior to surgery.

Anticholinesterases should be omitted on the morning of surgery as they interfere with both depolarizing and non-depolarizing neuromuscular blocking agents. In the absence of respiratory or bulbar involvement, sedative premedication is acceptable. MG is not a contraindication for peripheral nerve or neuraxial blockade.

Induction

Because of the reduced number of ACh receptors, patients with MG are relatively resistant to normal doses of succinylcholine, but large or repeated doses tend to produce a dual block. In contrast, MG patients are sensitive to the effects of non-depolarizing neuromuscular blockers and, if possible, these agents should be avoided. The muscle relaxation provided by the volatile agents is often sufficient to permit intubation. If muscle relaxants are used, neuromuscular function should be monitored. Patients should be ventilated through the procedure.

Postoperative

Most patients can be extubated at the end of the procedure, but those with bulbar dysfunction should be extubated when fully awake. Patients with respiratory or severe bulbar failure may benefit from a period of postoperative ventilation. Anticholinesterases must be reintroduced as soon as possible, though often at a lower dose. Adequate analgesia is essential and epidural analgesia may be considered.

Botulism

Aetiology

Botulism is the clinical manifestation of *Clostridium botulinium* infection. *C. botulinium* is a Gram-positive, spore-forming organism capable of producing a number of neurotoxins (A–G). Several of these target proteins in the presynaptic region of the human neuromuscular junction, preventing ACh release. Infection usually results from contaminated foods or wounds (increasingly common in intravenous/subcutaneous drug users).

Clinical features

Classically, botulism presents with bilateral cranial nerve palsies, which may be preceded by gastrointestinal upset if the toxin is ingested. Common symptoms and signs include:

- blurred vision, diplopia and ptosis
- expressionless face
- bulbar involvement: dysarthria, dysphagia and aspiration
- autonomic dysfunction: postural hypotension, dry mouth and constipation.

The disease can progress rapidly (hours to days) to a descending flaccid paralysis with loss of tendon reflexes. Ventilatory support may be required if there is respiratory muscle involvement. The sensory system is unaffected and the patient remains fully lucid. Patients are often apyrexial. CNS imaging and CSF values are normal, whereas EMG demonstrates NMJ blockade. Diagnostic confirmation requires the identification of the toxin in stool or plasma and, since it can take upwards of 48 hours to obtain a result, treatment should be initiated on clinical suspicion.

Treatment

The only effective treatment is the administration of botulism antitoxin and, as it only neutralizes unbound toxin, it should be given as early as possible. Wounds require surgical debridement. Antibiotics may accelerate toxin release and are not indicated. Patients should be managed in a critical care facility with careful monitoring of respiratory (including FVC) and bulbar function, and intubation should occur early. Patients may require ventilation for months before recovery. Meticulous attention to detail and modern intensive care techniques have reduced mortality after botulism to 3–5%.

Tetanus

Aetiology and pathology

Tetanus, though rare in the UK (10–15 cases per year), is still prevalent in many parts of the developing world. It is caused by the Gram-positive bacillus *Clostridium tetani*, which is ubiquitous within the environment. Inoculation is usually through a recognized deep wound, but tetanus can complicate surgery, snakebites or childbirth. The clinical effects are exerted through the expression of the exotoxin, tetanospasmin, which is taken up by the local nerve terminals and transported to the inhibitory interneurones in the brainstem and spinal cord, where it interferes with the release of inhibitory neurotransmitters (GABA and glycine). Motor neurones, preganglionic sympathetic neurones and parasympathetic centres are all affected.

Clinical features

The clinical picture is dominated by muscle spasms, rigidity and autonomic disturbance. Masseter and facial muscle spasm give rise to the characteristic 'lockjaw' and 'risus sadonicus'. Limb spasms may be severe enough to fracture bones and avulse tendons. Spasm of the laryngeal/pharyngeal muscles can occlude the airway while spasm and rigidity of the chest wall may result in respiratory failure. Spasms may occur spontaneously or in response to the slightest of visual, auditory or touch stimulation. Autonomic dysfunction is common. Resting tachycardia and hypertension are frequent but during 'autonomic storms' can rapidly convert to severe hypotension and bradycardia.

Management

An effective vaccination programme with booster doses after injury has almost eradicated tetanus from the developed world. In established disease, the aims of treatment are to:

- Neutralize free toxin with human tetanus immune globulin and enhance short-term immunity with tetanus toxoid.

- Eradicate the infection: metronidazole is the antibiotic of choice and wounds should undergo thorough surgical debridement.
- Control the spasms: nurse in a quiet environment keeping stimulation to a minimum. Midazolam is helpful initially but if spasms continue a propofol infusion may be required, necessitating intubation and ventilation. Neuromuscular blockade is used for those with refractory spasms. Other agents include magnesium, phenobarbitone, dantrolene and intrathecal baclofen.
- Control autonomic disturbance: β-blockers, vagolytics, clonidine and magnesium have all been used.

These measures, combined with fastidious supportive care, have significantly reduced mortality. Functional recovery is good in survivors.

Organophosphate poisoning

Organophosphates are commonly found in insecticides but are also used as chemical weapons. Intoxication, although rare in the UK, may be deliberate or accidental. Organophosphates can be absorbed by inhalation, by ingestion or through the skin and mucous membranes. They act by irreversibly inhibiting acetylcholinesterase, resulting in the overstimulation of muscarinic and nicotinic receptors. This produces a 'cholinergic crisis', characterized by:

- centrally mediated effects: agitation, convulsions, loss of consciousness and respiratory depression
- parasympathetic effects: bronchoconstriction, bradycardia, salivation, miosis, vomiting, abdominal cramps and diarrhoea
- neuromuscular junction effects: skeletal muscle fasciculations progressing to weakness.

A delayed polyneuropathy may develop weeks after the acute event. Diagnosis is initially clinical but may be supported by red blood cell anticholinesterase activity. Organophosphates can be detected in blood and urine.

Management

Depending on the situation, management initially involves decontamination of the patient and protection of healthcare workers. There is little evidence to guide treatment and initial supportive measures include:

- intubation and ventilation for respiratory failure or loss of consciousness
- haemodynamic support including fluid and vasoactive therapy, and treatment of dysrhythmias including temporary cardiac pacing
- control of seizures, initially with benzodiazepines.

Specific management includes:

- pralidoxime: an agent capable of reactivating acetylcholinesterase if given early, but it may be ineffective against certain organophosphates
- atropine: to reverse the muscarinic (parasympathetic)-mediated effects.

Therapies under investigation include magnesium and haemofiltration. If the patient is able to access healthcare services before respiratory compromise, outcome is usually good.

Bibliography

Benson CA, Harris AA. Acute neurologic infections. *Med Clin North Am* 1986; **70**: 987–1011.

Cannard K. The acute treatment of nerve agent exposure. *J Neurol Sci* 2006; **249**: 86–94.

Conti-Fine BM, Milani M, Kaminski HJ. Myasthenia gravis: past, present, and future. *J Clin Invest* 2006; **116**: 2843–54.

Goonetilleke A, Harris JB. Clostridial neurotoxins. *J Neurol Neurosurg Psychiatry* 2004; **75**(Suppl. 3): iii35–9.

Hirsch NP. Neuromuscular junction in health and disease. *Br J Anaesth* 2007; **99**: 132–8.

Peter JV, Moran JL, Graham PL. Advances in the management of organophosphate poisoning. *Expert Opin Pharmacother* 2007; **8**: 1451–64.

Sobel J. Botulism. *Clin Infect Dis* 2005; **41**: 1167–73.

Cross-references

Failure to breathe or wake up postoperatively, 749
Masseter muscle spasm, 772

Epilepsy

Ian Appleby

Epilepsy is a common disorder occurring in approximately 1 in 200 of the general population. It is a chronic illness due to an underlying disorder of neuronal activity, which is characterized by recurrent (two or more) seizures. Genetic, congenital and developmental conditions are commonly associated with epilepsy in the young; tumours are more likely in those over 40; and trauma and infective causes may occur at any age. Despite considerable progress in the medical management of epilepsy and the development of many new anticonvulsants, some patients, approximately 20–30%, remain refractory to drug therapy or develop intolerable side-effects. Many of these will be candidates for epilepsy surgery. Epilepsy is also the direct cause of approximately 1000 deaths per year in the UK as a result of status epilepticus, trauma from seizures or sudden unexpected death in epilepsy.

Causes

Most cases of epilepsy are idiopathic and a definite cause is found in only 25–35%. Specific causes include:

- genetic, e.g. juvenile myoclonic epilepsy
- trauma: depressed skull fractures or intracranial haemorrhage are predictors of post-traumatic epilepsy
- tumours: particularly with slow-growing frontal tumours
- infection: meningitis or encephalitis
- cerebrovascular disease: epilepsy occurs in 6–15% of stroke patients
- alcohol: lowers seizure threshold
- others, e.g. dementia, multiple sclerosis, metabolic disorders.

Pathophysiology

Electrical activity in the brain is normally well controlled, but in epileptogenic disorders normal brain regulatory functions are altered. Sudden and disordered neuronal activity is responsible for the clinical manifestations of epilepsy. In epilepsy there is:

- appearance of pacemaker neurones
- introduction of significant excitatory synaptic connections
- loss of postsynaptic inhibition.

Pacemaker neurones appear to be the centre of the epileptic focus and have the capacity to produce spontaneous burst discharges which are recognized as interictal spikes on the EEG. Increases in cellular activity and loss of normal inhibitory tone allow spread of these discharges to surrounding areas, resulting in uncontrolled neuronal firing and seizure activity. Changes in membrane flux, impaired γ-aminobutyric acid (GABA)-mediated synaptic inhibition and alterations in local neurotransmitter levels are implicated in this process.

Classification

Epilepsy may be generalized or partial (Box 1.3), but there are over 40 specific types of epilepsy recognized. Generalized epilepsies occur in 20% of epileptic patients, involve both hemispheres and are associated with an initial impairment of consciousness. Simple partial seizures are caused by a localized discharge and there is no impairment of consciousness. In complex partial seizures (CPSs), the initial focal discharge spreads widely and secondary loss of consciousness occurs. CPSs are the most common seizure disorder in adults and include temporal lobe epilepsy (TLE). In a high proportion of patients, high-quality MRI demonstrates hippocampal sclerosis in patients with TLE. Under such circumstances, extended temporal lobectomy may offer a reduction in seizure frequency and severity.

Anticonvulsant therapy

The aim of medical treatment is to achieve a seizure-free patient with minimal drug-related side-effects. Correct choice of anticonvulsant agent

Box 1.3 Classification of the epilepsies

- Generalized epilepsy
  - Generalized absence: *petit mal*
  - Generalized tonic-clonic: *grand mal*
  - Myoclonic
  - Tonic–clonic
  - Atonic
- Partial epilepsy
  - Simple
  - Complex partial: temporal lobe epilepsy
  - Partial onset with secondary generalization

Also, pseudoseizures and non-epileptic seizures

involves consideration of seizure type, seizure history, patient age and side-effects; there are now over 25 available drugs (Table 1.1). Therapy is initiated with a single agent given in a dose sufficient to produce therapeutic plasma levels. If seizures continue, or if unacceptable side-effects develop, a second agent is substituted for the first. Monotherapy is sufficient to control seizures in many patients but some require addition of second- or third-line agents. If a patient's epilepsy cannot be brought under control after adequate trials of two or three (expert opinion differs) anticonvulsant drugs, they are said to be medically refractory.

Preoperative assessment

The patient's history should be evaluated in relation to their epilepsy and other coexisting medical problems. Particular attention should be paid to:

- seizure frequency, type and pattern
- current anticonvulsant therapy (including plasma levels)
- complications of anticonvulsant therapy (Table 1.1)
- IQ – poorly controlled, chronic epilepsy may be associated with low IQ and thus may make informed consent problematic.

Anticonvulsant therapy must be continued up to and including the day of surgery. Plasma anticonvulsant levels should be checked and doses adjusted as necessary. Premedication may be prescribed as required, and benzodiazepines are appropriate. If there is any doubt as to how long the patient may remain nil by mouth postoperatively, consideration should be given to placement of a nasogastric tube to facilitate enteral administration of anticonvulsant drugs since, of the commonly prescribed drugs, only phenytoin, sodium valproate and lamotrigine are available in injectable form.

Anaesthetic agents and the EEG

The action of anaesthetic agents on the EEG is complex and usually dose related. Many agents have been reported to cause clinical seizure activity while also possessing anticonvulsant actions. Low doses generally have proconvulsant actions and higher doses anticonvulsant activity.

Table 1.1 Anticonvulsants: commonly prescribed drugs, first-line indication and side-effects

Drug	First-line indication	Side-effects
Phenytoin	Generalized tonic–clonic seizures Partial seizures	Skin rash, drowsiness, ataxia, slurred speech, gingival hypertrophy, excess hair growth, anaemias, neuropathy (blood levels essential to guide dosing)
Sodium valproate	Generalized tonic–clonic seizures Absence seizures	Tremor, drowsiness, weight gain, alopecia, raised hepatic transaminase, thrombocytopenia. Avoid in pregnancy
Carbamazepine	Generalized tonic–clonic seizures Partial seizures	Rash, double vision, ataxia, hyponatraemia, thrombocytopenia
Phenobarbitone	Generalized tonic–clonic seizures Partial seizures	Drowsiness, rash, osteomalacia, anaemia, folate deficiency
Ethosuximide	Absence seizures	Nausea, drowsiness, anorexia, photophobia
Lamotrigine	Generalized tonic–clonic seizures Partial seizures	Rash, drowsiness, double vision, headache, insomnia, tremor, flu-like symptoms
Levetiracetam	Partial seizures	Dizziness, drowsiness, insomnia, ataxia, tremor, headache, behavioural problems
Primidone	Generalized tonic–clonic seizures Partial seizures	Nausea, nystagmus, sedation, anaemias, ataxia
Vigabatrin	Partial seizures	Visual field defects, drowsiness, psychotic reactions
Gabapentin	Partial seizures	Drowsiness, dizziness, headache
Clobazam	Generalized tonic–clonic seizures Partial seizures	Drowsiness, tolerance

Barbiturates

Most barbiturates are anticonvulsants at normal clinical doses and thiopental may be used to control seizures. Thiopental infusion has also been used in the treatment of status epilepticus. Methohexitone activates the EEG, and should be avoided in epileptic patients.

Propofol

Propofol has been shown to activate the EEG in temporal lobe epilepsy and produce seizures and opisthotonos in non-epileptic patients, possibly via a glutaminergic mechanism. Conversely, however, anticonvulsant effects have also been reported and propofol is widely used in the treatment of status epilepticus resistant to other therapies. It is now clear that propofol has a profound dose-dependent effect on the EEG and causes activation at small doses and burst suppression (anticonvulsant action) at higher (clinical) doses.

Benzodiazepines

Diazepam and other benzodiazepines have anticonvulsant EEG effects and are widely used in the treatment of seizures.

Inhalational agents and nitrous oxide

The EEG effects of inhalational anaesthetic agents are dose dependent. EEG activity is maintained with sevoflurane, isoflurane and desflurane concentrations <1 MAC, although background epileptiform activity may be suppressed. Low-dose isoflurane has been used in the treatment of resistant status epilepticus. Higher inspired concentrations have profound effects on the EEG, and at levels >2 MAC the EEG becomes isoelectric. Of historical note, the effects of halothane are similar, with background epileptic activity being suppressed at clinically useful concentrations, while enflurane has a proconvulsant action which is exaggerated in the presence of elevated P_aco_2. Dose-dependent EEG changes occur with nitrous oxide, with anticonvulsant effects predominating at higher inspired concentrations.

Opioids

Opioids have minimal effect on the EEG at usual clinical doses, although marked EEG slowing occurs at high doses. Fentanyl at moderate doses (25 μg/kg) causes modest activation of the EEG, whereas high-dose opioid anaesthetic techniques result in EEG slowing. Alfentanil increases epileptiform activity and has been used to provoke seizure activity during electrocorticography (ECoG). Remifentanil appears to be safe in epileptic patients and may be used during epilepsy surgery with minimal impact on intraoperative EEG recording.

Local anaesthetics

Lidocaine has a biphasic effect on the EEG. At low plasma levels it has anticonvulsant-like actions, whereas at high levels it causes excitation of the central nervous system (CNS), including the provocation of seizures.

Anaesthetic technique

Patients with epilepsy may present for surgery for incidental conditions, following injury during a seizure or for neurosurgery for medically intractable epilepsy. General or local anaesthesia may be provided using standard techniques which avoid factors known to precipitate seizures (Box 1.4). Anaesthetic agents which are proconvulsant at usual clinical doses should be avoided.

Box 1.4 Causes of seizures in the perioperative period

- Pre-existing epilepsy
- Subtherapeutic anticonvulsant levels
- Hypoxia
- Hypercarbia
- Proconvulsant drugs/anaesthetic agents
- Electrolyte disturbances
  - Hyponatraemia
  - Hypoglycaemia
  - Uraemia
- Related disorders
  - Head injury
  - Eclampsia

Specific requirements for the management of a patient undergoing epilepsy surgery include the recording of intraoperative cerebral electrical activity (the ECoG) and/or activation of the epileptic focus. Knowledge of the effects of anaesthetic agents on the EEG allows a rational choice of technique to be made. Careful titration of end-tidal concentration of a volatile agent in combination with remifentanil infusion allows a depth of anaesthesia to be maintained which does not interfere with ECoG recording, while minimizing the risk of awareness. Alternatively, anaesthesia may be maintained by propofol infusion, although the effect on the ECoG is not yet fully characterized. Neuromuscular blockade should be maintained during the lighter stages of anaesthesia necessary for ECoG recording, and monitoring of neuromuscular function is essential because of interactions between muscle relaxant and anticonvulsants.

Intraoperative seizures during general anaesthesia are rare but may be masked by neuromuscular blockade. Unexpected tachycardia, hypertension or increases in $ETco_2$ are suspicious warning signs. An intravenous bolus of propofol or thiopental, followed by deepening of anaesthesia, is usually sufficient to bring seizures under control.

Postoperative care

Postoperative care is directed towards the nature of the surgery. It is essential to continue anticonvulsant therapy into the postoperative period, and anticonvulsant levels must be checked postoperatively.

Recurrent seizures, leading to status epilepticus, are more common in the postoperative period in patients with pre-existing epilepsy and have several precipitants (Box 1.3). Treatment of seizures in the postoperative period must be rapid and aggressive, and precipitating factors should be corrected. Seizures should be rapidly terminated with a short-acting anticonvulsant, such as propofol or a benzodiazepine. A top-up dose of the long-acting anticonvulsant should be added if plasma levels are low. If seizures occur after neurosurgery, a CT head scan is obligatory to rule out any potentially surgically treatable causes, e.g. extradural or subdural haematoma and pneumocephalus.

Bibliography

Chapman MG, Smith M, Hirsch NP. Status epilepticus. *Anaesthesia* 2001; **56**: 648–59.

Herrick IA, Gelb AW. Anesthesia for temporal lobe epilepsy surgery. *Can J Neurol Sci* 2000; **27**: S64–7.

Kofke WA, Tempelhoff R, Dasheiff RM. Anesthesia for epileptic patients and for epilepsy surgery. In: Cottrell JE, Smith DS (eds) *Anesthesia and Neurosurgery*. St Louis: Mosby, 2001.

Modica PA, Tempelhoff R, White PF. Pro- and anti-convulsant effects of anaesthetics (part 1). *Anesth Analg* 1990; **70**: 303–15.

Modica PA, Tempelhoff R, White PF. Pro- and anti-convulsant effects of anaesthetics (part 2). *Anesth Analg* 1990; **70**: 433–43.

National Society for Epilepsy. *Medication for Adults.* Chalfont St Peter: NSE, 2009.

Smith M. Anaesthesia in epilepsy surgery. In: Shorvon S, Dreifus F, Fish D, Thomas D (eds) *The Treatment of Epilepsy*. Oxford: Blackwell Scientific Publications, 1995.

Tellez-Zenteno JF, Dhar R, Wiebe S. Long-term seizure outcomes following epilepsy surgery: a systematic review and meta-analysis. *Brain* 2005; **128**: 1188–98.

Cross-references

Anaesthesia for supratentorial surgery, 326
Monitoring, 690
Neuromonitoring, 338

Head injury

Rashan Haniffa and Jeremy Radcliffe

Epidemiology

Up to 1 million people attend accident and emergency departments (A&E) in the UK each year with a history of head injury. Data from 2000/2001 identify 112978 admissions to hospitals (less than 20% of the attendees to A&E) in England with a primary diagnosis of head injury. Of these, 2446 underwent craniotomy for evacuation of an intracranial haematoma. Most head-injured patients are male (72%), and childhood injuries are common (30% of patients are under 15 years old). Falls (22–43%) and assaults (30–50%) are the most common cause of head injury in the UK, followed by road traffic accidents (~25%). Alcohol consumption is involved in up to 65% of adult head injuries.

Outcome

Although the incidence of traumatic brain injury (TBI) is high, the mortality rate is low (0.2% of people attending A&E), accounting for 6–10 deaths per 100000 population. This represents 1% of all deaths, but 15% of deaths in the 15–45 year age group. Outcome is correlated with patient age, post-resuscitation Glasgow Coma Scale (GCS) score (Table 1.2) on admission and pupillary responsiveness. The majority of poor outcome occurs after moderate (GCS 9–12) or severe (GCS 8 or less) head injuries, which account for only 10% of total A&E attendees. Half of all surviving head-injured patients have symptoms at 1 year, ranging from significant neurological disability to memory loss and difficulty with concentration. Mortality and long-term outcome can be significantly improved by aggressive treatment in the first few hours after severe TBI. Early rehabilitation also plays a crucial part in improving outcome.

TBI remains a major socioeconomic burden because it affects mainly children and young adults and contributes massively to the prevalence of long-term disability. The economic impact of head injury in the USA has been estimated to be $9.2 billion in lifetime medical costs and $51.2 billion in productivity losses.

Table 1.2 The Glasgow Coma Scale

Response	Score
Best motor response (observed in the upper limb)	
Obeys commands	6
Withdraws from painful stimuli	5
Localizes to painful stimuli	4
Flexes to painful stimuli	3
Extends to painful stimuli	2
No response	1
Best verbal response	
Orientated	5
Confused speech	4
Inappropriate words	3
Incomprehensible sounds	2
None	1
Eye-opening response	
Spontaneously	4
To speech	3
To pain	2
None	1

Pathophysiology

Primary brain injury occurs at the initial impact, causing a combination of focal contusions and haemorrhage (extradural, subdural, subarachnoid and intraventricular) as well as shearing of white matter tracts (in diffuse axonal injury). The focus here is on prevention via public and personal health education.

Secondary brain injury is essentially ischaemic in nature and occurs at any time after the primary injury as a result of intra- or extracranial factors. It may be exacerbated by modifiable events, such as hypotension, hypoxia, hypercarbia, fever, hyperglycaemia and seizures (Box 1.5). Potential mechanisms contributing to secondary cerebral ischaemia include reduced cerebral blood flow (especially in the first few hours after head injury) and impaired pressure autoregulation. Acute intracranial injury initiates a cascade of ionic and metabolic changes which render the brain susceptible to secondary systemic physiological insults. The identification, prevention and treatment of secondary brain injury is the principal focus of care for patients with severe head injury.

Box 1.5 Causes of secondary brain injury

- Intracranial factors
  - Expanding haematoma
  - Cerebral oedema
  - Seizures
- Extracranial factors
  - Hypotension
  - Hypoxaemia
  - Hypercapnia
  - Hypocapnia
  - Hyperthermia
  - Hyperglycaemia

Resuscitation

Prevention, recognition and treatment of conditions known to cause secondary brain injury (including surgically remedial compressive lesions) are the primary goals of acute care. The importance of securing the airway and maintaining adequate oxygenation and blood pressure in all patients with severe head injury cannot be overemphasized because secondary brain injury begins and continues from the moment of impact.

Airway

Severely head-injured patients are unlikely to be able to protect their airway and often have impaired gas exchange – hypoxaemia occurs in up to 65% of cases. Therefore, the airway must be cleared and protected. Indications for intubation and ventilation are shown in Box 1.6. Ventilation should aim to maintain adequate oxygenation and normal arterial carbon dioxide tension. To facilitate endotracheal intubation, a sleep dose of thiopental or propofol should be used to attenuate the rise in intracranial pressure (ICP) associated with laryngoscopy. Hypotension should, however, be avoided. A full stomach must be assumed and succinylcholine used as part of a rapid sequence induction technique. The small rise in ICP following administration of succinylcholine is of little concern compared with the risks of hypoxaemia and hypercapnia during prolonged intubation attempts with inadequate relaxation or sedation. The neck must be immobilized by in-line cervical stabilization or a Stiff Neck collar, as there is a high association between head injury and cervical spine fracture. Nasotracheal intubation should be avoided because of the risk of a skull base fracture. Following intubation, an orogastric tube may prevent acute gastric dilatation. A 30° head-up tilt, avoidance of tight tube-ties around the neck or venous canulation in the neck vessels, and prevention of raised intra-abdominal pressure (coughing, urinary retention) minimizes the risk of secondary rises in ICP.

Box 1.6 Indications for intubating the head-injured patient

- Airway protection
  - Loss of protective laryngeal reflexes
  - Unconscious patient (GCS ≤8)
  - Copious bleeding into the mouth
  - Facial injuries compromising the airway
- Hypoventilation and irregular respiration
  - Hypoxaemia (P_ao_2 <13 kPa on O_2 or <10 kPa on air)
  - Hypercapnia (P_aco_2 >6 kPa)
  - Spontaneous hyperventilation (P_aco_2, <4.0 kPa)
  - Associated chest injury
- In preparation for transfer
  - Unconscious patient (GCS ≤8)
  - If neurological deterioration is likely in transit
  - Anticipated difficult airway or copious bleeding into mouth
  - If seizures have occurred

Breathing

Inadequate ventilation or abnormal ventilatory patterns may be central (owing to cerebral damage and cervical cord injury) or peripheral (airway obstruction, aspiration and chest injury). Rapid correction of hypoventilation is essential to prevent secondary brain injury due to hypoxaemia and a rise in ICP secondary to hypercapnia. Following intubation, the lungs should be mechanically ventilated to maintain P_ao_2 >13 kPa and P_aco_2 between 4.5 and 5.0 kPa. Judicious moderate hyperventilation (P_aco_2 4.0–4.5 kPa) may be a useful means of emergency control of ICP pending definitive treatment, during which time the inspired oxygen concentration should be increased. Prolonged empirical hyperventilation, however, may precipitate cerebral ischaemia.

Circulation

Hypotension results in reduced cerebral perfusion, and maintenance of systemic blood pressure is a prerequisite for good neurological outcome after head injury. Guidelines produced by the National Institute for Health and Clinical Excellence (NICE) recommend that mean arterial pressure should be maintained at 80 mmHg or higher by infusion of fluid and vasopressors. Hypotension in an adult head-injured patient should always trigger a search for causes of blood loss. Volume replacement may be achieved with 0.9% saline (isotonic crystalloid) or colloid (although albumin may be associated with an increased mortality). Severe dilutional anaemia should be avoided with appropriate use of blood products. Studies of hypertonic saline have not proved definitively beneficial. Dextrose solutions should be avoided as the glucose is metabolized to lactate in the ischaemic brain and the free water augments cerebral oedema.

Dysfunction (neurological)

Conscious level is assessed using the GCS (Table 1.2), but localizing signs and pupillary reaction must also be recorded.

Examine

About 40% of head-injured patients have associated injuries which may affect outcome. These should be sought during a full trauma survey and appropriate investigations. Severe extracranial injuries should be dealt with immediately to avoid hypotension or ventilatory failure. Active bleeding and chest and abdominal injuries must be treated aggressively, but it is sufficient to stabilize non-life-threatening injuries.

Other management

- Treatment of an expanding intracranial haematoma may require urgent surgical intervention that should ideally be available within 4 hours; 20–30% of extradural haematomas present as rapid neurological deterioration following a lucid interval after the initial injury.
- Mannitol 20% (0.5 g kg^{-1}) may be used as a temporary means of reducing ICP following consultation with the neurosurgical centre.
- Anticonvulsants are used after post-traumatic seizures.
- Pyrexia is associated with worsened outcome, so rapid warming should be avoided in A&E.
- The timing of surgery for non-neurological injuries should ideally allow time for a period of stable neurological observation.

Investigations

Full blood count, urea and electrolytes, glucose, coagulation parameters, blood alcohol level and urine toxicology should be checked. Recommendations regarding CT imaging of the head are shown in Box 1.7.

Box 1.7 NICE recommendation of indication for CT scan of the head following injury

- GCS <13 on initial assessment
- GCS <15 at 2 hours after the injury
- Suspected open or depressed skull fracture
- Any sign of basal skull fracture*
- Post-traumatic seizure
- Focal neurological deficit
- More than one episode of vomiting
- Amnesia for events more than 30 minutes before impact
- **CT should also be performed immediately** for the following risk factors if loss of consciousness or amnesia since the injury:
  - Age 65 years or older
  - Coagulopathy†
  - Dangerous mechanism of injury‡

*Haemotympanum, 'panda' eyes, cerebrospinal fluid leakage from the ear or nose, Battle's sign.
†History of bleeding, clotting disorder, current treatment with warfarin.
‡A pedestrian or cyclist struck by a motor vehicle, an occupant ejected from a motor vehicle or a fall from a height of greater than 1 metre or five stairs.

Raised intracranial pressure

Patients receiving sedation should undergo ICP monitoring in a critical care environment or operating theatre when presenting GCS is ≤8 or has declined, or the CT scan shows evidence of mass effect from lesions, such as haematomas, contusions or cerebral oedema. A ventricular catheter connected to a strain gauge transducer is the most accurate method of ICP monitoring and has the therapeutic advantage of allowing for cerebrospinal fluid (CSF) drainage to treat rises in ICP. However, this method is not without risk, and ICP is most commonly monitored using solid-state intraparenchymal devices which are very safe and easy to insert. If ICP remains elevated despite adequate sedation, interventions include osmotic therapy (mannitol and hypertonic saline) and modest hyperventilation. In refractory cases, moderate hypothermia, barbiturates and decompressive craniectomy should be considered. Steroids have no role in the management of TBI.

Transfer

Head-injured patients frequently require interhospital and intrahospital transfer for neurosurgical management at short notice and outside normal working hours. Transfer is a hazardous procedure if poorly managed. The keys to successful transfer include:

- adequate resuscitation and stabilization prior to transfer
- adherence to monitoring standards during transfer, with the availability of appropriate equipment and drugs
- a doctor and assistant with suitable skills and experience of transfer of patients with head injury
- good communication between referring and receiving centres, including the development of joint protocols and collaboration between senior medical staff. See Box 1.8.

Box 1.8 Guidelines for transfer of head-injured patients

- The patient must be stabilized prior to transfer
- The doctor escorting the patient should be of appropriate seniority and have sufficient skill to recognize and treat deteriorations that may occur during transfer
- All equipment and drugs, including oxygen, should be checked prior to departure
- Patients with GCS ≤8 require intubation
- All intubated patients require:
  - Sedation (propofol), to prevent increases in ICP
  - Paralysis (vecuronium or atracurium), to prevent coughing and to facilitate mechanical ventilation
  - Analgesia (e.g. fentanyl), if indicated
- Monitoring should be of the same standard as expected in an operating theatre:
  - ECG, invasive blood pressure monitoring, $S_{p}O_2$ and temperature are the minimum acceptable
  - End-tidal CO_2 should be controlled
  - Urinary catheter, volume recorded

Bibliography

Association of Anaesthetists of Great Britain and Ireland. *Recommendations on Transfer of the Severely Head Injured Patient.* London: AAGBI, 2006.

Brain Trauma Foundation. Guidelines for the management of severe traumatic brain injury, 3rd edn. *J Neurotrauma* 2007; **24**: S1–106.

Moppett IK. Traumatic brain injury: assessment, resuscitation and early management. *Br J Anaesth* 2007; **99**: 18–31.

National Institute for Health and Clinical Excellence. *Head Injury: Triage, Assessment, Investigation and Early Management of Head Injury in Infants, Children and Adults.* Clinical Guideline 56. London: NICE, 2007.

Cross-references

Anaesthetic and ICU management of the head-injured patient, 334

Neuromonitoring, 338

Raised intracranial pressure/cerebral blood flow control, 791

Spinal cord injury, 36

Transport of the critically ill, 799

Inflammatory brain disease

Rohit Juneja and Jeremy Radcliffe

Although the blood–brain barrier is effective in reducing the exposure of the brain to many chemical effects, it is not able to prevent the chronic effects of neuroinflammation. The associated increased oxidative stress has been implicated in many neurological conditions. The inflammatory state is associated with structural change, disruption of neuronal communication and the accumulation of intra- and extracellular material. These changes may have a global or regional distribution and some functional structures may be more susceptible than others.

Dementia

Aetiology and pathophysiology

In the older patient, the most common cause of dementia is Alzheimer disease (AD). Other causes are shown in Table 1.3. There are currently about 750 000 people in the UK with a form of dementia, and it is estimated that this will rise to 940 000 by 2021. The incidence of dementia increases with age:

- 40–64 years: 1 in 1400
- 65–69 years: 1 in 100
- 70–79 years: 1 in 25
- >80 years: 1 in 6.

Table 1.3 Types of dementia

Type of dementia	Proportion of total cases (%)
Alzheimer disease (AD)	62
Vascular dementia (VaD)	17
Mixed dementia (AD and VaD)	10
Dementia with Lewy bodies	4
Frontotemporal dementia	2
Parkinson dementia	2
Other dementias	3

What is common between the various forms of dementia is the presence of a chronic neuroinflammatory state with reactive microglia-triggered release of inflammatory cytokines and increased oxidative stress, ultimately resulting in neurodegeneration and neuronal death. Accumulation of β-amyloid protein in AD, plaques and neurofibrillary tangles may represent the effects of ongoing inflammation. Similar inflammatory processes are thought to occur in multiple sclerosis and patients with Parkinson disease. Research is examining the use of non-steroidal anti-inflammatory drugs (NSAIDs) and antibiotics, such as minocycline, in the hope that neuronal dysfunction in dementia can be minimized with anti-inflammatory strategies.

Clinical features

Dementia is a complex of related signs and symptoms in which diverse areas of cognition, including memory, language and problem-solving, deteriorate. In contrast to delirium, which is an acute confusional state, dementia syndromes usually progress slowly and have often been present for at least 6 months before formal diagnosis, and manifest as increasing impairment of activities of daily living.

Drug treatment

Reversible anticholinesterase medications are the mainstay of the pharmacological management of dementia – they do not treat the disease but may slow the deterioration in some patients. Currently, donepezil, galantamine and rivastigmine are approved in the UK for the treatment of mild to moderate AD. They work by counteracting the deficiency in cholinergic neurones and increasing the concentration of neuronal acetylcholine. The glutamatergic agent memantine may also have a useful role in dementias. Frontotemporal dementia, in contrast, shows deficiencies in the serotonin and dopamine neurotransmitter systems.

Anaesthetic implications

Preoperative assessment includes a thorough physical examination of all systems since many patients with dementia are elderly, with unreported symptoms or comorbidities. In addition, an assessment of the degree of mental impairment should be made using the Abbreviated Mental Test Score or Mini-Mental State Examination – scoring under 6 or 23, respectively, is suggestive of dementia or delirium.

Consent

Patients with dementia may present difficulties regarding their ability to provide informed consent. The Mental Capacity Act 2005 states that there should be a default presumption of capacity: 'every adult has the right to make his or her own decisions and must be assumed to have capacity to do so unless it is proved otherwise'. Therefore, attempts to support the patient to make his or her own decisions should be made, and any actions or interventions must be in their best interests. It is advisable, wherever possible, to involve relatives in discussions and decisions.

Drug interactions

Sensitivity to, and delayed recovery from, sedative or anaesthetic agents may be encountered to an unpredictable extent. The failure in the cholinergic pathways in the brain renders patients suffering with AD very susceptible to the effects of anticholinergic drugs, in particular atropine, which is able to pass through the blood–brain barrier because of its tertiary structure. The administration of atropine may worsen a patient's neurological symptoms and be undesirably sedating. Anticholinesterase medication can antagonize the effects of non-depolarizing neuromuscular blocking drugs and potentiate succinylcholine.

Postoperative care

Pain assessment can be particularly difficult in patients suffering with dementia and often requires assessment using non-verbal cues or charting of visual analogue scales if cognitive status allows. Inadequate pain management is associated with delayed ambulation, loss of appetite, increased postoperative morbidity and worsening of the pre-existing cognitive impairment.

Chronic alcohol abuse can be a cause of dementia and is associated with the development of Wernicke's encephalopathy and Korsakoff's psychosis. In such patients, alcohol withdrawal needs to be anticipated in the perioperative period and prevented by the administration of thiamine preparations and benzodiazepines.

Creutzfeldt–Jakob disease

In contrast to the slowly progressing forms of dementia, the syndrome associated with Creutzfeldt-Jakob disease (CJD) develops over a period of a few months. Various forms of CJD are recognized. Sporadic CJD usually affects those over the age of 60; familial CJD displays autosomal dominant inheritance; and variant CJD (vCJD) can have an incubation period of many years and was until recently attributable solely to the ingestion of contaminated beef products. Between 1996 and 2006 there were 161 recorded cases of vCJD in the UK. Iatrogenic causes of CJD include transmission from the use of human-derived growth hormone, cadaveric dura mater grafts, and EEG and brain stereotactic needles.

Aetiology and pathophysiology

Although the exact detail is still poorly understood, CJD is caused by accumulation of a highly stable and resistant protein called the prion (PrP). The abnormal form has the designation PrP^{TSE} for transmissible spongiform encephalopathy. PrP^{TSE} accumulates in the brain and initiates an inflammatory cascade which eventually results in the formation of neuronal vacuoles and neuronal cell death. Testing for PrP^{TSE} is unreliable, and absence of the prion does not indicate absence of infectivity. PrP^{TSE} is resistant to standard chemical and physical methods of inactivation and even autoclaving is unreliable in removing all traces of the protein. Only incineration at 850°C or higher can guarantee PrP elimination.

Anaesthetic implications

For anaesthesia of known or suspected cases of CJD, single-use equipment, which is incinerated following use, should be employed. If single use laryngoscope handles are not available, they should be protected by a disposable sheath. Standard universal precautions should be taken, including the use of disposable gloves, waterproof apron, gown, mask and eye protection.

Samples should be clearly labelled 'biohazard' and the laboratory informed of the nature of the material before its arrival. Clinical waste from high- or medium-risk tissue (the CNS, posterior eye and pituitary gland) in a patient at 'increased risk' of vCJD should be incinerated. Where possible, procedures should be performed at the end of the operating list to allow adequate time for appropriate decontamination.

As PrP^{TSE} has been found to be concentrated in lymphoid tissue as well as the CNS, concerns have been raised regarding the anaesthetic management of patients for tonsillectomy. However, in 2008, the Association of Anaesthetists of Great Britain and Ireland published guidance on this matter and recommended that single-use laryngoscopes were not mandatory for such cases.

Blood transfusion

Since 2003, there have been three documented cases of vCJD transmission via blood transfusion, resulting in tighter restriction of blood products' usage. UK blood donors who received blood transfusion in the UK were removed from the donor pool and all plasma products are now imported into the UK (mainly from Germany and the USA).

Notification

Although not a statutory notifiable disease, any new cases of CJD (variant or otherwise) should be referred by the neurologist to the National Creutzfeldt–Jakob

Disease Surveillance Unit (NCJDSU) at http://www.cjd.ed.ac.uk/.

Bibliography

Association of Anaesthetists of Great Britain and Ireland. Safety guideline: infection control in anaesthesia. *Anaesthesia* 2008; **63**: 1027–36.

Department of Health. *Transmissible Spongiform Encephalopathy Agents: Safe Working and the Prevention of Infection.* Part 4. *Infection Control of CJD, vCJD and Other Human Prion Disease in Healthcare and Community Settings.* London: DH, 2010. See www.dh.gov.uk/prod_consum_dh/groups/dh_digitalassets/@dh/@ab/documents/digitalasset/dh_113959.pdf.

Fodale V, Quattrone D, Trecroci C, *et al.* Alzheimer's disease and anaesthesia: implications for the central cholinergic system. *Br J Anaesth* 2006; **97**: 445–52.

Frank-Cannon TC, Alto LT, McAlpine FE, Tansey MG. Does neuroinflammation fan the flame in neurodegenerative diseases? *Mol Neurodegen* 2009; **4**: 47.

National Institute for Health and Clinical Excellence. *Technology Assessment. Donepezil, Galantamine, Rivastigmine (Review) and Memantine for the Treatment of Alzheimer's Disease.* London: NICE, 2007 (updated 2009). See www.nice.org.uk/TA111.

Tang J, Eckenhoff MF, Eckenhoff RG. Anesthesia and the old brain. *Anesth Analg* 2010; **110**: 421–6.

Cross-reference

Neuromonitoring, 338

Multiple sclerosis

Ian Appleby

Multiple sclerosis (MS) is an autoimmune-mediated chronic inflammatory disease of the CNS. It is the most common cause of non-traumatic neurological disability in young adults in North America and Europe.

Aetiology

Although the exact cause is unknown, MS is thought to have an autoimmune aetiology mediated by complex interactions between genetic susceptibility and environmental insults. The inheritance is unclear, but there is increased concordance in monozygotic twins. There is an increased incidence in countries further from the equator and some evidence for viral triggers, as patients with MS report being affected by common viruses later than age-matched controls.

Epidemiology

The prevalence of MS is 2–150 per 100 000 population with regional variation. It is more common in the northern hemisphere, and migrants who move before age 15 take on the risk of the native population. Like many other autoimmune diseases it is more common in women than men, although in older people the sex distribution is 50:50. First presentation is usually in the third and fourth decades of life, although it can present at any age from early childhood.

Pathogenesis

MS is characterized by the formation of sclerotic plaques that represent the end-stage of a process of inflammation, demyelination and remyelination. Autoreactive lymphocytes cross the blood–brain barrier and deplete oligodendrocytes (myelin-forming cells). Remyelination can occur initially, but repeated attacks lead to plaques building up over the axon. Characteristically, the plaques are disseminated in space and time especially in the periventricular regions, optic nerve, brainstem and spinal cord white matter. Initially, the axons are preserved, but later demyelination is associated with irreversible axonal and neuronal degeneration.

Clinical features

Clinical manifestations reflect plaques in motor, sensory, visual and autonomic systems. There are few disease-specific features, and many symptoms and signs can occur (Box 1.9). Characteristic are Lhermitte's sign (an electrical sensation in the legs on neck flexion) and Uhthoff's phenomenon (transient worsening of symptoms on raising the body temperature, e.g. after exercise).

Box 1.9 Signs and symptoms of multiple sclerosis

- Cerebrum
  - Motor weakness
  - Sensory changes
  - Cognitive impairment
  - Affective disorders
- Optic nerve
  - Unilateral loss of vision
- Cerebellum
  - Diplopia
  - Vertigo
  - Ataxia
  - Impaired speech and swallowing
- Spinal cord
  - Weakness
  - Spasticity
  - Bladder dysfunction
- Other
  - Pain
  - Fatigue
  - Temperature insensitivity

Relapsing–remitting multiple sclerosis

Eighty per cent of patients present with an acute episode affecting one or several sites – known as the clinically isolated syndrome. Recovery from this and subsequent episodes is often complete. New episodes occur erratically but are rarely more than 1.5 per year. Relapses can be triggered by intercurrent illness, stress and hyperthermia, and are more common in the puerperium. Relapses are not usually triggered by surgery or anaesthesia, pregnancy or vaccinations.

Secondary progressive multiple sclerosis

Around 65% of patients enter this phase when recovery from each episode is incomplete and there is progressive neurological deterioration.

Primary progressive multiple sclerosis

In around 20% of patients the disease is progressive from the onset.

Diagnosis

Diagnosis is based on clinical, radiological (MRI) and laboratory criteria. Typically, there are two or more clinical episodes over 30 days apart, with a characteristic MRI to confirm the diagnosis.

Clinical

- History of exacerbation and remission.
- Clinical manifestations suggesting multiple lesions in different sites.
- Optic neuritis is the presenting sign in 20–30% of patients.

Laboratory

- Abnormal cerebral spinal fluid examination.
- Increased white cell count.
- Raised protein levels.
- Immunoglobulin (Ig) G oligoclonal bands on electrophoresis (found in 75–80%).

Radiological

Multifocal lesions are seen on MRI, especially involving the periventricular, cerebellum and spinal cord white matter. Gadolinium-enhanced scans demonstrate active MS lesions.

Treatment

There is no known treatment that predictably slows the course of MS. The aim of treatment is to return function after an attack and either prevent or increase the interval between further attacks.

Acute treatments

- Corticosteroids: high-dose methylprednisolone is used for acute relapses, and both oral and intravenous preparations have been shown to have equal efficacy. Prednisolone is usually introduced after 5 days.
- Plasmapheresis: can be used for steroid-resistant severe relapses.

Disease-modifying drugs

These drugs affect the relapsing–remitting stage of the disease and have no useful treatment effect either on the secondary progressive phase or in primary progressive MS.

- Beta-interferon: reduces the frequency of relapses by about 30% over 2–3 years, decreases the incidence of fixed disabilities but does not delay entry into the secondary progressive phase. It can be used early in the disease progress because of limited side-effects. Local injection site reactions and flu-like symptoms are relatively common.
- Glatiramer acetate: induces tolerance to myelin-reactive lymphocytes. It decreases the frequency of relapses in the early stages of the disease. There may be some benefit in combination therapy with β-interferon.
- Mitoxantrone: causes DNA and RNA inhibition. Its use is limited by toxic side-effects, including cardiotoxicity and acute leukaemia.
- Natalizumab: given by infusion as monotherapy in severe disease. It reduces the relapse rate and the chance of acquiring fixed disability.

Other therapies

- Baclofen and tizanadine are used to treat muscle spasm.
- Gabapentin is useful for painful symptoms.
- Amantidine is used to treat fatigue.
- Oxybutinin may help bladder function.
- Neurorehabilitation, including physiotherapy and occupational therapy.

Anaesthetic management

Anaesthetic implications of MS are unclear, and it is difficult to separate the effects of anaesthesia and surgery from spontaneous new lesion formation. However, stress can exacerbate MS symptoms and measures should be taken to relieve anxiety. The majority of patients undergoing surgery will be young and otherwise well, although some will be undergoing surgery for their symptoms (e.g. suprapubic catheter, intrathecal baclofen pump insertion).

Preoperative assessment

As well as a full medical history particular attention should be paid to:

- disease progression and history of relapses; current abnormal neurology should be documented
- evidence of infection: a rise in temperature of 0.5–1°C increases conduction block in demyelinated neurones
- respiratory reserve can be poor and respiratory function tests and blood gas analysis may be required
- bulbar function should be examined
- autonomic dysreflexia can occur in patients with extensive spinal cord demyelination
- steroid medication
- mental state: depression and fatigue are common
- the presence of any pressure sores or contractures which may affect surgical positioning.

Premedication

- All antispasmodic medication should be continued.
- H_2 receptor antagonists should be prescribed if there is any evidence of recurrent aspiration.
- Sedative premedication is usually avoided.

Intraoperative management

- There is no evidence for the benefits of one induction agent or maintenance technique over another.
- Tracheal intubation may be preferred if there is poor bulbar function.
- Succinylcholine should be avoided if there is extensive demyelination as it may cause hyperkalaemia.
- Non-depolarizing muscle relaxants are safe and response is normal, although monitoring of neuromuscular blockade is recommended.
- Temperature should be monitored and hypo- and hyperthermia should be avoided.
- Deep vein thrombosis prophylaxis is essential as there is an increased tendency to platelet aggregation.
- Careful attention should be paid to positioning, especially in patients with contractures and pressure sores.

Postoperative management

- Postoperative analgesia should take into account the patient's respiratory function.
- Respiratory physiotherapy may be required to remove pulmonary secretions.
- Normothermia should be maintained.
- Early mobilization and return to normal function should be encouraged.
- The stress of surgery may provoke a relapse.

General versus regional anaesthesia

There is no absolute contraindication to the use of regional anaesthesia in patients with MS, although it is sometimes avoided in patients with neurological signs and symptoms. Epidural and spinal anaesthesia can both be used in obstetric analgesia and anaesthesia, and in other circumstances a regional technique should be used if most appropriate for the patient and situation. There is no evidence that a regional technique leads to a symptomatic relapse, but the decision to proceed with either a general or a regional technique should be based on careful discussion with the patient. Before performing any regional blockade, careful note should be made of pre-existing signs and symptoms, and neurological assessment should be repeated after the blockade has worn off.

Bibliography

Compston A, Coles A. Multiple sclerosis. *Lancet* 2008; **372**: 1502–17.

Hebl J, Horlocker TT, Schroeder DR. Neuraxial anaesthesia and analgesia in patients with pre-existing nervous system disorders. *Anesth Analg* 2006; **103**: 223–8.

National Institute for Health and Clinical Excellence. *Management of Multiple Sclerosis in Primary and Secondary Care*. NICE Clinical Guideline CG08. London: NICE, 2003.

Cross-reference

Autonomic dysfunction and autonomic dysreflexia, 4

Parkinson disease

Chris Taylor

Parkinson disease (PD) is an idiopathic neurodegenerative condition and is the commonest cause of Parkinsonism – a syndrome characterized by tremor, rigidity and bradykinesia. Parkinsonism is the commonest movement disorder. PD affects approximately 0.3% of the UK population overall, increasing to 3% in those aged over 65 years. It is a worldwide disease, with a very slight male preponderance, and occurs in all ethnic groups.

Aetiology

The aetiology of PD is unknown, although the neurodegeneration may be induced by genetic, environmental or infectious factors. Increasing age is the most consistent risk factor. PD is distinguished from Parkinsonism, which has a number of specific causes (Box 1.10).

Pathophysiology

Parkinsonism occurs because of an imbalance of the antagonistic basal ganglion cholinergic and dopaminergic systems. In PD, pigmented cells in the substantia nigra are lost along with associated dopaminergic activity and replaced with glial cells. In addition, tyrosine β-hydroxylase, the rate-limiting step in dopamine synthesis, also diminishes. The remaining cells contain the pathological hallmark of eosinophilic Lewy bodies.

Box 1.10 Causes of Parkinsonism

- Genetic
  - Dominant, e.g. α-synuclein mutations (PARK 1) or gene duplications/triplications (PARK 4)
  - Recessive, e.g. parkin mutations (PARK 2) or DJ1 mutations (PARK 7)
- Drugs
  - Phenothiazines
  - Butyrophenones
  - Metoclopramide
- Toxins
  - Carbon monoxide
- Encephalitis
- Cerebrovascular disease
- Heavy metal poisoning and metabolic defects, e.g. Wilson disease
- Other degenerative CNS diseases
  - Supranuclear palsy
  - Multisystem atrophy

Clinical features

There are no specific diagnostic tests for PD and the diagnosis is made on clinical grounds. Patients exhibit the classic 'triad' of symptoms (usually asymmetrical):

- tremor at rest: 'pill rolling' at 4–6 Hz, improved by voluntary movement
- rigidity: 'cogwheel' in nature, juddering on passive extension
- bradykinesia: paucity of movement, monotonous speech, expressionless face, shuffling gait and abnormal posture.

Therapeutic trials offer confirmatory evidence, with over 90% of patients showing a good early improvement with levodopa (L-dopa).

PD is associated with a multitude of clinical features because of its multisystem effects (Box 1.11).

Management

Treatment is usually pharmacological, although surgical methods are useful for some patients.

Box 1.11 Organ systems affected by Parkinson disease

- Autonomic
  - Postural hypotension
  - Hyperhidrosis
  - Difficulty with micturition
  - Impotence
- Respiratory
  - Upper airway dysfunction
  - Excess bronchial secretions
  - Poor cough/retained secretions
- Cardiovascular
  - Postural hypotension
  - Dysrhythmias
- Gastrointestinal
  - Excessive salivation
  - Gastro-oesophageal reflux
- Neurological
  - Speech impairment
  - Dementia
  - Depression
  - Sleep disturbance

Drug treatment

- *L-Dopa and dopamine agonists* form the mainstay of pharmacological treatment of PD. L-Dopa, an inactive form of dopamine (which itself does not cross the blood–brain barrier), is converted by decarboxylases in the CNS. The addition of peripheral decarboxylase inhibitors, such as benserazide and carbidopa, which do not themselves cross the blood–brain barrier, reduces peripheral conversion, resulting in fewer side-effects. Ergot derivatives, such as bromocriptine, pergolide, lisuride, cabergoline, ropinirole and pramipexole, are dopamine receptor agonists; since they may cause nausea, hypotension and psychiatric disturbance, they are reserved as adjuvant therapy or for those with severe side-effects from L-dopa. Apomorphine is the only available parenteral dopaminergic drug and should be given with the antiemetic domperidone.
- *Monoamine oxide inhibitors*, such as selegiline (a monoamine oxidase type B inhibitor), reduce the central breakdown of dopamine.
- *Anticholinergic drugs*, such as procyclidine, benztropine, biperiden, benzhexol and orphenadrine, have limited efficacy and several side-effects, including confusion, urinary retention and glaucoma.
- *Catechol-O-methyl transferase inhibitors* (e.g. entacapone) improve the dopamine concentration profile, resulting in fewer on–off symptom fluctuations.

Surgical treatment

Stereotactic pallidotomy, thalamotomy and deep brain stimulation are increasingly used as treatment for PD. Fetal cell transplants remain experimental.

Anaesthetic implications of Parkinson disease

Preoperative assessment

The preoperative assessment should focus on identifying and optimizing the systemic complications of PD (Box 1.11). The severity of symptoms should be noted as well as the potential for cooperation with a regional technique. Although the normal timing of anti-Parkinsonian medication is disrupted by hospital admission and preoperative nil-by-mouth instructions, the continuation of medication up to 2 hours before surgery is usually beneficial. Regular treatment regimens should be modified when a subcutaneous apomorphine infusion is required for longer duration surgery.

Preoperative investigations include ECG, chest X-ray, spirometry (restrictive pattern often identified) and vital capacity measurement. Adequate preoperative hydration is essential to minimize the risk of cardiovascular complications. Patients with PD have a high incidence of gastro-oesophageal reflux, and this should be taken into consideration when planning the anaesthetic technique. A urinary catheter may be required, particularly for longer procedures.

Conduct of anaesthesia

L-Dopa therapy must be continued, by nasogastric tube if necessary. Regional anaesthesia may avoid some of the complications of general anaesthesia, but tremor, confusion and exaggerated hypotension may cause difficulties in awake patients. Potential drug interactions should be considered (Box 1.12 and Table 1.4). These are common but can be unexpected.

Box 1.12 Interaction of drug therapy for Parkinson disease with other therapy

- Amantadine: anticholinergics, L-dopa, CNS depressants and stimulants, diuretics
- Biperiden: antihistamines, CNS depressants, quinidine, metoclopramide
- L-Dopa/benserazide: MAOIs, potent opioids, antihypertensives, sympathomimetics, ferrous sulphate
- Benzhexol: MAOIs, phenothiazines, antihistamines, antidepressants, disopyramide, amantadine
- Benztropine: MAOIs, phenothiazines, antihistamines, antidepressants, disopyramide, amantadine
- Bromocriptine: erythromycin, metoclopramide, alcohol
- Cabergoline: neuroleptics, ergot alkaloids, dopamine antagonists, macrolides, hypotensive agents
- Entacapone: MAOIs, rimiterole, sympathomimetics, methyldopa, antidepressants, iron, bromocriptine
- L-Dopa/carbidopa: MAOIs, antihypertensives, sympathomimetics
- Orphenadrine: phenothiazines, antihistamines, antidepressants, amantadine, disopyramide, terodiline
- Pergolide: dopamine antagonists, antihypertensives, anticoagulants, competition for protein binding
- Pramipexole: amantadine, cimetidine, ranitidine, diltiazem, quinidine, quinine, verapamil, digoxin, procainamide, triamterene, sedatives, alcohol
- Procyclidine: phenothiazines, antihistamines, antidepressants, amantadine, disopyramide, ketoconazole, quinidine, MAOIs
- Ropinirole: antihypertensives, antiarrhythmics, neuroleptics, oestrogens, alcohol, drugs affecting P450
- Selegiline: fluoxetine, sertraline, paroxetine, pethidine, non-selective MAOIs, tricyclic antidepressants, anticoagulants, digitalis

MAOI, monoamine oxidase inhibitor.

Table 1.4 Interaction of commonly used drugs in patients taking treatment for Parkinson disease

Drug	Side-effects	Considerations
Antiemetics		
Metoclopramide Droperidol Prochlorperazine	Extrapyramidal side-effects or Parkinsonian symptoms	Use domperidone, 5-HT_3 (e.g. ondansetron) or antihistamine (e.g. cyclizine)
Analgesics		
Pethidine	↑BP and rigidity with selegiline	?Resemble malignant hyperpyrexia
Synthetic opiates	↑Rigidity	Dose related
Antidepressants		
Tricyclics	↑L-Dopa-induced dysrhythmias	
SSRIs	↑BP and cerebral excitation with selegiline	
Other		
Volatile anaesthetic agents	↑L-Dopa-induced dysrhythmias	Avoid halothane if ECG abnormal
Antihypertensives	Exaggerated drug effects ↑BP with indirect antihypertensives and selegiline	
Antipsychotics	Extrapyramidal side-effects or Parkinsonian symptoms	Use 'atypical' antipsychotics (e.g. clozapine or olazapine)

5-HT, 5-hydroxytryptamine; BP, blood pressure; SSRI, selective serotonin reuptake inhibitor.

Thiopental, etomidate and ketamine have been used in PD without harm, although there has been concern regarding a hypertensive reaction to ketamine in some patients. Despite reports of propofol causing exacerbation of dyskinesia, it generally reduces most symptoms and is safe to use. Volatile agents may potentiate treated PD-associated hypotension and dysrhythmias. NSAIDs and simple analgesics may be used as normal. Fentanyl, alfentanil and morphine may cause rigidity in some cases. The use of local and regional anaesthetic techniques minimizes potent opioid requirements. Depolarizing and non-depolarizing neuromuscular agents can be used safely in PD, as can neostigmine/glycopyrronium.

Direct-acting vasodilators are preferred for the treatment of intraoperative hypertension, but should be used with caution. Antiemetic and antipsychotic drugs (including chlorpromazine, droperidol and metoclopramide) may exacerbate Parkinsonian symptoms, whereas ondansetron and cyclizine are devoid of extrapyramidal actions and are therefore safe.

Postoperative care

Mobilizing may be delayed because of Parkinsonian symptoms and drug regimes should be reinstituted early to minimize this risk. Attention should be paid to pressure areas and thromboprophylaxis is necessary. Postoperative confusion can be treated with a benzodiazepine or 'atypical' antipsychotic while the cause is sought. Patient-controlled analgesia may be awkward for patients with PD and regional techniques should be continued as appropriate. Physiotherapy for chest (impaired cough, laryngeal function and increased secretions) and mobility facilitates early mobilization and minimizes postoperative complications.

Bibliography

Brennan K, Genever R. Managing Parkinson's disease during surgery. *BMJ* 2010; **341**: 990–3.

Lang A, Lozano A. Parkinson's disease: first of two parts. *N Engl J Med* 1998; **339**: 1044–53.

Lang A, Lozano A. Parkinson's disease: second of two parts. *N Engl J Med* 1998; **339**: 1130–43.

Nicholson G, Pereira A, Hall G. Parkinson's disease and anaesthesia. *Br J Anaesth* 2002; **89**(6): 904–16.

Severn A. Parkinsonism and the anaesthetist. *Br J Anaesth* 1988; **61**: 761–70.

Cross-references

Neuroleptic malignant syndrome, 774
The elderly patient, 607

Peripheral neuropathy

David Brealey and Nicholas Hirsch

Although generalized peripheral neuropathies are rare in general clinical practice, they pose a significant challenge to the anaesthetist, including:

- respiratory muscle weakness
- bulbar weakness
- sensitivity to neuromuscular blocking agents
- hyperkalaemia following succinylcholine.

Generalized peripheral neuropathies may be either acute or chronic, and may be related to demyelination or destruction of the nerve axons (Box 1.13).

Box 1.13 Causes of peripheral neuropathy

- Acute
  - Guillain–Barré syndrome
  - Porphyria
  - Toxins
  - Vasculitis
- Chronic
  - Chronic inflammatory demyelinating polyneuropathy
  - Paraneoplastic
  - Myeloma
  - Toxins/drugs, e.g. heavy metal intoxication, fluoroquinolones

Guillain–Barré syndrome

Aetiology

Guillain–Barré syndrome (GBS) is the commonest form of acute peripheral neuropathy in the UK, with an incidence of two per 100 000 population. Approximately two-thirds of patients have suffered from a preceding upper respiratory or gastrointestinal tract infection. GBS may also be triggered by other events, including surgery, but there is little evidence to link it to current vaccines. There are several well-recognized variants of GBS (Table 1.5).

Pathophysiology

GBS is an autoimmune disease of the peripheral nervous system in which there is immune-mediated destruction of the peripheral nerve myelin sheaths or, occasionally, the axons.

Clinical features

GBS presents with an ascending, symmetrical weakness typically starting in the lower limbs. It progresses over hours to days, reaching a nadir by 3–4 weeks. The weakness may ascend to affect muscles of respiration and bulbar function. In extreme circumstances all cranial and peripheral motor nerves may be affected, mimicking brainstem death. Examination demonstrates

Table 1.5 Variants of Guillain–Barré syndrome

Variant	Nerve pathology	Relative frequency in UK	Symptoms and signs
AIDP	Demyelination	90%	Predominantly motor involvement with pain and autonomic dysfunction
Fisher syndrome		5%	Ophthalmoplegia, ataxia, areflexia
Acute sensory and motor axonal neuropathy	Axonal degeneration	5% (65% in China)	Motor and sensory involvement. Autonomic dysfunction less severe than AIDP
Acute motor axonal neuropathy			Purely motor involvement
Acute sensory neuropathy			Primarily sensory, evidence of motor involvement on nerve conduction studies

AIDP, acute inflammatory demyelinating polyradiculoneuropathy.

a flaccid paralysis with loss of deep tendon reflexes. There are often associated sensory symptoms (e.g. pain, paraesthesia), although few (if any) demonstrable deficits. The majority of patients are severely affected and unable to walk without help, and 25% require ventilation for respiratory or bulbar failure.

Autonomic dysfunction is frequent, characterized by marked alterations in blood pressure, tachycardia, bradycardia (including asystole), urinary retention, ileus and sweating. ECG changes are also common.

Investigations

Lumbar puncture demonstrates a raised CSF protein (may be normal in the first week), with a normal CSF white cell count. Nerve conduction studies demonstrate either demyelination or axonal loss.

Treatment

Immunotherapy

Plasma exchange and intravenous Ig are equally efficacious in reducing time to recovery, autonomic dysfunction and the requirement for mechanical ventilation. Owing to its relative ease of use, intravenous Ig is now a standard of care. Steroids have no place in the treatment of GBS and may be deleterious.

Respiratory support

Twenty-five per cent of patients require intubation for respiratory failure. Regular FVC measurements are vital to detect deterioration in respiratory function, and intubation should occur before the patient is compromised. FVC <15 mL kg^{-1} is associated with the imminent need for ventilation, but earlier intubation may be necessary if bulbar weakness coexists. Tracheostomy is usually indicated as the period of ventilation may be prolonged.

Pain

The majority of patients suffer both nociceptive and neuropathic pain. Management combines regular analgesics, including opioid agents and adjuncts such as gabapentin or amitriptyline.

Thromboembolic prophylaxis

Graduated compression stockings and low-molecular-weight heparins should be used when possible.

Autonomic complications

Hypertension and tachycardia can be managed with β-blockers, whereas hypotension may require a norepinephrine infusion. Bradycardias can usually be managed with vagolytics, but may be severe enough to warrant temporary pacing. Ileus can be supported by nasogastric and rectal tubes and, if required, total parenteral nutrition.

Anaesthetic implications

Preoperative

Many patients will already be ventilated on the ICU. If not, assessment of bulbar and respiratory function including FVC (<20 mL kg^{-1}) will predict the need for postoperative ventilation. Ileus causes complications in up to 15% of patients with severe GBS and increases the risk of aspiration during induction. A rapid sequence induction may therefore be required.

Induction of anaesthesia

Succinylcholine can result in fatal hyperkalaemia, following excessive potassium release from the denervated muscles, and is contraindicated. Rocuronium is a suitable alternative if a rapid sequence technique is indicated. Autonomic dysfunction can make induction and intubation hazardous, resulting in a labile pulse and blood pressure.

GBS is not a contraindication to peripheral nerve or neuraxial blockade; however, very high blocks can impair respiratory muscle function further.

Intraoperative

Patients should be mechanically ventilated through the procedure if respiratory function is impaired. GBS patients are sensitive to the effects of non-depolarizing neuromuscular blocking agents and their use should be kept to a minimum. If appropriate, patients should be extubated fully awake once bulbar reflexes have returned.

Postoperative

Postoperative ventilation is often required. However, if patients are extubated, careful monitoring of respiratory function is vital, ideally in a critical care setting. Pain can be problematic since many patients are often not opiate naive, but needs rapid assessment and control.

Diphtheria

Aetiology

Diphtheria is caused by *Corynebacterium diphtheriae*, a Gram-positive bacillus. Although extremely rare in the UK, it is making a resurgence in parts of central and eastern Europe following the breakdown of immunization campaigns. It is easily spread through droplet transmission or touch. Its pathogenicity is related to the expression of an exotoxin.

Clinical features

Diphtheria usually presents as a pharyngitis, tonsillitis or laryngitis. Symptoms include low-grade fever, malaise, anorexia, hoarse voice and sore throat.

Examination demonstrates a grey/green membrane that may cover the soft palate or tonsils but can progress to cause airway obstruction. If the disease progresses, patients develop marked cervical lymphadenopathy and oedema, giving a characteristic bull-neck appearance. Absorption of the toxin leads to the systemic manifestations of diphtheria, including:

- myocarditis, dysrhythmias and heart failure
- demyelinating polyneuropathy: this principally affects bulbar and respiratory muscles, but also limbs and eyes. It tends to occur once the acute illness is resolving. The response is often biphasic, with patients deteriorating after an initial improvement. Recovery is variable but patients are often left severely disabled.

Diagnosis is clinical, but can be confirmed by isolating *C. diphtheriae* from the pharynx. Diphtheria carries a mortality of 5–10%.

Management

Treatment consists of antitoxin and benzylpenicillin (or erythromycin) and should be started once diphtheria is clinically suspected. Diphtheria is a notifiable disease.

The progressive neuropathy can result in respiratory failure, and approximately 20% of patients will require mechanical ventilation. Bulbar failure may require nasogastric feeding and, if severe, tracheostomy.

Anaesthetic implications

Patients with diphtheria may present with acute airway obstruction. Endotracheal intubation is hazardous as the pharynx and larynx are oedematous and the adherent membrane may obscure the view of the larynx entirely. Early recognition of airway compromise and close cooperation with ENT surgeons is vital.

The neuropathy usually develops after the acute infection, but puts the patient at risk of respiratory failure requiring postoperative ventilation. The chronically denervated muscles expose the patient to fatal hyperkalaemia if succinylcholine is used.

Porphyrias

Aetiology

The porphyrias are a group of diseases caused by an enzyme defect within the haem synthetic pathway, resulting in the overproduction of porphyrins. Porphyrias can be classified in several ways, e.g. site of defect (hepatic or erythropoietic), acute or non-acute (Box 1.14), or pattern of enzyme defect. It is the acute variety that has particular relevance to the anaesthetist.

Box 1.14 Types of acute and non-acute porphyria

- Acute
  - Acute intermittent porphyria (AIP)
  - Variegate porphyria (VP)
  - Hereditary coproporphyria (HCP)
- Non-acute
  - Erythropoietic porphyria
  - Porphyria cutanea tarda

Acute intermittent porphyria (AIP) affects about one in 20 000 Europeans, but is more common in northern Scandinavia. Variegate porphyria (VP) is less common, except in the Afrikaner community (1 in 250). Acute attacks are precipitated by events that decrease haem concentrations and thus stimulate the activity of δ-amino laevulinic acid (ALA) synthetase activity and accumulation of porphyrins within the tissues. These events include starvation, stress, dehydration, infection and certain drugs (Box 1.15).

Box 1.15 Drugs that precipitate porphyria

- Barbiturates
- Etomidate
- Phenytoin
- Sulphonamides
- Hydralazine
- Oral contraceptive pill

Clinical features

Acute attacks often present with severe abdominal pain (although often little is found on clinical examination), vomiting, electrolyte and autonomic disturbances (hypertension, tachycardia) and neurological involvement. Acute attacks often result in a severe neuropathy (predominantly motor) with the involvement of peripheral nerves, anterior horn cells, autonomic ganglia, brainstem and cerebellar pathways. Weakness commonly presents in proximal limb muscles but may progress, leading to tetraplegia and respiratory and bulbar failure. There are often associated sensory losses. Other manifestations include altered mental state, cranial nerve palsies, seizures and coma. Neurological recovery is often slow or incomplete. VP is also associated with bullous skin lesions on exposure to light during the acute episode. Hereditary coproporphyria (HCP) is also associated with photosensitivity but symptoms are usually less severe than in AIP and VP.

Management

Management of an acute attack involves managing the underlying precipitant, correcting electrolyte abnormalities, and treating pain, agitation and autonomic dysfunction. Intubation and ventilation will be required if there is bulbar or respiratory failure, or a significant decrease in level of consciousness.

Specific treatment is targeted at suppressing haem synthesis and includes carbohydrate and the administration of haematin, a haem compound that results in a negative feedback on ALA synthetase.

Anaesthetic considerations

Patients with porphyria can be anaesthetized safely providing trigger factors are avoided. Adequate hydration and correction of abnormal electrolytes is crucial, and preoperative starvation should be kept to a minimum. If starvation is unavoidable then intravenous glucose should be administered, although care needs to be taken to avoid hyponatraemia. Many modern anaesthetic drugs are definite or potential precipitants, but a simple and safe regimen includes:

- induction: propofol or possibly ketamine
- maintenance: propofol, nitrous oxide, halothane, isoflurane
- neuromuscular blockade: succinylcholine, vecuronium
- analgesia: morphine, fentanyl and paracetamol.

Porphyria is not a contraindication to neuraxial or peripheral nerve blocks and both bupivacaine and fentanyl are acceptable.

Postoperative care depends on accurate pain management and the avoidance of infection, dehydration and starvation.

Bibliography

Logina I, Donagh M. Diphtheritic polyneuropathy: a clinical study and comparison with Guillain-Barré syndrome. *J Neurol Neurosurg Psychiatry* 1999; **67**: 433–8.

Plasma Exchange/Sandoglobulin Guillain–Barré Syndrome Trial Group. Randomised trial of plasma exchange, intravenous immunoglobulin and combined treatments in Guillain-Barré syndrome. *Lancet* 1997; **349**: 225–30.

Puy H, Gouya L, Deybach JC. Porphyrias. *Lancet* 2010; **375**: 924–37.

Vucic S, Kiernan MC, Cornblath DR. Guillain-Barré syndrome: an update. *J Clin Neurosci* 2009; **16**: 733–41.

Cross-reference

Failure to breathe or wake up postoperatively, 749

Primary neuromuscular disease

David Brealey and Nicholas Hirsch

Destruction of upper motor neurones (UMNs) or lower motor neurones (LMNs) leads to paralysis of associated muscle groups. The process can be limited, producing minimal weakness and disability, or widespread and progressive, leading to paralysis, bulbar and respiratory failure and death. This patient group can present significant clinical and ethical challenges to the anaesthetist.

Motor neurone disease

Aetiology

Motor neurone disease (MND) describes a number of neurological disorders resulting from the degeneration of the anterior horn cells and motor cranial nuclei (Table 1.6). There is often considerable overlap between the different types of MND, making distinction difficult. The most common form is amytrophic lateral sclerosis (ALS), which is characterized by effects on both UMNs and LMNs. Affecting 1 or 2 per 100 000 population, its incidence peaks between 55 and 75 years. Survival is 2–5 years from diagnosis, with death usually resulting from respiratory failure.

Clinical presentation

The diagnosis is clinical, with investigations being used to exclude other causes of weakness. Patients usually present with progressive distal limb weakness, initially in the upper followed by the lower limbs. Weakness is often asymmetric, and patients notice wasting of affected muscle groups. Bulbar onset is less common, but presents with slurred speech progressing to dysphagia, nasal regurgitation and pulmonary aspiration. Respiratory muscle involvement rarely occurs at presentation, and leads to nocturnal hypoventilation with early morning headaches and hypersomnolence progressing to respiratory failure. As the disease progresses, patients are left paralysed, unable to swallow or communicate and eventually succumb to respiratory failure. Cognition remains intact in the majority of patients.

Examination usually demonstrates a combination of upper (spasticity and hyper-reflexia) and lower (wasting and fasciculation) motor neurone signs. There are no sensory signs and autonomic dysfunction occurs only late in the disease.

Management

Management is multidisciplinary and involves medical, symptomatic and non-pharmacological support.

Disease modifying

Riluzole is the only disease-modifying drug available and prolongs life by a median of 3 months. It is generally well tolerated but may cause liver dysfunction or neutropenia.

Respiratory

The majority of patients with MND die from respiratory failure. The use of non-invasive ventilation (in those without severe bulbar failure) improves both length and quality of life. Ventilation via tracheostomy, although rare in the UK, also prolongs life, particularly in patients with bulbar failure. Carbocisteine can be helpful in the management of thick secretions, whereas anticholinergic drugs are used in patients unable to manage their own secretions.

Pain

Pain is caused by immobility, cramps and spasticity and can be managed with analgesics, quinine sulphate, baclofen (oral or intrathecal) or injection of botulinum toxin into specific muscle groups. Physiotherapy may also be helpful.

Table 1.6 Motor neurone disease

	Motor neurone affected	Life expectancy	Proportion of MND (%)
Amytrophic lateral sclerosis	UMN and LMN	2–5 years	80
Progressive bulbar palsy	UMN and LMN	6 months to 3 years	15
Progressive muscular atrophy	Pure LMN	5–10 years	5
Primary lateral sclerosis	Pure UMN	May be normal	0.5%

UMN, upper motor neurone; LMN, lower motor neurone; MND, motor neurone disease.

Nutrition

Malnutrition is common and associated with a decreased survival. Early speech and language therapy and the insertion of a gastrostomy tube is vital.

Psychiatric

Patients often suffer from emotional lability, anxiety and depression, and a combination of behavioural and pharmacological therapies can be helpful. A small proportion of patients develop a frontal dementia.

Anaesthetic considerations

Preoperative

Patients with MND may present for incidental surgery or for procedures related to their condition, e.g. tracheostomy or baclofen pump insertion. A preoperative history of disease progress, symptoms and functional ability is important to predict postoperative course. Assessment of respiratory function, including details of recent chest infection or evidence of hypoventilation, is crucial. A 30% fall in vital capacity from standing to lying suggests significant diaphragm involvement and postoperative ventilation may be necessary. A history of drooling, choking and a nasal voice suggest bulbar impairment. Severe bulbar or respiratory impairment precludes sedation for procedures such as endoscopic gastrostomy insertion.

If the disease is advanced, information about advanced directives and limitations of care should complications occur must be sought.

Induction of anaesthesia

Succinylcholine may induce a fatal hyperkalaemia from the chronically denervated muscle and is contraindicated. Rocuronium is a suitable alternative if a rapid sequence induction is required.

Intraoperative

Patients with ventilatory impairment require ventilation throughout the procedure. Since patients with MND are sensitive to the effects of non-depolarizing neuromuscular blockers, the use of these agents should be minimized and their effects monitored. MND is not a contraindication to neuraxial blockade, although high blocks may further impair respiratory function.

Postoperative

Patients should be extubated only once fully awake and laryngeal reflexes have returned. Humidified oxygen, physiotherapy and early mobilization reduce postoperative respiratory complications. However, a period of postoperative ventilation may be required in those with respiratory failure. Adequate postoperative analgesia must be provided, and peripheral nerve blocks and epidurals reduce the need for opiates.

Rabies

Aetiology

Rabies is an acute encephalomyelitis following infection by a virus belonging to the *Lyssavirus* genus. Although eradicated in the UK, rabies is endemic in many parts of the developing world. Travellers returning from overseas may have been exposed to rabies through either an infected animal bite or, rarely, cuts contaminated with infected saliva.

Pathology

The rabies virus initially replicates in skeletal muscle before ascending, via the peripheral nerves, into the CNS. Once in the CNS, it replicates rapidly and disseminates around the body.

Clinical presentation

Symptoms are initially non-specific and include itching or pain at the wound site, and are followed by fever, myalgia and headache. The investigation of choice is polymerase chain reaction of skin biopsies to demonstrate viral RNA. The disease may progress in two distinct patterns.

Furious rabies

This accounts for 80% of cases and is associated with periods of agitation, delirium, autonomic disturbances, and upper motor neurone/cranial nerve lesions. It is associated with the classic hydrophobia in which drinking or even the thought of water causes intense laryngeal spasm. Patients may die of acute cardio/respiratory arrest or progress to paralysis, coma and respiratory failure.

Paralytic rabies

Patients develop a progressive flaccid paralysis eventually resulting in bulbar and respiratory failure. Hydrophobia is rare.

Treatment and anaesthetic implications

As rabies is almost invariably fatal, management is aimed at prophylaxis or postexposure prophylaxis. Advice should always be taken from the virology department.

By the time the patient starts to show symptoms death is almost invariable, with most patients dying of multiorgan failure. Although there have been some notable successes, survival is often associated with significant neurological impairment. There is no evidence base to guide management but expert consensus guidance recommends:

- patients should be barrier nursed
- critical care facilities should be capable of dealing with the respiratory, bulbar and autonomic dysfunction and the ensuing multiorgan failure

- combination antiviral therapy, including:
  - rabies vaccine
  - human rabies immunoglobulin
  - intravenous and intraventricular ribavirin and interferon α
  - intravenous ketamine (reduces rabies replication and blocks access of virus to the *N*-methyl-D-aspartic acid receptor).

Some have also advocated the use of sedatives to induce burst suppression on the EEG. Whatever the critical care response, death is to be expected and arguably palliative care would be more appropriate, particularly for those presenting late in the disease.

Poliomyelitis

Aetiology

Since the introduction of effective vaccination programmes, polio has been eradicated from the developed world, including in the UK, but is still endemic in parts of the Indian subcontinent and sub-Saharan Africa. It is the result of the highly infectious poliovirus and the usual route of infection is via the gastrointestinal tract.

Clinical features

The majority of infections are either asymptomatic or present as a 'flu-like illness'. Fewer than 1% of patients develop the 'classical' paralytic polio. Paralytic polio follows the viral destruction of the motor neurones within the anterior horn cells, producing a flaccid paralysis and loss of associated reflexes. It usually affects the lower limbs and the weakness is often asymmetric, with proximal muscle groups being more affected than distal.

Poliovirus may invade the brainstem, destroying the lower cranial nerves and giving rise to bulbar polio. In this situation, patients have difficulty swallowing, speaking and suffer from recurrent aspiration. A combination of bulbar and cervical cord involvement produces bulbospinal polio, in which a combination of bulbar weakness and diaphragmatic involvement can severely impair respiratory function, rendering the patient ventilator dependent.

Following a period of stability, some patients notice a further deterioration in function, associated with fatigue and joint and muscle pains. This is known as the post-polio syndrome and, although poorly understood, is not due to 'reactivation' of polio virus.

Treatment

There is no treatment for polio, so management is supportive. Initially, this involves analgesics, treating intercurrent infections and nutritional and ventilatory support. As a large proportion of patients with paralytic polio recover, these measures are often temporary. However, a few are left with long-standing weaknesses requiring ongoing rehabilitation, callipers, braces and recurrent surgery for progressive deformity. Ongoing domiciliary ventilatory support may also be required.

Anaesthetic implications

Polio survivors may present to the anaesthetist for incidental surgery, corrective orthopaedic surgery or occasionally for tracheostomy as a result of bulbar/respiratory failure. Key points in their management include:

- the avoidance of sedation in those with respiratory or bulbar failure
- the avoidance of succinylcholine because of the risk of hyperkalaemia
- ventilation throughout the procedure in patients with respiratory failure
- awake extubation in patients with bulbar failure
- postoperative management in a critical care environment for those with significant respiratory/bulbar failure.

Bibliography

Howard RS. Poliomyelitis and the postpolio syndrome. *Br Med J* 2005; **330**: 1314–18.

Jackson AC, Warrell MJ, Rupprecht CE, *et al.* Management of rabies in humans. *Clin Infect Dis* 2003; **36**: 60–3.

Miller RG, Mitchell JD, Lyon M, Moore DH. Riluzole for amyotrophic lateral sclerosis (ALS)/motor neuron disease (MND). *Cochrane Database Syst Rev* 2007; (1): CD001447.

Radunovic A, Annane D, Jewitt K, Mustfa N. Mechanical ventilation for amyotrophic lateral sclerosis/motor neuron disease. *Cochrane Database Syst Rev* 2009; (4): CD004427.

Willoughby RE, Tieves KS, Hoffman GM, *et al.* Survival after treatment of rabies with induction of coma. *N Engl J Med* 2005; **352**: 2508–14.

Spinal cord injury

Katharine Hunt

Aetiology

The incidence of spinal trauma is approximately 50 per million of the population per year. The cervical spine is most susceptible to injury as it is the least supported, although thoracolumbar junction injuries are also relatively common. Injuries to the vertebral bodies, discs and soft tissue/ligaments may all occur. Up to 50% of spinal cord injuries are associated with systemic injuries, with traumatic head injury and major chest trauma being the most common.

Pathophysiology

In acute spinal cord injury, primary injury is often caused by stretching or tearing of the cord as a result of hyperflexion or hyperextension of the spinal column. The cord may also be damaged by direct, penetrating trauma or by disrupted bony structures. These mechanisms all lead to a disruption of neural tissue and ischaemia. Ongoing or secondary ischaemic injury may follow as a result of hypotension, hypoxaemia and progressive cord oedema. This ultimately leads to an inflammatory cascade that results in free radical formation, cellular oedema and apoptosis, resulting in further destruction of neural tissue.

The hallmarks of chronic spinal cord injury, namely the return of reflex activity resulting in hyper-reflexia and hypertonia, appear 6–8 weeks following the initial insult. Spinal cord injury not only results in neurological dysfunction but also affects other organ systems.

Clinical features

Central nervous and neuromuscular systems

Following acute spinal cord injury, the interruption of both somatic and visceral sensation results in an immediate loss of somatic and autonomic reflexes coupled with the development of a flaccid paralysis. This is termed 'spinal shock' and may last anywhere between 24 hours and 6 weeks after injury. It is eventually replaced by disinhibited cord function, resulting in spasticity and augmented reflexes below the level of the injury.

Cardiovascular system

Although hypertension is often present immediately after injury, this is swiftly replaced by hypotension owing to loss of sympathetic pathways. Compensatory reflexes are lost, particularly if the lesion is above T1, and a profound bradycardia may ensue as a result of unopposed parasympathetic activity. These symptoms may be exacerbated by bleeding from other systemic injuries. In chronic spinal cord injury, the most common cardiovascular manifestation is autonomic dysreflexia. Cardiac arrhythmias, including vagally mediated bradycardia, and orthostatic hypotension may also continue.

Respiratory system

The degree of airway and respiratory compromise in spinal cord injury is governed by the level of the cord lesion and the presence or absence of any systemic injuries, such as head or chest trauma. In cervical cord injuries, cord oedema may ascend, resulting in the need for respiratory support. Lesions above C4 result in loss of both diaphragmatic and intercostal function with the possible additional loss of accessory muscle function. Such patients require immediate ventilatory support. Diaphragmatic function is often spared in lesions below C5, and, although spontaneous ventilation may be possible, an ineffective cough is often present.

Patients with chronic spinal cord injury frequently suffer from retained secretions, recurrent chest infections and chronic respiratory failure, resulting in the need for whole-time or night-time ventilatory support.

Gastrointestinal and genitourinary systems

Spinal cord injury results in bowel and bladder atony, with gastric dilatation, paralytic ileus and urinary retention. These lead to an increased risk of regurgitation and pulmonary aspiration, constipation, recurrent urinary tract infections and renal calculi.

Other

Profound cutaneous dilatation and an inability to initiate sweating result in loss of the ability to regulate temperature after spinal cord injury. In addition, those with chronic spinal cord injury have a high incidence of pressure sores because of immobility coupled with poor nutrition, hypoalbuminaemia and osteoporosis. The incidence of venous thromboembolic disease is also high in this population.

Acute management

As with any patient with major trauma, an immediate assessment of airway, breathing and circulation should be carried out. The patient should be immediately immobilized in a rigid cervical collar, and if it is anticipated that the patient will be moved, placed on a spinal board. However, care should be taken during movement since no device guarantees stability. The patient should be examined for areas of tenderness and deformity over the area of the spine, and the degree of sensory, motor and reflex function should be ascertained and documented using the American Spinal Injury Association (ASIA) chart as soon as possible. Given the high incidence of associated injury in patients with spinal cord injury, a thorough systemic examination should be performed at the earliest opportunity. Imaging either with plain films or, better, with CT should be carried out to screen the vertebral column for injury. Negative findings do not exclude ligamentous or soft-tissue damage and further investigations such as MRI may need to be sought.

Airway and breathing

The airway should be secured and supplemental oxygen given as soon as possible. Frequently, intubation will be required (Box 1.16) and this should be carried out either with manual in-line stabilization or, if the patient is cooperative, with awake fibreoptic intubation. Problems that should be considered prior to intubation of a patient with spinal cord injury include:

- inability to extend neck
- associated maxillofacial injuries
- full stomach/risk of regurgitation.

Box 1.16 Indications for consideration of tracheal intubation after spinal cord injury

- P_ao_2 <10.0 kPa
- P_aco_2 >6.5 kPa
- Vital capacity <20 mL kg^{-1}
- Aspiration risk
- Associated chest/lung or facial injuries
- Associated traumatic brain injury

With injury of less than 24 hours, succinylcholine can be administered safely without risk of hyperkalaemia. Cricoid pressure may be administered, but there is a risk of exacerbation of cervical spine subluxation.

Circulation

Hypotension and bradycardia are common after acute spinal cord injury. Hypotension should be treated with aggressive fluid resuscitation coupled with the diagnosis and treatment of systemic injuries that might be causing haemorrhage and hypovolaemia. Volume replacement is best guided by central venous pressure measurements. If hypotension persists after adequate fluid replacement, vasoconstrictors and inotropes should be considered. Bradycardia should be treated with atropine.

Other

A nasogastric tube and urinary catheter should be inserted to manage bowel and bladder atony. Venous thromboprophylaxis should be considered, although the exacerbation of haemorrhage from systemic injuries and future surgical interventions may negate the use of pharmacological therapy in the acute phase.

Management of the spinal injury

Spinal injuries may be managed conservatively or with surgery. In conservative treatment, the cervical spine can be immobilized using traction applied using skull tongs. This often entails prolonged bed rest, although application of a halo body jacket allows some mobilization. Surgical treatment involves an open reduction and stabilization of spinal fractures, along with spinal decompression.

Following several large trials that appeared to demonstrate improved neurological outcome after high-dose methylprednisolone (National Acute Spinal Cord Injury Studies (NASCIS) I, II and III), use of this drug became commonplace in the treatment of acute spinal cord injury. However, criticisms surrounding the results of these studies, coupled with the known risks of administering high-dose steroids, such as increased infection risk and poor glycaemic control, have led to a decrease in the popularity of this treatment. Use of steroids is now an individual clinician's choice and should be made in the knowledge that side-effects from their administration are likely to outweigh any potential benefits.

Anaesthetic implications

Preoperative assessment

In both acute and chronic spinal cord injury, careful assessment of both the respiratory and cardiovascular systems must be carried out, with particular attention to lung function tests and arterial blood gas analysis. Respiratory depressant drugs should be avoided in patients who are self-ventilating. Because this population of patients undergo multiple procedures, they are at increased risk of latex allergy. An antisialagogue may be given if fibreoptic intubation is required.

Monitoring

In addition to standard anaesthetic monitoring, invasive blood pressure and central venous pressure monitoring should be carried out. Urinary catheterization is also required. Procedures involving spinal cord manipulation may require somatosensory or motor-evoked potential monitoring.

Anaesthetic technique

Patients undergoing spinal surgery usually require general anaesthesia and no one technique is superior to another. Succinylcholine should be avoided beyond 3 days after injury.

Patients with spinal cord injuries requiring non-spinal surgery may have their operation performed either with no anaesthesia (dependent upon operation and sensory level) or under regional or general anaesthesia. Both general and regional techniques diminish autonomic dysreflexia.

Bradycardias, which may occur as a result of intubation and pain, should be treated with atropine and fluid challenges and, when given prior to the induction of anaesthesia, these interventions may prevent the hypotension which is common in this group of patients.

Some patients with high spinal cord lesions will require postoperative ventilation, and others aggressive physiotherapy to prevent postoperative chest infection.

Patients with chronic spinal cord lesions in labour provide a particular challenge to the anaesthetist. This group are highly susceptible to autonomic dysreflexia, which can be induced by uterine contractions, instrumental delivery and perineal distension. Life-threatening episodes of dysreflexia may continue for up to 48 hours after delivery, and it is recommended that epidurals are continued during this period. If an epidural is technically impossible then the dysreflexia should be controlled with systemic drugs such as hydralazine or nifedipine.

Bibliography

Bhardwaj A, Kirsch J, Mirski M, Stevens R. Critical care and perioperative management in traumatic spinal cord injury. *J Neurosurg Anesthesiol* 2003; **15**: 215–29.

Hunt K, Laing R. Spinal cord injury. In: Gupta A, Gelb A (eds) *Essentials of Neuroanaesthesia and Neurointensive Care*, 2nd edn. Philadelphia: WB Saunders, 2008, pp. 211–17.

Cross-reference

Autonomic dysfunction and autonomic dysreflexia, 4
Head injury, 16

Subarachnoid haemorrhage

Tamsin Gregory and Sally Wilson

Subarachnoid haemorrhage (SAH) is defined as bleeding into the subarachnoid space. It is a devastating neurological disease with multisystem sequelae.

Types of subarachnoid haemorrhage

Rupture of an intracranial (Berry) aneurysm is the commonest cause of spontaneous SAH. Other causes of SAH, including head injury-related traumatic SAH (tSAH), are shown in Box 1.17.

Box 1.17 Causes of subarachnoid haemorrhage

- Intracerebral saccular aneurysms (75%)
- Arteriovenous malformations (5%)
- Carotid dissection
- Vasculitis
- Bleeding diatheses
- Recreational drug use (cocaine/ecstasy)
- Bleeding into meningeal tumours
- Amyloid angiopathy
- Unknown (20%)

Spontaneous subarachnoid haemorrhage

- The incidence of spontaneous (non-traumatic) SAH is 8–10 per 100 000 population per year, with the highest rates in the Finnish and Japanese populations. It occurs most frequently between ages 45 and 60. Women have a higher incidence than men after the sixth decade.
- The incidence has declined slightly over the past four decades.
- Risk factors include hypertension, smoking and familial tendency. There may be an association with alcohol excess and oral contraceptive pill usage.
- 1–2% of patients who present to A&E with headache have SAH, although 25% of those with 'the worst headache of their lives' and abnormal neurology have SAH.
- SAH is a notable cause of maternal mortality, contributing to a number of deaths in the Confidential Enquiry into Maternal Deaths triennial reports.

Traumatic subarachnoid haemorrhage

- The incidence of tSAH is around 100 per 100 000 population per year.
- Up to 40% of patients with moderate to severe head injury have evidence of subarachnoid blood on CT scan.
- tSAH is associated with an increased incidence of hypoxia, hypotension, skull fractures, cerebral contusions and raised ICP.
- Associated vasospasm is less common than in spontaneous SAH.
- When the history preceding the head injury is unclear, cerebral angiography should be performed to exclude spontaneous SAH and secondary trauma.

Intracranial aneurysms

The natural history of intracranial aneurysms is incompletely understood, but the annual rupture rate is thought to be 0.5–2%. Aneurysms more than 10 mm in diameter are at particular risk of haemorrhage. The majority of aneurysms (80–90%) are in the anterior (carotid) circulation – posterior and anterior communicating arteries or middle cerebral artery – and 10–15% in the posterior (vertebrobasilar) circulation. Aneurysms typically develop at bifurcations because of turbulent blood flow.

As the pressure within the aneurysm or the radius of the aneurysm increases and the wall thickness reduces, the tension within it, and therefore propensity to rupture, increases (Laplace's law). After rupture, blood is released under arterial pressure into the subarachnoid space, causing a massive and sudden rise in ICP. Blood then spreads throughout the CSF in the subarachnoid space around the brain and spinal cord. This is often associated with intracerebral and more rarely subdural haematoma.

Presentation

The most common presentation of aneurysmal SAH is sudden onset, severe (thunderclap) headache with associated photophobia, nausea, vomiting and meningism. Other presentations include loss of consciousness due to a rise in ICP, seizures, focal neurological deficits and isolated cranial nerve palsies. Drowsiness, agitation and restlessness are also common. A total of 15–30% of patients die on aneurysm rupture, secondary to sustained rise in ICP.

The SAH may be preceded by a prodromal headache days or weeks prior to the ictus. This is caused by a 'sentinel bleed' and probably represents extravasation of blood into the aneurysmal wall or subarachnoid space. The breakdown products of blood in the subarachnoid space cause meningeal irritation with neck stiffness. Back pain and bilateral radicular leg pain may also occur.

Clinical grading scales (e.g. World Federation of Neurosurgeons; Table 1.7) are used to standardize clinical assessment and estimate prognosis.

Table 1.7 World Federation of Neurosurgeons classification of subarachnoid haemorrhage and associated morbidity and mortality

Grade	Glasgow Coma Scale score	Motor deficit
I	15	Absent
II	14–13	Absent
III	14–13	Present
IV	12–7	Absent or present
V	6–3	Absent or present

Diagnosis

Computed tomography

- Thin-slice (3 mm) non-contrast CT scans are highly sensitive (>95%) for blood in the subarachnoid space within 24 hours of acute haemorrhage.
- The location and distribution of the blood may suggest the site of bleeding.
- The amount of blood on the CT scan is described by the Fisher scale (Table 1.8).
- Blood is rapidly cleared from the subarachnoid space and the diagnostic sensitivity of CT decreases to 30% at 2 weeks.
- The increased density of blood on the CT scan is a function of haemoglobin concentration and SAH may not be apparent in anaemic patients.
- CT scans may also detect associated intracranial haematoma and hydrocephalus.

Table 1.8 Fisher grading of CT appearance of subarachnoid haemorrhage (SAH)

Grade	Finding on CT
1	No subarachnoid blood detected
2	Diffuse or vertical layers <1 mm
3	Localized clot and/or vertical layer >1 mm
4	Intracerebral or intraventricular clot with diffuse or no SAH

Angiography

- Intra-arterial catheter digital subtraction angiography (DSA) remains the gold standard for confirming the presence of an aneurysm or arteriovenous malformation.
- CT angiography (CTA) is now used in many centres as the primary investigation to identify an aneurysm.
- Magnetic resonance angiography (MRA) may be used as an alternative to CTA or DSA.
- Improved imaging technology over the past decade has allowed greater endovascular access to the brain, allowing aneurysm treatment during the same procedure as diagnosis.

Lumbar puncture

- A lumbar puncture is indicated in patients with a suspected SAH in the presence of a normal CT scan.
- Blood-stained CSF that does not clear or the presence of xanthochromia suggests SAH.

Management

The main aims of treatment are to:

- optimize perfusion in the area of the aneurysm
- reduce the risk of rebleeding prior to definitive treatment (surgical clipping or coil embolization)
- reduce the risk of vasospasm, which may cause delayed ischaemic deficit and subsequent cerebral infarction
- maintain a high index suspicion for the development of hydrocephalus.

Airway assessment and management

Tracheal intubation and mechanical ventilation should be undertaken in patients in coma or with a decreasing level of consciousness. Agitated patients may also need early elective intubation to facilitate angiography or transfer to a neurosurgical centre.

Blood pressure control

Blood pressure is often elevated secondary to pain, anxiety and sympathetic activation and should be treatment promptly to minimize the risk of further aneurysmal bleeding. Analgesia may be sufficient, but, if not, rapidly acting antihypertensive agents are required. Labetalol infusions, β-blockers and calcium channel antagonists are all commonly used.

Serial assessment of neurological function

A drop in GCS may signify an extension of the bleed or development of hydrocephalus and may require further imaging or ICP control.

Intracranial pressure control

General measures, including ensuring endotracheal tubes are taped not tied, nursing at 30° head-up and prevention of obstruction of cerebral venous drainage should be observed. Additional measures include:

- external ventricular drain insertion if the CT shows enlarged ventricles
- mannitol 0.25–0.5 mg kg^{-1}
- furosemide 0.25–0.5 mg kg^{-1}.

Vasospasm

After aneurysmal SAH, about two-thirds of patients have vasospasm demonstrable on angiography, and half of these develop clinically significant vasospasm. This results in cerebral ischaemia and remains an important cause of morbidity and mortality. Symptoms include alteration in conscious level, disorientation and focal neurological deficits.

Vasospasm is more common in patients with poor initial grades and those with larger clots in the basal cisterns. It usually develops 3–10 days after the SAH, with a peak incidence at day 7. Without treatment the mortality is 30–50%.

Pathophysiology

This remains unclear, although vasoactive substances in the subarachnoid blood result in severe vasoconstriction. Breakdown products of oxyhaemoglobin are believed to play a major role by producing superoxide free radicals that inactivate nitric oxide. Intracellular calcium stores are released which produce prolonged smooth muscle contraction. There may also be a calcium-mediated imbalance between prostaglandins. In addition, histological changes, such as adventitial inflammation and intimal hyperplasia, are part of the complex pathophysiology of cerebral vasospasm.

Diagnosis

- Angiography.
- Transcranial Doppler ultrasonography.
- Both methods have limitations and a diagnosis is often made on clinical grounds, i.e. altered conscious level or focal deficit.

Treatment

Triple H therapy

Triple H therapy – hypertension, hypervolaemia and haemodilution – has been the mainstay of treatment of cerebral vasospasm, although haemodilution is not now commonly applied. Triple H therapy reverses the clinical symptoms of vasospasm in up to 70% of patients, but does not reduce the incidence of delayed ischaemic neurological deficit.

- A vasopressor (usually norepinephrine) is used to increase mean arterial blood pressure, usually above 90 mmHg. This is most safely achieved following definitive treatment of the aneurysm, when the risk of rebleeding is low. Invasive monitoring of arterial blood pressure is needed and a non-invasive measure of cardiac output may be useful especially in patients with cardiac dysfunction.
- There is little evidence that volume loading is helpful beyond correction of hypovolaemia, and volume expansion is less important than induced hypertension. A central venous pressure of 12–15 mmHg is the usual target.
- Haemodilution is the least understood part of triple H therapy. The rationale is that reduction of the haematocrit to below 30% decreases blood viscosity. However, at these levels, the oxygen-carrying capacity of blood is also reduced, which may worsen outcome.

Nimodipine

- Nimodipine, a specific antagonist of the L-type voltage-gated calcium channel, administered orally (60 mg 4 hourly) decreases the incidence of cerebral infarction and poor outcomes. Since it has minimal side-effects it is used prophylactically in all patients with SAH. Hypotension is rarely a problem in well-hydrated patients. Nimodipine is thought to provide benefit by inhibiting calcium entry into smooth muscle cells and vasoactive substance release from platelets and endothelial cells. It does not reduce the incidence of angiographic vasospasm, so its beneficial effects may also occur because of more general brain protective mechanisms.

Angioplasty

- Balloon angioplasty is effective for the treatment of discrete lesions in large proximal arteries. The optimal timing is uncertain and major complications include vessel rupture, dissection, occlusion and haemorrhagic infarction.
- Chemical angioplasty using intra-arterial papaverine has an immediate, but short-lived, effect and has been abandoned by most centres. Other agents used include intra-arterial nicardipine, nimodipine and milrinone.

Rebleeding

- The rate of rebleeding following the initial SAH is 4% during the first 24 hours and then 1–2% per day for the following 2 weeks. Without definitive treatment 50% of patients will rebleed within 6 months. The mortality rate from a rebleed is 50–60%, mainly because of vasospasm.
- Rebleeding is related to variations and changes in blood pressure, rather than the absolute pressure. Bed rest, analgesia and stabilization of blood pressure are recommended to minimize the risk of rebleeding. Aggressive BP reduction should not

be attempted as it may lead to reduced cerebral perfusion in the presence of raised ICP.

Hydrocephalus

- Acute obstructive hydrocephalus (within 72 hours) is common, particularly after poor-grade SAH. It is caused by subarachnoid clot in the basal cisterns and is managed with external ventricular drainage.
- Any signs of a falling GCS are an indication for immediate CT scan since it may represent impending hydrocephalus.
- Late communicating hydrocephalus (after 30 days) occurs in 25% of patients and may require a permanent ventricular shunt.

Seizures

- Occur in up to 25% of patients after SAH.
- Prophylactic anticonvulsant treatment is not usually recommended.

Cardiac dysfunction

- ECG abnormalities (e.g. QT prolongation, ST segment changes) are common and may be associated with a small troponin rise. They are usually transient but may persist for up to 8 weeks.
- Neurogenic stunned myocardium (NSM) is a reversible, neurologically mediated syndrome characterized by ECG changes and left ventricular dysfunction. NSM may be asymptomatic but in severe cases can result in cardiogenic shock and pulmonary oedema.
- Cardiac abnormalities are probably the result of excessive local release of norepinephrine from myocardial sympathetic nerve terminals causing physiological myocardial denervation in the presence of normal myocardial perfusion.
- Cardiac arrhythmias occur in 35% of patients, of which 5% are life-threatening. These include sinus tachycardia, atrial fibrillation, torsades de pointes and ventricular fibrillation.
- Myocardial dysfunction, ECG changes and biomarker rises correlate with the degree of neurological injury but do not require change in management.
- If there is any doubt as to whether these changes are a result of SAH or primary myocardial injury, coronary angiography is diagnostic.

Electrolyte disturbances

- Hyponatraemia complicates up to 30% of cases of SAH owing to the syndrome of inappropriate secretion of antidiuretic hormone or the cerebral salt-wasting syndrome. Cerebral salt wasting is due to secretion of atrial natriuretic peptide causing excessive natriuresis, hyponatraemia and hypovolaemia.
- Other electrolyte disturbances, including hypokalaemia, hypomagnesaemia and hypocalcaemia, are also common.

Respiratory complications

Respiratory dysfunction or failure accounts for 23% of non-neurological causes of death after SAH. Common complications include:

- pneumonia
- pulmonary oedema – neurogenic or cardiogenic
- pulmonary embolus.

Bibliography

Macmillan CSA, Grant IS, Andrews PJD. Pulmonary and cardiac sequelae of subarachnoid haemorrhage: time for active management? *Intensive Care Med* 2002; **28**: 1012–23.

Molyneux AJ, Kerr RSC, Yu L-M, *et al.* International subarachnoid aneurysm trial (ISAT) of neurosurgical clipping versus endovascular coiling in 2143 patients with ruptured intracranial aneurysms: a randomized comparison of effects on survival, dependency, seizures, rebleeding, subgroups, and aneurysm occlusion. *Lancet* 2005; **366**: 809–17.

Priebe H-J. Aneurysmal subarachnoid haemorrhage and the anaesthetist. *Br J Anaesth* 2007; **99**: 102–18.

Smith M. Intensive care management of patients with subarachnoid haemorrhage. *Curr Opin Anaesthesiol* 2007; **20**: 400–7.

Cross-references

Anaesthesia for interventional neuroradiological procedures, 304
Anaesthesia for intracranial neurovascular surgery, 308
Anaesthesia for non-craniotomy neurosurgery, 315
Neuromonitoring, 338

2 Endocrine system

Thomas A Crozier

Acromegaly

Thomas A Crozier

Excessive secretion of growth hormone (GH) in adults causes hypertrophy of soft tissues and bone, particularly in the tips (Greek *akros*, meaning extremities), leading to the name of the disease. The effects are mediated directly by GH and insulin-like growth factor-1 (IGF-1). Treatment for the condition may be surgical (hypophysectomy) or medical (dopamine antagonists or somatostatin analogues).

Pathophysiology

GH and IGF-1 stimulate cell growth. Soft tissues, including viscera such as kidneys, heart and muscles, ligaments and cartilage are enlarged: large hands are often the first visible sign of acromegaly. Bones cannot grow in length, so changes lead to deformity. Heart and kidney failure contribute to the two- to threefold increase in morbidity and mortality of patients with acromegaly. GH induces hepatic gluconeogenesis and reduces glucose tolerance. IGF-1 is involved in the regulation of tumour growth, and epidemiological studies suggest that patients with acromegaly have a higher risk for malignancies, particularly of the thyroid, breast, prostate and probably colon. The patients complain of fatigue and headaches, arthralgias and hyperhidrosis.

An elevated IGF-1 level in peripheral blood is the most sensitive laboratory test for acromegaly. Single GH determinations are of little value, since GH secretion is pulsatile and the blood levels vary widely. However, the failure of GH levels to decrease in response to a 75 g oral glucose tolerance test is helpful in confirming the diagnosis.

The pathological changes seen in acromegaly affect virtually every system (Box 2.1).

Box 2.1 Signs and symptoms of acromegaly

- Cardiovascular
  - Hypertension and cardiomegaly
  - Cardiomyopathy
  - Angiopathy (diabetic)
- Respiratory system
  - Obstructive sleep apnoea due to partial upper respiratory tract obstruction resulting from hypertrophy of the tongue and pharyngeal and nasal mucosa
  - Lower and rougher voice, from vocal cord involvement
  - Possible glottic stenosis or vocal cord paresis
- Soft tissues and skeleton
  - Hypertrophy of hands and feet
  - Macroglossia and prognathism
  - Coarse facial features
  - Carpal tunnel syndrome
- Neuromuscular system
  - Peripheral neuropathy
  - Myopathy with reduced strength
- Endocrine system
  - Impaired glucose tolerance, diabetes mellitus
  - Hypercalcaemia and hypercalciuria
  - Goitre (diffuse or nodular) with tendency to autonomy
  - Deficiency of other pituitary hormones owing to pressure of adenoma (adrenocorticotropic hormone, hypocortisolism; thyroid-stimulating hormone, hypothyroidism; arginine vasopressin, diabetes insipidus)

Preoperative assessment

The primary anaesthetic concerns in the patient with acromegaly are potential difficulties in securing the airway and cardiovascular complications. A careful assessment of the airway is essential, including a history of snoring, intermittent nocturnal apnoea and daytime drowsiness. Preparations should be made for a difficult intubation, and the patient should be informed of a possible awake fibreoptic intubation. Attention should be paid to possible concomitant cardiovascular, respiratory, neuromuscular and endocrine disorders. Continuous postoperative respiratory monitoring in the ITU should be arranged beforehand, especially for the patient with obstructive sleep apnoea.

Premedication might be with a moderate dose of an oral benzodiazepine, but opiates should be avoided in patients with upper airway involvement. If relevant glucose intolerance is present, the patient might require management as a diabetic.

Investigations in patients with acromegaly

- Blood tests: creatinine, electrolytes, glucose, calcium, thyroid hormones.
- Neck X-rays: for glottic involvement, pharyngeal tissue overgrowth.

- Indirect laryngoscopy may reveal vocal cord involvement.
- Cardiovascular investigations should include:
  - History of exercise capacity, chest X-ray, 12-lead ECG, echocardiography (if cardiomyopathy or valvular involvement is suspected).
- Consider a baseline arterial blood gas analysis.
- Consider cardiopulmonary exercise testing.

Perioperative management

Airway

Because of the facial deformity, it may be difficult to obtain a tight seal with the face-mask and ventilation may be difficult. Intubation is the safest option for securing the airway, particularly for longer procedures or when access to the head is impaired.

Skilled assistance is mandatory whenever intubation is required, particularly if there is upper airway involvement. Videolaryngoscopes (e.g. Glidescope) can be useful, but awake fibreoptic intubation should be considered the safest option. Orotracheal intubation should be preferred since the nasal mucosa may be hypertrophied. If there are no signs of upper airway involvement, intravenous induction and intubation under direct laryngoscopy should be preferred. The neuromuscular blocking drug is administered only after one has ascertained that the patient can be ventilated by bag and mask. In the rare case that the patient's glottis cannot be visualized by video or fibreoptic laryngoscopy, elective tracheostomy under local anaesthesia should be considered.

Monitoring

The invasiveness of intraoperative monitoring depends on the planned surgery and the coexisting diseases of the patient. Basic monitoring includes ECG, non-invasive blood pressure, pulse oximetry and neuromuscular function. If the fingers are too large for the $S_{p}o_{2}$ probe, an ear lobe clip can be used.

One should consider additional monitoring with an arterial cannula, central venous catheter and cardiac output measurement (e.g. pulse contour cardiac output (PiCCO) or thermodilution) in patients with relevant cardiovascular impairment, particularly for extensive surgery.

Laboratory tests should include serum electrolytes, acid–base status and blood sugar.

Postoperative management

Extubation should only be performed when muscle relaxation has completely resolved (train-of-four (TOF) ratio >0.9). Patients with airway obstruction should be closely monitored with pulse oximetry and serial arterial blood gases during the first 24 hours postoperatively, preferably in the ITU. Supplemental oxygen should not be necessary in the absence of pulmonary complications. Drugs that reduce muscular tone (e.g. benzodiazepines) must be administered with great caution to avoid inducing loss of pharyngeal muscle control and upper airway obstruction. Forced inspiration against the occluded airway can precipitate negative pressure pulmonary oedema.

Hypophysectomy will terminate the excessive GH production with associated gluconeogenesis and hyperglycaemia. Insulin therapy must thus be carefully adapted to the reduced requirements. The operation can also cause a deficiency of other pituitary hormones, such as vasopressin, adrenocorticotropic hormone (ACTH) or thyroid-stimulating hormone (TSH) that will require appropriate treatment (see below).

Some of the clinical features of acromegaly may resolve slowly following treatment (e.g. vocal cord changes, left ventricular hypertrophy) but osseous hypertrophy will be permanent.

Bibliography

Schmitt H, Buchfelder M, Radespiel-Troger M, Fahlbusch R. Difficult intubation in acromegalic patients: incidence and predictability. *Anesthesiology* 2000; **93**: 110–14.

Seidman PA, Kofke WA, Policare R, Young M. Anaesthetic complications of acromegaly. *Br J Anaesth* 2000; **84**: 179–82.

Cross-references

Adrenocortical insufficiency, 46
Anaesthesia for trans-sphenoidal hypophysectomy, 332
Cardiomyopathy, 136
Diabetes mellitus, 60
Difficult airway: prediction, 664
Hypertension, 151

Adrenocortical insufficiency

Thomas A Crozier

Adrenocortical insufficiency, characterized by inadequate cortisol secretion and low serum concentrations of the hormone, is classified as primary, secondary or tertiary depending on whether the disturbance is in the adrenal cortex itself, the pituitary or the hypothalamus. Differentiation of the last two is of academic interest only for the anaesthetist and will be both referred to as secondary.

Primary adrenocortical insufficiency is the inability of the adrenal cortex to secrete cortisol and aldosterone owing to destruction of the gland. Classical Addison disease is caused by an autoimmune process and is important because it is frequently part of the autoimmune polyendocrine syndrome type 2 (APS-II, Schmidt's syndrome) that includes Hashimoto thyroiditis hypothyroidism and type 1 diabetes mellitus. Patients should therefore undergo appropriate endocrine screening. Other causes of primary adrenocortical insufficiency are given in Box 2.2.

Box 2.2 Aetiology of primary adrenocortical insufficiency

- Idiopathic
- Autoimmune (Addison disease)
- Congenital adrenal hyperplasia (mainly adrenal 21-hydroxylase deficiency)
- Infection (e.g. tuberculosis, meningococcal)
- Surgical removal
- Haemorrhage/infarction (e.g. Waterhouse–Friderichsen syndrome)
- Infiltration, malignant destruction, amyloid
- Adrenal leukodystrophy (rare)

Secondary adrenocortical insufficiency is due to a lack of ACTH stimulation. The most common cause is suppression of corticotropin-releasing hormone (CRH) and ACTH secretion by exogenous glucocorticoids (see Iatrogenic adrenocortical suppression, p. 72). Under normal circumstances these patients do not suffer from lack of cortisol and, in fact, may present with typical signs of hypercortisolism. Insufficiency becomes manifest when glucocorticoid administration is stopped or not adapted to increased perioperative requirements (see Iatrogenic adrenocortical suppression, p. 72). Further causes of secondary adrenocortical insufficiency are damage to the pituitary or hypothalamus, e.g. by tumours, postpartum or by surgery (see Pituitary disorders and hypopituitarism, p. 78). If untreated, these patients are likely to show signs and symptoms of adrenocortical insufficiency.

Determining the cause of abnormally low serum cortisol concentrations requires testing the various components of the hypothalamic–pituitary–adrenal (HPA) axis. A normal response to stimulation with synthetic ACTH (Synacthen test) virtually rules out primary insufficiency, but further testing is required if secondary insufficiency with involution of the adrenal cortex is likely, such as in chronic glucocorticoid therapy. Low circulating ACTH concentrations and a lack of response to CRH stimulation can indicate pituitary dysfunction and consequently secondary adrenal insufficiency. Insulin-induced hypoglycaemia ('insulin tolerance test') tests the integrity of the HPA axis as a whole, but is hazardous and restricted to specialist facilities.

For clinical purposes, one must differentiate between patients with non-functioning adrenal cortex glands who are on glucocorticoid substitution therapy and those who are not, because the former are compensated and can basically be treated as normal patients, whereas the latter tend to suffer circulatory collapse and develop symptoms of manifest insufficiency in periods of stress and illness.

Signs and symptoms of manifest adrenocortical insufficiency are:

- muscle weakness, myalgia, easy fatigability
- loss of appetite, weight loss (in part due to fluid losses)
- disorientation, confusion, dizziness
- postural hypotension
- nausea, vomiting and diarrhoea.

Pathophysiology

Cardiovascular system

Aldosterone increases sodium reabsorption in the distal tubule, and its lack leads to sodium wasting and fluid loss with hypovolaemia. Cortisol upregulates β-adrenergic receptors and facilitates the effects of circulating catecholamines. Its prolonged absence leads to catecholamine-refractory hypotension.

Skin

Patients with Addison disease have a typical dark pigmentation, particularly in the mouth and on skin creases (hand lines). This is caused by melanocyte-stimulating hormone (MSH), which is derived from the same polypeptide precursor and is co-secreted with ACTH. MSH levels increase together with ACTH owing to the absence of negative cortisol feedback control.

Biochemical/metabolic

- Sodium loss, potassium retention (hyponatraemia, hyperkalaemia, high urinary sodium excretion).
- Hyperuricaemia.
- Hypoglycaemia on fasting in isolated adrenocortical insufficiency.
- Hyperglycaemia if associated with diabetes mellitus as part of APS-II.
- Hypercalcaemia.

Blood count

- Haematocrit normal to elevated owing to dehydration.
- Normochromic normocytic anaemia, low haematocrit (after rehydration).
- Eosinophilia, leukocytosis.

Preoperative assessment

Previously undiagnosed adrenocortical insufficiency is difficult to detect, since the symptoms are non-specific and can be attributed to more likely causes. The typical hyperpigmentation and blood chemistry are the most helpful clues to the diagnosis. The stress of surgery, infection or trauma can cause the condition to decompensate and precipitate an Addisonian crisis with its high mortality.

Prolonged steroid therapy can suppress the HPA axis without causing symptoms, since these are prevented by the exogenous steroid. In these patients, symptoms will become manifest if the steroids are withheld or the dose not adapted to increased requirements.

In addition to routine laboratory investigations (electrolytes, fasting blood glucose, full blood count, creatinine or urea), patients with adrenocortical insufficiency should be screened for hypothyroidism and diabetes mellitus. A chest X-ray for signs of pulmonary or cardiac disease and an ECG should be performed.

Preoperative measures

Patients with adrenocortical dysfunction maintained on adequate corticosteroid substitution therapy are not necessarily at any additional risk. However, they will require perioperative increase of the glucocorticoid dose to compensate for the increased requirements posed by the trauma of surgery. The required amount depends on the invasiveness of the surgical procedure (see below).

Patients with untreated adrenocortical insufficiency should not be scheduled for elective surgery until corticosteroid therapy has been given for a sufficient length of time, as determined by the endocrinologists. This can take days to weeks.

Patients with untreated manifest adrenocortical insufficiency or Addisonian crisis presenting for emergency surgery are high-risk patients who require invasive intraoperative monitoring and must be managed postoperatively in an ITU. Preoperative measures are aimed at stabilizing the circulation, correcting fluid deficits and electrolyte disturbances, and initiating glucocorticoid therapy. Infusion pumps with norepinephrine and/or vasopressin should be immediately available.

Perioperative management

Patients on stable long-term glucocorticoid substitution therapy

These patients will generally not require more invasive measures for any given operation than a comparable patient with functioning adrenal glands. There is no particular requirement for the choice of anaesthetic.

The patient will require additional glucocorticoid doses to meet the increased demands after the surgical trauma. There is no truly evidence-based therapy; the recommended regimens are given in Table 2.1.

Patients with latent adrenocortical insufficiency

Patients with poorly controlled adrenocortical insufficiency are at a higher risk and will require a more invasive approach. These patients are frequently dehydrated, hypoglycaemic and have a tendency to cardiovascular instability, in part because of the downregulation and desensitization of the catecholamine receptors associated with cortisol deficiency.

In addition to routine monitoring (ECG, capnometry, pulse oximetry), the following measures are recommended:

- arterial cannula for continuous invasive blood pressure recording
- urinary catheter (renal function, fluid balance)
- central venous catheter (estimation of right atrial filling pressure, inotrope infusions)
- cardiac output measurement for haemodynamically unstable patients.

Depending on the extent of surgery and the patient's tolerance of the procedure, the patient can be

● **Table 2.1** Steroid treatment regimens

Patients on long-term steroid therapy (prednisolone equivalent dose)		
<10 mg day^{-1}	Assume normal HPA response	Usual daily steroid dose; additional cover not required
>10 mg day^{-1}	Minor surgery	Usual daily steroid dose plus 25 mg hydrocortisone at induction or Twice the usual daily steroid dose
	Moderate surgery	Usual daily steroid dose plus 25 mg hydrocortisone at induction plus 100 mg day^{-1} for 24 hours
	Major surgery	Usual daily dose plus 25 mg hydrocortisone at induction plus 100 mg day^{-1} for 48–72 hours
High-dose immunosuppression	Usual immunosuppressive dose in perioperative period	
Patients who have stopped taking steroids		
<3 months		Treat as if on steroids
>3 months		No perioperative steroids necessary

HPA, hypothalamic–pituitary–adrenal.

managed in a post-anaesthetic care unit, but might require transfer to an ITU.

Patients with manifest adrenocortical insufficiency

A patient presenting with manifest adrenocortical insufficiency or Addisonian crisis who requires emergency surgery should be prepared and stabilized as long as possible in the ITU.

The preparations will have included large-bore venous cannulae for rapid fluid infusions, an arterial cannula for invasive blood pressure monitoring and measuring blood gases and acid–base status, and a central venous catheter (preferably multilumen) for estimating right atrial filling pressure and infusing vasopressors and inotropic agents. Cardiovascular function monitoring can be essential (pulmonary artery catheter, cardiac output, transoesophageal echocardiography (TOE)). A urinary catheter is placed for monitoring renal function and assessing fluid balance.

Extravascular dehydration and hyponatraemia are treated with normal saline (0.9% NaCl), and plasma expanders can be given to correct hypovolaemia. Glucose infusions are given to correct hypoglycaemia as well as an adjunct to an insulin infusion to lower elevated serum potassium concentrations.

Fluid replacement

- Sodium chloride 0.9%, 1 litre rapidly, then more slowly (hypernatraemia must be corrected very slowly to avoid pontine myelinosis and permanent neurological damage).
- Glucose (10% intravenous (i.v.) infusion) to correct hypoglycaemia.
- Plasma volume expanders.

Adrenocorticoid hormone replacement

- Hydrocortisone (200 mg i.v.) or equivalent dose of other glucocorticoid, such as prednisolone (50–100 mg i.v.) as a bolus injection.
- Continuing therapy with hydrocortisone infusion (100 mg in normal saline in 24 hours) (or equivalent).
- Fludrocortisone (0.1 mg once a day) for mineralocorticoid deficiency.

Cardiovascular support

- Norepinephrine infusions are used to counteract hypotension due to vasodilatation.
- Vasopressin infusions can be effective when the response to norepinephrine is insufficient.

General anaesthesia

Anaesthesia should be induced in theatre with full monitoring. Induction should be performed cautiously with small doses of the hypnotic repeated at delayed intervals to allow for increased sensitivity, hypovolaemia and prolonged circulatory times. Blood pressure control can be impaired in these patients and they can be overly sensitive to negative inotropic effects and suppression of the baroreceptor reflex. There is no particular indication for any one anaesthetic technique, but a balanced technique with an opioid will reduce the required concentration of volatile anaesthetic. Ketamine is a suitable intravenous agent. The induction agent etomidate is not contraindicated, since its transitory inhibitory effect on steroid synthesis is irrelevant in these patients, whereas its reduced or absent effects on vascular tone, myocardial inotropy and baroreceptor reflex are beneficial.

The infusion of vasoconstrictors (norepinephrine, vasopressin) and inotropic agents may be required. Continuous infusions of crystalloid solutions will be necessary to correct preoperative fluid deficits and replace perioperative losses. Colloids may be necessary to replace blood loss.

Local anaesthesia

Cardiovascular instability during surgery under local anaesthesia may require additional intravenous fluid replacement and inotropic support.

Postoperative management

Postoperative measures will include invasive haemodynamic monitoring, balancing fluid intake and output, correcting electrolyte abnormalities (may have postoperative hypokalaemia), monitoring renal function and continuing corticosteroid therapy.

Bibliography

Fraser CG, Preuss FS, Bigford WD. Adrenal atrophy and irreversible shock associated with cortisone therapy. *JAMA* 1952; **149**: 1542–3.

Nicholson G, Burrin JM, Hall GM. Peri-operative steroid supplementation. *Anaesthesia* 1998; **53**: 1091–104.

Salem M, Tainsh RE Jr, Bromberg J, *et al.* Perioperative glucocorticoid coverage. A reassessment 42 years after emergence of a problem. *Ann Surg* 1994; **219**: 416–25.

Weatherill D, Spence AA. Anaesthesia and disorders of the adrenal cortex. *Br J Anaesth* 1984; **56**: 741–9.

Cross-references

Iatrogenic adrenocortical suppression, 72
Water and electrolyte disturbances, 633

Carcinoid syndrome

Brian J Pollard

Carcinoid syndrome is caused by peptides, particularly serotonin (5-hydroxytryptamine (5-HT)) and bradykinin, which reach the systemic circulation in abnormally high concentrations after release by carcinoid tumours. The incidence is approximately 8 in 100 000 population.

Carcinoid tumours are derived from argentaffin cells and may occur in several locations, e.g. bronchus and pancreas, although 75% are found in the gastrointestinal tract, most commonly in the appendix. Appendiceal tumours are usually benign. The amines and peptides responsible for the symptoms of carcinoid syndrome may be produced by both benign and malignant tumours. Up to 20 peptides and amines have been isolated, including 5-HT, bradykinin, histamine, somatostatin, prostaglandins, vasoactive intestinal peptide (VIP) and substance P. Only about 7–18% of patients with carcinoid tumours exhibit the carcinoid syndrome, as only 25% of malignant tumours produce peptides and these are normally cleared from the portal circulation by the liver if the tumour is in the gastrointestinal tract. Carcinoid syndrome usually results from the presence of liver secondaries that secrete peptides directly into the hepatic veins and thus into the systemic circulation. Bronchial tumours release peptides which bypass the portal circulation, resulting in symptoms at an earlier stage.

Preoperative evaluation

Patients should have had a CT or MRI scan to determine the site of the tumour and the possible existence of metastases. Symptoms may be caused by the primary tumour, e.g. intestinal obstruction, haemoptysis, or from the systemic effects of peptides released by the tumour, e.g. right heart valve lesions.

5-Hydroxytryptamine

The following symptoms may be caused by 5-HT:

- Watery diarrhoea (75% of patients) associated with cramps. This may be severe, resulting in dehydration, hyponatraemia, hypokalaemia, hypochloraemia and metabolic acidosis due to bicarbonate loss.
- Malabsorption with steatorrhoea and hypoproteinaemia.
- Pallor.
- Hypertension (5-HT stimulates the release and inhibits the uptake of norepinephrine and potentiates the response of α_1-adrenoreceptors to catecholamines).
- Tachycardia (5-HT is a positive chronotrope).
- Hyperglycaemia.
- Right heart failure (33% of patients) due to pulmonary stenosis and tricuspid regurgitation resulting from subendocardial fibrosis.
- Raised urinary 5-hydroxyindoleacetic acid (5-HIAA) levels, which are diagnostic of carcinoid syndrome. A 24 hour urinary collection is usually undertaken.

Bradykinin

This may cause the following symptoms:

- flushing (90% of patients) of the face and upper body, increasing in duration as the disease progresses
- hypotension
- bronchospasm (20% of patients), especially in previous asthmatics and in the presence of cardiac disease.

Histamine

This may cause the following symptoms:

- flushing
- hypotension
- bronchospasm.

Preoperative drug therapy

Preoperative drug therapy is aimed at antagonizing the mediators of the carcinoid syndrome or preventing their release from carcinoid tumours.

Serotonin antagonists

Cyproheptadine and methysergide are effective against gastrointestinal manifestations. Ketanserin blocks the effects of serotonin mediated by the 5-HT_2 receptor, i.e. vasoconstriction, bronchoconstriction and platelet aggregation. It also has adrenergic antagonist activity and reduces central sympathetic outflow, and is therefore used to treat hypertension in patients with carcinoid.

Bradykinin antagonists

Aprotinin inhibits the kallikrein cascade. By infusion, it is used to control flushing and treat hypotension. Steroids reduce the synthesis of prostaglandins, which mediate the action of bradykinin.

Histamine antagonists

H_2 antagonists or combination antihistamines are more effective than H_1 blockers on their own.

Inhibitors of mediator release

Somatostatin inhibits the release of mediators from carcinoid tumours. It has a short half-life and must be given by infusion. Octreotide, a long-acting synthetic octapeptide somatostatin analogue, is used as a sole agent to treat diarrhoea, hypertension, hypotension and bronchospasm in patients with carcinoid syndrome. It reduces the plasma levels of mediators by inhibiting their release from carcinoid tumours.

Anaesthetic considerations

- Hypovolaemia and electrolyte abnormalities may be significant in patients with severe diarrhoea.
- Prevent the release of mediators, i.e. give somatostatin or somatostatin analogues.
- Avoid factors which can trigger a carcinoid crisis by causing the release of mediators:
  - catecholamines: release peptides from carcinoid tumours
  - anxiety, hypercapnia, hypothermia and hypotension: release catecholamines
  - drugs which release histamine, e.g. morphine, atracurium, succinylcholine and mivacurium
  - hypertension: causes the release of bradykinin.
- Prepare for a carcinoid crisis: resistant bronchospasm and sudden variations in arterial pressure, particularly at induction of anaesthesia and when the tumour is handled.

Preoperative management

- Correct fluid and electrolyte abnormalities secondary to severe diarrhoea, and consider nutritional support if malabsorption is severe.
- Echocardiography may be valuable to investigate right heart and tricuspid valve function.
- Octreotide, 100 μg subcutaneously two or three times a day for 2 weeks prior to surgery followed by 100 μg intravenously at induction of anaesthesia and a slow postoperative wean over a few days, reduces mediator release.
- Continue antagonists of serotonin, bradykinin and histamine to minimize symptoms and maintain haemodynamic stability.
- All antimediator drugs, e.g. ketanserin, cyproheptadine, somatostatin, antihistamines and aprotinin, should be available for immediate administration if required perioperatively.
- Premedication should include an anxiolytic drug and a sedative antihistamine, e.g. benzodiazepine and promethazine.

Perioperative management

Monitoring starts prior to induction and should include:

- intra-arterial blood pressure (BP)
- ECG
- central venous pressure
- blood gases
- blood sugar
- airway pressure
- in patients with right-sided heart lesions, pulmonary hypertension must be avoided and pulmonary artery catheterization should be considered
- oesophageal Doppler recording may be useful.

Regional anaesthesia is relatively contraindicated, as hypotension may occur. General anaesthesia should be induced with drugs which maintain haemodynamic stability, obtund the hypertensive response to laryngoscopy and tracheal intubation, and do not release histamine. Succinylcholine and ketamine should be avoided. Volatile agents may delay recovery and cause myocardial depression but are often used. A technique including high-dose narcotics has been used successfully. An anaesthetic machine with different ventilatory modes may be required to compensate for episodes of bronchospasm.

Hypotension should be treated with fluid guided by the central venous pressure, oesophageal Doppler or with an infusion of aprotinin. Angiotensin and vasopressin have also been used. Catecholamines should not be given as they cause the release of peptides. Hypertension is controlled with intravenous ketanserin and cyproheptadine. Adrenergic receptor antagonists and clonidine have also been used, but can precipitate hypotension. Somatostatin and its analogues prevent pre- and perioperative episodes of hypertension, hypotension and bronchospasm that may be resistant to other forms of drug therapy. An intravenous dose of octreotide may be useful in the treatment of an intraoperative carcinoid crisis.

Postoperative management

As recovery from anaesthesia in this group of patients may be delayed and close monitoring should continue, the patient should be sent to either a high-dependency unit (HDU) or ITU in the immediate postoperative period. If octreotide has been used preoperatively it should be reduced slowly over the first postoperative week.

The severity of symptoms does not predict the severity of perioperative complications, so that patients with minor preoperative symptoms may have significant intraoperative complications. Perioperative preparation and vigilance is of great importance in the anaesthetic management of these patients. The introduction of somatostatin and its analogues has shifted the emphasis of treating perioperative carcinoid crises from antagonizing mediators which have been released to inhibiting their release from carcinoid tumours altogether.

Bibliography

Holdcroft A. Hormones and the gut. *Br J Anaesth* 2000; **85**: 58–68.

Hughes EW, Hodkinson BP. Carcinoid syndrome: the combined use of ketanserin and octreotide in the management of an acute crisis during anaesthesia. *Anaesth Intensive Care* 1989; **17**: 367–70.

Quinlivan JK, Roberts WA. Intraoperative octreotide for refractory carcinoid-induced bronchospasm. *Anesth Analg* 1994; **78**: 400–2.

Veall GR, Peacock JE, Bax ND, Reilly CS. Review of the anaesthetic management of 21 patients undergoing laparotomy for carcinoid syndrome. *Br J Anaesth* 1994; **72**: 335–41.

Cross-references

Intraoperative bronchospasm, 762
Intraoperative hypertension, 765
Obstruction or perforation, 447
Pulmonary hypertension, 164

Conn syndrome

Thomas A Crozier

Hypersecretion of aldosterone leads to a characteristic clinical condition referred to as Conn syndrome or hyperaldosteronism. Excess aldosterone production can be classified as primary, due to an adrenal adenoma (Conn syndrome in the strict sense in 30%), bilateral adrenal hyperplasia (70%) or adrenal carcinoma (rare), or as secondary caused by an overactive renin–angiotensin system resulting from, e.g. renal artery stenosis, congestive heart failure or hypoalbuminaemia, as in liver cirrhosis or nephrotic syndrome.

Primary (hyporeninaemic) hyperaldosteronism was thought to be rare, but more recent epidemiological studies have shown it to be responsible for up to 20% of the cases of moderate to severe hypertension. Adrenal hyperplasia, the most common cause, has its highest prevalence in men over the age of 60.

Signs and symptoms

Primary hyperaldosteronism can be asymptomatic but usually presents as hypertension. The patient might complain of muscle weakness, muscle spasms or intermittent paralysis, fatigue and headaches. Polyuria, polydipsia and nocturia are described. Laboratory investigations show normal to low serum potassium, low renin levels, hypernatraemia and metabolic alkalosis. Aldosterone levels are useful in the diagnosis but aldosterone antagonists, angiotensin-converting enzyme (ACE) inhibitors, angiotensin II (AT-II) receptor antagonists and β-receptor blockers must be discontinued for up to 4 weeks prior to testing to avoid false-positive or false-negative results. Renal function may be abnormal, and the chest X-ray might show a widened heart silhouette owing to hypokalaemic cardiomyopathy. The hypertension of hyperaldosteronism predisposes to cardiovascular complications.

Cardiovascular system

- Hypertension, moderate to severe.
- ECG signs of hypokalaemia and hypomagnesaemia (U waves and flattening of T wave).
- Congestive heart failure, cardiomyopathy.

Laboratory

- Low renin.
- High aldosterone.
- Hypokalaemic alkalosis from renal tubular loss of potassium and magnesium.
- Hypernatraemia.
- Possible abnormal glucose tolerance test.

Treatment

Treatment is based on the results of MRI and possibly selective adrenal vein sampling. Primary hyperaldosteronism due to an adenoma (unilateral, aldosterone in adrenal venous sample) is treated by surgical removal. Hyperaldosteronism due to adrenal hyperplasia (bilateral) is treated with spironolactone or potassium canrenoate, both of which are aldosterone antagonists.

Preoperative evaluation

Investigations

- Creatinine (or urea), electrolytes, haemoglobin and blood glucose.
- Acid–base status (alkalosis).
- ECG (arrhythmias, left ventricular hypertrophy).
- Chest X-ray (cardiomegaly).
- Blood typing.

Preparations

- Restore potassium losses: infusion of up to 20 mmol K^+ per hour. Replacing the deficit will require at least 24 hours. Normalization of ECG changes (flattened T waves, U waves) indicates therapeutic success.
- Blood pressure control with aldosterone antagonist (if not already part of the treatment regimen), e.g. oral spironolactone or eplerenone, or intravenous canrenoate potassium.
- Control of hyperglycaemia with insulin infusions, if necessary.

Perioperative management

Premedication

Moderate sedation with hypnotic (benzodiazepine) to prevent hypertensive episodes.

Induction and maintenance

Induction in customary manner (etomidate could be used and its inhibitory effect on steroid synthesis may be exploited to reduce aldosterone production).

A balanced technique with opioids and controlled ventilation is the method of choice.

Continuous thoracic epidural anaesthesia continued in the postoperative period helps to prevent hypertensive episodes, but may require a perioperative infusion of norepinephrine to counteract vasodilatation with hypotension.

Special points for adrenalectomy

The technique used for adrenalectomy (laparoscopic or open) and the patient's position (supine or lateral decubitus) depends on the size of the tumour, its location and the surgeon's preference.

Intraoperative blood loss is generally minimal, but can be considerable if major adjacent blood vessels are injured. Muscle relaxation must be adequate to ensure easy surgical access. The diaphragm may be breached with resulting pneumothorax.

Intraoperative monitoring

- Arterial cannula for close monitoring of blood pressure and to monitor acid–base balance.
- Central venous line for monitoring fluid requirements (inaccurate in patients with cardiomyopathy).
- ECG monitoring during induction and intubation (high risk of arrhythmia, ischaemia).
- Capnography (note that hyperventilation exacerbates alkalosis).
- Urinary catheter to monitor renal function.
- Peripheral nerve stimulation (increased sensitivity to neuromuscular blocking agents).
- Hypertensive episodes can occur during initial inflation of pneumoperitoneum or surgical manipulation of the gland. Treat with vasodilators (e.g. labetolol, urapidil, glyceryl trinitrate, phentolamine). Avoid β-blockers except to treat reflex tachycardia.

Postoperative care

- Monitored bed or ITU for possible postoperative cardiovascular instability and electrolyte disturbances. Potassium, sodium and blood pressure return slowly to normal.
- Effective analgesia, e.g. thoracic epidural or patient-controlled analgesia, after open surgery.
- Postoperative respiratory support for impaired ventilation (dorsolumbar or abdominal incision; pre-existing myopathy).
- Watch for: cardiac arrhythmias, abnormal glucose tolerance, impaired renal function, residual pneumothorax.
- Necessity of glucocorticoid or mineralocorticoid supplementation must be decided in each individual case, e.g. after bilateral adrenalectomy.

Bibliography

Gockel I, Heintz A, Kentner R, *et al.* Changing pattern of the intraoperative blood pressure during endoscopic adrenalectomy in patients with Conn's syndrome. *Surg Endosc* 2005; **19**: 1491–7.

Quack I, Vonend O, Rump LC. Familial hyperaldosteronism I-III. *Horm Metab Res* 2010; **42**: 424–8.

Schirpenbach C, Reincke M. Primary aldosteronism: current knowledge and controversies in Conn's syndrome. *Nat Clin Pract Endocrinol Metab* 2007; **3**: 220–7.

Strauch B, Zelinka T, Hampf M, *et al.* Prevalence of primary hyperaldosteronism in moderate to severe hypertension in the Central Europe region. *J Hum Hypertens* 2003; **17**: 349–52.

Walz MK, Gwosdz R, Levin SL, *et al.* Retroperitoneoscopic adrenalectomy in Conn's syndrome caused by adrenal adenomas or nodular hyperplasia. *World J Surg* 2008; **32**: 847–53.

Winship SM, Winstanley JH, Hunter JM. Anaesthesia for Conn's syndrome. *Anaesthesia* 1999; **54**: 569–74.

Cross-references

Hypertension, 151
Intraoperative hypertension, 765
Laparoscopy, 458
Water and electrolyte disturbances, 633

Cushing syndrome (hypercortisolism)

Thomas A Crozier

This term refers to a typical set of symptoms caused by high circulating levels of cortisol or other glucocorticoids that can be of endogenous or exogenous origin. Endogenous Cushing syndrome can be secondary to excess ACTH production: the eponymous Cushing disease is caused by an ACTH-secreting pituitary tumour. ACTH secretion can be part of the paraneoplastic syndrome seen with bronchial or pancreatic carcinoma. Primary Cushing syndrome is caused by hormone-secreting tumours or hyperplasia of the adrenal cortex that have escaped ACTH control. Exogenous Cushing syndrome is seen in patients on long-term glucocorticoid treatment, e.g. for rheumatoid arthritis, asthma, autoimmune diseases or immunosuppression.

Classification and causes of Cushing syndrome

Primary (non-ACTH dependent)

- Adrenal tumours (adenoma, carcinoma).
- Adrenal hyperplasia.

Secondary (ACTH-dependent, 60% of non-iatrogenic cases)

- Pituitary adenoma (Cushing disease).
- Ectopic ACTH-producing tumours (bronchial, pancreatic carcinoma).

Iatrogenic

- Glucocorticoid administration.

Other

- Pseudo-Cushing syndrome (alcoholism, polycystic ovarian syndrome, depression).

Pathophysiology and surgical therapy

The disease features of Cushing syndrome are a direct result of the physiological effects of glucocorticoids. The symptoms of Cushing syndrome with the greatest relevance for the anaesthetist are arterial hypertension, impaired glucose tolerance, susceptibility to infections, fragile skin, fat deposits on the back of the neck (positioning), osteoporosis, facial obesity and hypokalaemia. In hypercortisolism due to exogenous glucocorticoid treatment, ACTH secretion is suppressed and cortisol secretion from the adrenal glands might not be sufficient to meet the demands of stressful situations.

Cushing disease is treated surgically by removal of the pituitary, preferably using a minimally invasive technique such as an endoscopic trans-sphenoid procedure. The standard surgical therapy of primary hypercortisolism is laparoscopic adrenalectomy, which has a very low perioperative mortality rate.

Preoperative assessment and preparation

The anaesthetist can encounter one of two scenarios involving patients with Cushing syndrome: those with surgery undertaken to cure the condition (e.g. hypophysectomy, bilateral adrenalectomy) or those whose hypercortisolism is not related to the surgical procedure (most common). Both groups will require similar intraoperative care but postoperative management will differ considerably.

In addition to standard preoperative assessment, note must be taken of the severity and treatment of hypertension, presence and treatment of diabetes mellitus, the patient's ability to recline their head, presence of skin lesions and serum potassium. These conditions and not cortisol levels themselves will determine the necessity of extended intraoperative monitoring (arterial cannulation, central venous catheter) and intensive postoperative care.

History

- Metabolic: diabetes.
- Cardiopulmonary: hypertension, dyspnoea.
- Skin: tendency to bruising, fragile skin, poor wound healing.
- Muscles/bones: weakness, osteoporosis, pathological fractures.
- Central nervous system (CNS): depression, psychiatric symptoms.
- Glucocorticoid therapy: drug, dose, duration.
- Medication: antihypertensives, antidiabetics, diuretics.

Examination

- Skin and subcutaneous tissue: oedema, veins for venous access, skin infection, moon face, nuchal fat.
- Airway: mouth opening, obstructions.
- Bone: kyphosis, reclination of head.
- Muscle: proximal muscle wasting, endocrine myopathy.

Laboratory and technical investigations

- Full blood count, renal function parameters, electrolytes, blood glucose.
- ECG: ischaemia, arrhythmias.
- Chest X-ray: cardiomegaly, pulmonary congestion, pulmonary masses or atelectasis (bronchial carcinoma and paraneoplasia).
- Respiratory function test (myopathy affecting respiratory muscles).

Perioperative management

No alteration of normal premedication is required. Concomitant medications should be continued as usual. Patients taking glucocorticoids should be given their morning dose and may require augmented intraoperative supplementation (see Iatrogenic adrenocortical suppression, p. 72). Patients with diabetes should be treated appropriately. Careful positioning is crucial to avoid damage to the fragile skin and fractures of the osteoporotic bones.

No particular anaesthetic technique is required, but intubation with positive pressure ventilation is generally recommended. Anaesthetic agents should be administered slowly in patients with impaired cardiovascular function. Distribution volumes and protein binding of anaesthetic drugs may be altered and sensitivity to neuromuscular blocking agents may be increased.

Induction of anaesthesia may be complicated by difficulties in establishing venous access and by a difficult airway. Appropriate equipment should be immediately available.

Intraoperative monitoring is tailored to the surgical procedure and the pre-existing diseases, but is generally more invasive.

Monitoring

Basic

- ECG (with ST segment analysis), non-invasive blood pressure, pulse oximetry, capnometry, neuromuscular blockade.

Supplemental

- Central venous pressure, invasive arterial pressure, arterial blood gases, urine output.

Invasive

- Pulmonary arterial pressures, cardiac function (PiCCO, TOE or thermodilution).

Postoperative management

Except for minor procedures, the patient should be admitted to an ITU postoperatively, particularly after intra-abdominal or thoracic surgery. Respiratory and cardiovascular complications are the primary concern. Electrolyte imbalance and hyperglycaemia may persist or reappear and there is an increased risk of cardiovascular events and deep vein thrombosis (DVT) with pulmonary thromboembolism. Muscle weakness and obesity can interfere with mobilization. Stress ulcer prophylaxis is mandatory.

Postoperative therapy

Basic

- Adequate analgesia (e.g. patient-controlled analgesia).
- Respiratory care (e.g. incentive spirometry).
- Stress ulcer prophylaxis.
- Anticoagulation (DVT prophylaxis).
- Electrolyte balancing (reduce sodium load, additional potassium).
- Early mobilization.

Specific

- Blood glucose control with insulin for diabetes mellitus.
- Glucocorticoid therapy in patients with iatrogenic Cushing syndrome or surgical removal of the source of excess cortisol (see Iatrogenic adrenocortical suppression, p. 72).

Bibliography

Barzaghi LR, Losa M, Giovanelli M, Mortini P. Complications of transsphenoidal surgery in patients with pituitary adenoma: experience at a single centre. *Acta Neurochir (Wien)* 2007; **149**: 877–85.

Chow JT, Thompson GB, Grant CS, *et al.* Bilateral laparoscopic adrenalectomy for corticotrophin-dependent Cushing's syndrome: a review of the Mayo Clinic experience. *Clin Endocrinol (Oxf)* 2008; **68**: 513–19.

Newell-Price J, Trainer P, Besser M, Grossman A. The diagnosis and differential diagnosis of Cushing's syndrome and pseudo-Cushing's states. *Endocr Rev* 1998; **19**: 647–72.

Weatherill D, Spence AA. Anaesthesia and disorders of the adrenal cortex. *Br J Anaesth* 1984; **56**: 741–9.

Cross-references

Adrenocortical insufficiency, 46
Diabetes mellitus, 60
Iatrogenic adrenocortical suppression, 72

Diabetes insipidus

Thomas A Crozier

Diabetes insipidus (a Greek–Latin composite meaning 'passing through without taste', as opposed to diabetes mellitus, with similar symptoms but with sweet urine) is characterized by polyuria (up to 1 L h^{-1}) with dilute urine (50–100 mOsm kg^{-1}), excessive thirst and polydipsia. Untreated diabetes insipidus (DI) leads to dehydration with hypernatraemia and hypokalaemia; plasma osmolality and sodium concentrations may be in the normal range if the patient is allowed to drink *ad libitum*.

There are several forms of DI (Table 2.2), but the one most common and most relevant in this context is neurogenic, or central, DI resulting from reduced or absent vasopressin secretion from the posterior pituitary.

In nephrogenic DI, which can be hereditary or drug induced and is the second most common form of DI, the kidneys do not respond to the water-retaining action of vasopressin, whereas in gestational DI circulating vasopressin is degraded by vasopressinase produced in the gravid uterus. DI in pregnancy may also be a symptom of pre-eclampsia or gestational liver disease, conditions that are treated by delivery of the baby to avoid maternal or neonatal mortality.

Central DI is not affected by fluid restriction but does respond to the vasopressin analogue desmopressin, which differentiates it from nephrogenic DI.

A form known as dipsogenic DI is caused by exaggerated fluid intake, either habitual or due to psychiatric disturbances, or to a defect in hypothalamic thirst control. Desmopressin is ineffective in dipsogenic DI and is even likely to increase the sense of thirst, but fluid restriction should reduce diuresis and increase urine osmolality.

About 25% of the cases of central DI have no obvious cause and are classified as idiopathic. The form most likely to occupy the anaesthetist is acquired and results from brain damage due to tumour, trauma or during neurosurgery. This form may be transient or permanent, but most frequently tends to run a triphasic course. The initial phase is polyuria that can begin intraoperatively and last for up to 5 days. This is followed by an antidiuretic phase of approximately the same duration. A third phase of permanent DI can follow depending on the extent of damage to the hypothalamus and pituitary.

Patients with concomitant untreated cortisol and vasopressin deficiencies (e.g. after hypophysectomy) may not present with polyuria, since hypocortisolism reduces

Table 2.2 Forms of diabetes insipidus

Form	Pathophysiology	Cause	Treatment
Central	Lack of vasopressin	Idiopathic (25%) Hereditary (rare) Acquired: trauma, neurosurgery, tumour (brain, lung), infection	Vasopressin analogue desmopressin (DDAVP) Carbamazepine
Nephrogenic	Insensitivity of kidney to vasopressin	Hereditary: vasopressin receptor defect (V_2), aquaporin 2 defect Acquired: kidney disease, drugs (e.g. lithium, demeclocycline, methoxyflurane, amphotericin B) Electrolyte imbalance: e.g. hypercalcaemia, hypokalaemia	Hydrochlorothiazide Amiloride
Gestational	Lack of vasopressin	Increased degradation of vasopressin by vasopressinase	DDAVP
Dipsogenic	Polydipsia	Disturbed thirst sensation Psychiatric disorders	Fluid restriction

renal free water clearance. Treatment with cortisol will demask the vasopressin deficiency and induce polyuria.

Preoperative assessment

Patients with preoperative DI are usually already being treated for the disorder. No patient with suspected DI should undergo scheduled surgery until it is either ruled out or confirmed and successfully treated, preferably by an endocrinologist.

The ongoing therapy should be recorded and noted how it is to be continued. Patients with central DI will usually be taking desmopressin (DDAVP) as nasal spray (5–20 μg twice a day) or orally (0.1–0.4 mg three times a day). This should be given on the day of surgery.

Patients should not be subjected to prolonged periods without fluids, and those managed with *ad libitum* oral fluid intake will require an infusion to be established several hours before surgery in order to avoid a full stomach at induction.

Preoperative assessment should include signs of dehydration and low cardiac filling pressures, serum electrolytes and osmolality, and renal function parameters (urea, creatinine). Information on urine volume should be elicited from the patient, and serum and urine osmolalities should be determined.

Hypernatraemia and hypovolaemia should be treated gradually. Too rapid changes of serum osmolality or acute volume loading can precipitate cardiac decompensation or cerebral oedema.

Perioperative management

One of the challenges in managing a patient with DI is maintaining fluid and electrolyte balance. This task is easier if diuresis is controlled with titrating doses of DDAVP (e.g. 1 μg i.v. doses). In addition to the standard monitoring for the procedure, particular attention should be given to urine output and serum concentrations of sodium and potassium. If possible, serum and urine osmolalities should be controlled frequently, and DDAVP given if serum osmolality exceeds 290 mOsm L^{-1}.

One should be aware of the fact that DI can arise without warning at any time during neurosurgical procedures. The diagnosis should be considered if diuresis continuously exceeds 200–300 mL h^{-1} without volume loading or diuretics (e.g. mannitol).

Fluid and electrolyte balance must continue in the postoperative period and DDAVP be administered as necessary. Urine output, vascular filling pressures and serum osmolality should be monitored in the ITU following major surgery or significant blood losses.

Bibliography

Hayanga AJ, Kohen R, Egeland B, *et al.* Central diabetes insipidus: a rare perioperative cause of severe hypernatraemia. *Anaesth Intensive Care* 2008; **36**: 235–41.

Kassebaum N, Hairr J, Goldsmith W, *et al.* Diabetes insipidus associated with propofol anesthesia. *J Clin Anesth* 2008; **20**: 466–8.

Lacassie HJ, Muir HA, Millar S, Habib AS. Perioperative anesthetic management for Cesarean section of a parturient with gestational diabetes insipidus. *Can J Anaesth* 2005; **52**: 733–6.

Moug SJ, McKee RF, O'Reilly DS, *et al.* The perioperative challenge of nephrogenic diabetes insipidus: a multidisciplinary approach. *Surgeon* 2005; 3: 89–94.

Smith M, Hirsch NP. Pituitary disease and anaesthesia. *Br J Anaesth* 2000; **85**: 3–14.

Wise-Faberowski L, Soriano SG, Ferrari L, *et al.* Perioperative management of diabetes insipidus in children. *J Neurosurg Anesthesiol* 2004; **16**: 220–5.

Cross-reference

Pituitary disorders and hypopituitarism, 78

Diabetes mellitus

Brian J Pollard

Type 1 (insulin-dependent diabetes mellitus)

An autoimmune disorder of the pancreas characterized by β-cell destruction.

Characteristics

- Onset usually in younger age group.
- Absolute insulin deficiency.
- Abrupt onset of symptoms.
- Tendency to ketosis.

Diagnosed by consistently raised random plasma glucose >11.1 mmol L^{-1} (venous whole blood glucose >10 mmol L^{-1}) or fasting plasma glucose >7.0 mmol L^{-1} (blood glucose >6.1 mmol L^{-1}).

There is a type of diabetes known as 'latent autoimmune diabetes in adults', which was first described in the early 1990s. It refers to adults who present with a slowly progressive form of diabetes that is autoimmune in nature and resembles type 1 diabetes but in an older age group. It may be treated initially without insulin but insulin may be needed later on in the course of the condition. Complication rates appear to be similar to those of type 2 diabetes.

Complications

Long term

- Retinopathy.
- Ischaemic heart disease: 2–4 times higher than in the general population.
- Hypertension: BP increased in 30–60% of diabetics.
- Nephropathy: 30–40% of type 1 diabetics.
- Neuropathy: peripheral and autonomic (autonomic found in up to 40% of type 1 diabetics).
- Respiratory disease: poor glycaemic control in type 1 diabetics has been associated with impaired lung function.
- Stiff joint syndrome: may cause difficulty with intubation.
- Skin: foot ulcers.

Short term

- Hypoglycaemia: this is potentially the most serious acute complication.
- Hyperglycaemia with metabolic disturbance; may be exacerbated by the 'stress response' during surgery.
- Gastric stasis is common, especially with hyperglycaemia and ketoacidosis.

Preoperative assessment

History

- Diabetes:
  - duration
  - control
  - type, quantity and timing of insulin dosage.
- Assess presence of coexisting disease:
  - renal: nephropathy (mild-severe)
  - cardiovascular system (CVS):
    - ischaemic heart disease with decreased exercise tolerance
    - hypertension
  - respiratory system
  - CNS: peripheral and autonomic neuropathy.
- Other drugs.

Examination

Full physical examination, with attention to cardiac, respiratory and renal disease according to any positive indicators in the history.

Investigations

- Glycaemic control:
  - short term: fasting blood glucose
  - long term: glycosylated haemoglobin (HbA_1C); this should be within normal limits. An HbA_1C >9% is indicative of poor control, and hyperglycaemia, hypovolaemia and electrolyte abnormalities should be anticipated and corrected preoperatively.
- Full blood count.
- Renal function: urinalysis, plasma urea, creatinine and electrolyte concentration.
- Chest X-ray, if clinically indicated.
- ECG or exercise ECG: silent ischaemia.
- HbA_1C >7% can be used as a predictor of coronary heart disease. If associated with other risk factors such as a poor exercise tolerance, age over 55, obesity or physical inactivity a 'stress ECG' to evaluate for silent ischaemia may be indicated before major surgery. An inability to climb two flights of stairs has a positive predictive value of 89% for postoperative cardiopulmonary complications in these patients.

Aims of perioperative management

Maintenance of normoglycaemia

Blood glucose should stay within the range 6–11 mmol L^{-1}. Hyperglycaemia causes dehydration, electrolyte disturbance, acidosis, poor tissue perfusion and organ ischaemia, impaired wound healing and increased susceptibility to infection. Cerebral or myocardial ischaemia will be aggravated by hyperglycaemia. Hypoglycaemia may cause cerebral damage.

Appropriate management of coexisting disease

This is a greater cause of morbidity than the diabetes itself. Cardiovascular drugs, including β-blockers, should be continued in the preoperative period, as they may be protective. Fluid and electrolytes should be optimized preoperatively.

Autonomic neuropathy may cause cardiovascular instability during anaesthesia.

General principles of management

Major surgery

Ideally, the patient is admitted 24 hours preoperatively. With the increasing use of preassessment clinics, advice can be given about the management of insulin preoperatively, and well-controlled diabetic patients can be safely admitted on the evening before surgery or on the morning of surgery. Long-acting insulins should be omitted the night before surgery. Ideally, patients with diabetes should be operated on at the beginning of a list. If this is not possible, a sliding scale should be started in the morning.

Glucose

Glucose should be started when calories or fluids are required and cannot be obtained by the enteral route. Sufficient glucose is supplied to prevent hypoglycaemia and to provide basal energy requirements. It is recommended that 5–10 g h^{-1} of glucose be given. This usually works out at about 100–200 mL h^{-1} of 5% dextrose for an average person. For longer term infusions, 0.9% sodium chloride is also needed to prevent hyponatraemia.

Insulin

It is important to consult the local hospital guidelines for management of the diabetic patient. The following regime will provide satisfactory management in the absence of any local guidelines. Whichever regime is chosen, it is important to measure the blood glucose regularly (every 1–2 hours) using a point-of-care capillary glucose monitor.

The morning dose of insulin may be omitted if the patient is starved; alternatively, a reduced dose of one-third of the regular morning dose (as a rapid-acting variety) together with an intravenous glucose infusion may be given to prevent fasting ketoacidosis in brittle diabetics. However, if the patient is due to have surgery in the afternoon, either (1) set up an infusion of glucose + insulin + potassium in the morning or (2), if allowed to eat, give half the usual dose of insulin with a light breakfast, then set up an infusion mid-morning when the effects of the insulin are wearing off.

Insulin should be given by an intravenous infusion, following a sliding scale regimen (Table 2.3). Intravenous boluses have too short a half-life and they may cause deterioration of metabolic control. Absorption of subcutaneous insulin is variable, especially in the perioperative period, and this route is not recommended for patients undergoing major surgery. Strict monitoring of blood glucose must be performed.

Table 2.3 Typical sliding scale for insulin

Blood glucose (mmol L^{-1})	Insulin infusion* (units h^{-1})
0–5	0
6–10	1–2
11–15	2–3
16–20	3–4
>20	Medical intervention needed

*Infusion: make up 50 units insulin to 50 mL with saline (1 U mL^{-1}). No need to add colloid, provided the first few millilitres are flushed through the giving set.

Insulin may be also added to a bag of glucose (the Alberti regimen; see Box 2.3). The usual requirements are 0.25–0.35 U g^{-1} glucose.

Box 2.3 The Alberti regimen

Glucose 10%	500 mL
Insulin (actrapid)	15 U
Potassium	10 mmol

- Add together
- Infuse this at 100 mL h^{-1}
- Blood glucose is monitored 2 hourly and the insulin content of a bag adjusted by 5 U if the blood glucose falls outside the range 6–11 mmol L^{-1}

Insulin requirements are increased with steroid therapy, sepsis, liver disease, obesity and during cardiopulmonary bypass.

Potassium

Potassium should be added as required; usually, 20 mmol L^{-1} of glucose.

Minor surgery/day cases

Type 1 diabetic patients commonly present for day-case surgery. Ideally, the procedure should be performed in the morning, should be minor, should be unlikely to cause much pain and should have a low incidence of postoperative nausea and vomiting. The patients should be able to demonstrate a good understanding of how to alter their insulin dose, and they must have good support at home. The HbA_1C should be <7%. Facilities must exist to admit these patients postoperatively, if necessary.

A sliding scale insulin infusion and/or glucose should be started if the fasting glucose is outside the range 6–11 mmol L^{-1}, or if there is any delay to the start of surgery, and should be started if, postoperatively, the patient suffers with nausea and vomiting. The infusion should then continue until a normal diet is resumed. Nausea and vomiting may indicate the development of ketoacidaemia.

Monitoring

Both hypoglycaemia and hyperglycaemia are harmful. Under anaesthesia, symptoms of hypoglycaemia are masked.

Blood glucose should be checked every 0.5–1 hours preoperatively and in theatre using a capillary blood glucose meter. Periodically confirm with laboratory blood glucose tests for longer procedures. Postoperatively, check hourly until a normal diet is established. Plasma potassium should be monitored 3–4 hourly, or more frequently if clinically indicated.

Anaesthesia

No technique has been shown to be superior. Regional techniques, where appropriate, are preferable to general anaesthesia, as they usually allow a swifter return to normal eating patterns. They may partially decrease the 'stress response' associated with surgery.

Type 2 (non-insulin-dependent diabetes mellitus)

This is more common than type 1. It is characterized by either hepatic or extrahepatic insulin resistance or both, is probably due to decreased stimulation of glycogen synthesis in muscle by insulin and is related to impaired glucose transport. Insulin secretion and/or insulin action are thought to be deficient with excessive hepatic glucose production.

The age of onset is variable. It is usually a disease of adults. They have a slow onset and the development of ketoacidosis is unlikely.

There is an increased incidence of macrovascular disease, especially peripheral vascular and cardiovascular disease, irrespective of age at diagnosis. Silent myocardial ischaemia is common, particularly if there is poor glycaemic control and in the presence of other risk factors such as obesity, physical inactivity and age >55 years. Nephropathy is common and is associated with cardiovascular disease.

The mainstays of management are diet, exercise and drugs. The following families of drugs exist:

- Sulphonylureas (e.g. gliclazide) increase pancreatic β-cell sensitivity to glucose, thereby enhancing insulin release. Long-acting drugs (e.g. chlorpropamide) may exacerbate hypoglycaemia during fasting and are now rarely used.
- Biguanides (e.g. metformin) reduce hepatic glucose production and enhance glucose uptake in muscles.
- Thiozolidinediones (e.g. pioglitazone and rosiglitazone) improve peripheral glucose uptake in the muscle and fat and inhibit hepatic glucose production. They are not associated with lactic acidosis but may cause hepatotoxicity.
- Prandial glucose regulators, such as nateglinide and repaglinide, stimulate release of insulin from the pancreas. They have a fast onset and short duration of action and are therefore taken just before meals. They are less likely to cause hypoglycaemia than sulphonylureas.
- Acarbose inhibits α-glucosidases in the brush border of small intestinal mucosa and thus delays absorption of glucose.
- The 'gliptins' (e.g. sitagliptin and vildagliptin) increase insulin secretion and reduce glucagon secretion.

Preoperative assessment

This should follow the same lines as for type 1 diabetes mellitus.

Perioperative management

These patients are still able to secrete some insulin; however, they are insulin resistant.

Minor surgery/day surgery

Well-controlled, diet-managed patients do not usually need special treatment apart from regular monitoring of the blood glucose. For those on oral hypoglycaemic agents, their treatment should continue as normal up to the day before surgery and then omit any oral hypoglycaemics on the day of surgery. Ideally, surgery should be undertaken in the morning. If the patient is scheduled for afternoon surgery, regular monitoring of blood glucose should take place. As most patients are allowed fluids up to 2 hours preoperatively, give glucose-containing drinks if the blood glucose decreases. If blood glucose is <11 mmol L^{-1} it is usually sufficient to just monitor the blood glucose. Start a sliding scale infusion of insulin if the patient is an inpatient and the fasting blood glucose is >11 mmol L^{-1}.

The most important feature is careful, frequent monitoring of blood glucose and early corrective measures if the blood glucose goes outside the range 6–11 mmol L^{-1}.

Major surgery

Treat as type 1 diabetic patients. Hyperosmolar, hyperglycaemic, non-ketotic coma may occur postoperatively. There is some evidence against the use of Hartmann's solution, but it is unlikely to be deleterious if given slower than 1 L h^{-1}.

Anaesthesia

Many of these patients will be presenting for surgery for complications of their diabetes. Careful management of pre-existing medical problems is important. Anaesthesia should cause minimal metabolic disturbance. Regional techniques are usually preferable to general anaesthesia, unless there is severe cardiovascular disturbance. Local hospital guidelines for the management of diabetic patients should be followed if possible.

Bibliography

Fourlanos S, Dotta F, Greenbaum CJ, *et al.* Latent autoimmune diabetes in adults (LADA) should be less latent. *Diabetologia* 2005; **48**: 2206–12.

Gugutkov D, Smilov I. Anaesthetical approaches to patients with diabetes. *Anesthesiol Intensive Care* 2009; **39**: 42–46.

Killen J, Tonks K, Greenfield JR, Story DA. New insulin analogues and perioperative care of patients with diabetes mellitus. *Anaesth Intensive Care* 2010; **38**: 244–9.

McAnulty GR, Robertshaw HJ, Hall GM. Anaesthetic management of patients with diabetes mellitus. *Br J Anaesth* 2000; **85**: 80–90.

Schernthaner G, Hink S, Kopp HP, *et al.* Progress in the characterization of slowly progressive autoimmune diabetes in adult patients (LADA or type 1.5 diabetes). *Exp Clin Endocrinol Diabetes* 2001; **109**(Suppl. 2): S94–108.

Scherpereel P. Perioperative care of diabetic patient. *Minerva Anestesiol* 2001; **67**: 258–62.

Scherpereel PA Tavernier B. Perioperative care of diabetic patients. *Eur J Anaesthesiol* 2001; **18**: 277–94.

Cross-reference

Fluid and electrolyte balance, 754

Hyperparathyroidism

Thomas A Crozier

The parathyroid glands are small organs, usually between four and six, located directly behind the thyroid gland, that secrete the polypeptide parathyroid hormone (parathormone (PTH)).

PTH acts to increase serum calcium concentrations. It directly increases renal tubular reabsorption of calcium and decreases that of phosphate. It indirectly increases calcium concentrations by stimulating osteoclast activity to release calcium from bones, and by increasing calcium absorption from the gut through activation of vitamin D in the kidney. Excess PTH can cause hypercalcaemia, whereas PTH deficiency causes hypocalcaemia.

Hyperparathyroidism refers to excessive secretion of PTH from the parathyroid glands that may or may not be associated with hypercalcaemia. The aetiological classification is complicated and differentiates primary, secondary and tertiary disease.

Primary hyperparathyroidism

Primary hyperparathyroidism is associated with hypercalcaemia owing to unstimulated PTH secretion from parathyroid glands caused by:

- single adenoma (80%) or multiple gland hyperplasia (10–15%)
- adenoma (e.g. multiple endocrine neoplasia syndromes MEN1 or MEN2A)
- parathyroid carcinoma (1–3%).

Secondary hyperparathyroidism

Secondary hyperparathyroidism is the physiological regulatory response to hypocalcaemia or hyperphosphataemia, e.g. in chronic renal failure. PTH is elevated but serum calcium is low to normal.

Tertiary hyperparathyroidism

Tertiary hyperparathyroidism is essentially a primary dysfunction arising when chronic stimulation leads to the formation of an autonomous adenoma. Serum calcium is elevated.

The hypercalcaemia of malignancy is induced by various mechanisms, among which is the secretion of parathyroid hormone-related protein (PTHrP) with PTH activity by the tumour. Ectopic PTH secretion is rare.

Clinical presentation

Most of the signs and symptoms of hyperparathyroidism are due to hypercalcaemia, and their severity is related to the level of serum calcium. Patients with mild hypercalcaemia (serum calcium <3.0 mmol L^{-1}) are often asymptomatic. Serum calcium concentrations above 4 mmol L^{-1} can cause coma and cardiac arrest and require emergency therapy.

General signs and symptoms

- Fatigue.
- Mental symptoms, especially psychosis and depression.

Renal system

- Polyuria, dehydration, polydipsia, renal calculi, nephrocalcinosis, renal failure.

Gastrointestinal tract

- Anorexia, nausea and vomiting, dyspepsia, peptic ulcers, abdominal pain, constipation.

Cardiovascular system

- Tachycardia, arrhythmias, hypertension, shortened QT interval, widened T wave.

Preoperative assessment

History

Search for the symptoms and signs of hypercalcaemia. A mnemonic for these is groans (abdominal pain), moans (depression, confusion), bones (bone pain) and stones (kidney stones).

Investigations

- Serum calcium, electrolytes, creatinine, urea.
- ECG (shortened QT interval, widened T wave).

Patients with severe hypercalcaemia may present with hypovolaemia and coma. Emergency treatment consists of hydration with intravenous saline and forced diuresis (furosemide), intravenous phosphate replacement, inhibition of osteoclast activity with biphosphonates and calcitonin and, possibly, glucocorticoids; emergency parathyroidectomy.

Perioperative management

Perioperative management for parathyroidectomy will follow the recommendations for thyroid surgery:

- protect the eyes against accidental opening and mechanical damage
- reinforced endotracheal tube
- secure airway connections
- balanced anaesthesia.

A urinary catheter and arterial cannulation may be necessary in patients with critically elevated serum calcium concentrations.

A central venous catheter is occasionally requested by the surgeon to draw blood samples for intraoperative PTH measurements in order to determine whether the overactive glands have been correctly removed.

Postoperative complications

Most complications of parathyroid surgery are similar to those of thyroidectomy.

Oedema of the glottis and pharynx may occasionally follow parathyroid surgery.

The characteristic complication of parathyroidectomy is hypocalcaemia due to excessive resection, or traumatic or ischaemic damage to the remaining glands. Hypocalcaemia increases neuromuscular irritability. Symptoms of hypocalcaemia are paraesthesiae in the hands, perioral tingling, carpal spasms, hyperactive tendon reflexes, positive Chovstek and Trousseau's signs, laryngospasm, long QTc with the risk of malignant cardiac arrhythmias. Calcium gluconate or calcium chloride is given intravenously to treat symptomatic hypocalcaemia.

Repeated determinations of serum calcium, phosphate, magnesium and parathyroid hormone will be required for several days postoperatively.

Bibliography

Bilezikian JP. Management of acute hypercalcemia. *N Engl J Med* 1992; **326**:1196–1203.

Fraser WD. Hyperparathyroidism. *Lancet* 2009; **374**: 145–58.

Cross-references

Acute kidney injury, 196
Chronic kidney disease, 203

Hyperthyroidism

Thomas A Crozier

Hyperthyroidism is caused by the excessive secretion of thyroid hormones. This occurs most frequently in women between the ages of 20 and 40 years, often within 6 months postpartum. The female to male sex ratio is 5:1 to 10:1.

The main cause of hyperthyroidism is autoimmune multinodular diffuse enlargement (toxic nodular goitre) caused by thyroid-stimulating immunoglobulins (TSIs) that act as a 'long-acting thyroid stimulator' (LATS) and thyroid growth immunoglobulins (TGIs) that induce the growth of thyroid follicles.

Other causes of hyperthyroidism are early-stage Hashimoto thyroiditis, choriocarcinoma, TSH-secreting pituitary tumours and autonomous thyroid adenoma ('hot nodule'). The last is the most frequent cause in elderly patients. Iatrogenic causes of hyperthyroidism are prolonged treatment with amiodarone or thyroxine overdosing.

Most clinical features of hyperthyroidism are directly related to the effects of serum triiodothyronine (T_3) and thyroxine (T_4), but the myxoedema that presents as exophthalmus and pretibial oedema in patients with Graves disease is a subcutaneous deposition of glycosaminoglyans caused by antibody stimulation of the TSH receptor and is unrelated to thyroid hormone action.

Diagnosis is confirmed by elevated serum concentrations of free and total T_4 and T_3 and undetectable serum TSH. However, high levels of thyroxine are seen in clinically euthyroid patients during fasting, or during treatment with β-blockers or glucocorticoids because of reduced conversion of T_4 to T_3 ('high T_4 syndrome'). A high total T_4 level with normal response to TSH stimulation is also seen under opiate therapy as a result of the increased concentration of thyroxine-binding globulin (TBG) that reduces the fraction of free T_4(FT_4).

Signs and symptoms

General and metabolism

Nervousness, tremor, mental impairment, heat intolerance, warm moist skin, weight loss despite increased appetite, fatigue, diarrhoea, menstrual disturbances and impaired glucose tolerance. The presentation is different in older patients, with constipation, apathy, depression and loss of appetite prevailing.

Cardiovascular

Tachycardia, systolic hypertension, hyperdynamic circulation, arrhythmias, atrial fibrillation, dyspnoea and congestive heart failure.

Neuromuscular

Muscular weakness, proximal myopathy, hyperreflexia, nerve entrapment syndromes and increased central neuronal apoptosis.

Laboratory

Anaemia, thrombocytopenia and elevated liver enzymes.

Serum catecholamine concentrations are not increased and the signs of sympathetic stimulation are due to thyroid hormone-induced sensitization and upregulation of β-adrenergic receptors. Hyperplasia of the adrenal cortex is frequently observed.

Preoperative assessment

Manifest hyperthyroidism increases the risk of perioperative complications and is a contraindication for elective surgery, with the exception of thyroidectomy as a measure of last resort when conservative treatment has failed to control the condition. Other patients should be treated with antithyroid drugs, e.g. carbimazole or propylthiouracil, until euthyroid. Iodide is given to reduce the vascularity of the gland. Symptoms can be alleviated with β-receptor antagonists.

Patients with manifest hyperthyroidism requiring emergency surgery have a high risk of perioperative, particularly cardiovascular, complications and require special care.

History and examination

Thyroid hormone status should be evaluated in patients with goitre. Goitre alone is most often associated with iodine-deficiency hypothyroidism, but may also be present in patients with hyperthyroidism. The patient must be examined for signs and symptoms of increased thyroid function. The neck should be inspected and the presence of stridor on forced inspiration noted. Engorged jugular veins can indicate retrosternal goitre.

Investigations

Patients with suspected hyperthyroidism require determination of T_4, FT_4, T_3 and TSH, in addition to routine laboratory data. Elevated hormone levels may exist without clinical signs of hyperthyroidism. Chest and neck X-rays will show the position of the trachea and reveal any compression or deviation caused by a goitre. Retrosternal goitre usually does not interfere with intubation even when the trachea is displaced. Indirect laryngoscopy is performed preoperatively by many surgeons to document vocal cord function. CT and MRI scans are occasionally ordered, and can reveal the magnitude and extent of tracheal stenosis.

Perioperative management

Premedication may be necessary to reduce anxiety. Antithyroid drugs, including β adrenergic receptor blockers, should be continued on the day of surgery. The perioperative management of patients undergoing non-thyroid surgery who are euthyroid under medication does not differ in any relevant manner from patients without a thyroid disorder, except for possible difficulties in airway management.

Airway management

Equipment for a difficult intubation should always be available. Minor tracheal involvement is usually of little import, but awake fibreoptic intubation or inhalation induction should be considered in patients with severe displacement of the trachea, tilting of the glottis or when the trachea is compressed by a fibrotic Riedel's struma.

Thyroidectomy

A reinforced oral tracheal tube is used to prevent kinking and occlusion under pressure during surgical dissection. Special endotracheal tubes are available that allow intraoperative localization of the superior laryngeal and recurrent nerve and monitoring of their integrity. These must be positioned with the sensor area in the correct location.

The use of a laryngeal mask airway has been advocated for thyroid surgery, but the risk of intraoperative dislodgement cannot be ignored, particularly since correction is difficult because of the obstructed access to the patient's head.

The tip of the tube should be advanced beyond the distal edge of tracheal compression and firmly taped in position with all connections secured, as access to the airway is limited when surgery has commenced.

Thyroidectomy can be performed under deep or superficial cervical plexus block, but general anaesthesia is the usual practice. There is no evidence that the choice of anaesthetic agent is important, and none of the newer volatile anaesthetics have been associated with organ dysfunction in hyperthyroid subjects. There is some concern regarding the use of drugs that can precipitate or worsen tachycardia. Among these are anticholinergics, neuromuscular blocking agents with significant vagolytic activity (e.g. pancuronium) and ketamine.

The eyelids should be taped and the eyes protected against mechanical damage, particularly in patients with the exophthalmus associated with Graves disease.

The patient is positioned with the neck fully extended, and this may be the source of postoperative discomfort. The surgical site is elevated to reduce venous bleeding, but this position can predispose to venous air embolism. If epinephrine-containing local anaesthetic solutions are used to infiltrate the wound, the maximum doses should be observed.

Bradycardia and hypotension are complications of carotid sinus manipulation and can be treated with intravenous atropine, if necessary. Infiltration of the area with lidocaine can suppress the glossopharyngeal nerve afferents and prevent recurrence. Persisting tachycardia and hypertension can result from manipulation of the gland.

Vocal cord motility can usually be visualized by direct laryngoscopy immediately after extubation. Otherwise, have the patient speak and listen for hoarseness or aphonia.

The management of surgery in hyperthyroid patients is summarized in Box 2.4, and the eligibility of patients for surgery is summarized in Table 2.4.

Box 2.4 Management of thyroid surgery in hyperthyroid patients

- General anaesthesia with balanced technique (avoid anticholinergics)
- Prepare for difficult intubation
- Non-kinking reinforced endotracheal tube advanced beyond any stenosis
- Secure connections
- Protect eyes
- Prepare for cardiac responses (brady/tachycardia, hypo/hypertension)
- Prepare for exacerbated hyperthyroid symptoms in non-euthyroid patients
- Assess voice after extubation

Non-thyroid surgery

Hyperthyroid patients

In general, only emergency surgery is performed on patients with manifest hyperthyroidism. Anaesthetic management is designed to control the symptoms of hyperthyroidism and prevent a further worsening.

Monitoring is more invasive and can require arterial and central venous cannulation. Large-bore venous

Table 2.4 Hyperthyroidism and eligibility for surgery

	Type of surgery	
	Elective	Emergency
Subclinical (only suppressed TSH)	+	+
Elevated T_3, T_4, no symptoms	(+)	+
Clinically manifest	–	With supportive therapy and aggressive thyroid suppressive measures

TSH, thyroid-stimulating hormone; T_3, serum triiodothyronine; T_4, serum thyroxine.
Iodine and substances containing iodine should be avoided in patients with active hyperthyroidism (contrast medium, amiodarone, disinfectants such as iodoform, povidone–iodine).

cannulae should be inserted to allow adequate and rapid fluid replacement. Temperature monitoring is mandatory.

Treatment of the tachycardia with a β-blocker should begin before induction and continue throughout the entire perioperative period. Cardiac arrhythmias may require treatment with lidocaine.

Regional anaesthesia should be considered whenever feasible. Care is required in treating associated hypotension, since the hyperthyroid patient has an exaggerated sensitivity to adrenergic stimulation. Direct-acting vasoconstrictors, such as phenylephrine or metaraminol, should be preferred to indirectly acting drugs.

A balanced technique is recommended for general anaesthesia with an opioid and either propofol or a volatile anaesthetic. Muscle relaxation, when required, should be adapted to the muscular weakness of the hyperthyroid patient, and neuromuscular monitoring is mandatory. A possible exaggerated response to atropine must be anticipated when reversing neuromuscular blockade. Glycopyrrolate may be a better choice because of its weaker chronotropic effects. Relaxation with rocuronium and reversal with sugammadex might be a suitable choice. Vasopressors must be used cautiously owing to the increased sensitivity to catecholamines.

Fluid infusions must be adequate to replace the loss due to elevated temperature.

Postoperative complications

Nerve injury

Nerve injury is a recognized complication of thyroid surgery and can affect the recurrent and the superior laryngeal nerves. The lesion is frequently caused by nerve distension and is reversible within a few days, but permanent damage will result if the nerve is severed.

Unilateral injury to the recurrent laryngeal nerve is well tolerated because abduction of the contralateral vocal cord is not affected, but after bilateral injury both cords remain in a paramedian position with an extremely narrow glottic opening that requires reintubation.

Injury to the superior laryngeal nerve interrupts the function of the cricothyroid muscle and causes a hoarse voice. It also disrupts the sensory input from the larynx above the vocal folds that triggers reflex closure of the glottis and prevents aspiration.

Thyrotoxicosis (thyroid storm)

Thyroid storm is the result of the sudden release of thyroid hormones, causing the exacerbation of the symptoms of hyperthyroidism, particularly in inadequately treated or untreated hyperthyroid patients. The result is tachycardia, cardiac arrhythmias, hyperthermia, altered consciousness, congestive heart failure, dehydration and shock. The tachycardia and elevated temperature can initially be mistaken for malignant hyperthermia. Thyroid storm can appear intraoperatively, but usually becomes manifest between 6 and 18 hours after surgery. The condition is not common but has a high mortality rate.

The mainstays of therapy are symptomatic support with a β-blocker to reduce heart rate, high-dose corticosteroids, aggressive intravenous fluid therapy and cooling, and suppression of thyroid hormone synthesis and secretion with sodium iodide and thyrostatic drugs. The long-standing β-blocker of choice was propranolol, but the shorter acting esmolol has been recommended to avoid the occasional cardiovascular collapse that has been described with propranolol.

Other complications

Haematoma with compression of the trachea is a postoperative emergency requiring immediate reintubation to prevent asphyxia. The cause is usually a slipped arterial ligature, but some see a connection with postoperative coughing and thus advocate extubation while the patient is deeply anaesthetized. Opening the wound might relieve the pressure and stitch cutters or clip removers should be immediately available.

Long-standing goitre can cause tracheomalacia that allows the trachea to collapse during inspiration once the supporting surrounding structure is removed. Reintubation or tracheotomy is often required.

Less common surgical complications are tracheal laceration with or without subcutaneous emphysema, tracheo-oesophageal fistula leading to aspiration, and recurring pneumonia, pneumothorax and pneumomediastinum. Injury to the phrenic nerve can present as postoperative hypoxaemia or respiratory distress. Accidental removal of the parathyroid glands will lead to postoperative hypocalcaemia with its associated symptoms.

Bibliography

Farling PA. Thyroid disease. *Br J Anaesth* 2000; **85**: 15–28.

Hobbiger HE, Allen JG, Greatorex RG, Denny NM. The laryngeal mask airway for thyroid and parathyroid surgery. *Anaesthesia* 1996; **51**: 972–4.

Kalra S, Williams A, Whitaker R, *et al.* Subclinical thyroid dysfunction does not affect one-year mortality in elderly patients after hip fracture: a prospective longitudinal study. *Injury* 2010; **41**: 385–7.

Kaplan JA, Cooperman LH. Alarming reactions to ketamine in patients taking thyroid medication: treatment with propranolol. *Anesthesiology* 1971; **35**: 229–30.

Cross-reference

Difficult airway: overview, 647

Hypothyroidism

Thomas A Crozier

Hypothyroidism is found in about 5% of the population in most surveys and is endemic in some areas. In patients over 65, the prevalence of manifest hypothyroidism (elevated TSH, low T_4) is 7% and a further 5–10% have subclinical hypothyroidism with elevated TSH and normal T_3 and T_4. About one-third of patients with subclinical hypothyroidism develop manifest disease within 4 years. Hypothyroidism is usually a primary disease of the thyroid gland and the main causes are iodine deficiency, chronic autoimmune thyroiditis (Hashimoto), previous radioiodine therapy and thyroidectomy. Over-abundant intake of iodine (amiodarone, dietary iodide) or lithium therapy can induce hypothyroidism. Patients with Hashimoto hypothyroidism are at increased risk for concomitant Addison disease as well as type 1 diabetes mellitus. Secondary hypothyroidism is caused by a lack of TSH owing to pituitary or hypothalamic dysfunction, and its diagnosis must be based on the circulating levels of thyroid hormones alone.

Signs and symptoms

The typical symptoms of hypothyroidism result from decreased metabolism and include lethargy, hypothermia, intolerance to cold, cool dry skin, coarse features, hoarse voice and brittle hair.

Cardiovascular system

Cardiac output is reduced, with bradycardia, reduced stroke volume and hypotension. The baroreceptor reflex is obtunded. Cardiomegaly with pericardial effusion may be present. The myocardium is overly sensitive to the negative inotropic effects of anaesthetics.

Respiratory system

The ventilatory response to hypoxia and hypercapnia is decreased. Oedema can reduce diffusion capacity measured by carbon monoxide transfer, and can progress to pleural effusions that further reduce ventilatory capacity.

Nervous system

Lethargy, depression, confusion, ataxia, myalgia, delayed relaxation of deep tendon reflexes (Woltman sign) and increased sensitivity to the respiratory depressive effects of opioids.

Laboratory

Anaemia (association of Hashimoto thyroiditis with pernicious anaemia) and hyponatraemia.

Gastrointestinal tract

Loss of appetite, constipation, paralytic ileus and ascites.

The most severe manifestation of hypothyroidism is myxoedema coma (not identical to myxoedema as a symptom) with impaired consciousness, myopathy, hypothermia, hypoglycaemia, hypotension, hyponatraemia and hypoventilation.

Mild hypothyroidism can prolong the recovery period, and, in the course of serious illness or major surgery, even subclinical hypothyroidism can decompensate to myxoedema coma with a mortality rate of up to 80%. On the other hand, subclinical hypothyroidism appears to have a protective effect. Elderly men with high TSH and low normal FT_4 have a lower overall mortality rate, and subclinical hypothyroidism presenting only with elevated TSH but normal serum concentrations of T_3 and T_4 does not appear to be a risk factor for minor to moderately invasive surgery.

Preoperative assessment

Because of its high prevalence, an active search for signs and symptoms of hypothyroidism is indicated. Elective surgery is not advisable in patients with symptomatic hypothyroidism. These patients should be treated with oral thyroxine, ideally until serum T_3 and T_4 levels are normal and TSH is no longer elevated. Cortisol substitution will be required for concomitant adrenal cortex dysfunction.

Patients with severe symptomatic hypothyroidism and emergency surgery can be treated with intravenous T_3 and glucocorticoids in an ITU under full monitoring. Myocardial ischaemia and congestive heart failure are the most serious complications of this therapy.

Investigations

In addition to thyroid parameters, the laboratory work-up should include haemoglobin, renal function parameters and serum electrolytes. The ECG should be evaluated for low voltage (pericardial effusions) and pathological T waves. The chest X-ray should be checked for signs of cardiomegaly, pulmonary vascular

Table 2.5 Hypothyroidism and eligibility for surgery

	Type of surgery	
	Elective	Emergency
Subclinical (only elevated TSH)	+	+
Low T_3, T_4	(+)	+
Clinically manifest	–	With supportive therapy, intravenous T_3, glucocorticoids

TSH, thyroid-stimulating hormone; T_3, triiodothyronine; T_4, serum thyroxine.

congestion and pleural effusions. Additional X-rays of the neck and thoracic inlet should be obtained in patients with goitre.

Perioperative management

Hypothyroidism is virtually always a concomitant disease and not the indication for surgery. Patients who are euthyroid under thyroxine substitution therapy are no different from patients without thyroid dysfunction.

The untreated or insufficiently treated patient presents a high perioperative risk, in part because of the frequently coexisting adrenocortical insufficiency. A dose of glucocorticoid (e.g. prednisolone 25–50 mg i.v.) should be administered as a pragmatic prophylactic measure.

The dose of the oral premedication should take into account the increased CNS sensitivity with greater risk of respiratory depression.

Blood pressure and ECG must be monitored closely during induction and continued into the postoperative period. Insertion of an arterial cannula under local anaesthesia before induction for continuous blood pressure monitoring should be considered. A central venous catheter can be useful in all but very minor procedures, and cardiac output monitoring should be considered for major surgery. Temperature monitoring is mandatory, since hypothyroid patients are at risk of hypothermia.

Intravenous induction agents must be given in small doses at larger intervals, since intravascular volume is reduced and cardiac output decreased. Rapidly injecting a standard dose will critically suppress the impaired myocardial function and the baroreceptor reflex with severe consequences. Thiopental is probably preferable to propofol, but etomidate should be seriously considered for intravenous induction. The problems inherent in intravenous induction can be avoided by inhalational induction with sevoflurane.

The airway should be secured and ventilation controlled since the respiratory responses to hypoxia and hypercapnia are reduced. Forced air heating and infusion warmers should be used to prevent intraoperative heat losses.

Recovery can be delayed and a prolonged period of postoperative ventilation may be necessary because of the slow elimination of the anaesthetic drugs. Patients should be cared for in an intensive care facility and monitored for a worsening of their condition and the occurrence of myxoedema coma.

The management of surgery in hypothyroid patients is summarized in Table 2.5.

Bibliography

Farling PA. Thyroid disease. *Br J Anaesth* 2000; **85**: 15–28.

Ladenson PW, Levin AA, Ridgeway EC, Daniels GH. Complications of surgery in hypothyroid patients. *Am J Med* 1984; **77**: 261–6.

Levelle JP, Jopling MW, Sklar GS. Perioperative hypothyroidism: an unusual postanesthetic diagnosis. *Anesthesiology* 1985; **63**: 195–7.

Murkin JM. Anaesthesia and hypothyroidism: a review of thyroxine physiology, pharmacology and anaesthetic implications. *Anesth Analg* 1982; **61**: 371–83.

van den Beld AW, Visser TJ, Feelders RA, *et al.* Thyroid hormone concentrations, disease, physical function, and mortality in elderly men. *J Clin Endocrinol Metab* 2005; **90**: 6403–9.

Vretzakis G, Ferdi E, Papaziogas B. Insidious hypothyroidism unmasked after operation. *Eur J Anaesthesiol* 2002; **19**: 532–4.

Cross-reference

Thyroidectomy, 392

Iatrogenic adrenocortical suppression

Thomas A Crozier

Iatrogenic adrenocortical suppression is commonly the result of glucocorticoid hormone therapy. Glucocorticoids are prescribed for a wide variety of diseases from hay fever and arthritis to lupus erythematosus and Crohn disease or immunosuppression after an organ transplant. Perioperative complications can arise in these patients depending on the steroid dose and the duration of therapy.

Pathophysiology

Glucocorticoids administered in higher doses and over a prolonged period suppress cortisol secretion from the adrenal cortex and cause involution of the gland. The mechanism is activation of the negative cortisol feedback loop with suppression of CRH secretion from the hypothalamus and ACTH from the pituitary.

Aside from the complications associated with hypercortisolism, patients with glucocorticoid therapy are asymptomatic. Infection, stress or trauma place increased physiological demands on cortisol secretion. The patient with steroid-suppressed adrenocortical function is unable to respond adequately and can develop cardiovascular symptoms if the glucocorticoid dose is not suitably adapted. In analogy to patients with endogenous Cushing syndrome undergoing adrenalectomy, patients with glucocorticoid therapy are at risk of developing an Addisonian crisis if the steroid therapy is terminated or not increased adequately to meet the physiological demands in the perioperative period.

Preoperative assessment

Degree of adrenal suppression

The indication for glucocorticoid therapy as well as the dose and duration of administration are the two major concerns when taking the history. The indication may be of little relevance for the anaesthetist, but might be highly relevant, e.g. a severe autoimmune disease such as systemic lupus erythematosus or rheumatoid arthritis with atlanto-occipital subluxation.

The degree of adrenal suppression is correlated with the dose and duration of the glucocorticoid therapy. This is difficult to assess and is usually not attempted prior to surgery. There is some dispute with regard to the duration of administration and dose of glucocorticoid that is required to suppress adrenal cortical function to an extent relevant to surgery and anaesthesia. The general consensus is that short-term use (less than 1 month) and doses of less than the equivalent of 7.5 mg prednisolone per day carry little risk of suppressing the HPA axis (Table 2.6). Suppression may also occur after topical, oral, parenteral, nebulized or inhaled preparations, but less consistently.

The basic perioperative management of patients with possible iatrogenic adrenocortical suppression but without symptoms of hypercortisolism is identical to that described previously for patients with adrenocortical insufficiency on long-term corticoid substitution therapy.

Patients with high-dose glucocorticoid therapy exhibiting signs and symptoms of iatrogenic Cushing syndrome must be treated with the caution described in Cushing syndrome (hypercortisolism), p. 55. Glucocorticoid

Table 2.6 Potency of adrenocortical hormones compared with cortisol

Steroid	Glucocorticoid	Mineralocorticoid
Cortisol (hydrocortisone)	1	1
Prednisolone	4	0.7
Dexamethasone	40	2
Aldosterone	0.1	400
Fludrocortisone	10	400

therapy must also be continued and adapted to the stress situation in these patients, as described in Table 2.6.

Bibliography

Fraser CG, Preuss FS, Bigford WD. Adrenal atrophy and irreversible shock associated with cortisone therapy. *JAMA* 1952; **149**: 1542–3.

Nicholson G, Burrin JM, Hall GM. Peri-operative steroid supplementation. *Anaesthesia* 1998; **53**: 1091–104.

Salem M, Tainsh RE Jr, Bromberg J, *et al.* Perioperative glucocorticoid coverage. A reassessment 42 years after emergence of a problem. *Ann Surg* 1994; **219**: 416–25.

Weatherill D, Spence AA. Anaesthesia and disorders of the adrenal cortex. *Br J Anaesth* 1984; **56**: 741–9.

Cross-references

Adrenocortical insufficiency, 46
Asthma, 105
Rheumatoid disease, 255
Sarcoidosis, 118

Muscular dystrophies

Brian J Pollard

The muscular dystrophies are a group of genetically determined primary degenerative myopathies. They are best classified by their mode of inheritance.

- X-linked:
  - Duchenne (most common and most severe)
  - Becker.
- Autosomal recessive:
  - limb girdle
  - childhood
  - congenital (? associated with arthrogryposis).
- Autosomal dominant:
  - facioscapulohumeral
  - oculopharyngeal.

All demonstrate atrophy and weakness of muscle to differing degrees. The onset and groups of muscles involved varies according to the specific dystrophy. Their names often define the muscles involved. Involvement of organs other than muscles is uncommon except in Duchenne muscular dystrophy, which is by far the most common and severe.

Duchenne muscular dystrophy

Striated, smooth and cardiac muscle fibres may be affected.

Respiratory failure is common owing to:

- muscle weakness
- oropharyngeal muscle weakness allowing repeated aspiration
- spinal deformities, causing restrictive lung disease.

Obstructive cardiomyopathy occurs, but cardiac failure is often masked by immobility. Arrhythmias are common; tachycardia and ventricular fibrillation have been reported on induction. Severe bradycardia may occur in the facioscapulohumeral variant. There is a particular ECG pattern with Duchenne dystrophy, namely sinus tachycardia, tall R wave in V_1, deep Q wave in the lateral leads and a short P–R interval.

Hypomotility of the gastrointestinal tract and weak pharyngeal muscles predispose to aspiration. Acute gastric dilatation has been reported.

In the musculoskeletal system, pseudohypertrophy of affected muscles occurs and contractures can be problematic. Kyphoscoliosis occurs early on in the disease and further diminishes respiratory reserve. There may be an association with malignant hyperthermia; a malignant hyperthermia (MH)-like syndrome has been reported following succinylcholine and halothane.

Preoperative assessment

History

- Review of respiratory function.
- Previous anaesthetic history (MH).
- Swallowing difficulties.

Investigations

- Respiratory function tests.
- Arterial blood gases.
- ECG.
- Echocardiography if significant CVS disease.
- Chest X-ray (aspiration, cardiac failure).

Premedication

- Avoid respiratory depressants.
- Acid aspiration prophylaxis and at least 6 hours' starvation.
- If positive history of MH-type reaction, use non-triggering anaesthetic agents.

Perioperative management

Monitoring

- ECG.
- End-tidal CO_2 ($ETco_2$).
- Temperature.
- Peripheral nerve stimulator.

Induction and maintenance

Positioning may be difficult because of contractures and kyphoscoliosis.

The association with MH is unproven, and succinylcholine and volatile agents have been given uneventfully. However, succinylcholine has been associated with hyperkalaemia, cardiac arrest, muscle rigidity and rhabdomyolysis and should be avoided. If there is significant CVS disease then minimal volatile agents should be used with opioids. Total intravenous anaesthesia provides a safe alternative to a volatile anaesthetic technique. Sensitivity to non-depolarizing muscle relaxants has been reported; small doses of vecuronium seem to be safe with continued neuromuscular monitoring. Watch $ETco_2$, ECG and temperature for early signs of MH, and have dantrolene available in theatre.

Local or regional techniques will avoid the risks of general anaesthesia, but may be difficult because of contractures and kyphoscoliosis.

A nasogastric tube should be passed as a precaution against gastric dilatation.

Postoperative management

- Observation on ITU/HDU for at least 24 hours.
- Ventilate prophylactically if any doubt about respiratory function.
- Physiotherapy will reduce postoperative respiratory complications.
- Acute gastric dilatation occurs up to 48 hours postoperatively, so leave nasogastric tube *in situ*.

Bibliography

Sethna NF, Rockoff MA, Worthen HM, Rosnow JM. Anesthesia related complications in children with Duchenne's muscular dystrophy. *Anesthesiology* 1988; **68**: 462–5.

Smith CL, Bush GH. Anaesthesia and progressive muscular dystrophy. *Br J Anaesth* 1985; **57**: 1113–18.

Cross-reference

Cardiomyopathy, 136

Myotonia

Brian J Pollard

A myotonic response in a muscle is where there is a sustained contraction of the muscle which persists after the cessation of voluntary effort or stimulation. It is an abnormality of the muscle itself and not of the neuromuscular junction. It appears in three hereditary syndromes, all of which are of autosomal dominant inheritance:

- dystrophia myotonica
- myotonia congenita
- paramyotonia.

The last two are essentially benign myotonic disorders of skeletal muscle only, which do not shorten life. Dystrophia myotonica (myotonic muscular dystrophy or myotonia atrophica) is a form of muscular dystrophy with myotonic symptoms which precede atrophy and weakness. However, atrophy and weakness, particularly of facial, sternomastoid and distal muscles, are the major complaints. Incidence is 1:20000, with onset between the second and fourth decades. The diagnosis is often made late in the clinical course.

Respiratory failure is common because of:

- muscle weakness and myotonia
- CNS-mediated respiratory failure
- oropharyngeal muscle weakness allowing repeated aspiration.

There is a reduced response to carbon dioxide.

Smooth muscle involvement in the gut leads to difficulty in swallowing and decreased gastric motility. Both of these predispose to aspiration. There is a high incidence of gallstones.

Presenile cataracts can be the earliest presenting feature.

In the CVS, rhythm and conduction abnormalities both occur; first-degree heart block is the commonest. Cardiomyopathy has been noted, and arterial pressure is usually low but rises with worsening congestive heart failure. Cor pulmonale may occur as a result of respiratory failure.

Abnormal glucose tolerance tests are common.

Preoperative assessment

History

- Review of respiratory disease.
- Swallowing difficulties.
- Cardiovascular history (pacemaker for heart block?).
- Drugs for myotonia: quinine, procainamide, phenytoin, steroids.

Investigations

- Respiratory function tests and arterial blood gases.
- Chest X-ray (bronchiectasis/infection from aspiration).
- Fluoroscopy will detect diaphragmatic myotonia.
- ECG and 24 hour tape if rhythm disorder suspected.
- Echocardiography if significant CVS involvement.

Premedication

- Avoid respiratory depressants.
- Acid aspiration prophylaxis is advisable.
- Intravenous potassium supplementation may make myotonia worse.

Perioperative management

Monitoring

This must commence in the anaesthetic room:

- ECG
- arterial cannula for pressure and blood gas monitoring is desirable
- invasive CVS monitoring is advisable if there is significant CVS impairment
- peripheral nerve stimulator (note that this may give a false sense of security regarding muscle power)
- temperature.

Induction and maintenance

Cardiovascular and respiratory depression may be profound with the induction of anaesthesia. A minimal dose of induction agent should be used. Gaseous induction may be preferable.

Pulmonary ventilation is usually required and tracheal intubation will protect the airway. Because of muscle atrophy, intubation can usually be performed without muscle relaxation. Succinylcholine should be avoided as widespread myotonia may occur, making intubation very difficult. Short-acting non-depolarizing muscle relaxants may provide relaxation but often do not; minimal doses with close monitoring should be used. Reversal of non-depolarizing block with neostigmine may increase myotonia, therefore it is safest to allow the block to wear off spontaneously.

Opioids should be restricted owing to respiratory depression.

Normothermia should be maintained to decrease postoperative shivering, which will increase myotonia.

Myotonia may occur with diathermy and surgical handling. This will be refractory to neuromuscular blockade and both regional and peripheral nerve blockade. Myotonia may be treated with intravenous procainamide (note: heart block) or phenytoin. Intravenous regional anaesthesia or direct infiltration of the muscle with local anaesthetic may reduce the myotonia.

Regional techniques

These avoid general anaesthesia and its complications; unfortunately, myotonia is not abolished and paralysis of the abdominal muscles may precipitate respiratory failure. Epidural block may be helpful for pain relief, particularly after upper abdominal surgery, and avoids opioids postoperatively.

Local anaesthetic injected directly into the muscle will relieve myotonia and may be used at the surgical site.

Postoperative management

- Patients should be closely monitored in the ITU/HDU.
- Postoperative ventilation is advisable.
- Oxygen therapy should only be used with extreme caution and under monitoring in patients with chronic hypoxic drive.
- Early physiotherapy.
- Tracheostomy/minitracheostomy may be required if bronchial secretions are troublesome.
- ECG monitoring should be continued, as arrhythmias and sudden death have been reported.

Bibliography

Imison AR. Anaesthesia and myotonia: an Australian experience. *Anaesth Intensive Care* 2001; **29**: 34–7.

Russell SH, Hirsch NP. Anaesthesia and myotonia. *Br J Anaesth* 1994; **72**: 210–16.

Cross-references

Cardiomyopathy, 136
Disorders of the oesophagus and of swallowing, 177
Open and laparoscopic cholecystectomy, 451
Pacing and anaesthesia, 777

Pituitary disorders and hypopituitarism

Thomas A Crozier

The pituitary gland or hypophysis is two separate organs: the glandular anterior pituitary derived from Rathke's pouch, an invagination of the oral ectoderm, and the posterior pituitary, an extension of the hypothalamus. Hormones of the anterior pituitary are synthesized and stored in specific pituitary cells, whereas the posterior pituitary stores and releases hormones that are synthesized in the hypothalamus and transported through the pituitary stalk.

Pathophysiology

Pituitary dysfunction refers to either hypersecretion or deficiency of one or several pituitary hormones owing to a congenital defect or to lesions in the hypothalamus, in the pituitary stalk or in the pituitary itself. The clinical features depend on the hormones involved and on the degree of disruption. Patients presenting with symptoms attributable to inappropriate secretion of one pituitary hormone should be evaluated carefully with regard to dysfunction of other endocrine functions under pituitary control.

Hypopituitarism is used by some as a synonym for GH deficiency, but the term should be reserved for hyposecretion of more than one pituitary hormone; the term panhypopituitarism is used when both the anterior and posterior pituitary are affected.

Hypopituitarism is a common sequel of pituitary surgery, but can also be due to pressure from a primary pituitary tumour. Other causes include brain surgery, postpartum pituitary necrosis (Sheehan syndrome), extrasellar tumours, infection, hypoperfusion or radiotherapy. Hypopituitarism is such a common and clinically relevant complication of traumatic brain injury that it should be actively searched for in these patients. Diagnosis may be confirmed by circulating hormone levels, or by functional tests such as lack of response of GH to hypoglycaemia, of ACTH to CRH, of TSH to thyrotrophin-releasing hormone (TRH) or alleviation of polyuria by desmopressin. Hyperpituitarism is nearly always due to tumours or hyperplasia of the secretory cells.

Preoperative assessment

Patients with pituitary tumours or reasons to suspect pituitary dysfunction must be evaluated with regard to endocrine function. The preoperative work-up should include serum concentrations of ACTH, cortisol, TSH and thyroid hormones (see Adrenocortical insufficieny, p. 46 and Cushing syndrome (hypercortisolism), p. 55, and Hyperthyroidism, p. 66 and Hypothyroidism, p. 70). Patients with hypopituitarism due to intracranial tumours or head injuries must be evaluated with regard to accompanying conditions, such as elevated intracranial pressure (see Neurosurgery, p. 299, Raised intracranial pressure/cerebral blood flow control, p. 791). The field of vision should be noted, since the optic nerves pass through the immediate vicinity of the pituitary and can have suffered preoperative damage.

Perioperative management

Patients with pituitary tumours, but with confirmed normal endocrine function and without accompanying problems such as raised intracranial pressure, require no special treatment, unless they are scheduled for hypophysectomy (see Neurosurgery, p. 299). The management of patients with adrenal or thyroid disorders secondary to pituitary dysfunction or with posterior pituitary dysfunction is described in the appropriate sections.

Anterior pituitary

Anterior pituitary secretion is regulated by hypothalamic releasing hormones or inhibitory factors. The main hormones of the anterior pituitary are:

- ACTH (adrenocorticotropin; corticotroph cells)
- TSH (thyroid-stimulating hormone, thyrotropin; thyrotroph cells)
- GH (growth hormone, somatotropin; somatotroph cells)
- prolactin
- follicle-stimulating hormone (FSH)
- luteinizing hormone (LH)
- β-endorphin and MSH are co-secreted with ACTH from the same precursor peptide.

Although any or all of the anterior pituitary hormones can be affected by pituitary dysfunction, those with the greatest direct relevance for the anaesthetist are ACTH, TSH and GH, either through their control of other endocrine organs (ACTH, TSH) or through their action on tissue growth. These effects will be dealt with in separate chapters (Adrenocortical insufficieny, p. 46 and Cushing syndrome (hypercortisolism), p. 55, Hyperthyroidism, p. 66, Hypothyroidism, p. 70 and Acromegaly, p.44).

Thyroid-stimulating hormone

TSH is the principal regulator of thyroid function. Its release from the pituitary is controlled by hypothalamic hormones; stimulated by TRH and inhibited by somatostatin, and also modulated by the negative feedback effect of the thyroid hormones. TSH levels will, therefore, be unphysiologically high in patients with primary hypothyroidism (see above) and low in patients with primary hyperthyroidism.

Isolated pathologically elevated TSH is rare and can be due to a thyrotropic adenoma or congenital thyroid hormone resistance. Thyroid hormone levels are usually normal in the former and elevated in the latter.

Patients with low TSH levels due to pituitary dysfunction will have symptoms and signs of hypothyroidism (see above), with low serum thyroxine (T_4) and a blunted TSH response to TRH stimulation. Isolated TSH deficiency is rare and patients are more likely to present with combined endocrine deficiency. Unphysiologically low TSH levels may also be caused by corticosteroid medication, TSH receptor antibodies, disturbed day–night rhythm (shift workers) or endogenous depression.

Adrenocorticotropin

ACTH stimulates cortisol and aldosterone secretion from the adrenal cortex. Its release is stimulated by hypothalamic CRH and suppressed by the negative feedback action of glucocorticoids. Benzodiazepines and opioids reduce CRH secretion.

Pituitary hypersecretion of ACTH from a corticotropic adenoma induces the secondary hypercortisolism known as Cushing disease. The non-responsiveness of the adenoma to negative glucocorticoid feedback control is the rationale behind the dexamethasone suppression test used to differentiate pituitary hypersecretion from other causes of Cushing syndrome. Non-suppressible ACTH secretion is also seen in paraneoplastic syndromes, particularly associated with pancreatic carcinoma and small-cell lung tumours (see Adrenocortical insufficiency, p. 46 and Cushing syndrome (hypercortisolism), p. 55).

ACTH deficiency of either hypothalamic or hypophyseal origin leads to cortisol hyposecretion. Aldosterone secretion will usually be normal, since it is also controlled by other pathways. Serum cortisol concentrations will be low but will usually respond to stimulation with synthetic ACTH (Synacthen®) in primary hypopituitarism, and to CRH stimulation in hypothalamic dysfunction. The clinical picture is that of cortisol deficiency (see above).

Growth hormone

GH (somatotropin) is secreted by the somatotrophic cells of the anterior pituitary. It stimulates the production of IGF-1 in the liver. Regulation of growth hormone secretion is complex and under both stimulatory and inhibitory control. Secretion is stimulated by the hypothalamic hormones' growth hormone-releasing hormone (GHRH) and ghrelin as well as androgens during puberty. Dopaminergic mechanisms contribute to the regulation of GHRH secretion; L-dopa increases and bromocriptine suppresses secretion. GH secretion is inhibited by the hypothalamic hormone somatostatin and is also under negative feedback control of circulating GH and IGF-1. Hyperglycaemia and glucocorticoids also inhibit GH secretion. To illustrate the complex interactions: hypoglycaemia, the standard clinical test of somatotroph function, does not directly stimulate GH release but acts indirectly by inhibiting somatostatin and thus removing its inhibitory effect on GH secretion.

Patients with untreated GH deficiency during childhood are of short stature but otherwise normally proportioned (pituitary dwarfism). Adult-onset GH deficiency is rare, and associated with a wide variety of effects and a tendency to increased cardiovascular morbidity and mortality. The effects of most immediate interest to the anaesthetist are insulin resistance, diastolic cardiac dysfunction and increased levels of fibrinogen and plasminogen activator inhibitor.

Excessive GH secretion is usually due to an adenoma of the somatotroph cells or, in rare cases, from an ectopic tumour. The adenoma can cause headaches, impaired vision and deficiencies of other pituitary hormones in late stages, but its primary clinical relevance is due to the high levels of GH. In the rare instance of a somatotroph adenoma occurring in childhood, one would see the very large stature referred to as pituitary gigantism. Somatotrophic adenomas in adults cause the impressive features of acromegaly (see above). Self-administration of excessive doses of GH over a long period can also cause similar symptoms.

Posterior pituitary

The hormones of the posterior pituitary or neurohypophysis, vasopressin (AVP or antidiuretic hormone (ADH)) and oxytocin, are synthesized in the hypothalamus, transported along the pituitary stalk and stored in the posterior pituitary until they are secreted.

Vasopressin/antidiuretic hormone

Vasopressin (arginine vasopressin (AVP)) is the most relevant of these two to anaesthetic practice because of its effects on blood pressure and fluid homeostasis. AVP acts through V_2 receptors on the collecting duct cells in the kidney tubules to facilitate water reabsorption along the concentration gradient formed by the AVP-stimulated reabsorption of sodium and chloride in the thick ascending limb of the loop of Henle.

AVP deficiency causes diabetes insipidus and compromises intraoperative blood pressure control, particularly during epidural or spinal anaesthesia and in patients with hypovolaemia. The hypersecretion seen in the SIADH manifests itself in hyponatraemia (see below).

Disorders of the pituitary

The pathology of pituitary dysfunction can be directly mediated by the involved pituitary hormones, such as GH or AVP, and are described below. In other cases, the disease process is due to the subsequent dysfunction of the endocrine glands under pituitary control. These are dealt with in the appropriate chapters.

Bibliography

Klose M, Feldt-Rasmussen U. Does the type and severity of brain injury predict hypothalamo-pituitary dysfunction? Does post-traumatic hypopituitarism predict worse outcome? *Pituitary* 2008; **11**: 255–61.

Kristof RA, Rother M, Neuloh G, Klingmuller D. Incidence, clinical manifestations, and course of water and electrolyte metabolism disturbances following transsphenoidal pituitary adenoma surgery: a prospective observational study. *J Neurosurg* 2009; **111**: 555–62.

Smith M, Hirsch NP. Pituitary disease and anaesthesia. *Br J Anaesth* 2000; **85**: 3–14.

Cross-references

Adrenocortical insufficiency, 46
Anaesthesia for trans-sphenoidal hypophysectomy, 332
Anaesthetic and ICU management of the head-injured patient, 334
Conn syndrome, 53
Cushing syndrome, 55
Diabetes insipidus, 58
General principles of anaesthesia, 300
Hypertension, 151
Hyperthyroidism, 66
Hypothyroidism, 70

Syndrome of inappropriate antidiuretic hormone hypersecretion

Thomas A Crozier

The syndrome of inappropriate antidiuretic hormone hypersecretion (SIADH) is characterized by the excessive release of vasopressin despite low plasma osmolality. The condition is frequently seen in patients with CNS lesions (trauma, tumour, infections), but can also occur as a result of ectopic vasopressin secretion, e.g. in pulmonary tuberculosis or as a paraneoplastic syndrome in small-cell bronchial carcinoma. SIADH can also be caused by drugs, such as neuroleptics, antidepressants (tricyclic, selective serotonin reuptake inhibitors), amiodarone, chlorpropramide, anticonvulsants (carbamazepine), ecstasy and others. It must be differentiated from the hypo-osmolar hyponatraemia that can occur as a complication of hypothyroidism or adrenal insufficiency.

The water retention and natriuresis caused by vasopressin leads to dilutional hyponatraemia, occasionally but not always with fluid overload. The patient complains of headache, nausea and vomiting and can be confused. Serum sodium concentrations below 120 mmol L^{-1} can cause convulsions and coma.

Management should include treating the cause whenever possible. SIADH is usually asymptomatic and restricting fluids to 800–1000 mL per day usually suffices to increase serum sodium. Demeclocycline, a tetracycline antibiotic, is a potent vasopressin receptor antagonist that can be used off-label when fluid restriction is difficult to enforce. Severe symptomatic hyponatraemia requires treatment with intravenous hypertonic saline. Correction of the serum sodium concentration should not be more than 12 mmol L^{-1} day^{-1} since a more rapid increase can cause central pontine myelinolysis.

Bibliography

Bartter FC, Schwartz WB. The syndrome of inappropriate secretion of antidiuretic hormone. *Am J Med* 1967; **42**: 790–806.

Hannon MJ, Thompson CJ. The syndrome of inappropriate antidiuretic hormone: prevalence, causes and consequences. *Eur J Endocrinol* 2010; **162**(Suppl. 1): S5-S12.

Palmer BF. Hyponatremia in patients with central nervous system disease: SIADH versus CSW. *Trends Endocrinol Metab* 2003; **14**: 182–7.

Sherlock M, Thompson CJ. The syndrome of inappropriate antidiuretic hormone: current and future management options. *Eur J Endocrinol* 2010; **162**(Suppl. 1): S13–S18.

Cross-references

Fluid and electrolyte balance, 754

Water and electrolyte disturbances, 633

Uncommon endocrine tumours

Brian J Pollard

The acronym 'APUD' describes groups of cells which are capable of the synthesis of certain biologically active amines and peptides. The letters APUD come from the description *a*mine *p*recursor *u*ptake and *d*ecarboxylation. APUDomas are groups or tumours of cells with APUD properties. The clinical manifestation of each tumour is characterized by overproduction of particular hormones and/or peptides. APUD cells may be found in the pituitary gland, adrenal medulla, peripheral autonomic ganglia, gastrointestinal tract, pancreas, lung, gonads and thymus. Tumours may occur as part of the multiple endocrine neoplasia (MEN) syndrome. The management of patients with phaeochromocytoma, insulinoma and carcinoid tumours is dealt with elsewhere.

Gastrinoma

Gastrinoma is a very rare gastrin-producing tumour. The incidence is 1:1 000 000 per year. It is the second common most functional islet cell tumour. Gastrin stimulates acid production from gastric parietal cells. Gastrinomas present with peptic ulcer disease; the Zollinger–Ellison syndrome is characterized by gastric acid hypersecretion with recurrent peptic ulceration and diarrhoea. Between 20 and 60% of patients with gastrinoma have coexisting MEN1; 60% of gastrinomas are malignant, and 50% of patients have metastases at diagnosis.

Perioperative management

Initial treatment is medical and involves:

- proton pump inhibitors, e.g. omeprazole
- H_2 antagonists, e.g. ranitidine, cimetidine
- octreotide (octapeptide analogue of somatostatin).

Surgery is considered if medical therapy does not suppress gastric acid hypersecretion, and usually involves resection of tumours. Pre- and intraoperative tumour localization is important. Patients with MEN1 may have multiple tumours with a tendency towards duodenal wall location.

Acute presentation may occur with gastrointestinal bleeding and perforation. Diarrhoea may lead to fluid volume depletion, electrolyte disturbance and dysrhythmias. Invasive cardiovascular monitoring is required and surgery is prolonged.

Postoperative management

- HDU or ITU management.
- Continue cardiovascular and biochemical monitoring.
- Mortality is high in emergency procedures.

VIPomas

These extremely rare tumours release *v*asoactive *i*ntestinal *p*eptide. Patients present with severe, large-volume secretory diarrhoea. Potassium and bicarbonate are lost from the gut, resulting in hypokalaemia and metabolic acidosis. The WDHA syndrome refers to the association of *w*atery *d*iarrhoea, *h*ypokalaemia and *a*chlorhydria.

Preoperative management

- Symptom control with octreotide and correction of electrolyte abnormalities.
- Aggressive management of fluid volume status and metabolic acidosis.

Perioperative management

- Invasive cardiovascular monitoring.
- VIPomas are vascular tumours.
- Frequent blood sampling for pH and electrolytes.

Insulinoma

This is the most common type of islet cell tumour. Most (90%) are benign, intrapancreatic, small and solitary. Up to 10% are multiple, associated with MEN. Incidence is 4:1 000 000 per year.

Tumours secrete insulin or proinsulin, causing hypoglycaemia. If undiagnosed, or symptoms uncontrolled, patients may present with:

- cerebral dysfunction, focal neurological deficits
- abnormal behaviour, confusion
- visual disturbance, weakness, sweating.

Medical therapy may include the following:

- diazoxide: inhibits release of insulin from tumour
- diuretics: treat oedema associated with use of diazoxide
- glucagon infusion: maintenance of blood sugar
- β-blockers: blood pressure control
- calcium channel blockers: blood pressure control
- cytotoxic drugs: antitumour effect.

Preoperative assessment

Most cases are diagnosed and the patient prepared for surgery. Assessment for other endocrine tumours (MEN) should be made. Patients may be obese and hypertensive. Tumour localization may be done pre- and/or intraoperatively to allow selective removal of the adenoma and avoid blind subtotal pancreatectomy. Techniques include spiral CT, endoscopic and intraoperative ultrasound, angiography and selective venous hormone sampling. Bimanual palpation of the pancreas at surgery is useful.

Perioperative management

- Patients having wide fluctuations in blood glucose may require dextrose infusion up to 2–3 hours before surgery.
- Generous premedication.
- Prepare for major laparotomy.
- Direct cardiovascular monitoring.
- Continuous or intermittent glucose, insulin and potassium sampling.
- 50% glucose available to treat hypoglycaemic response to tumour manipulation.
- Likely intraoperative tumour localization.
- Continue glucose and insulin monitoring postoperatively.

Multiple endocrine neoplasia

This occurs with tumours involving two or more endocrine organs. The usual tumour sites in the various subtypes of MEN are as follows:

- MEN1 (rare, complex, dominant inheritance)
  - parathyroid
  - pancreatic islets
  - anterior pituitary.
- MEN2 (autosomal dominant inheritance, incomplete penetrance, variable expression)
  - medullary thyroid carcinoma: this can occur alone or as a separate syndrome
  - adrenal (phaeochromocytoma)
  - parathyroid.
- MEN2A
  - tumour sites as above
  - affected patients have normal physical appearance.
- MEN2B
  - thyroid
  - adrenal (phaeochromocytoma)
  - patients have marfanoid habitus, mucosal neuromas, gut ganglioneuromatosis.

Perioperative management

Presentation depends on the clinical syndrome resulting from the particular tumours involved. Usually, patients are diagnosed and prepared for major surgery. In emergency surgery, the possibility of endocrine tumours should be remembered:

- generous premedication
- invasive cardiovascular monitoring
- frequent blood sampling for hormones, glucose, electrolytes, etc.
- continue cardiovascular and biochemical monitoring postoperatively.

Bibliography

Azimuddin K, Chamberlain RS. The surgical management of pancreatic neuroendocrine tumours. *Surg Clin North Am* 2001; **81**: 511–25.

Gagel R. Multiple endocrine neoplasia. In: Gagel R (ed.) *Endocrinology and Metabolism Clinics of North America*, vol. 23. Philadelphia: WB Saunders, 1994.

Owen R. Anaesthetic considerations in endocrine surgery. In: Lynn J, Bloom SR (eds) *Surgical Endocrinology*. Oxford: Butterworth-Heinemann, 1993, pp. 71–84.

3

Respiratory system

Neil Soni

- Anaesthesia and bronchogenic carcinoma — *Suveer Singh and Neil Soni*
- Anaesthesia and chronic obstructive pulmonary disease — *Suveer Singh and Neil Soni*
- Anaesthesia and sleep apnoea syndrome — *Suveer Singh and Neil Soni*
- Asthma — *Suveer Singh and Neil Soni*
- Bronchiectasis — *Rick Keays and Neil Soni*
- Cystic fibrosis — *Rick Keays and Neil Soni*
- Restrictive lung disease — *Suveer Singh and Neil Soni*
- Sarcoidosis — *Rick Keays and Neil Soni*
- Smoking and anaesthesia — *Rick Keays and Neil Soni*

Anaesthesia and bronchogenic carcinoma

Suveer Singh and Neil Soni

Lung cancer is the most common cause of cancer mortality worldwide for men and women, causing approximately 1.2 million deaths per year (Table 3.1). The most common symptoms are shortness of breath, unexplained cough, haemoptysis, chest pain, bone pain and weight loss. They develop from the airways or parenchyma.

The main types of lung cancer are *non-small-cell lung carcinoma* and *small-cell lung carcinoma*. Early stage (stage 1 or 2) non-small-cell lung carcinoma (NSCLC) is treated with surgery, while small-cell lung carcinoma is treated by chemotherapy and radiation. Other tumours, such as large-cell, neuroendocrine (carcinoid), bronchioloalveolar cell type and rarer forms can all present as lung malignancies. The most common cause of lung cancer is long-term exposure to tobacco smoke. The occurrence of lung cancer in non-smokers, who account for as many as 15% of cases, is often attributed to a combination of genetic factors, radon gas, asbestos, air pollution and passive exposure to cigarette smoke.

Derived from the epithelium, squamous cell carcinomas are the most common NSCLC. They are usually centrally located, at the carina or in the first- to third-generation bronchi, hence proximal. Adenocarcinoma is less common. The peak incidence is in men in their fifties.

Presentation may be with airway obstruction and lung collapse, or through spread via the peribronchial tissues with subsequent invasion of the mediastinum. It spreads by both lymphatic and haematological routes, and distal metastasis is common in the liver, adrenals, bone and brain.

Treatment of lung cancer, whether with surgery, chemotherapy, radiation therapy or a combination of these, can be associated with notable toxicity. It may not be feasible for patients with significant impairment because of their lung cancer or comorbid conditions to undergo resection or even aggressive chemoradiotherapy. Performance status can be assessed by a variety of methods, including the Karnofsky Performance Status or the World Health Organization (WHO) status.

Anaesthetic involvement is mainly for lung resection (i.e. lobectomy, pneumonectomy). However, newer indications for palliative interventional bronchoscopic procedures are increasing. Debulking/disobliteration of central symptomatic obstructive lesions followed, if necessary, by tracheobronchial stents can ameliorate some of the symptoms of advancing disease. This may be done by rigid bronchoscopy or flexible bronchoscopy, using a number of different modalities, such as electrocautery, laser, cryotherapy/cryoextraction, argon plasma coagulation or mechanical debulking.

Preoperative assessment

Patients may present with a range of symptoms and signs including:

- Local: chest pain, cough, dyspnoea, haemoptysis, hoarseness and pleural effusion
- Distal: metastasis with associated problems
- Paraneoplastic: ectopic hormonal activity, such as adrenocorticotrophic hormone (ACTH), parathyroid hormone and antidiuretic hormone (ADH), insulin

Table 3.1 Lung cancer and its incidence

Characteristic	Squamous cell (epidermoid)	Adenocarcinoma	Large cell	Small cell
Approximate incidence	25–30%	30–35%	15–20%	20–25%
Five year survival	25%	12%	13%	1%
Operability	43–50%	35%	35–43%	Rare
Potential for metastasis	Low to moderate	Moderate	Moderate	High
Response rate to systemic treatment	Low	Low	Low	Moderate

and glucagon. Cushing syndrome can occur from ectopic ACTH production with hypokalaemia. The clinical features of full-blown Cushing syndrome are rarely identifiable as they do not have time to develop. Muscle weakness with Lambert–Eaton syndrome produces a myasthenia-like weakness, which has however, differences from myasthenia. The weakness is more pronounced in the mornings and can improve with exercise, but does not affect facial or respiratory muscles. It affects voltage-gated calcium channels on the presynaptic membrane of the neuromuscular junction. The inhibition of the voltage-gated calcium channels prevents acetylcholine from being released from the presynaptic terminal and the subsequent stimulation of the postsynaptic terminal, which would lead to muscle contraction. Adenomas occur which may be carcinoid, secreting 5-hydroxytryptamine. The carcinoid syndrome may present as episodic sweating, wheeze and breathlessness.

These patients are usually smokers and so chronic obstructive pulmonary disease (COPD) is a common concomitant problem.

Investigations

- Chest X-ray often may not reveal the tumour but will show signs of concomitant problems such as chronic obstructive airways disease. It is useful to demonstrate pleural effusions or, with an enlarged heart shadow, pericardial effusion, which would suggest mediastinal invasion.
- ECG is useful, as thoracic surgery can result in rhythm disturbance, especially atrial fibrillation. Moreover, these smokers have a high incidence of asymptomatic ischaemic heart disease.
- Electrolytes may be the only sign of ectopic ADH secretion with a low sodium, which will eventually produce clinical signs of confusion and weakness. Ectopic ACTH secretion can lead to symptoms related to a high cortisol; in particular, hypokalaemia and adrenocortical failure can lead to hyperkalaemia with or without hypernatraemia. Parathyroid hormone produces hypercalcaemia, but so do widespread bony metastases with elevated alkaline phosphatase. Glucose values can be adversely influenced by ectopic insulin or glucagon.
- Lung function tests are important if any significant lung resection is planned. FEV_1 and FVC are the most commonly available and useful, whereas low gas transfer (below ~30%) may have implications for risk of postoperative respiratory failure. Exercise testing may be extremely helpful and baseline arterial blood gases on air should be taken.

Patients probably will have presented through a lung multidisciplinary team. A chest CT and/or CT-PET scan, and tissue sampling by bronchoscopy, transbronchial needle aspiration (conventional or endobronchial ultrasound guided), mediastinoscopy or interventional radiology, will have staged the disease, enabling appropriate management.

Inoperability

The new TNM (tumour, node, metastasis) staging system of the International Union Against Cancer will determine which primary lung cancers are theoretically operable (Table 3.2). As part of the staging system, in general, stage 1 and stage 2 disease are operable. There are some classical indicators of inoperability which indicate stage 3 or 4 advanced disease. These include superior vena caval obstruction or other great vessel involvement, nerve palsies including left recurrent laryngeal and phrenic nerve damage, carinal or tracheal involvement, oesophageal invasion, vertebral involvement and Pancoast syndrome.

Table 3.2 TNM staging system for lung cancer (7th edition)

Primary tumour (T)	
T1	Tumour ≤3 cm diameter, surrounded by lung or visceral pleura, without invasion more proximal than lobar bronchus
T1a	Tumour ≤2 cm in diameter
T1b	Tumour >2 cm but ≤3 cm in diameter
T2	Tumour >3 cm but ≤7 cm, or tumour with any of the following features: Involves main bronchus, ≥2 cm distal to carina Invades visceral pleura Associated with atelectasis or obstructive pneumonitis that extends to the hilar region but does not involve the entire lung
T2a	Tumour >3 cm but ≤5 cm
T2b	Tumour >5 cm but ≤7 cm

(Continued on next page)

● **Table 3.2** (*Continued*)

T3	Tumour >7 cm or any of the following: Directly invades any of the following: chest wall, diaphragm, phrenic nerve, mediastinal pleura, parietal pericardium, main bronchus <2 cm from carina (without involvement of carina) Atelectasis or obstructive pneumonitis of the entire lung Separate tumour nodules in the same lobe		
T4	Tumour of any size that invades the mediastinum, heart, great vessels, trachea, recurrent laryngeal nerve, oesophagus, vertebral body, carina, or with separate tumour nodules in a different ipsilateral lobe		
Regional lymph nodes (N)			
N0	No regional lymph node metastases		
N1	Metastasis in ipsilateral peribronchial and/or ipsilateral hilar lymph nodes and intrapulmonary nodes, including involvement by direct extension		
N2	Metastasis in ipsilateral mediastinal and/or subcarinal lymph node(s)		
N3	Metastasis in contralateral mediastinal, contralateral hilar, ipsilateral or contralateral scalene, or supraclavicular lymph node(s)		
Distant metastasis (M)			
M0	No distant metastasis		
M1	Distant metastasis		
M1a	Separate tumour nodule(s) in a contralateral lobe; tumour with pleural nodules or malignant pleural or pericardial effusion		
M1b	Distant metastasis		
Stage groupings			
Stage IA	T1a–T1b	N0	M0
Stage IB	T2a	N0	M0
Stage IIA	T1a, T1b, T2a	N1	M0
	T2b	N0	M0
Stage IIB	T2b	N1	M0
	T3	N0	M0
Stage IIIA	T1a, T1b, T2a, T2b	N2	M0
	T3	N1, N2	M0
	T4	N0, N1	M0
Stage IIIB	T4	N2	M0
	Any T	N3	M0
Stage IV	Any T	Any N	M1a or M1b

Pancoast syndrome is an apical carcinoma invading the eighth cervical and first thoracic nerves. Severe pain and wasting in the upper limb occurs with stellate ganglion involvement. The patient has Horner syndrome (ptosis, enophthalmos, miosis, impaired sweating on face).

Very often these patients can now have palliative stents placed for debulked endobronchial disease or symptomatic compressive extrinsic disease. They appear to be safe and are manufactured from silicon or a metal–nitinol alloy (placed via rigid bronchoscopy or interventional radiology), requiring general anaesthesia. Nitinol bronchial stents can be placed via flexible bronchoscopy under general anaesthesia or conscious sedation, or through endobronchial tubes. Complications, such as migration, misplacement, infection, biofouling and stent fractures (in older generation stents) can occur and are explained as part of informed consent. However, these procedures usually offer immediate relief of symptoms and at least short-term benefit in the acute setting. They have even been attributed to liberation from mechanical ventilation after acute respiratory failure in selected case series.

Preoperative preparation

Optimize respiratory function

This will include optimizing the pharmacological approach, such as β_2-adrenergic agonists, anticholinergics, active physiotherapy and steroids for inadequately controlled COPD.

Any effusions should be drained. Electrolytes and haemoglobin should be corrected. Although a restrictive approach to transfusion should be adopted, bear in mind that these patients are at risk of ischaemic heart disease, so aiming for a haemoglobin level >10 g dL^{-1} is not unreasonable.

In patients undergoing debulking techniques or stenting, careful consideration of the anatomical placement of the stent should be discussed with the operator prior to anaesthesia. Modern imaging provides useful information that often correlates with functionality. These patients will often be dyspnoeic and may have partial collapse of parts of the lung. In theory, they will be dramatically improved by the procedure; however, if the collapse has been long-standing, it may not be recoverable, but it will predispose to infection. Careful planning is required.

Premedication

This is determined by the clinical situation. Minimize stress to the patient with an anxiolytic if necessary; sometimes a drying agent will help.

Anaesthetic technique

In patients with tracheal or bronchial compromise, coughing may become problematic and threaten airway patency. Inhalational techniques are likely to precipitate problems whereas the inability to intubate and then to ventilate is unlikely. Therefore, for major surgical interventions or for significant procedures on the central airways, a full general anaesthetic with relaxation and mechanical ventilation is usually required. Remifentanil during induction has advocates. Almost any induction technique is suitable. Short- to medium-acting relaxants which do not accumulate are ideal with neuromuscular monitoring. Volatile agents are bronchodilating by nature. Some advocate the use of heliox during induction if there is significant airway narrowing.

For lung resection, the use of double-lumen endotracheal tubes, to allow single-lung ventilation, has largely been superseded by endobronchial blocking balloons. These are placed under bronchoscopic visualization and are effective for isolating major airway haemorrhage when in position prophylactically.

Partial or complete central airway obstruction or symptomatic tracheobronchial–oesophageal fistulae can sometimes be palliated by debulking and/or stenting, respectively. Stents require appropriate and careful planning with regards position, size and type. Bronchial stents may be deployed when awake. Others will require general anaesthesia as described. A range of techniques can be used. Rigid bronchoscopy with a Sanders injector is a well-established technique, as is the suspension laryngoscope, favoured by ENT/head and neck surgeons. Always be very careful as the Sanders injector can easily result in high-pressure air trapping if there is partial obstruction. At the end of the case, ensure that the patient has a good cough reflex prior to leaving the relatively safe theatre environment.

Patients with pre-existing stents needing anaesthesia

If a patient has a stent, ensure the position is known, image if possible, seek an opinion from whoever placed the stent and, ideally, view the stent bronchoscopically before placing an endotracheal tube. The aim is to avoid dislodging the stent. In an emergency, be aware of the stent and try to visualize it before intubation, if possible.

Acute postoperative central airway obstruction

In this situation, it is difficult to re-establish spontaneous breathing. The appearance has been likened to inadequate reversal of the muscle relaxant with an ineffective breathing pattern that is largely abdominal. Desaturation ensues, often associated with a deteriorating level of consciousness, which may be in part due to hypercarbia. Blood gases will demonstrate hypercarbia and hypoxia. Assume airway obstruction. Control the airway and go to rigid bronchoscopy as secretions at the carina or in the trachea are the most likely cause. The differential diagnosis is tension pneumothorax after airway instrumentation, but that is very rare from stent placement.

Postoperative care

This will be determined by the nature of the surgery and the requirement for ventilation. This may be determined in part by the surgery, respiratory function and also the other comorbidities often present in this population. Even without ventilation, these patients will often require specialist postoperative care.

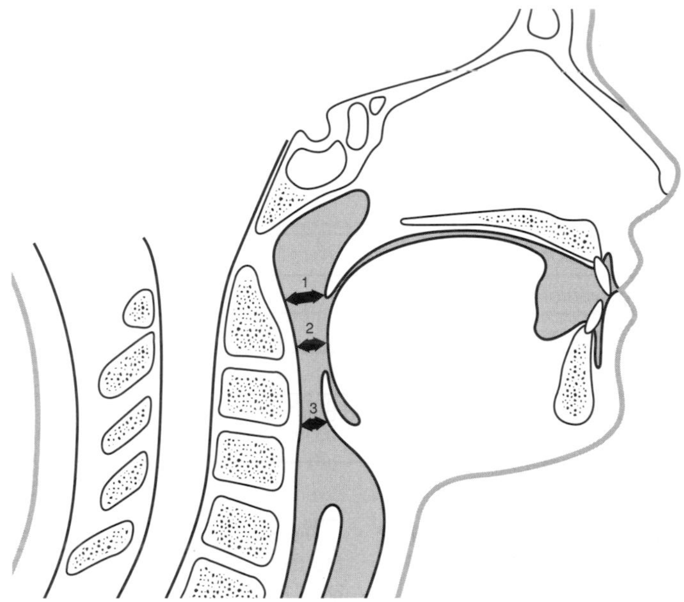

Figure 3.2 Airway obstruction in sleep apnoea. 1, Nasopharynx – tensor palatine; 2, oropharynx – tongue enlargement and posterior tissues; 3, laryngopharynx – tissues around epiglottis and base of tongue.

Immediate effects during an apnoea may be seen in patients and include:

- low P_ao_2 associated with tachycardia or, more concerningly, bradycardia
- associated nocturnal angina, and myocardial infarction
- diurnal pulmonary and systemic hypertension.

The consequences of SAS are seen symptomatically as excessive daytime sleepiness, impaired concentration, mood changes, morning headache, waking with a choking sensation, dry mouth and many more. Signs include snoring, excessive daytime sleepiness, nocturnal sweating and witnessed apnoea. Secondary effects include polycythaemia, pulmonary hypertension and right heart failure. In patients with excess weight there are likely to be other significant comorbidities. Other non-specific effects include gastro-oesophageal reflux, hypertension and ischaemic heart disease, and patients with diabetes have increased instability. There is an increased incidence of sudden death in untreated patients with SAS compared with age-matched controls.

Sleep, anaesthesia and apnoea

REM sleep is the time with most influence on sleep apnoea. In neonates it accounts for up to 50% of sleep, whereas by middle age it is about 20% of all sleep and takes some time to develop through the preceding phases. It diminishes with age or with medications such as antidepressants.

The perioperative impact of sleep apnoea

The repetitive episodes of upper airway obstruction during sleep, with sleep disruption, hypoxaemia and autonomic arousals, contribute to the cardiovascular risk. Furthermore, anatomic narrowing in the pharynx due to excess tissue, tonsillar hypertrophy or craniofacial variations can lead to airway difficulties. Desaturations of sufficient intensity may precipitate arrhythmias or acute coronary syndrome in susceptible individuals. Moreover, the central nervous depressant effects of sedatives, analgesics and anaesthetics can suppress the natural arousal mechanism induced by hypoxaemia or hypercapnia in patients with SAS. This may lead to prolongation of the apnoeic episode in the postoperative period. Another potential concern is the impact of restoration of sleep after a period of customary yet involuntary perioperative sleep deprivation. The phenomenon of rebound REM sleep, with its associated profound desaturations, may be under-recognized in the postoperative setting, conceivably occurring in a general ward setting with low-level monitoring or even after discharge.

Although there have been no prospective randomized trials of anaesthetic risk in patients with SAS, there are several reports of postoperative cardiac arrhythmias, myocardial infarction, cerebrovascular events and hypoxaemia-induced organ dysfunction occurring in those with OSA in the postoperative period. Furthermore, there have been sporadic reports of fatalities in patients with OSA in the postoperative period.

The effect of sedation and anaesthesia on patients with sleep apnoea

The use of sedatives and sedating analgesics (i.e. opioids) has effects on the upper and lower respiratory tracts that mimic those in sleep. They can produce a reduction in the FRC and cause atelectasis. This has potential implications for preoxygenation during general anaesthetic induction, as FRC is considered an 'oxygen reservoir'. In patients with OSA associated with obesity, this reduced pharyngeal anatomical space, together with the functional disturbance of the dilator muscles (particularly genioglossus), is accompanied by a reduction in lung volume as a result of fat distribution around the diaphragm in central obesity. This is suggested to reduce the traction on the pharynx exerted by the trachea. The usual neural mechanisms in wakefulness, to compensate for these anatomical imbalances, are lost during sleep. The pharynx is more susceptible to closure in these patients, potentially exacerbating the upper airway risk further in that subgroup with OSA.

Sedatives also reduce the phasic activity of pharyngeal muscles just prior to inspiration, mimicking the response to REM sleep in patients with OSA. Thus, during general anaesthesia, there is a loss of the protection against upper airway collapse (caused by the lower respiratory tract muscles generating negative pressure on the airway). Moreover, sedatives depress the compensatory arousal responses to hypoxia, hypercapnia and upper airway collapse that characterize the repeated sleep–wake cycle in OSA (Fig. 3.3). The risk of prolonged apnoeas and desaturation then increases, as has been noted in many patients with OSA undergoing sedation.

In the postoperative period, the residual central depressant effects of these agents may cause prolonged apnoeas and desaturation at a time and place when reduced monitoring is present. The disruption of sleep architecture and quality has also been documented in the postoperative period following surgery. Thus, reduced total sleep time (owing to various environmental and extraneous factors, such as noise, nursing protocols, anxiety, pain and supine positioning) and less REM sleep and non-REM slow wave sleep are reported, which may take several days for normalization. Indeed, a REM sleep rebound, following this phase of sleep debt, could lead to profound desaturation in patients with OSA, even after discharge.

Assessment

History

It is still predominantly under-recognized. Look for a history of snoring, daytime sleepiness or lethargy, and witnessed apnoeas. Identify other features, such as depression or neurocognitive or functional decline.

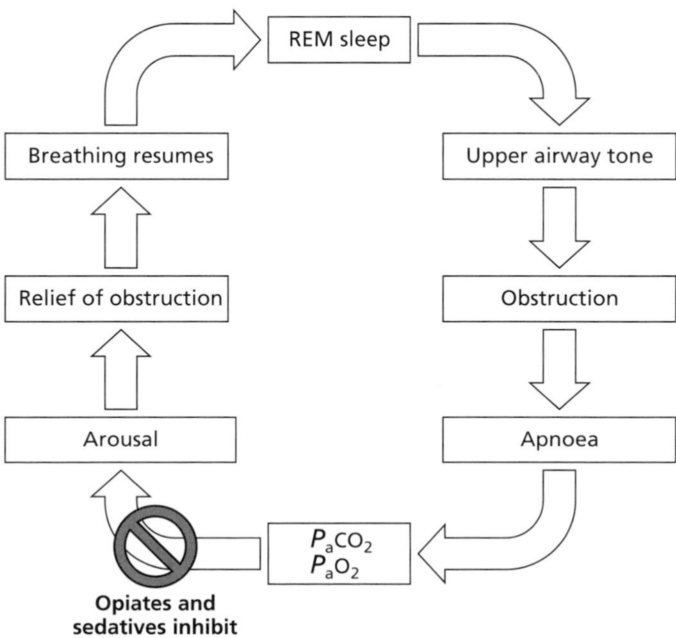

Figure 3.3 The pathophysiology of obstructive sleep apnoea and how sedatives can suppress the natural arousal responses of hypoxaemia and hypercapnia. REM, rapid eye movement.

Jain S, Dhand R. Perioperative treatment of patients with obstructive sleep apnoea. *Curr Opin Pulmonary Med* 2004; **10**: 482–8.

Khajehdehi, Shapiro CM. STOP questionnaire: a tool to screen patients for obstructive sleep apnea. *Anesthesiology* 2008; **108**: 812–21.

Loadsman JA, Hillman DR. Anaesthesia and sleep apnoea. *Br J Anaesth* 2001; **86**: 254–66.

Meoli AL, Rosen CL, Kristo D, *et al.*; Clinical Practice Review Committee, American Academy of Sleep Medicine. Upper airway management of the adult patient with obstructive sleep apnea in the perioperative period: avoiding complications. *Sleep* 2003; **26**: 1060–5.

Renotte MT, Baele P, Aubert G, Rodenstein DO. Nasal continuous positive airway pressure in the perioperative management of patients with obstructive sleep apnoea submitted to surgery. *Chest* 1995; **107**: 367–74.

Shahar E, Whitney CW, Redline S, *et al.* Sleep disordered breathing and cardiovascular disease: cross sectional results of the Sleep Heart Health Study. *Am J Respir Crit Care Med* 2001; **163**: 19–25.

Tung A, Rock P. Perioperative concerns in sleep apnea. *Curr Opin Anaesthesiol* 2001; **14**: 671–8.

www.sign.ac.uk/pdf/sign73.pdf.

Cross-references

Difficult airway: management, 651
Difficult airway: prediction, 664
Failure to breathe or wake up postoperatively, 749
Preoperative assessment of pulmonary risk, 625

Asthma

Suveer Singh and Neil Soni

Asthma is a very common respiratory disorder which may be defined as recurrent attacks of paroxysmal dyspnoea, characterized by variable airflow obstruction and increased bronchial hyper-responsiveness to a range of stimuli. Aetiology, pathology and clinical presentation are all heterogeneous, but an underlying inflammatory response is usually present. There is an immense range of clinical pathology from children with reversible bronchospasm through to elderly patients in whom the bronchospasm is superimposed on chronic respiratory disease. The incidence of intraoperative bronchospasm is remarkably low, and occurs in the older asthmatics and those with active asthma at the time.

Epidemiology

Variable geographical distribution, affecting about 5% of the population as a whole but up to 10% of children.

Morbidity

Increased risk of postoperative respiratory complications, especially in the older patient with chronic airways disease in whom cardiac problems may also be present.

Pathophysiology

Non-specific hyper-responsiveness is a common feature. This may be demonstrated by increased response to methacholine, exercise, histamine, cold-air challenge or hyperventilation. Airway obstruction is due to constriction of airway smooth muscle, mucus secretion and oedema of the airway wall. Mechanisms include neural and cellular pathway activation. The neural pathway involves afferent irritant receptors in airways, causing reflex stimulation of postganglionic parasympathetic fibres, resulting in smooth muscle constriction and mucus secretion. C-fibre stimulation releases local neuropeptides; substance P changes membrane permeability and mucus secretion; and neurokinin A causes bronchoconstriction. Cellular pathway activation is known to involve immunoglobin E-mediated histamine release from mast cells, but eosinophils, neutrophils, macrophages and lymphocytes CD8 and Th1 may also release mediators.

Mediators (Table 3.7) include the leukotrienes (LTB_4) and the cysteinyl leukotrienes (CysLTs). LTB_4 is a proinflammatory mediator that acts as a potent neutrophil chemotaxin while CysLTs are potent bronchoconstrictors that increase vascular permeability, cause mucus secretion and mucociliary dysfunction, stimulate eosinophil recruitment and also increase bronchial responsiveness. At a cellular level, smooth muscle tone is controlled by intracellular levels of cyclic adenosine monophosphate and possibly cyclic guanosine monophosphate, low levels leading to bronchoconstriction. The effect on ventilatory function is ventilation/perfusion (V/Q) mismatch, leading to hypoxia, and air trapping, leading to hypercapnia.

An early acute phase leads into a late-phase reaction, which is associated with cellular infiltration and may be sustained for several days.

Preoperative assessment

Asthmatics should be offered preoperative assessment, ideally a week before surgery so that treatment can be optimized (Table 3.8). The history of their illness, the severity of attacks in terms of frequency, hospital admissions, exercise tolerance and current medication need to be known, and likewise any identified trigger factors. In particular, frequency of use of the inhaler

Table 3.7 Mediators implicated in asthma

Mediator	Bronchospasm	Oedema	Mucus secretion
Histamine	+	+	+
Prostaglandin	+	+	
Leukotrienes C_4, D_4, E_4	+	+	+
Thromboxane	+	+	
Platelet-activating factor	+	+	

Table 3.8 Preoperative management suggestions

Clinical	Preoperative intervention
Asymptomatic No medications No recent asthma episodes No obstruction on spirometry	Nothing needed
Occasional bronchodilators; no steroids	Probably nil; consider inhaled steroids
On inhaled steroids	Continue inhaled steroids
Spirometry is below baseline	Consider short course of steroids
On oral steroids	Same or increased dose preoperatively Extra dose before induction Continue hydrocortisone postoperatively

may give an indication of both severity and stability of their asthma. If, when and how much steroid is being used and when the last exacerbation occurred, whether it has required hospital admission and when should also be determined.

Factors that might indicate an increased propensity to bronchospasm include recent upper respiratory tract infection, those on steroids and patients who have required ventilation in the past; clearly, any past history of respiratory complications related to surgery. In non-asthmatics a family history of atopy or of asthma should alert the anaesthetist to the possibility of intraoperative bronchospasm.

Some patients with COPD may have a significant reversible or asthmatic component to their chest problems. On physical examination the presence of wheezes might indicate inadequate control and that current medication requires review. The presence of a respiratory tract infection is a relative contraindication to anaesthesia.

Investigations

- Chest X-ray may show elements of hyperinflation. In the older patient, chronic lung changes or concomitant cardiac problems may be identified. Look for evidence of right ventricular predominance, suggesting long-standing and major problems.
- An ECG may also provide evidence of long-standing right ventricular hypertrophy or cor pulmonale in patients with chronic disease. These patients constitute a very high-risk group.
- Lung function tests: forced expiratory volume in 1 second (FEV_1) reduced more than forced vital capacity (FVC) (FEV_1 normally 50 mL kg^{-1}, and 70–80% FVC).
- Blood gases: baseline blood gases in asthmatics with COPD may be of value in postoperative management.

Maintenance drugs

The most significant change in the management of asthmatics over the last few years is the range of agents which can maintain control of the asthma (Table 3.9). Many of these are now long acting. Patients should continue on their maintenance therapy throughout their hospital stay if possible.

Premedication

Sedation is often useful as anxiety may provoke an attack in some patients. Atropine will inhibit vagally mediated spasm. If an intramuscular opioid is required, pethidine is probably the least undesirable. Both preoperative bronchodilators and steroids reduce the likelihood of postoperative complications, so an additional dose of bronchodilator may be given by inhaler or nebulizer with the premedicant drugs. Patients on steroids should be given steroids, and if on high doses (>1500 μg day^{-1} in adults; less in children), will require peri- and postoperative replacement as adrenal suppression may be present. The limited information available does not highlight either wound healing or infection problems with these short periods of increased steroid use.

Choice of anaesthesia

Regional anaesthesia may be both feasible and acceptable to the patient, but anxiety can trigger bronchospasm and so patient acceptance is important. If general anaesthesia is necessary, avoid stimulation of the respiratory tract and, when possible, drugs known to cause bronchospasm. The advent of sevoflurane has made inhalational induction a possibility.

Induction

Any induction agent or carrier agent, such as Cremophor EL, which may release histamine should be avoided.

Table 3.9 Agents used to maintain control of asthma

Drug type	Examples of agents	Side-effects
Stabilizing agents	Sodium cromoglycate	
Bronchodilators β_2-agonist (short-acting 4–6 h)	Salbutamol/levosalbutamol Terbutaline	Tremor, anxiety, tachycardia Hypokalaemia/hypomagnesaemia
β_2-agonist (long-acting >12 h)	Arformoterol Salmeterol	Fewer side-effects No anti-inflammatory action
Phosphodiesterases	Aminophylline	Tachycardia/arrhythmias
Inhaled steroids	Becotide, flixotide, budesonide	
Inhaled anticholinergics	Ipratropium	
Leukotriene antagonists	Zileuton, montelukast, pranlukast	
IgE immunotherapy	Omalizumab	
Others	Ketamine Magnesium	Sympathomimetic Smooth muscle relaxation
Gases	Volatile agents Heliox	Bronchodilation Reduced airway resistance F_iO_2 <1

F_iO_2, fraction of inspired oxygen.

Both thiopentone and propofol have been implicated, albeit rarely, but generally thiopentone is a safe agent to use although it can cause histamine release and does not block airway reflexes. Similarly, propofol can cause problems, but usually has bronchodilator actions with a beneficial effect in suppressing airway reflexes. Etomidate is safe to use. Ketamine has not only been used to treat status asthmaticus but also has a place in the asthmatic patient with bronchospasm requiring emergency anaesthesia. It is not an ideal induction agent.

Intubation

Although spraying the larynx with lidocaine, prior to intubation, has its advocates, some reports and studies confirm the ability of sprayed lidocaine to stimulate bronchospasm (not histamine mediated). The place of the laryngeal mask has yet to be established. Nebulized albuterol preintubation has been reported to be helpful.

Maintenance

The volatile agents halothane, enflurane, isoflurane and sevoflurane are all potent bronchodilators. They have been used in the treatment of refractory asthma and they are ideal for maintaining anaesthesia.

Muscle relaxants

Succinylcholine is a potent histamine releaser so avoid if possible. Atracurium and mivacurium, like the older tubocurarine, are associated with bronchospasm as a result of histamine release. Pancuronium and vecuronium enjoy a better reputation whereas rocuronium has been associated with some reactions. Be aware that reversal with anticholinesterases can trigger bronchospasm. Atracurium has the advantage of Hofmann degradation, so there is less need for anticholinesterase. Anticholinesterases can induce bronchospasm, although the atropine given concurrently should inhibit this.

Analgesia

Local and regional techniques are recommended, but are not always feasible. Morphine and diamorphine release histamine and so should be avoided. There is controversy as to the histamine-releasing potential of pethidine, but it has been widely used. Fentanyl and alfentanil are probably the safest of the opioids commonly used. Aspirin is known to cause bronchospasm in one group of asthmatic patients and is best avoided. The place of other non-steroidal anti-inflammatory drugs (NSAIDs) is less clear.

The role of heliox

In theory, this mixture should reduce the work of breathing, and this has been shown, to a limited degree, in older asthmatics, possibly because of the reduction in resistance to gas flow as a result of the lower density of the gas.

Postoperative management

Analgesia must be effective, whether using systemic drugs or regional techniques. The problems of chronic asthmatics refer to the problems of chronic lung disease. Effective analgesia and the ability to tolerate physiotherapy and cough adequately prevents the development of atelectasis. Warm, humidified air and the use of bronchodilators should minimize the impact of mucus retention and plugging.

The emergency case with symptomatic bronchospasm

This is a potentially disastrous situation, but fortunately rare. Surgery must be absolutely essential to warrant proceeding. The normal methods for treating bronchospasm should be employed aggressively, with the use of steroids if indicated. There is potentially a role for magnesium sulphate, 2 g intravenously, which may assist bronchodilatation. The induction agent of choice is probably ketamine. Succinylcholine does release histamine in some patients but its use may be difficult to avoid. An opiate, such as fentanyl, can be used. Inhalational agents, such as isoflurane or halothane, are effective in treating bronchospasm and should assist induction. Once induced and deep on these agents, the patient may be better controlled than prior to induction. Continued bronchospasm with high airway pressure may require the use of β-agonists and, if required, epinephrine (either by nebulizer or intravenously).

Ventilation may pose problems, as airway pressures are likely to be high. Manipulation of tidal volume, rate and inspiratory/expiratory (I/E) ratios can be used to minimize peak airway pressure with due attention to the maintenance of an adequate minute ventilation. Permissive hypercapnia has been employed sometimes out of necessity and is reasonably tolerated. The possibility of a pneumothorax must be considered throughout the case. Postoperative management should be in an ICU.

Development of intraoperative asthma

It must be remembered that not all wheezing is necessarily asthma. Tube placement at the carina or in a main bronchus can produce wheezing. Airway obstruction may result from tube blockage, secretions or blood, while aspiration, tension pneumothorax or an anaphylactic or anaphylactoid reaction may all produce spasm. Treatment consists of eliminating these possibilities and the use of deep inhalational anaesthesia and bronchodilators to gain relief of the problem.

Salbutamol (2–5 μg kg^{-1} slowly i.v.) or aminophylline (5 mg kg^{-1}) may be given. Steroids or hydrocortisone (100 mg) will not have an immediate effect but may assist in gaining control. Airway pressures may have been very high (see above), so beware of pneumothorax developing.

The end of the case is a critical time when bronchospasm may be invoked in an awakening patient. Extubation deep may reduce the likelihood of bronchospasm, but, in many cases, this would be inappropriate. Reversal with neostigmine can provoke bronchospasm, so liberal use of a vagolytic such as glycopyrrolate can reduce the risk.

Drugs to avoid

- Tubocurarine.
- Morphine, diamorphine and other histamine-releasing opiates.
- β-Blockers.
- Aspirin, and probably other NSAIDs which are prostaglandin mediated.

Bibliography

Burburan SM, Xisto DG, Rocco PR. Anaesthetic management in asthma. *Minerva Anestesiol* 2007; **73**: 357–65.

Colebourn CL, Barber V, Young JD. Use of helium-oxygen mixture in adult patients presenting with exacerbations of asthma and chronic obstructive pulmonary disease: a systematic review. *Anaesthesia* 2007; **62**: 34–42.

Doherty GM, Chisakuta A, Crean P, Shields MD. Anesthesia and the child with asthma. *Paediatr Anaesth* 2005; **15**: 446–54.

Tirumalasetty J, Grammer LC. Asthma, surgery, and general anesthesia: a review. *J Asthma* 2006; **43**: 251–4.

Woods BD, Sladen RN. Perioperative considerations for the patient with asthma and bronchospasm. *Br J Anaesth* 2009; **103**(Suppl. 1): i57–65.

Cross-references

Intraoperative hypertension, 765

Pulmonary hypertension, 164

Bronchiectasis

Rick Keays and Neil Soni

Bronchiectasis is characterized by long-standing abnormal dilatation of the bronchi, with chronic inflammation. It is a chronic inflammatory process and tends to be extremely productive of sputum with a predisposition to either chronic infection or colonization with intermittent acute episodes of infection.

Historically, bronchiectasis was a consequence of chronic recurrent infection. Pneumonias, measles, whooping cough, tuberculosis and fungal infections were the main causes. Now, with antibiotics, vaccination and better nutrition it is far less common and cystic fibrosis is the main cause. Sometimes patients will present for surgical treatment of their bronchiectasis. There are some specific syndromes associated with it, such as Kartagener syndrome (described in 1933), which is the combination of situs inversus, sinusitis and bronchiectasis.

Diagnosis is by high-resolution CT scan; therefore, anaesthesia for bronchography has been relegated to history.

Pathophysiology

Causes of bronchiectasis

- Following childhood pneumonia.
- Congenital:
  - cystic fibrosis
  - bronchial cartilage deficiency
  - abnormal ciliary motility (Kartagener syndrome)
  - hypogammaglobulinaemia.
- Distal to bronchial obstruction:
  - inhaled foreign body
  - tumour.

The clinical features of bronchiectasis are variable. In severe bronchiectasis there is up to 500 mL of purulent sputum per day, which becomes dramatically worse during an acute exacerbation. Other features include haemoptysis, which arises from bronchial and intercostal arteries, from the areas of severe inflammation with altered local circulation. In long-standing disease, the pulmonary changes can lead to pulmonary hypertension and cor pulmonale. Metastatic abscess formation can occur. Amyloidosis is a rare complication.

Management

Chest physiotherapy with percussion and postural drainage is key, but early intervention with antibiotics may prevent acute exacerbations. These patients are often chronically colonized with resistant organisms owing to their antibiotic exposure. *Pseudomonas aeruginosa* is particularly common as is *Haemophilus influenzae*.

Preoperative assessment

A detailed history should elicit the severity of the problem in terms of exercise tolerance compared with the patient's usual state, sputum production and acute exacerbations. Any information about colonizing organisms is useful. An antibiotic history is important.

Tests include blood gases as a baseline but ordinary chest X-ray is probably not of benefit, whereas a recent CT scan would be helpful.

Other respiratory function tests are generally not very helpful.

Cardiovascular system

It is important to look for any signs of right ventricular strain or cor pulmonale on X-ray. An echocardiogram may be more helpful.

Preoperative management

The patient will need extensive physiotherapy and be exacerbation free prior to surgery. Discussion with the chest physician and the microbiologist should determine the appropriate antibiotic to be given for several days preoperatively.

Premedication

Minimize, but be aware that anticholinergic drugs may make the secretions thicker and harder to shift. Respiratory depressant drugs should be used with caution.

Anaesthetic management

The surgery will determine the most appropriate form of anaesthesia. If possible, use regional techniques, however, this is clearly not always possible. Monitoring should be commensurate with the anaesthetic and surgery, and should be commenced in the anaesthetic room. Pulse oximetry and ECG are basic prerequisites.

Key points regarding the anaesthetic

There are no particular agents that are contraindicated. Try to keep the oxygen saturations high (>90%) to maintain a safety margin. The end-tidal CO_2 ($ETco_2$) is likely to be different from the arterial value, but nevertheless should provide trend measurements.

Sputum retention is likely to be a problem and will predispose to secondary infection, so use humidification and persist with regular tracheal suction. It may be necessary to use a bronchoscope to remove inspissated secretions and sputum. In patients with very severe localized bronchiectasis, it may be feasible to try to isolate that part of the lung with a bronchial blocker.

Proper attention to sterile technique is important in such patients, particularly in those with Kartagener syndrome as they also have a defect in neutrophil chemotaxis. Also, nasal tubes should be avoided in view of the accompanying sinusitis.

Postoperative care

- Arrange early postoperative physiotherapy before the case. In patients with cystic fibrosis, high-dependency care may be helpful to ensure mobilization and physiotherapy. Good analgesia is essential and patient-controlled devices, epidural analgesia or NSAIDs are all useful. Entonox may also be helpful.
- Avoid postoperative ventilation whenever possible.

Bibliography

Gavai M, Hupuczi P, Berkes E, *et al.* Spinal anesthesia for cesarean section in a woman with Kartagener's syndrome and a twin pregnancy. *Int J Obstet Anesth* 2007; **16**: 284–7.

Hopkin JM. The suppurative lung diseases. In: Weatherall DJ, Ledingham JGG, Warrell DA (eds) *Oxford Textbook of Medicine*, 2nd edn. Oxford: Oxford University Press, 1987, pp. 15.100–15.103.

Howell PR, Kent N, Douglas MJ. Anaesthesia for the parturient with cystic fibrosis. *Int J Obstet Anesth* 1993; **2**: 152–8.

Katz J. *Anaesthesia and Uncommon Diseases*, 5th edn. Philadelphia: WB Saunders, 1998.

Lamberty JM, Rubin BK. The management of anaesthesia for patients with cystic fibrosis. *Anaesthesia* 1985; **40**: 448–59.

Yim CF, Lim KS, Low TC. Severe pulmonary hypertension in a patient with bronchiectasis complicated by cor pulmonale and a right-to-left shunt presenting for surgery. *Anaesth Intensive Care* 2002; **30**: 467–71.

Cross-references

Cystic fibrosis, 111
Lobectomy, 415
Intraoperative hypertension, 765

Cystic fibrosis

Rick Keays and Neil Soni

Cystic fibrosis (CF) is the most common genetic Caucasian disease with an incidence in northern Europeans of about 1 in 3000 births. The gene involved encodes CF transmembrane conductance regulator protein (CFTR). It functions as a chloride channel on the apical border of epithelial cells lining most exocrine glands and affects many transport systems including sodium, ATP channels, intracellular vesicle transport and bicarbonate–chloride exchange, which is critical to mucin structure and activities. There have been at least 1500 mutations identified that affect CFTR function in a variety of ways, but the genotype is a poor predictor of disease severity and outcome.

Diagnosis is usually made in infancy and the sweat test is easy and reliable. A chloride concentration greater than 60 mmol L^{-1} is diagnostic. With improved intensive management of affected individuals, the median age of survival is now 38 years.

In infancy and childhood gastrointestinal problems are common, such as meconium ileus, intussusception and pancreatic insufficiency. Respiratory problems arise slightly later and infections commence during childhood. Later in childhood and adulthood the full panoply of gastrointestinal, respiratory and renal manifestations may be seen (Table 3.10). The respiratory problems are chronic infection, with recurrent acute exacerbations leading to bronchiectasis, and chronic colonization often with resistant organisms (Table 3.11). *Pseudomonas* is particularly likely to develop in the uncleared plaques of mucus, especially with impairment of the normal mechanisms that inhibit bacterial binding to epithelium combined with faulty immunological responses to the bacteria, which then go on to form resistant biofilms. Airway inflammation is a notable finding in CF. An allergic response to *Aspergillus fumigatus* occurs in some patients.

Endocrine problems include diabetes.

Despite this plethora of problems modern treatment is continually improving. Nebulized hypertonic saline, macrolide antibiotics, β-agonists and ibuprofen are useful in disease management. Hypertonic saline helps by pulling fluid into the airways and helps hydrate the periciliary layer and improve mucociliary clearance.

Table 3.10 Clinical manifestations and surgical presentation

Infancy	Childhood	Adulthood
Infection	Sinusitis Polyposis; polypectomy Allergic aspergillosis Intravenous access	Haemoptysis Pneumothorax Infection Sinusitis and nasal polyposis Allergic aspergillosis Need for lung transplant
Meconium ileus/peritonitis; intestinal atresia Pancreatitic insufficiency Rectal prolapse	Distal intestinal obstruction Intussusception Biliary fibrosis Hepatic steatosis Malabsorption Diabetes	Biliary fibrosis; obstructive jaundice – need for cholecystectomy Cirrhosis; varices, coagulopathy Distal intestinal obstruction Adenocarcinoma bowel Diabetes
Hyponatraemic hypochloraemic alkalosis Dehydration	Renal calculi Hyponatraemic hypochloraemic alkalosis	Renal calculi Renal failure Hyponatraemic hypochloraemic alkalosis Vasculitis Hypertrophic pulmonary osteoarthritis Osteoporosis, fractures

Table 3.11 Respiratory pathophysiology

Mechanism	Therapeutic approach
Reduced mucociliary clearance Mucus plugging Atelectasis	Physiotherapy, multidisciplinary team care Mucolytics
Colonization; *Pseudomonas, Staphylococcus, Haemophilus, Stenotrophomonas, Burkholderia cepacia* and *Aspergillus*	Aerosolized antibiotics, such as tobramycin, colistin Targeted treatment of acute infection
Obstructive airway pattern, reduced FEV_1, reduced peak flow and increased residual volumes Bronchiectasis, emphysema, fibrosis Apical blebs – pneumothorax	β-adrenergic agents Oral or inhaled steroids
Pulmonary hypertension Cor pulmonale	Oxygen therapy NIV/CPAP ?biPAP

biPAP, bilevel positive airway pressure; CPAP, continuous positive airway pressure; FEV_1, forced expiratory volume in 1 second; NIV, non-invasive ventilation.

Preoperative assessment

Patients are always under a specialist unit and always have insight into and are well informed about their disease state. Ask about the normal level of function and exercise capacity, cough, sputum quality and quantity, or wheezing and whether there are any current infective problems. It is important to be cognizant of pancreatic and bowel dysfunction, and also any endocrine problems such as diabetes.

Key features are:

- current chest status of the CF
- exercise tolerance
- recent hospitalization
- current or recent antibiotics, including any intravenous antibiotics.

Investigations

Chest X-ray looking for hyperinflation, extent of bronchovascular markings and evidence of cysts or bronchiectasis; CT scan may be more informative.

Lung function tests may show an obstructive pattern.

Measure blood gases, if indicated. As the disease progresses, chronic hypoxia and hypercapnia predispose to raised pulmonary artery pressures and vascular resistance, which leads to right ventricular strain and cor pulmonale. These patients may require home oxygen or may be on NIV. This needs to be known so that access to their devices postoperatively is possible.

Renal and liver function should both be checked as these may deteriorate insidiously. In advanced disease there may be abnormal clotting.

Preparation

The chest condition must be optimized. Engage physiotherapists, who will have a plan to ensure that the patient is as well as he or she can be – the physiotherapists and the patient will know. Request physiotherapy immediately prior to going to theatre. Bronchodilators, steroids as required and hydration are all important. Use current antibiotics or those recommended by microbiology for the surgery.

Use bowel preparation to avoid constipation, and H_2 antagonists or similar as reflux is common.

Plan the anaesthetic technique to suit the surgery. Use regional anaesthesia when possible, either as the entire technique (difficult in children) or as an adjunct to general anaesthesia so emergence is rapid and pain free at the end of surgery. Try to have a minimal impact on respiratory function and also plan to be able to commence physiotherapy immediately postoperatively if possible. Use humidified gases, and care should be taken with any nasal tubes, as most patients have hypertrophic sinonasal mucosa with or without polyps.

Monitoring

To fit the surgery and the patient. If there is evidence of pulmonary hypertension or impaired myocardial function, invasive monitoring may be appropriate. Watch the airway pressure as it may be an indicator of plugging or collapse. $ETco_2$ and oximetry are both useful but may need to be supplemented by arterial blood gases and, if the patient is diabetic, the blood sugar should be monitored. In neonates, transcutaneous monitors can be used.

Tailor the anaesthetic to the patient and the surgery.

Induction

If the patient has reflux, a rapid sequence technique should be used, but otherwise a standard induction. Use preoxygenation followed by propofol as it wears off rapidly. Some anaesthetists will avoid nitrous oxide as there is a small risk of pneumothorax, and a high F_iO_2 is often required. A volatile agent that is non-irritant is ideal. Sevoflurane has the advantage of bronchodilation and will also facilitate intubation when a minimal but adequate dose of a non-histamine-releasing relaxant such as vecuronium or cisatracurium can be used.

Positive pressure ventilation is usually not a problem unless there is very severe disease. Suctioning may be necessary to clear the secretions perioperatively. The role of intraoperative physiotherapy has been discussed in the literature and there may be occasions when this could be useful. Only extubate when the patient will breathe well and be able to cough, as avoiding atelectasis is important. Prior to extubation, instillation of saline may be helpful for the physiotherapy following extubation.

Postoperative management

Rapid emergence and good analgesia, with a combination of opioids, NSAIDs and local anaesthetic, when appropriate, will enable early physiotherapy and mobilization. These patients are at high risk of postoperative complications, particularly pulmonary complications from sputum retention, plugging and consequent atelectasis. An enhanced recovery area is ideal unless patients need more intensive monitoring and care. If necessary, CPAP and NIV can be used. Positive pressure ventilation can produce significant problems in these patients with barotraumas and a tendency to air trapping, detrimental changes in V/Q and increasing dead space, so it is best avoided if possible.

Proper hydration and opiate-sparing techniques may avoid the complication of distal intestinal obstruction.

Pregnancy

The normal physiological changes of pregnancy, such as increased minute ventilation and oxygen requirements, may stress respiratory function whereas fluid shifts may exacerbate problems with right ventricular strain. Prognostic factors include weight gain <4.5 kg, FVC <50%, colonization with *Burkholderia cepacia*, frequent respiratory infections and hospitalizations, diabetes and pancreatic insufficiency. If there is evidence of cor pulmonale this is likely to become much worse with pregnancy and there is a recognized mortality.

Regional techniques are clearly preferable, in particular combined techniques in which a good block can provide postoperative analgesia. There are circumstances in patients with severe disease when this may not be feasible, but the decision to use general anaesthesia should not be taken lightly, in particular if it may exacerbate the incipient respiratory infection and failure.

Bibliography

Della Rocca G. Anaesthesia in patients with cystic fibrosis. *Curr Opin Anesthesiol* 2002; **15**: 95–101.

Edenborough FP, Mackenzie WE, Stableforth DE. The outcome of 72 pregnancies in 55 women with cystic fibrosis in the United Kingdom 1977–1996. *Br J Obstet Gynaecol* 2000; **107**: 254–61.

Geller DE, Rubin BK. Respiratory care and cystic fibrosis. *Respir Care* 2009; **54**: 796–800.

Huffmyer JL, Littlewood KE, Nemergut EC. Perioperative management of the adult with cystic fibrosis. *Anesth Analg* 2009; **109**: 1949–61.

Karlet MC. An update on cystic fibrosis and implications for anesthesia. *AANA J* 2000; **68**(2): 141–8.

Nunn JF, Milledge JS, Chen D, Dore C. Respiratory criteria for fitness for surgery and anaesthesia. *Anaesthesia* 1988; **43**: 543–51.

O'Sullivan BP, Freedman SD. Cystic fibrosis. *Lancet* 2009; **373**(9678): 1891–904.

Tannenbaum E, Prasad SA, Dinwiddie R, Main E. Chest physiotherapy during anesthesia for children with cystic fibrosis: effects on respiratory function. *Pediatr Pulmonol* 2007; **42**: 1152–8.

Cross-references

Bronchiectasis, 109
Lobectomy, 415
One-lung anaesthesia, 714
Intraoperative hypertension, 765
Rigid bronchoscopy, 423

Restrictive lung disease

Suveer Singh and Neil Soni

These are a range of conditions producing a restrictive picture on lung function with reduced total lung capacity, reduced resting volume yet often with normal airways resistance and airflow (Table 3.12).

The restrictive lung diseases may be classified as intrinsic or extrinsic. Intrinsic restriction is characteristic of a group of over 200 diverse conditions affecting the pulmonary interstitium (i.e. the space bounded by the alveolar epithelium and the pulmonary capillary bed and including the perivascular and perilymphatic tissues) and encompassed by the term diffuse parenchymal lung disease (DPLD) (Fig. 3.4). These are usually characterized by an impaired gas transfer factor and a reduced gas transfer coefficient (*K*co), as a result of impaired exchange between alveolar-capillary units within the interstitium.

The most commonly encountered DPLDs in clinical practice are the so-called idiopathic interstitial pneumonias (IIPs), which separate into idiopathic pulmonary fibrosis (IPF), which was previously recognized as cryptogenic fibrosing alveolitis, and the non-IPF diseases, which generally have a better prognosis. Other DPLDs are subclassified as granulomatous, exposure related (organic or inorganic), drug and radiation induced, associated with collagen, vascular or rheumatological diseases, pulmonary–renal and vasculitides, and rare orphan diseases (e.g. histiocytosis X, lymphangioleiomyomatosis).

Extrinsic restriction of lung function is usually associated with a reduced gas transfer, but a normal or increased *K*co corrected for lung volume. Essentially, the reduced lung volumes are the result of limited excursion of the chest wall, pleura or neuromuscular impairment of the respiratory system. Note that left ventricular dysfunction is also a cause.

Pathophysiology

The volume of the functional residual capacity (FRC) is determined by the balance of inward elastic recoil of the lungs and the outward elastic recoil of the chest wall. Impairment of either will restrict movement and result in a lower FRC. Total thoracic compliance is the combined compliance of the lung and chest wall, which is reduced. Particularly in advanced DPLD, there is V/Q mismatch and oxygen transfer reduction, leading to hypoxaemia. This is often apparent earlier following exercise.

The restrictive nature of the system means that smaller tidal volumes necessitate a higher respiratory rate to maintain effective minute ventilation and acid–base homeostasis. This is generally true in intrinsic disease, but extrinsic restrictive conditions, such as neuromuscular disease or obesity, have a propensity to respiratory muscle fatigue and alveolar hypoventilation, which may over time lead to type 2 or hypercapnic respiratory failure and pulmonary hypertension. The efficiency of ventilation is reduced by the smaller volumes as the effective dead space rises in relation to the tidal volume. The underlying disease process will further add to lung dysfunction.

Anaesthesia

The problems posed are the restricted lung volumes which reduce the ability of the lung to respond to stress. There is limitation of gas transfer and a predisposition to infection. Compliance is reasonable over a limited range of lung volumes above which it reduces dramatically, so ventilation must remain within these limited volumes.

Table 3.12 Restrictive lung diseases

Type	Mechanism	Condition
Intrinsic	DPLD	See Fig. 3.2
Extrinsic	Limitation of chest wall excursion	Kyphoscoliosis, ankylosing spondylitis, thoracoplasty, pleural effusion, obesity
	Respiratory muscles/neuromuscular	Polio, Guillain–Barré syndrome, muscular dystrophy
	Pleural thickening	

DPLD, diffuse parenchymal lung disease.

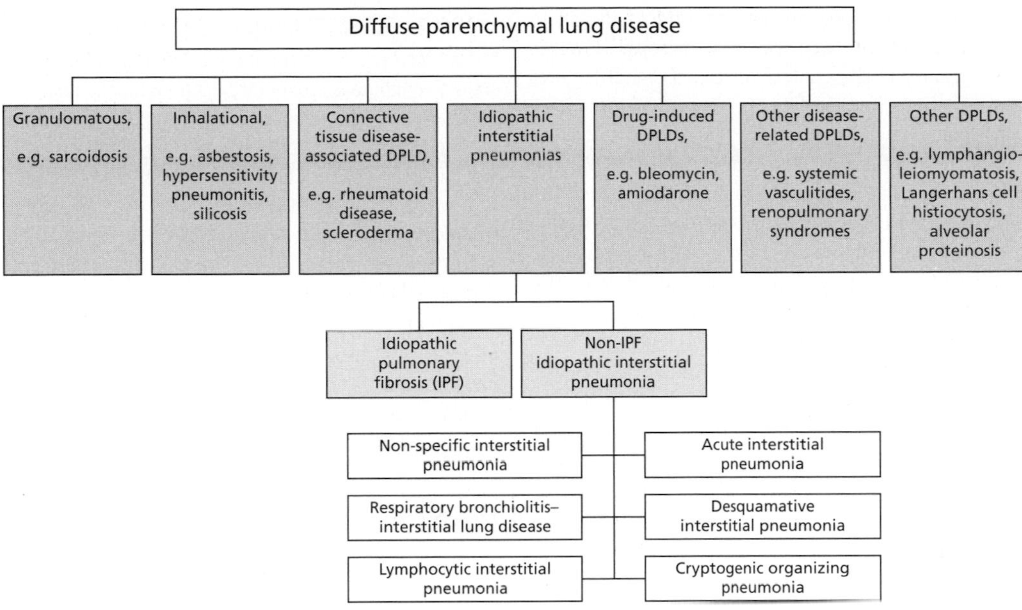

Figure 3.4 A classification scheme for diffuse parenchymal lung disease (DPLD).

Preoperative preparation

It is important to elicit the underlying cause of the restrictive picture.

History

With likely DPLD, exertional breathlessness, cough and reduced exercise tolerance may be apparent depending on the type and severity of disease. The history should elucidate the exercise tolerance and the degree of dyspnoea at rest and on exercise. Features of pulmonary hypertension and right ventricular failure such as ankle oedema may be present. Viral prodromal-like respiratory illnesses often characterize the clinical history and may be difficult to distinguish from respiratory tract infections. The past medical history should identify disorders associated with DPLD (e.g. rheumatoid arthritis and connective tissue disease). Radiotherapy for breast or thoracic malignancy can result in pulmonary fibrosis. Patients with a past history of granulomatous disease, e.g. ulcerative colitis, are at increased risk of developing sarcoidosis.

Chemotherapy such as bleomycin and other drugs such as amiodarone, methotrexate, gold, and homeopathic or complementary medications can cause DPLD.

The occupational history of exposures (organic and inorganic) and systemic features that may indicate connective tissue, vasculitis or rheumatological disease should be determined.

With suspected extrinsic diseases, weight-related problems, sleep-disordered breathing, left ventricular failure and neuromuscular weakness should be asked about.

Examination

On examination, assess the degree of dyspnoea, look for cyanosis and evidence of finger clubbing (indicative of IPF). Features of systemic disease such as Raynaud's or polyarthropathy are sought. There may be fine, bilateral 'Velcro-like' crackles heard on auscultation. Evidence of pulmonary hypertension, right heart dysfunction (i.e. loud pulmonary second heart sound, tricuspid regurgitation, raised jugular venous pressure and ankle swelling), oropharyngeal indicators of sleep apnoea and left ventricular dysfunction should be excluded.

Investigations

Chest X-ray often shows a reticulonodular appearance, with characteristically small lung fields. The distribution of changes is indicative of the aetiology. Upper zones are associated with granulomatous or acute exposure-related DPLD. Lower zone predominance is usually related to the IIPs. Honeycombing and loss of clarity of the heart borders is generally a sign of advanced disease.

High-resolution CT scan is the diagnostic investigation of choice in suspected DPLD. The patterns of distribution of ground glass, interstitial thickening, traction bronchiectasis and consolidative conglomerates are often sufficient to allow diagnosis without need for lung biopsy. However, this is usually in the context of secure clinical features and ultimately the profile of longitudinal functional behaviour.

Respiratory function tests show decreased VC and FEV_1, so the ratio remains normal. FRC is reduced. The diffusing lung capacity for carbon monoxide (DLco) is reduced in intrinsic lung disease, as is the gas transfer coefficient *K*co. Progressive decline in DLco (<40% predicted) is an independent predictor of poor prognosis in IIP. Preserved or high *K*co associated with low DLco is evidence of extrinsic disease. In neuromuscular disease, the maximum inspiratory pressures (both volitional 'sniff' and non-volitional diaphragm studies) are dramatically reduced. The VC is a helpful serial measure of progression of DPLD (especially if >10% change). In neuromuscular weakness, a serial fall in VC may warrant a discussion about assisted ventilation in the acute or postoperative setting.

In patients with coexistent emphysema, lung volumes may be preserved. A mixed obstructive/restrictive defect may sometimes be seen in sarcoidosis, lymphangioleiomyomatosis, respiratory bronchiolitis interstitial lung disease and hypersensitivity pneumonitis.

Arterial blood gases may show hypoxaemia. CO_2 rises in extrinsic disease and sometimes with advanced DPLD.

Exercise tests, such as the 6 minute walk test, are useful in IPF. Desaturation to 88% or 200 metres portend a poor prognosis. Exercise tolerance is reduced, so exercise testing with oximetry will indicate oxygen requirement and can be used to follow disease progression.

Preoperative optimization

Reverse any airflow limitation with bronchodilators, and steroids may be needed. Treat cardiac failure appropriately, well in advance of surgery. Treat any possibility of infection. If there are limiting factors such as pleural effusions then drainage may be very helpful. Assessment and treatment by physiotherapy. A cardiological opinion is essential if it is thought that there is pulmonary hypertension best elicited by echocardiography preoperatively.

The anaesthetic

Plan the anaesthetic in terms of the procedure and the limitations of the patient in particular if the procedure is amenable to regional technique. If a regional technique is used then beware that the height of the block may impair ventilatory muscle function, both chest and abdomen, so should not go above the level of T10 depending on the patient.

General anaesthesia

Some advocate anticholinergic agents. Monitoring should encompass oximetry, capnography and the ability to carry out blood gas sampling. Cardiovascular monitoring will be defined by the cardiovascular stability of the patient and the nature of the procedure. In patients with kyphoscoliosis, or ankylosing spondylitis, difficult intubation should be anticipated. A further problem in these patients with chest wall abnormalities is surgical positioning.

Ventilation may be difficult. Small tidal volumes will be necessary and, if exceeded, can result in very high airway pressures and a risk of pneumothorax. Oxygenation may also be problematic despite ventilation, so high inspired oxygen may be necessary.

Postoperative management

As with other severe lung diseases the postoperative period is a potential source of problems. Sputum retention and basal atelectasis will both contribute to the restrictive picture and may have significant effects on the already poor lung function. Extubation is best in a compliant awake patient so that coughing, mobilization and physiotherapy are possible early. Adequate analgesia is essential, with the usual difficult balance between analgesia and sedation. A high-dependency area is ideal postoperatively.

Beware of hypoxia and of insidious hypercapnia. NIV, either CPAP or bilevel, can be used to facilitate postoperative lung volume recruitment and relieve the work of breathing as necessary.

The physiotherapists are key to the management for several days postoperatively, until the patient is fully mobile. Adjuncts such as incentive spirometry, intermittent CPAP or intermittent positive pressure breathing may be helpful as bridges to recovery.

Summary

The recognition of intrinsic and extrinsic lung diseases is an important distinction, although easily made clinically. The intrinsic diseases are predominantly the DPLDs, characterized by the IIPs, in which pulmonary fibrosis usually progresses. Identifying the severity of disease from previous work-up allows appropriate planning of the perioperative course. Those with established progressive fibrosis and reduced DLco are at significant risk of postoperative respiratory complications. The usual principles of optimizing current cardiorespiratory status, offering regional anaesthetic techniques when possible, recognizing the ventilatory adjustments needed for smaller, non-compliant lungs and managing the postoperative period in a high-dependency setting with physiotherapy and analgesic support hold.

Bibliography

Bradley B, Branley HM, Egan JJ, *et al.*; British Thoracic Society Interstitial Lung Disease Guideline Group, British Thoracic Society Standards of Care Committee; Thoracic Society of Australia; New Zealand Thoracic Society; Irish Thoracic Society. Interstitial lung disease guideline: the British Thoracic Society in collaboration with the Thoracic Society of Australia and New Zealand and the Irish Thoracic Society. *Thorax* 2008; **63**(Suppl. 5): v1–58.

Hughes JM, Lockwood DN, Jones HA, Clark RJ. DLCO/QAM diffusion limitation at rest and on exercise in patients with interstitial fibrosis. *Respir Physiol* 1983; **2**: 155–66.

http://emedicine.medscape.com/article/301760-diagnosis

Quigley M, Hansell DM, Nicholson AG. Interstitial lung disease: the new synergy between radiology and pathology. *Histopathology* 2006; **49**: 334–42.

West JB. *Restrictive Diseases in Pulmonary Pathophysiology: the Essentials*, 3rd edn. Baltimore: Williams & Wilkins, 1987, pp. 92–111.

www.pneumotox.com

www.uptodate.com/online/content/search/diseases+of+the+chest+wall

Cross-reference

Preoperative assessment of pulmonary risk, 625

Sarcoidosis

Rick Keays and Neil Soni

Sarcoidosis is a systemic, granulomatous disease of unknown aetiology. It seems likely that the granulomas form through an interaction between antigens, as yet unknown, and T cells. It has geographical variation. Slightly more common in women, its peak onset is in patients in their twenties and thirties. Presentation is variable, but 90% of patients have lung involvement, often with bilateral hilar adenopathy or pulmonary infiltrates. Skin, lymph node, eye and liver are the next most affected organs in that order. Cardiac involvement is less common but potentially fatal. There may be radiological appearances, particularly involving the small bones of the hand and feet, or symmetrical arthritis of large joints. Occasionally, there is neurological involvement.

While imaging and a plethora of tests can imply sarcoidosis, such as elevated angiotensin converting enzyme levels, a raised calcium, raised immunoglobulins and 'gallium-lit' lesions, the only way to definitively diagnose the condition is by biopsy, which will show non-caseating granulomas. Tuberculosis and fungal infection are often the differential diagnosis.

The implications to the anaesthetist mainly relate to the pulmonary involvement, which may involve fibrotic lung changes and a restrictive pattern, usually with a reduction in diffusing capacity. Most patients will have an abnormal chest X-ray at some stages in the disease and usually hilar lymphadenopathy. Occasionally, there may be obstructive lesions in the airways themselves.

There may be nasopharyngeal and laryngeal involvement affecting the arytenoids and supraglottic area, and patients occasionally present with dysphonia, then stridor and dyspnoea, which may necessitate emergency tracheostomy.

Cardiovascular involvement is an uncommon manifestation in clinical practice at 2%, but 25% of postmortem examinations of known cases of sarcoidosis have cardiac involvement. Preferential granulomatous involvement of the conduction system is manifest as a variety of dysrhythmias, including complete heart block. Congestive cardiac failure with features of a dilated cardiomyopathy may also be present.

Renal involvement is uncommon at less than 2%, but has a protean presentation. It may occur through hypercalcaemia or nephrocalcinosis or both. It may also cause either interstitial or membranous nephritis.

Hepatic and pancreatic involvement have been reported.

The neurological system may be affected in 5–15% of patients with sarcoidosis, although, again, the postmortem evidence suggests far more. Most common are cranial nerve palsies, which account for 65% of the neurological manifestations. Headache is also common, but fitting is uncommon. Rarely, mono- or polyneuropathies can develop, which may cause sensory or motor deficit, or a combination of both. Cerebellar symptoms can also occur. Neuropsychological disturbance is also uncommon. Spinal involvement is rare, but may present with various forms of paresis including cauda equina syndrome.

Preoperative assessment

In such a protean disease, it is hard to suggest a universal approach (Table 3.13). A clear history of the

Table 3.13 Investigations and results

Investigations	Results (if system involved)
Chest X-ray	Bilateral hilar lymphadenopathy, reticulonodular shadowing, pleural effusions, cardiomegaly, atelectasis
Electrocardiogram	Conduction defects, ventricular hypertrophy
Arterial blood gases	Reduced Po_2 on room air
Lung function tests	Restrictive/obstructive defects
Electrolytes	Raised calcium/potassium
Echocardiography	Ventricular hypokinesis, mitral valve involvement, septal thickening and bright echoes (consistent with fibrogranulomatous infiltration)

Po_2, partial pressure of oxygen.

range of problems that are known should be elicited, but awareness of occult cardiology and neurology should be borne in mind.

The prevalence of respiratory system involvement indicates careful respiratory assessment. Specific attention is focused on a history of stridor (suggesting laryngeal involvement), swallowing difficulties (hinting at neurological problems), or any breathlessness indicating the more common interstitial-type lung disease. A chest X-ray and blood gases will be useful to identify any overt respiratory issues. Pulmonary function tests may help clarify degrees of restrictive lung injury defects. The covert nature of cardiac involvement mandates taking a history of any palpitations or fainting episodes and an ECG to look for any signs of actual or potential heart block. Pacing may be indicated.

Renal function is relatively easy to assess, as is the measurement of calcium looking for hypercalcaemia. Neurological involvement needs to be elicited, especially if it is intended to use a regional technique.

Perioperative management

Ophthalmic problems are common, but most of these can, at least in theory, be dealt with under local anaesthesia. This should focus on the problems that have been elicited. The most common problem is the respiratory system. As with other respiratory conditions, caution with sedation is advised. Avoiding and preventing hypoxia is the aim and the liberal use of supplemental oxygen is obviously recommended. These patients may already be on steroids but, if not, steroids may be of benefit.

Anaesthesia

Given the massive range of potential problems that may be an issue, it is vital to tailor the anaesthetic to the patient. If feasible, the use of a regional technique may be advantageous in the presence of significant respiratory disease but may be difficult if there is neurological involvement. Clearly, laryngeal involvement with stridor is a special case that needs careful planning.

Postoperative management

If the predominant area of risk is respiratory, the focus should be on good analgesia, mobilization and physiotherapy. Renal issues may need attention to avoid pre-renal insults. With such a myriad of presentations and potential problems there is no specific area in which sarcoidosis is different from its component parts. The role of steroids and other agents needs careful attention as these may need to be continued and probably increased in the postoperative phase.

Bibliography

Bonfioli AA, Orefice F. Sarcoidosis. *Semin Ophthalmol* 2005; **20**(3): 177–82.

Butler CR, Nouraei SA, Mace AD, *et al.* Endoscopic airway management of laryngeal sarcoidosis. *Arch Otolaryngol Head Neck Surg* 2010; **136**: 251–5.

Carmichael P, O'Donnell JP. The protean face of renal sarcoid. *J Nephrol* 2003; **16**: 721–7.

Dubrey SW, Falk RH. Diagnosis and management of cardiac sarcoidosis. *Prog Cardiovasc Dis* 2010; **52**(4): 336–46.

Harder H, Büchler MW, Fröhlich B, *et al.* Extrapulmonary sarcoidosis of liver and pancreas: a case report and review of literature. *World J Gastroenterol* 2007; **13**: 2504–9.

Hoitsma E, Faber CG, Drent M, Sharma OP. Neurosarcoidosis: a clinical dilemma. *Lancet Neurol* 2004; **3**: 397–407.

Parrish S, Turner JF. Diagnosis of sarcoidosis. *Dis Mon* 2009; **55**: 693–703.

Pierre-Louis B, Prasad A, Frishman WH. Cardiac manifestations of sarcoidosis and therapeutic options. *Cardiol Rev* 2009; **17**(4): 153–8.

Cross-references

Cardiac conduction defects, 132
Pacing and anaesthesia, 777
Preoperative assessment of pulmonary risk, 625
Restrictive lung disease, 114

Smoking and anaesthesia

Rick Keays and Neil Soni

Recognition of the problems of smoking has taken a long time and is only just beginning possibly to alter behaviour; as a result, a significant proportion of patients will be smokers or will have a long, but recently stopped, smoking history.

Pathophysiology

The preoperative effects of smoking on the respiratory system are well known:

- airway hyper-reactivity, especially small airways
- reduced mucociliary clearance
- increased mucus secretion
- a change in epithelial permeability
- altered surfactant and hence compliance
- small airway narrowing
- V/Q mismatch.

The effects on the cardiovascular system include a tendency to hypertension, in part because of chronic nicotine exposure and in part because of atherosclerotic change. Nicotine itself increases catecholamine values at the levels seen in smokers (15–50 ng L^{-1}). Carboxyhaemoglobin blocks oxygen uptake and shifts the oxygen dissociation curve to the left. There is also a tendency to increased haemoglobin values in long-standing smokers secondary to relative hypoxaemia and carboxyhaemoglobin. This forms part of a predisposition to thrombosis, although this is not clear-cut in all studies. It causes damage to the vascular endothelium, releases endothelin, has a negative effect on nitric oxide dynamics and alters superoxide production. It acutely affects clot dynamics and thrombin structure, and thus is thrombogenic. Curiously, cigarette smoke may have a synergistic effect with clopidogrel, reducing platelet aggregation; but, in general, it should be considered thrombogenic.

The immunological effects of smoking are diverse, but include reduced phagocytic and cytotoxic T-cell activity. There is some evidence for impaired immune defences.

Smoking is associated with enzyme induction, so there may be an altered response to some drugs; however, the clinical relevance of these effects is questionable.

In the postoperative phase, smokers are more prone to hypoxaemia, have slightly higher $P\text{CO}_2$ and have more change in pulmonary function tests, with a reduction in FEV_1/FVC ratio suggesting greater small airway obstruction. Pulmonary complications were doubled in one series. Also, in major surgery, the time to extubation, intensive care and hospital stays were all increased.

Preoperative assessment

The issues around giving up smoking preoperatively will be discussed below, but, ideally, patients should have stopped some weeks previously. There is a range of associated diseases which should be assessed. These include chronic respiratory disease, cardiovascular disease and, especially, hypertension and ischaemic heart disease. There is also association with excess alcohol intake. In heavy smokers with airways disease, the nutritional state may be affected.

Investigations

Any organ system that may be affected should be assessed from a history and an examination, and these should guide investigation. The presence of cardiovascular disease, real or potential, should lead to consideration of an ECG and, if there is any suggestion of failure, an echocardiogram may be instructive. Respiratory function should be assessed; exercise tolerance is important and may be more helpful than respiratory function tests, which may need to include blood gases as a baseline. This will be more relevant if patients have chronic airways disease. Clearly, any signs of infection should be sought (Table 3.14).

Premedication

These patients will probably have irritable airways. They may be hypersecretory. An anticholinergic may be helpful. In those who have given up there may be signs of nicotine withdrawal with agitation, so anxiolytics may be considered. H_2 antagonists or antacids should be considered.

Perioperative management

Monitoring that is appropriate for the nature of the procedure and the comorbidities of the patient. Saturation monitoring may overestimate whether

Table 3.14 Possible preoperative investigations and results in (heavy or long-term) smokers

Investigation	Result
Full blood count	Increased haematocrit
ECG	Signs of ischaemic heart disease
Chest X-ray	Chronic airways limitation
	Infection
	Malignancy
Arterial blood gases	Hypoxaemia/hypercarbia
Lung function tests	Decreased FEV_1
	Diminished FVC
	Decreased PEFR

FEV_1, forced expiratory volume in 1 second; FVC, forced vital capacity; PEFR, peak expiratory flow rate.

there is significant carboxyhaemoglobin content. Smoking more than 20 cigarettes per day is associated with a carboxyhaemoglobin level of <4%, and this will fall fairly rapidly after stopping smoking, so the P_{50} will return to normal at 12 hours or faster if the patient receives an increased inspired oxygen concentration. If there is evidence of impaired respiratory function or heavy smoking right up to anaesthesia then an increased $F_{I}O_2$ would be sensible.

Choice of anaesthetic technique

This should be appropriate to the patient and the procedure. In the presence of airway problems associated with smoking, a regional technique may be preferred when feasible and may allow more effective physiotherapy postoperatively.

General anaesthesia

The main considerations are the irritable airways, and there may be a nicotine-mediated exaggerated pressor response to intubation. This may be obtunded with lidocaine applied locally. Spontaneous breathing, unless deep, may be problematic with coughing.

Postoperative management

This again should reflect the comorbidities. Early active physiotherapy should be instigated if there are chronic lung problems. The risk of secondary infection is increased, as is the likelihood of postoperative complications generally. It is wise to continue enhanced oxygen by mask for 24 hours. The incidence of postoperative nausea and vomiting is reduced among smokers.

Stopping smoking and postoperative outcome

The issue of smoking and complications is more contentious than it appears. The vast majority of studies show that current smokers have higher complication rates than non-smokers or previous smokers. The complication rate in some series among smokers is effectively doubled. Wound healing is also impaired. Not all studies show this; for example, in lung resection for carcinoma, the incidence of complications was not different between those who stopped smoking and those who did not. This was seen as a reason not to delay surgery. It is reasonable to assume that smoking is associated with more postoperative complications and also impaired wound healing.

More difficult is the issue of advice as to when to stop smoking (Table 3.15). It is clear that stopping 6–8 weeks before surgery is beneficial in terms of reduced complication rates (52% to 18%), but there was a suspicion that stopping for less time might be detrimental. Current thinking has moved on. Benefit has been demonstrated for stopping smoking 3–4 weeks before surgery. Furthermore, a single study showed no benefit but no detriment from cessation for 1–3 weeks before surgery. Current advice should be that postoperative complications are reduced and wound healing improved by stopping smoking even for as little as 3 weeks. Shorter intervals may not be helpful but have no detriment. This was not seen in a recent paper in patients undergoing thoracotomy.

Outcome

In 1944, Morton reported a sixfold increase in the incidence of postoperative respiratory morbidity in smokers compared with non-smokers. These findings

Table 3.15 Benefits of stopping smoking in the perioperative period

Time before surgery	Benefit
2 h	Nicotine blood levels fall
12 h	Carbon monoxide blood levels fall
Days	Sputum volume reduced; haematocrit falls
Weeks	Ciliary activity restored towards normal; epithelial permeability returns towards normal
Months	Immune system recovery; drug metabolism restored towards normal

have been confirmed in several other studies more recently. Every opportunity should be taken to discourage smoking in the perioperative period.

Bibliography

Al-Sarraf N, Thalib L, Hughes A, *et al.* Effect of smoking on short-term outcome of patients undergoing coronary artery bypass surgery. *Ann Thorac Surg* 2008; **86**: 517–23.

Barrera R, Shi W, Amar D, *et al.* Smoking and timing of cessation: impact on pulmonary complications after thoracotomy. *Chest* 2005; **127**: 1977–83.

Edmonds MJ, Crichton TJ, Runciman WB, Pradhan M. Evidence-based risk factors for postoperative deep vein thrombosis. *ANZ J Surg* 2004; **74**: 1082–97.

Egan TD, Wong KC. Perioperative smoking cessation and anesthesia: a review. *J Clin Anesth* 1992; **4**: 63–72.

Kotani N, Hashimoto H, Sessler DI, *et al.* Smoking decreases alveolar macrophage function during anesthesia and surgery. *Anesthesiology* 2000; **92**: 1268–77.

Kuri M, Nakagawa M, Tanaka H, *et al.* Determination of the duration of preoperative smoking cessation to improve wound healing after head and neck surgery. *Anesthesiology* 2005; **102**: 892–6.

Myles PS, Iacono GA, Hunt JO, *et al.* Risk of respiratory complications and wound infection in patients undergoing ambulatory surgery: smokers versus nonsmokers. *Anesthesiology* 2002; **97**: 842–7.

Rock P, Rich PB. Postoperative pulmonary complications. *Curr Opin Anaesthesiol* 2003; **16**: 123–31.

Sweeney BP, Grayling M. Smoking and anaesthesia: the pharmacological implications. *Anaesthesia* 2009; **64**: 179–86.

Cross-reference

Anaesthesia and chronic obstructive pulmonary disease, 91

4

Cardiovascular system

Stefan De Hert

- General considerations — *Stefan De Hert*
- Aortic valve disease — *Jan Fräßdorf*
- Atrial septal defect — *Susanne Eberl*
- Cardiac conduction defects — *Peter Meijer*
- Cardiomyopathy — *Stefan De Hert*
- Children with congenital heart disease for non-cardiac surgery — *Susanne Eberl*
- Congenital heart disease in adult life — *Veronika Evers*
- Coronary artery disease — *Quanhong Zhou and Stefan De Hert*
- Hypertension — *Peter Meijer*
- Ischaemia–reperfusion injury — *Stefan De Hert and Benedikt Preckel*
- Mitral valve disease — *Jan Fräßdorf*
- Patients with heart failure — *Quanhong Zhou and Stefan De Hert*
- Patients with pacemakers and implantable defibrillators — *Benedikt Preckel*
- Pulmonary hypertension — *Benedikt Preckel*
- Surgery after heart transplantation — *Stefan De Hert*
- Tetralogy of Fallot — *Veronika Evers*

General considerations

Stefan De Hert

Heart disease may be a potential source of perioperative complications. The risk of such complications depends on the patient's condition prior to surgery, the prevalence of comorbidities and the type of surgical procedure. Perioperative cardiac complications may specifically arise in patients with documented or asymptomatic ischaemic heart disease, left ventricular dysfunction and valvular heart disease when the perioperative period is associated with increased cardiac stress owing to haemodynamic disturbances. It is, therefore, of utmost importance that such patients are identified and adequately prepared for, and carefully treated during the perioperative period.

In the absence of national registries, data on cardiac outcome have to be derived from the few large-scale clinical trials performed in a patient population undergoing non-cardiac surgery. The Dutch Echocardiographic Cardiac Risk Evaluating Applying Stress Echo (DECREASE) I, II and IV trials included 3893 intermediate- and high-risk surgical patients over the period 1996–2008. In this patient population the incidence of perioperative cardiac death or myocardial infarction was 3.5%. The Perioperative Ischaemic Evaluation (POISE) trial enrolled 8351 non-cardiac surgical patients throughout 2002–7. Total perioperative mortality was 2.7%, and 1.6% was due to cardiovascular death. Non-fatal myocardial infarction was observed in another 4.4% of the study population. Although differences in incidences between studies may be related to variability in study population and definition of cardiovascular complications, it seems that major non-cardiac surgery is associated with an incidence of cardiac death between 0.5 and 1.5% and of major cardiovascular complications between 2.0 and 3.5%.

Both the American and European Cardiology Societies have recently published – in close collaboration with the respective anaesthesiology societies – guidelines for preoperative cardiac risk assessment and perioperative cardiac management in patients undergoing non-cardiac surgery. However, owing to the lack of large prospective randomized trials on different issues, a considerable amount of recommendations on the topic have only level of evidence B (data derived from a single randomized clinical trial or large non-randomized studies) or even level of evidence C (consensus of opinion of the experts and/or small studies, retrospective studies, registries). Nevertheless, these guidelines may be helpful for decision-making in the perioperative treatment of each individual patient, more specifically with regard to the preoperative evaluation and the potential discontinuation of chronic medication and the use of perioperative monitoring techniques.

It is important to note that a number of cardiac disease states may profoundly affect normal cardiovascular physiology. Therefore, knowledge of these alterations is of prime importance for adequate perioperative care of such patients.

In cardiac surgery, the choice of the anaesthetic regimen has been suggested to influence postoperative outcome. It has indeed been reported that the use of a volatile anaesthetic regimen during coronary surgery was associated with a shorter hospital length of stay and a lower incidence of perioperative myocardial infarction and mortality. To date, no such data are available for patients undergoing non-cardiac surgery. In the absence of strong evidence favouring a specific anaesthetic regimen, it seems that the choice of anaesthetic technique or agent seems to be less important than the maintenance of a stable haemodynamic status resulting in a favourable myocardial oxygen supply/demand ratio. This is especially true for patients with known or suspected cardiac disease. Specific anaesthetic considerations will be addressed in the different topics dealing with the various cardiac conditions. However, as a general rule, it can be stated that most modern anaesthetic drugs provide a fairly good cardiovascular stability and that with careful titration no major anaesthesia-related haemodynamic disturbances are to be expected. Finally, the anaesthetist should have thorough knowledge of the various inotropic and vasoactive drugs and be experienced with their use.

Bibliography

Fleisher LA, Beckman JA, Brown KA, *et al.* ACC/AHA 2007 guidelines on perioperative cardiovascular evaluation and care for noncardiac surgery: a report of the American College of Cardiology/American Heart Association Task Force on Practice Guidelines (writing committee to revise the 2002 guidelines on perioperative cardiovascular evaluation for noncardiac surgery). *Circulation* 2007; **116**: e418–e500.

Fräβdorf J, De Hert S, Schlack W. Anaesthesia and myocardial ischaemia/reperfusion injury. *Br J Anaesth* 2009; **103**: 89–98.

Poldermans D, Bax JJ, Boersma E, *et al.* Task Force for Preoperative Cardiac Risk Assessment and Perioperative Cardiac Management in Non-cardiac Surgery of European Society of Cardiology (ESC); European Society of Anaesthesiology (ESA). Guidelines for pre-operative cardiac risk assessment and perioperative cardiac management in non-cardiac surgery: the Task Force for Preoperative Cardiac Risk Assessment and Perioperative Cardiac Management in Non-cardiac Surgery of the European Society of Cardiology (ESC) and endorsed by the European Society of Anaesthesiology (ESA). *Eur J Anaesthesiol* 2010; **27**: 92–137.

Aortic valve disease

Jan Fräßdorf

Aortic stenosis

Epidemiology

Senile calcification, rheumatic heart disease, congenital abnormalities and infectious endocarditis are the main aetiologies of aortic stenosis. With increasing age the risk of aortic stenosis increases. Whereas approximately 25% of people aged over 65 have only a thickening of the aortic valve ('sclerosis'), 3% of those older than 75 have severe aortic stenosis. Rheumatic disease is nowadays a rare condition in the Western population, but remains worldwide the most common cause of aortic stenosis. In Western populations 'calcific degenerative disease' is the leading cause for aortic stenosis. This may lead in the seventh or eighth decade of life to severe aortic stenosis. One exception is subjects with a bicuspid aortic valve. These patients suffer earlier from severe aortic stenosis, mostly in their fourth or fifth decade of life.

Severe aortic stenosis remains asymptomatic for a long time. In asymptomatic patients the risk of death is less than 1% per year. When clinical symptoms such as dyspnoea on exertion, angina pectoris and syncope occur, the mortality increases and the median survival is 4.5 years (patients with dyspnoea on exertion), 2.6 years (patients with dizziness on exertion) and 1 year if overt heart failure occurs

Pathophysiology

A normal aortic valve has an orifice of 2–4 cm^2. Severe aortic stenosis is diagnosed if one or more of the following features are present:

- blood flow velocity through the aortic valve is more than 4 $m\ s^{-1}$
- the mean pressure gradient is more than 50 mmHg
- the aortic valve orifice is less than 1 cm^2
- the relation of aortic valve orifice and area of the left ventricular outflow tract is <0.25.

Because of the narrowing of the valve orifice, the resistance of blood flow through the valve increases and consequently a pressure gradient across the valve occurs. This pressure gradient will induce concentric hypertrophy of the left ventricle. In this condition higher left ventricular filling pressures are necessary to maintain preload and adequate stroke volume of the ventricle. This increases wall tension, and in conditions when diastolic blood pressure decreases subendocardial ischaemia may occur. In addition, relaxation of the left ventricle is impaired, leading to a shorter diastole and less time for coronary perfusion.

When the compensatory mechanisms start to fail, filling pressures will increase further and the left ventricle is no longer capable of overcoming the pressure gradient over the aortic valve and maintaining adequate cardiac output. The atrial contribution to left ventricular filling becomes more essential and may increase up to 40%. Therefore, maintaining sinus rhythm is essential to maintain cardiac output in these patients.

Anaesthesia

Preassessment

It is not unusual that during preanaesthetic evaluation a *de novo* murmur of the heart is discovered. Every new murmur should be evaluated with echocardiography. Mild to moderate aortic stenosis is usually asymptomatic and is not considered to be an active cardiac condition, as defined in the practice guidelines of the AHA/ACC. However, even a moderate pressure gradient between 25 and 49 mmHg is associated with an increased perioperative cardiovascular risk.

This risk increases further if clinical symptoms such as syncope, heart failure and angina occur. Therefore, patients' history and physical status should be carefully evaluated to detect these signs of decompensated aortic stenosis. Special attention should be paid to concomitant comorbidities. Coronary artery disease adds an additional risk for cardiovascular events in non-cardiac surgery in this patient population.

The intraoperative risk depends on the severity of the aortic stenosis and the extent of the surgical intervention. Vascular surgery is considered to be associated with a high cardiovascular risk, namely caused by huge volume shift perioperatively. However, even minor surgery can be associated with occult volume shifts through preoperative fasting, bowel preparation prior to surgery or unexpected blood loss. Haemodynamic changes due to pneumoperitoneum or due to stress (inappropriate anxiolysis preoperatively or pain control postoperatively) are less well tolerated in patients with aortic stenosis. However, risk stratification should be done on an individual basis.

In general, it is recommended that severe aortic stenosis should be treated with aortic valve replacement prior to elective surgery.

Intraoperative management

The main goals of anaesthetic management are maintaining adequate coronary perfusion pressure (adequate afterload and diastolic blood pressure), cardiac output, relatively slow heart rate (longer diastole, more filling and coronary perfusion time) and sinus rhythm.

As maintaining preload is crucial for these patients, monitoring of the intravascular volume status is mandatory. Pressure correlates of filling, as measured with the pulmonary artery catheter, are unreliable in this setting as a measure of volumes and preload. In addition, the risk of rhythm disturbances associated with the introduction of a pulmonary artery catheter may aggravate the already compromised haemodynamic status in these patients. Volume-based measurements, such as pulse pressure variation or pulse contour analysis, are not validated in this setting. The most useful tool seems to be transoesophageal echocardiography. Besides analysis of the structural changes of the aortic valve, also the function of the heart and an estimation of the volume status of the heart can be obtained. However, application of this technology requires skilled observers.

Tachycardia is poorly tolerated in patients with aortic stenosis. With increased heart frequency, diastolic filling, coronary perfusion time and systolic ejection time decrease, resulting in decreasing cardiac output. This may lead to a vicious circle, leading to haemodynamic instability, acute cardiac decompensation and cardiac arrest. A heart frequency between 60 and 70 b.p.m. should be aimed at.

Dysrhythmias are not well tolerated and should be promptly treated. It is important to maintain sinus rhythm, and cardioversion possibilities should be available in the operating room.

There is no evidence that neuraxial anaesthesia is associated with a reduced morbidity or mortality compared with general anaesthesia. A reduction in the SVR is not well tolerated in patients with aortic stenosis as this leads to a reduction in coronary artery perfusion pressure. Therefore, careful titration of anaesthetic medication is mandatory.

Postoperative management

The same considerations regarding volume management, pain therapy and monitoring apply to the postoperative period. As the staff on a normal ward are usually not trained and/or used to handling patients with severe aortic stenosis, it is justified to transfer patients with severe aortic stenosis postoperatively to an ICU, even after minor surgery.

Aortic regurgitation

Epidemiology

Worldwide, rheumatic fever still is the main cause of aortic regurgitation. However, this condition has become rare in the Western hemisphere, where congenital or degenerative diseases are the main cause for aortic regurgitation.

Aortic regurgitation may occur because of abnormalities of the aortic valve (i.e. rheumatic fever, bicuspid valve, Marfan syndrome, infectious endocarditis or trauma) or because of abnormalities of the aortic tissue (dissecting aneurysm, arthritis, systemic hypertension or trauma). Also in patients with aortic stenosis, aortic regurgitation is a common observation. The prevalence of severe aortic regurgitation in the overall population is estimated to be less than 1%.

Pathophysiology

Structural changes of the cusps or dilatation and distortion of the aortic annulus will prevent efficient closure of the aortic valve and lead to regurgitation of a part of the stroke volume back into the left ventricle. This provokes a volume load to the left ventricle, resulting in an increased left ventricular end-diastolic volume and wall stress.

The regurgitant orifice is the main determinant of the regurgitation volume. The diastolic transvalvular pressure difference between the aorta and left ventricle has less influence on this volume. In severe aortic regurgitation the regurgitant fraction can be up to 60% of the stroke volume. To maintain cardiac output, heart rate is increased. Bradycardia is less tolerated in aortic regurgitation; as diastolic time increases, the time of regurgitation increases as well. The increased heart rate, in combination with shorter coronary perfusion time, increased end-diastolic pressure and low diastolic aortic pressure, may lead to myocardial ischaemia, thereby further impairing myocardial function. In chronic, slow progressive, aortic regurgitation, however, oxygen balance is maintained for a long period owing to dilatation of the left ventricle and consequent decrease in wall tension.

Mild to moderate aortic regurgitation is well tolerated in patients and these are, most of the time, asymptomatic. Even severe aortic regurgitation can remain unrecognized for a long period. Symptoms occur as an imbalance occurs between diastolic left ventricular distension (preload), myocardial mass (hypertrophy) and systolic wall tension (afterload).

Anaesthesia

Preassesment

Symptoms differ between an acute onset in severe aortic regurgitation due to trauma or aortic dissection (acute chest pain, shortness of breath, cardiogenic shock) and the chronic form (initially asymptomatic, later exertional dyspnoea or at rest, tachycardia, palpitations caused by arrhythmias and angina).

On auscultation a high pitched diastolic murmur can be heard; bounding pulses due to widened pulse pressure are found in severe aortic regurgitation; on the ECG signs of left ventricular hypertrophy can be seen; and an X-ray of the chest may show left ventricular enlargement.

There is only limited evidence on the perioperative risk of patients with aortic regurgitation undergoing non-cardiac surgery. Asymptomatic patients probably do not have an additional risk. However, if patients with severe aortic regurgitation become symptomatic (New York Heart Association (NYHA) classification of III or higher), the perioperative risk increases significantly. Generally speaking, patients with aortic insufficiency tolerate anaesthesia better than those with aortic stenosis.

Diagnosis and classification is usually done non-invasively with echocardiography. In severe aortic regurgitation, a regurgitant fraction of more than 60%, a diastolic flow reversal in the descending aorta and a large regurgitant jet can be seen. To assess functional capacity of the patient, exercise stress testing can be useful. Antihypertensive treatment should be continued perioperatively to prevent rebound hypertension.

Intraoperative management

There are no specific considerations regarding the use of anxiolytic drugs prior to non-cardiac surgery. Drugs prescribed by the cardiologist should be continued, taking care of the possible interactions between antihypertensive drugs and the haemodynamic effects of anaesthetic agents. Regarding a possible anticoagulation of the patient and a scheduled neuraxial blockade, the international or national guidelines should be followed.

There is no evidence that any anaesthetic technique or drug is to be preferred. The main goal during the procedure is to maintain a higher heart rate and a low afterload to minimize the regurgitant fraction. In severe aortic regurgitation or in the presence of signs of congestive heart failure, the use of continuous, invasive, arterial blood pressure monitoring is justified. Continuous measurement of the ST segment of at least two ECG leads (II and V5) should be established to detect early possible myocardial ischaemia.

Neither a central venous catheter nor a pulmonary artery catheter are able to give an accurate indication of the filling status of the patient. However, in severe aortic regurgitation, a central venous catheter can be justified to administer vasoactive medication in a safe manner.

Echocardiographic monitoring can be useful in haemodynamically unstable patients to assess the filling of the left ventricle, detect regional wall motion abnormalities and other structural changes of the heart. Especially the possible additional presence of aortic stenosis has to be excluded, as this may change the management of the patient.

Postoperative management

Especially after procedures with large volume shifts, the patient has to be monitored carefully to detect early any sign of congestive heart failure.

Bibliography

Dujardin KS, Enriquez-Sarano M, Schaff HV, *et al.* Mortality and morbidity of aortic regurgitation in clinical practice: a long-term follow-up study. *Circulation* 1999; **99**: 1851–7.

Goldbarg SH, Halperin JL. Aortic regurgitation: disease progression and management. *Nat Clin Pract Cardiovasc Med* 2008; **5**: 269–79.

Groban L, Butterworth J. Perioperative management of chronic heart failure. *Anesth Analg* 2006;**103**: 557–75.

Horstkotte D, Loogen F. The natural history of aortic valve stenosis. *Eur Heart J* 1988; **9**(Suppl. E): 57–64.

Kertai MD, Boersma E, Klein J, *et al.* Aortic stenosis: an underestimated risk factor for perioperative complications in patients undergoing noncardiac surgery. *Am J Med* 2004; **116**: 8–13.

Supino PG, Borer JS, Preibisz J, Bornstein A. The epidemiology of valvular heart disease: a growing public health problem. *Heart Fail Clin* 2006; **2**: 379–93.

Torsher LC, Shub C, Rettke SR, Brown DL. Risk of patients with severe aortic stenosis undergoing noncardiac surgery. *Am J Cardiol* 1998; **81**: 448–52.

Cross-references

Aortic valve disease, 126
Cardiopulmonary exercise testing, 600
Patients with heart failure, 159
Preoperative assessment of cardiovascular risk in non-cardiac surgery, 621

Atrial septal defect

Susanne Eberl

Atrial septal defect (ASD) is a common heart defect in children, occurring in 1 in 1500 live births and accounting for approximately 10% of all congenital heart diseases.

Embryology

The formation of two septa – the primum and the secundum – divides the atria into left and right sides. First, the truncus presses down on the roof of the atria, causing an indentation that marks the beginning of the growth of the septum primum. This indentation forms a crescent of tissue that folds in and actively grows downward towards the ventricles to meet the endocardial cushion tissue, which is simultaneously developing there. The septum primum then develops perforations in its centre to allow blood to continue to pass to the left atrium during intrauterine life. Meanwhile, an enfolding of the atrial walls produces a crescent of tissue that covers the perforations in the septum primum and forms the septum secundum.

Anatomic types

Primum atrial septal defect

Persistence of the ostium primum is due to faulty fusion of the anterior and posterior endocardial cushions; it is located in the inferior part of the atrial septum and is often associated with a cleft in the anterior leaflet of the mitral valve. This is a variant of an atrioventricular (AV) septum defect.

Secundum atrial septal defect

An unusually large ostium secundum or failure of the septum secundum to approximate with the septum primum results in a secundum defect. Defects of the septum secundum can be classified as follows.

Patent foramen ovale

A patent foramen ovale (PFO) is a normal fetal communication between the two atria that usually closes soon after birth. In up to 30% of people the PFO remains patent.

Sinus venosus atrial septal defect

This occurs high in the atrial septum, often close to the opening of the superior vena cava. It may be associated with partial anomalous pulmonary venous drainage.

Coronary sinus atrial septal defect

A coronary sinus defect is characterized by an unroofed coronary sinus and persistent left superior vena cava that drains into the left atrium. A dilated coronary sinus often suggests this defect. This can result is desaturation owing to a right-to-left shunt into the left atrium. The diagnosis can be made by injecting contrast agent into the left upper extremity.

Pathophysiology

The degree of shunting of blood across an ASD is related to the relative compliance of the two ventricles and the cross sectional area of the defect. In the neonate, right- and left-sided cardiac pressures are approximately equal and little or no shunting occurs. As PVR falls, left-to-right shunting develops. Symptoms are related to the ratio of the pulmonary to systemic flow (Q_p/Q_s). A ratio of less than 1.5 is well tolerated with minimal symptoms, whereas a ratio greater than 3 results in fatigue, dyspnoea and heart failure. An increase in pulmonary blood flow leads to increased pulmonary artery pressures and PVR. This, in turn, results in right ventricular hypertrophy and further elevations in pulmonary artery pressures. Eventually, the ventricular pressures may equalize, which causes bidirectional shunting across the defect. Uncommonly, in severe cases, the raised PVR can cause right-to-left shunting. This manifests as cyanosis, and is a type of Eisenmenger syndrome. Surgery will halt the progression to cyanotic disease, but, if it is delayed until PVR is fixed and irreversible, closure can precipitate acute right heart failure.

Natural history

ASDs do not often close spontaneously. Small, haemodynamically insignificant defects have no effect on life span, although there is a small increase in infective endocarditis and paradoxical embolism. Therefore, intravenous tubing and connectors must be rigorously checked for the presence of air.

Most individuals with an uncorrected ASD do not have significant symptoms through early adulthood. Left-to-right shunt and right ventricular volume overload may manifest in the third or fourth decade. About 70% develop symptoms by this time. Symptoms are typically decreased exercise tolerance, easy fatiguability, palpitations and syncope; 14% of adults with large ASDs manifest signs of congestive heart failure.

Large defects cause pulmonary vascular disease and decrease life expectancy. Patients who have defects repaired after 40 years of age have decreased survival compared with controls.

Atrial septal defect closure

The decision to repair any kind of ASD is based on clinical and echocardiographic information, including the size and location of the ASD, the magnitude and haemodynamic impact of the left-to-right shunt, and the presence and degree of pulmonary arterial hypertension. In general, elective closure is advised for all ASDs with evidence of right ventricular overload or with a clinically significant shunt (Q_p/Q_s >1.5). Lack of symptoms is not a contraindication for repair. In childhood, spontaneous closure of a secundum ASD may occur. However, in adulthood, spontaneous closure is unlikely. Patients may be monitored relatively conservatively for a period before intervention is advised.

Percutaneus atrial septal defect closure

With the development of specifically designed closure devices, this endovascular therapy for closure of an ASD is now one of the most commonly performed procedures. The technique is intended for closing secundum ASDs. Defects falling outside this area are not suitable for percutaneus closure. The choice of closure device depends on both the size and the margins of the defect. In general, there are two design types for closure. Daily aspirin in a dose of 3–5 mg kg^{-1} is recommended for a minimum period of 6 months after implantation of either type of device. The main complications associated with ASD closure include vessel injury, cardiac arrhythmia, cardiac perforation and device embolization.

Surgical atrial septal defect closure

Operative closure of ASDs prevents late complications and increases life expectancy. Closure is preferably carried out at 4–5 years of age.

Besides residual intracardiac shunts, children may rarely demonstrate persistent right ventricular dilation and abnormal ventricular septal motion postoperatively. Pulmonary venous obstruction, mitral valve problems and development of atrial arrhythmias could be other sequelae.

Diagnosis and preoperative evaluation

Uncomplicated defects are asymptomatic and are detected by auscultation of pulmonary flow murmurs and echocardiography. Significant defects are associated with frequent respiratory infections in children and fatigue and dyspnoea in adults. Patients with large defects present in early infancy with symptoms of increased pulmonary flow and heart failure, whereas smaller defects may remain undetected until adulthood. Examination reveals a pulmonary systolic murmur and fixed splitting of the second heart sound. There may be a tricuspid flow murmur.

Cardiac catheterization is not necessary for the preoperative evaluation of ASD repair, and is rarely carried out before surgery. If it has been performed, an increase in oxygen saturation will be apparent at the atrial level. There may be a small systolic gradient in the right ventricular outflow tract (RVOT) owing to increased blood flow.

Atrial septal defect and Eisenmenger syndrome

Patients with right-to-left shunts will appear cyanotic and have finger clubbing. Auscultation reveals an increased component to the second heart sound. Pulmonary regurgitation, if present, will cause a decrescendo diastolic murmur. Chest X-ray shows right ventricular hypertrophy, prominent pulmonary arteries and increased lung markings. Cardiac catheterization will confirm increased right ventricular and pulmonary artery pressures.

Anaesthetic technique

The choice of premedication assumes importance only in those patients with significant heart failure, low cardiac output and right-to-left shunting. In these patients, caution with sedatives is necessary as profound decompensation may occur with small doses.

The alveolar concentration of moderately soluble agents (e.g. sevoflurane) increases more rapidly in patients with left-to-right shunts during induction. Insoluble agents, such as nitrous oxide, are little influenced by the shunt.

Intravenous induction is relatively slower owing to the additional dilution by recirculating blood. An increased dose of induction agent may be necessary, with attention paid to the risks of overdosage. However, these theoretical concerns on the rate of induction are of relatively minor clinical importance compared with the nature of premedication and the adequacy of alveolar ventilation. Standard hypnotic agents (thiopentone, propofol) are used for intravenous induction. Opioids, such as fentanyl, are preferred for patients with advanced disease. Inhalational agents are usually used for maintenance of anaesthesia.

Potent inhalational agents depress cardiac output and decrease SVR and could potentially reverse a left-to-right shunt. However, this is unusual in the absence of marked pulmonary hypertension, when intravenous agents may be preferable.

The monitoring required does not differ from that appropriate for patients without ASDs. Invasive monitoring is indicated for repair of the defect itself.

Bibliography

Baum VC, Perloff JK. Anaesthetic implications of adults with congenital heart disease. *Anesth Analg* 1993; **76**: 1342–58.

Coté CJ, Lerman J, Todres ID (eds). *A Practice of Anesthesia for Infants and Children*, 4th edn. Philadelphia: WB Saunders, 2009.

Konstantinedes S, Geibel A, Olschewski M, *et al.* A comparison of surgical and medical therapy for atrial septal defect in adults. *N Engl J Med* 1995; **333**: 469–73.

Cross-references

Cardiac conduction defects, 132
Congenital heart disease in adult life, 141
Patients with heart failure, 159
Patients with pacemakers and implantable defibrillators, 161
Pulmonary hypertension, 164

Cardiac conduction defects

Peter Meijer

During anaesthesia, many conditions may induce cardiac arrhythmias, which are usually benign in the normal heart. In the presence of heart diseases, such as hypertrophic or dilated cardiomyopathy, myocarditis, congenital heart lesions, ischaemic heart disease and primary electrical abnormalities, the risks increase, and arrhythmias can be easily exacerbated by haemodynamic impairment, sympathetic tone modulation, adrenergic stimulation and the use of anaesthetic drugs.

Atrioventricular block

Atrioventricular (AV) block can be defined as a delay or interruption in the transmission of an impulse from the atria to the ventricles owing to an anatomical or functional impairment in the conduction system. The conduction disturbance can be transient or permanent, and can have many causes.

Conduction can be delayed, intermittent or absent. The commonly used terminology includes first-degree (slowed conduction without missing beats), second-degree (intermittent conduction, often in a regular pattern, e.g. 2:1, 3:2 or higher degrees of block), and third-degree or complete AV block.

First-degree atrioventricular heart block

This is caused by a delay in conduction through the AV node, which results in a P–R interval of greater than 0.2 s. This may be caused by ageing, ischaemia, myocarditis, cardiomyopathy, aortic regurgitation or any cause of increased vagal tone. This heart block is usually asymptomatic, and can easily be treated with atropine or glycopyrollate.

Second-degree atrioventricular heart block

Mobitz type I (Wenckebach) is caused by a delay in the conduction through the AV node and is characterized by progressive prolongation of the P–R interval until there is a dropped beat. This rhythm is usually asymptomatic and requires no specific therapy.

Mobitz type II is caused by a block below the AV node (usually in the His–Purkinje fibres). The ECG shows sudden block of conduction without progressive elongation of the P–R interval. The failure of one or more P waves to conduct to the ventricles can lead to dizziness, presyncope or syncope (called Stokes–Adams attacks).

An increase in heart rate as a result of exercise, atropine or atrial pacing can worsen the AV block. Conversely, vagal manoeuvres may slow the sinus rate, allowing for more time for excitability to recover in or below the bundle of His, and facilitate conduction.

A type II block is permanent and may progress to higher or even complete heart block. Therapy of Mobitz type II AV block begins by looking for and correcting reversible causes of slowed conduction, such as myocardial ischaemia, increased vagal tone and drugs that depress conduction.

If no reversible causes are present, the treatment of AV block involves the avoidance of medications that impair AV conduction (when possible) and permanent pacemaker placement in selected patients.

Right bundle branch block

Right bundle branch block (RBBB) is characterized by a QRS of >120 ms and RSR complexes in V1–V3 and wide S waves in V6. An RBBB is found in 1% of all hospitalized adults and does not necessarily imply serious cardiac disease. In patients with heart disease, new onset of an RBBB does predict a higher rate of coronary artery disease, congestive heart failure and mortality. There are no special anaesthetic concerns for patients with RBBB.

Left bundle branch block

The left bundle branch is made up by the smaller anterior fascicle with a blood supply from the septal branches of the left anterior descending artery and the larger posterior fascicle that usually has a dual blood supply from the left anterior descending and the right coronary artery.

A *left anterior fascicular block* causes delayed activation of the anterosuperior left ventricular wall and is characterized by left axis deviation of more than 60° with minimal prolongation of the QRS complex.

A *left posterior fascicular block* is less common than a left anterior fascicular block and results in delayed activation of the inferoposterior left ventricular wall. On the ECG a right-axis deviation greater than 120° with minimal prolongation of the QRS complex is present. Both hemiblocks are associated with coronary artery disease and, therefore, such patients should have a thorough preoperative evaluation.

Complete *left bundle branch block* (LBBB) presents with a QRS of >0.12 s and notched R waves in all leads. Incomplete LBBB shows a similar pattern of wide R waves in all leads, but the QRS complex is 0.10–0.12 s. These two blocks are also associated with coronary artery disease.

Bifascicular heart block

Bifasicular heart block is defined as a hemiblock and RBBB. This is also associated with coronary artery disease and this block may over time progress to complete heart block. However, in the absence of symptoms there is no evidence to support the placement of a prophylactic pacemaker prior to elective surgery with general or regional anaesthesia.

Implications for anaesthesia

In patients with a newly acquired RBBB or LBBB, there is an increased likelihood for development of coronary artery disease and congestive heart failure. Overall, the mortality rate is higher than in the general population. Although a bundle branch block is not an independent predictor of perioperative cardiac mortality, there is a risk of progression to a complete block. Anaesthetics, interaction of antiarrythmic drugs and anaesthetics, regional anaesthesia, disturbances of electrolytes and blood gases, intubation, venous or pulmonary catherization, surgical manipulation, hypothermia and myocardial ischaemia may initiate such a progression. The risk of progression is higher if a first- or second-degree AV block is also present.

Indications for temporary transcutaneous pacing are presented in the most recent guidelines of the American Heart Society. During administration of general anaesthesia, first-degree AV block with bifascicular block and first-degree AV block and LBBB are recommended as elective indications for temporary pacing, although there is little evidence to support the need for this approach. The use of isoprenaline and atropine may be useful.

A number of drugs may induce transient bradycardia that may require temporary pacing until the drug has been stopped. Some commonly used medications that may cause sinus node dysfunction or AV block are:

- digitalis (especially in the setting of hypokalaemia)
- older central acting antihypertensive agents (e.g. clonidine, methyldopa, guanethidine)
- β-Adrenergic blockers (e.g. metoprolol, atenolol)
- calcium channel blockers (e.g. verapamil, diltiazem)
- type 1A antiarrhythmic drugs (e.g. quinidine, procainamide, disopyramide)
- type 1C antiarrhythmic drugs (e.g. flecainide, propafenone)
- type III antiarrhythmic drugs (e.g. amiodarone, sotalol)
- tricyclic antidepressants (e.g. phenothiazines, lithium, phenytoin)
- cholinesterase inhibitors.

It is important that vagal stimulation and any combination of drugs likely to cause bradycardia are avoided while administering anaesthesia to these patients. Atropine, epinephrine and isoprenaline should be prepared prior to induction of anaesthesia in any case.

Third-degree (complete or trifascicular) atrioventricular heart block

This is present when there is no conduction from the atria to the ventricles. If the block is above the AV node the rate is 45–55 b.p.m. and the QRS complex is normal. If the block is below the AV node the rate will be 30–40 b.p.m. and the QRS complex will be wide in all leads. This block should always be treated with a temporary or permanent pacemaker. Isoprenaline (1–4 μg kg^{-1} min^{-1}) may be used while the pacemaker is being placed.

Atrioventricular dissociation

AV dissociation is not a diagnosis, but a symptom that is due to one of four causes:

1. Slowing of the dominant pacemaker of the heart, which allows the escape of a latent pacemaker.
2. Acceleration of a latent pacemaker that takes over control of the ventricles.
3. Block that prevents normal impulse conduction and allows the ventricles to beat under the control of a secondary pacemaker.
4. Any combination of these three.

Paroxysmal supraventricular tachycardia

Paroxysmal supraventricular tachycardia (PSVT) is characterized by a rapid regular rhythm with a narrow QRS complex and absence of the P wave. PSVT rhythms are usually abrupt in onset and termination. PSVT is easily distinguished from *rapid atrial fibrillation*, which is irregular, and from *rapid atrial flutter*, which has flutter waves.

PSVT is observed in 5% of normal adults and in patients with a pre-excitation syndrome, such as Wolff-Parkinson-White syndrome. There is no association with intrinsic heart disease. Changes in autonomic nervous system tone, anaesthetics and volume shifts can precipitate a PSVT.

In the Wolff-Parkinson-White syndrome the supraventricular tachycardia is caused by activation of accessory AV conduction pathways, which leads to early and rapid ventricular contractions. The ECG typically shows a short P–R interval (<0.12 s), a wide QRS (>0.12 s) and a delta wave.

Cardiomyopathy

Stefan De Hert

Cardiomyopathies consist of a group of conditions characterized by a progressive failure of ventricular function. Based on the cause of the disease, cardiomyopathies can be classified as intrinsic cardiomyopathies (the cause of the disease lies in the myocardium itself) or extrinsic cardiomyopathies (the cause of the disease lies outside the myocardium).

Intrinsic cardiomyopathies

Formerly, when no identifiable external cause for the cardiomyopathy could be found, it was classified as idiopathic cardiomyopathy. Nowadays, a number of causes of intrinsic cardiomyopathies have been identified including drug and alcohol toxicity, viral infections and genetic causes, but still cases of cardiomyopathy remain without identifiable cause (idiopathic).

Extrinsic cardiomyopathies

These include cardiomyopathies in which the primary pathology is outside the myocardium itself. These include:

- ischaemic heart disease
- hypertension
- valve disease
- congenital heart disease
- diabetes
- metabolic disease (e.g. amyloidosis, haemochromatosis).

In the Western world, ischaemic heart disease is the prime cause for cardiomyopathy. Of note, in South America, an important cause of cardiomyopathy is Chagas disease.

Independent from the cause, cardiomyopathies are also classified according to their morphological appearance, which is also related to the pathophysiological process.

Hypertrophic cardiomyopathy

Hypertrophic cardiomyopathy is characterized by an uneven myocardial hypertrophy. As thickening progresses, the heart stiffens. Hypertrophic cardiomyopathy can occur at any age, but the condition tends to be more severe with earlier onset. Most affected people have a family history of the disease and there are some genetic mutations that have been linked to hypertrophic cardiomyopathy.

A specific clinical entity is the *hypertrophic obstructive cardiomyopathy (HOCM),* which constitutes a pronounced hypertrophy at the level of the left ventricular outflow tract and may lead to left ventricular outflow obstruction. This pathology mimics severe aortic stenosis and may lead to catastrophic haemodynamic disturbances during anaesthesia if not anticipated and treated adequately.

Factors that increase outflow obstruction are:

- increased myocardial contractility
- tachycardia
- decreased preload
- decreased afterload.

Factors that decrease outflow obstruction are:

- decreased myocardial contractility
- slower heart rate
- increased preload
- increased afterload.

Dilated cardiomyopathy

This is the most common type of cardiomyopathy, which is characterized by a progressive dilatation of the ventricles leading to heart failure. The disease can occur at any age but is most frequently observed in middle-aged people and affects more men.

Restrictive cardiomyopathy

In the course of restrictive cardiomyopathy the heart muscle becomes progressively more rigid and less elastic. This will lead to severe impairment of the ventricular compliance and results in a clinical picture resembling constrictive pericarditis or tamponade. The impaired diastolic filling will ultimately lead to cardiac failure. While the disease may occur at any age, it is most frequently observed in older people.

Anaesthetic considerations

Preoperative evaluation

At the early stage of the disease patients with cardiomyopathy may have no signs and symptoms. However, with the progression of the disease the classical clinical symptoms of cardiac failure will present. These include breathlessness with exertion or even at rest, peripheral oedema, fatigue and rhythm disturbances. Since cardiomyopathy can be hereditary, an evaluation of the family history may offer valuable information.

Preoperative evaluation usually consists of a complete cardiological work-up including ECG, cardiac imaging (echocardiogram, MRI), blood tests and also cardiac catheterization with biopsy for diagnosis.

Intra- and postoperative management

Basically, patients with cardiomyopathy are patients with heart failure and they should be treated as such (see Patients with heart failure, p. 159). Special attention should be paid to the patient with a hypertrophic obstructive cardiomyopathy. In these patients it is of utmost importance that adequate filling of the ventricle is preserved and tachycardia is avoided at any stage of the perioperative period. Hypotension in these patients should primarily be treated by volume administration and control of the heart rate and *not* by the use of inotropic drugs. In these patients, the use of transoesophageal echocardiography may be of great value to guide therapy.

Bibliography

Amour J, Kersten JR. Diabetic cardiomyopathy and anesthesia. *Anesthesiology* 2008; **108**: 524–30.

Elliott P, Andersson B, Arbustini E, *et al.* Classification of the cardiomyopathies: a position statement of the European Society of Cardiology working group on myocardial and pericardial diseases. *Eur Heart J* 2007; **29**: 270–85.

Fontaine G, Gallais Y, Fornes P, *et al.* Arrhythmogenic right ventricular dysplasia/cardiomyopathy. *Anesthesiology* 2001; **95**: 250–4.

Kipps AK, Ramamoorthy C, Rosenthal DN, Williams GD. Children with cardiomyopathy: complications after noncardiac procedures with general anesthesia. *Pediatr Anesth* 2007; **17**: 775–81.

Poliac LC, Barron ME, Maron BJ. Hypertrophic cardiomyopathy. *Anesthesiology* 2006; **104**: 183–92.

Richardson P, McKenna W, Bristow M, *et al.* Report of the 1995 World Health Organization/ International Society and Federation of Cardiology Task Force on the definition and classification of cardiomyopathies. *Circulation* 1996; **93**: 841–2.

Cross-reference

Preoperative assessment of cardiovascular risk in non-cardiac surgery, 621

Children with congenital heart disease for non-cardiac surgery

Susanne Eberl

The global incidence of congenital heart diseases is approximately 9 in 1000 live births. Even in patients with corrected congenital heart disease, significant residual problems may remain. It is, therefore, very important for the anaesthetist to conduct a thorough preoperative evaluation and preparation, understand the pathophysiology of the disease and use proper anaesthetic agents.

Pathophysiology

Shunt lesions

With large defects, the direction and magnitude of shunting (Q_p/Q_s) is determined by the ratio of PVR and SVR. As defects become smaller, shunting becomes largely independent of changes in vascular resistance and is primarily determined by defect size. An arterial saturation of about 80% reflects an even shunt distribution between pulmonary and systemic circulation.

Right-to-left shunts

This means shunting of unsaturated blood from the right side to the left side of the heart and systemic circulation (cyanotic defect) with increased risk of (paradoxical) systemic air embolization. Therefore, careful attention must be paid to clear air from intravenous infusions and to use air and particle filters.

Tetralogy of Fallot, complete transposition of the great arteries, truncus arteriosus, single ventricle, aortopulmonary shunts, total anomalous pulmonary venous connection and Eisenmenger syndrome belong to this category.

Hypoxaemia and cyanosis are the most important consequences. This also means that each anaesthetic manoeuvre that increases PVR or decreases SVR additionally increases right-to-left shunt and thus adversely affects saturation. Inhalation induction may be delayed; intravenous induction accelerated.

Other problems include polycythaemia with an increased risk of cerebral/renal thrombosis, increased blood volume and viscosity, and coagulopathy with impaired platelet aggregation.

Because of the permanent hypoxic conditions and the enhanced pressure load of the right ventricle with increased cardiac work, this results in decreased cardiac reserve with stress.

Left-to-right shunts

Acyanotic congenital heart disease is associated with the shunting of blood from the left side to the right side of the heart and pulmonary circulation. This results in pulmonary overperfusion and volume overload of the right ventricle. This may progress to pulmonary hypertension with an increased risk of pulmonary hypertensive crisis and, because of the decreased cardiopulmonary reserve, to congestive heart failure. A pulmonary hypertensive crisis is characterized by a rapid increase in PVR to the point where pulmonary arterial pressure exceeds systemic blood pressure. The resulting right heart failure leads to a decrease in pulmonary blood flow, decreased cardiac output, hypoxia and biventricular failure.

ASD, VSD, AV septum defect and patent ductus arteriosus belong to this category.

Obstructive lesions

Obstructive lesions result in cardiac hypertrophy (either the right or the left ventricle) with the danger of potential myocardial ischaemia (especially subendocardial). Owing to a fixed cardiac output, the ventricle is unable to compensate for changes in vascular resistance. Complete obstructive lesions are dependent upon patency of the ductus arteriosus. Obstruction may be fixed or dynamic.

Right ventricular outflow tract obstructions

These include pulmonary stenosis or atresia, tricuspid atresia and Ebstein anomaly with intact ventricular septum.

Left ventricular outflow tract obstructions

These include coarctation of the aorta, interrupted aortic arch, aortic stenosis and atresia, and mitral stenosis.

Patients with ischaemic left myocardium can easily develop sudden serious arrhythmias that can lead to an unsuccessful reanimation setting.

Complex shunt lesions

These consist of outflow obstruction(s) plus central communication(s).

Preoperative management

Patient assessment also requires consideration of the physiological trespass imposed by anaesthesia and surgery. Children undergoing major procedures, as well as those with congestive heart failure, pulmonary hypertension or complex congenital heart disease are best managed in a specialized facility.

Patients may present with unrepaired, palliated or repaired lesions. Repairs may be physiological, but not anatomical, and may be followed by residual problems such as arrhythmias (especially atrial repairs), ventricular dysfunction, residual shunts, valvular stenosis or regurgitation, and pulmonary hypertension (especially in patients with Down syndrome).

It is essential to obtain all possible information (history and physical examination), especially that concerning previous cardiac evaluations, catheterizations and surgical procedures. Special attention should be directed towards cyanosis, dyspnoea, and symptoms and signs of congestive heart failure (poor feeding, perspiring while feeding, failure to thrive, hepatomegaly, tachypnoea and peripheral oedema).

Current medications should be reviewed and careful note taken of other medical problems, such as developmental delay, seizure disorders, reactive airway disease and other associated extracardiac congenital anomalies. It is important to record the patient's baseline oxygen saturation and its expected fluctuation range as well as exercise intolerance.

Investigations should be directed by the history and physical findings and may include chest X-ray, electrocardiogram, complete blood count, blood urea, creatinine, electrolytes, coagulation, cardiology consultation, echocardiogram and possible cardiac MRI or catheterization.

Premedication

Dehydration due to prolonged fasting should be avoided, especially in children with polycythaemia, to decrease the risk of thrombotic complications.

The utility of sedative premedication should be assessed on an individual basis. While it may be beneficial in certain instances (e.g. TOF, catecholamine-induced arrhythmias), it may be hazardous in children with decreased cardiopulmonary reserve or with significant increased PVR. Most centres use a dose of 0.5 mg kg^{-1} oral midazolam. A combination of midazolam and ketamine in syrup seems to increase sedation and anxiolysis without increasing side-effects such as salivation or excitation.

According to the AHA, endocarditic prophylaxis is recommended only for cyanotic congenital heart defects that have not been fully repaired, defects that have been completely repaired with prosthetic (artificial) material or a device (either placed by surgery or by catheter intervention) for the first 6 months after the repair procedure, and repaired congenital heart disease with residual defects (persisting leaks or abnormal flow) at the site or adjacent to the site of a prosthetic patch or prosthetic device.

For children, the recommended doses are: amoxicillin, 50 mg kg^{-1} initially and 25 mg kg^{-1} subsequently; or clindamycin, 10 mg kg^{-1} initially and 5 mg kg^{-1} subsequently (for other antibiotics, read the guidelines).

Induction

In most children intravenous access is established after inhalational induction. However, in children considered at high risk, such as those with severe left ventricular or right ventricular obstruction, severe cardiac dysfunction or pulmonary hypertension, consideration should be given for placement of intravenous access before induction.

Inhalational and volatile anaesthetics dilate the vascular bed and lower sympathetic responsiveness. Therefore, a reduced dosage and careful titration of any anaesthetic agents is required, especially in patients with decreased cardiac reserve or right-to-left shunts.

Thiopental and propofol are reasonable options for children who can tolerate mild decreases in myocardial contractility and SVR. They should be used with caution in those children with limited cardiac reserve, cyanotic defects or high sympathetic tone.

Etomidate is a useful agent in critically ill children. Ketamine as sole induction agent or in combination with etomidate may be advantageous when preservation of heart rate, blood pressure and ejection fraction seem to be important; it should be used in combination with an antisialagogue (e.g. glycopyrrolate). Opioids in combination with benzodiazepines provide excellent cardiovascular stability in children with congenital heart disease. An increased dose of muscle relaxants may be required if the circulatory time is prolonged.

Maintenance

Whether inhalational agents, additional opioids, regional blocks or other intravenous agents are used for maintenance depends on the patient's pathophysiology, the destabilizing effect of surgery and the individual preference of the anaesthetist.

Volatile anaesthetics are suitable in children with less severe disease. Ketamine or opioids may be used in children at risk of excessive myocardial depression with volatile anaesthesia.

Regional anaesthesia has been demonstrated to be safe and effective in children with congenital heart disease. Dealing with hypovolaemic children, those with a fixed cardiac output or children with coagulation abnormalities could be a contraindication for regional anaesthesia. Careful fluid management is essential.

Hypotension will lead to hypoxaemia in patients dependent upon shunts for pulmonary perfusion or to cardiac failure in those with outflow obstruction. A fluid challenge combined with a pure adrenergic agent such as phenylephrine helps in restoring perfusion and blood pressure.

Intraoperative monitoring

Standard paediatric anaesthetic monitoring is used. In children with cyanotic congenital heart disease the end-tidal CO_2 underestimates arterial carbon dioxide and the difference between the two is not constant. Invasive monitoring is indicated for children with advanced disease or for major surgery.

Airway and ventilation

Ventilation should be adjusted to maintain an optimum PVR by control of lung volume, end-expiratory pressure, carbon dioxide and oxygen tensions.

Hypoxaemia, and thus a drop in oxygen saturation, is mainly a problem of vascular resistances. Two possible solutions are: decreasing PVR (hyperventilation with 100% oxygen, low PEEP, alkalosis, reducing stress, deepen anaesthesia, muscle relaxants, pulmonary vasodilatation (NO, Flolan, iloprost, phosphodiesterase inhibitors)) or increasing SVR (volume, vasoconstrictors).

In patients with tetralogy of Fallot, increased catecholamine levels secondary to stress or stimulation may cause RVOT spasm and right-to-left shunting (hypercyanotic spells). The additional treatment consists of β-blockers.

Postoperative management

Monitoring and supplemental oxygen administration should be used until the child has fully recovered. The provision of adequate analgesia and careful fluid management are essential. Elective admission to a paediatric ICU should be considered for major procedures and for children with advanced cardiac disease or complex medical problems.

Bibliography

Carmosino MJ, Friesen RH, Doran A, Ivy DD. Perioperative complications in children with pulmonary hypertension undergoing noncardiac surgery or cardiac catheterization. *Anesth Analg* 2007; **104**: 521–7.

Diaz LK. Anesthesia and postoperative analgesia in pediatric patients undergoing cardiac surgery. *Paediatr Drugs* 2006; **8**: 223–33.

Poortmans G. Anaesthesia for children with congenital heart disease undergoing diagnostic and interventional procedures. *Curr Opin Anaesthesiol* 2004; **17**: 335–8.

Sümpelmann R, Osthaus WA. The pediatric cardiac patient presenting for noncardiac surgery. *Curr Opin Anaesthesiol* 2007; **20**: 216–20.

Vener DF, Tirotta CF, Andropoulos D, Barach P. Anaesthetic complications associated with the treatment of patients with congenital cardiac disease: consensus definitions from the Multi-Societal Database Committee for Pediatric and Congenital Heart Disease. *Cardiol Young* 2008; **18**(Suppl. 2): 271–81.

Walker A, Stokes M, Moriarty A. Anesthesia for major general surgery in neonates with complex cardiac defects. *Paediatr Anaesth* 2009; **19**: 119–25.

Cross-references

Cardiac conduction defects, 132
Congenital heart disease in adult life, 141
Patients with heart failure, 159
Patients with pacemakers and implantable defibrillators, 161
Pulmonary hypertension, 164

Congenital heart disease in adult life

Veronika Evers

The Euro Heart Survey estimated that currently approximately 1.2–2.7 million patients with congenital heart disease have reached adulthood, most of them after corrective or palliative surgery. Many have associated abnormalities as part of a syndrome.

Only a few types of congenital heart disease will offer in adulthood minimal or no significant residual problems. Less intricate forms of lesions may include patent ductus arteriosus ligation, uncomplicated repair of secundum or sinus atrial septal defect and uncomplicated repair of isolated ventricular septal defect (VSD) within the first years of life.

All more complex forms carry substantial risk of remaining and potentially progressive structural, electrophysiological, contractile, haemodynamic and end-organ abnormalities. As a result, most patients with congenital heart disease require lifelong care because the long-term outcome of the complex surgical procedures is often complicated by atrial or ventricular arrhythmias, heart failure, pulmonary hypertension or endocarditis.

Basic approach to congenital cardiac lesions

Adults with congenital heart disease can generally be divided into three groups:

1 patients who have never been operated on
2 patients who have received palliative treatment
3 patients who have undergone complete anatomical repair.

All these patients require a thorough preoperative history, physical examination and cardiological evaluation. It is crucial to understand that physiology and anatomy can vary significantly among patients who superficially carry identical diagnoses.

Most of the congenital cardiac defects can be classified into one of three groups:

1 those resulting in increased pulmonary blood flow
2 those resulting in decreased pulmonary blood flow
3 those resulting in obstruction of blood flow.

Cardiovascular impairment in these patients can usually be traced to one of these causes: arrhythmias, cardiac failure, pulmonary disease and hypoxaemia.

Arrhythmias

One of the most significant long-term problems for patients with congenital heart disease is the occurrence of arrhythmias or any other rhythm at a non-appropriate rate. These can be entirely asymptomatic, but may also cause haemodynamic deterioration and even sudden death.

Disorders of the conduction system are more common than disorders of impulse generation. Contributors to impaired conduction include altered anatomy and physiology, direct surgery-related injury and the presence of chronic hypoxaemia and haemodynamic stress.

Anaesthetic considerations

Drugs or combinations of medications that slow nodal pacemaker activity or myocardial conduction by decreasing sympathetic tone or by increasing vagal tone should be avoided. Premedication is useful to prevent anxiety-related excessive sympathetic activity preoperatively.

Atropine and isoprenaline increase the heart rate by increasing the automaticity of the nodal pacemaker, while AV conduction is significantly influenced. Atropine also protects against vagal and drug-induced bradycardia. Therefore, atropine administration should precede a dose of neostigmine or succinylcholine, but its routine use as premedication should be avoided.

The use of muscle relaxants without significant vagolytic activity such as the benzylisoquinolines (atracurium > mivacurium > cisatracurium), which do not block cardiac vagal (muscarinic) receptors, is recommended.

Although the placement of a permanent pacemaker is not indicated, a temporary pacing device should be readily available. Hypovolaemia must be avoided in patients with poor exercise tolerance or a demonstrated inability to increase heart rate, as cardiac output solely depends on stroke volume.

Cardiac failure

Cardiac failure can be defined as the metabolic imbalance of supply and demand caused by a low cardiac output and may be present in this patient population. Anaesthetic considerations are similar to those for patients with heart failure.

Pulmonary disease

Apart from their congenital heart defect, these patients also frequently present with congenital airway abnormalities, which places additional demands on the cardiovascular system. Pulmonary disorders in adults with congenital heart disease can generally be divided into three groups:

1 involvement of airway anatomy
2 altered pulmonary blood flow
3 nerve palsy.

An acute pulmonary disease may stress an already marginal compensated cardiovascular system as an additional burden to the point of failing.

Airway anatomy

Adults born with a complex form of congenital heart disease mostly have endured frequent and prolonged intubation and ventilation and have undergone extensive surgical or interventional manoeuvres. This predisposes them to acquired pathological subglottic or glottic pathologies.

Tracheal or bronchial stenosis can be caused by vascular rings or an enlarged heart, pulmonary artery or aorta. As artificial prosthetic conduits do not grow, adults with palliated or corrected congenital heart disease may, therefore, present with the sequelae of scar strictures of the airway.

Altered pulmonary blood flow

Pulmonary stenosis complicates many different forms of congenital cardiac lesions and generates an increased volume and/or pressure workload to the right heart.

Persistent elevation of pulmonary blood flow and/or pulmonary hypertension leads to a progressive increase in PVR. Furthermore, the large and small airways become obstructed, consecutively impairing gas exchange and altering pulmonary mechanics.

Nerve palsy

As a consequence of anatomical relations, the phrenic and recurrent laryngeal nerve can easily be compressed or stretched by the pathology of the aorta, pulmonary artery and/or atria. Similarly, surgical corrections of congenital heart disease carry a high risk for injury to these nerves. An ipsilateral Horner syndrome can be found as the result of sympathetic chain damage.

Anaesthetic considerations

The preoperative evaluation process should address three main issues relating to pulmonary alterations in patients with congenital heart disease:

1 associated abnormalities of the anatomy of the airway
2 the characteristics of pulmonary blood flow
3 intrinsic pulmonary disease must be differentiated from subsequent damage secondary to the cardiac disease.

Perioperatively, the problems of fixed pulmonary hypertension may present a major challenge to the anaesthetist. Anaesthetic considerations regarding choices of drugs and monitoring are similar to those for all patients with fixed pulmonary hypertension, with the exception that the altered anatomy and physiology with corrected congenital heart disease may offer an additional challenge. It is, therefore, suggested that care of such patients should primarily be done by anaesthetists with specific experience in this pathology.

Abnormal haemostasis may be present in these patients and appears to correlate with the degree of hypoxaemia and erythrocytosis. The mechanisms of the haemostatic defects, however, have not yet been fully defined. The coagulation deficits include thrombocytopenia, platelet dysfunction, hypofibrinogenaemia and accelerated fibrinolysis. Finally, patients with congenital heart disease with synthetic vascular conduits are often maintained on pharmacological anticoagulation.

Patients with cyanotic congenital heart disease are at risk for the development of perioperative thrombosis, because the increased red blood cell mass and abnormal platelet function induce sludging in the microcirculation. As peripheral venous blood directly accesses the systemic arterial circulation via a right-to-left shunt in patients with cyanotic congenital heart disease, paradoxical emboli originating in the lower extremities or pelvic veins may reach the brain. Also, air or particles injected in peripheral or central venous lines can be sources of paradoxical emboli.

The overall anaesthetic aim in patients with a cyanotic disease is to manage the shunt direction (Table 4.1), whereas the choice of anaesthetic comes second:

- ensure adequate hydration
- maintain systemic arterial blood pressure
- avoid increasing oxygen demand
- minimize PVR; optimize pulmonary blood flow.

Table 4.1 Factors affecting pulmonary vascular resistance (PVR)

Decrease in PVR	Increase in PVR
Increasing P_aO_2	Sympathetic stimulation Light anaesthesia Pain
Hypocarbia	Hypoxia
Alkalaemia	Acidaemia
Reduced intrathoracic pressure Spontaneous ventilation Normal lung volumes High frequency and jet ventilation	Increased intrathoracic pressure Controlled ventilation Atelectasis PEEP
Avoidance of sympathetic stimulation Deep anaesthesia	Hypercarbia
Pharmacological methods Isoprenaline Phosphodiesterase III inhibitors PG infusion (PGE_1 and PGI_2) Inhaled nitric oxide	Hypothermia

PEEP, positive end-expiratory pressure; PG, prostaglandin.

Hypoxaemia

In patients with congenital heart disease, chronic as opposed to acute hypoxaemia is a common symptom and is usually associated with reduced pulmonary blood flow and/or right-to-left shunting. Hypoxaemia is a concomitant feature of arrhythmias, concurrent cardiac failure and pulmonary disease.

Anaesthetic management

Preoperative assessment

The following questions should be answered:

1 Has the patient undergone corrective or palliative surgery, and, if so, what is the resulting anatomy and are there residual defects?
2 What is the patient's current status?
3 Is the patient cyanotic, with either obligatory right-to-left intracardiac shunting or mixing lesions? Does the patient have a functional single ventricle?
4 If acyanotic, is this a left-to-right shunting lesion or an obstructive lesion?
5 What is the proposed procedure and what anticipated effects will the procedure have on the patient's pathophysiology?
6 Does this patient need infective endocarditis prophylaxis?
7 Are there associated anomalies?

Preoperative fasting

Permitting patients to drink water preoperatively should be encouraged, especially in cyanotic and polycythaemic patients. There seems to be no evidence to suggest that a shortened fluid fast results in an increased risk of aspiration, regurgitation or related morbidity compared with the standard 'nil by mouth from midnight' fasting policy. Commencement of a preoperative intravenous infusion should be considered to avoid dehydration and decrease risk for thrombosis.

Preoperative medication

The use of sedation to alleviate preoperative anxiety must be individualized, in particular with regard to cyanotic and hypoxic or hypoxaemic patients.

Endocarditis prophylaxis

The 2007 AHA guidelines recommend endocarditis prophylaxis only in those settings associated with the highest risk of developing this complication, which are:

- prosthetic heart valves, including bioprosthetic and homograft valves
- prosthetic material used for cardiac valve repair
- prior history of endocarditis
- unrepaired cyanotic congenital heart disease, including palliative shunts and conduits
- completely repaired congenital heart defects with prosthetic material or device, whether placed by surgery or by catheter intervention, during the first 6 months after the procedure
- repaired congenital heart disease with residual defects at the site or adjacent to the site of the prosthetic device
- in the presence of substantial leaflet pathology and regurgitation in a transplanted heart.

Monitoring

- Clear all infusion lines of bubbles.
- Five-lead ECG, blood pressure (invasive is recommended), pulse oximetry.
- Capnography.
- Temperature.
- Defibrillator stand-by.

More invasive monitoring should be considered in patients with congenital heart disease undergoing large operations or in patients in a critical state.

Induction, maintenance and types of anaesthesia

Anaesthesic management relies on the complete understanding of the anatomical and pathophysiological impact of the cardiac malformation. The choice of the narcotic drug in general is of less importance than achieving the inevitable physiological goals in terms of contractility, preload and systemic and PVR. Once the goals are defined, appropriate agents, dosages and routes of administration can be selected.

The uptake of inhalational anaesthetics is influenced by the degree of intracardiac shunting and the patient's cardiac output. A right-to-left shunt causes a slow rate of uptake into the blood, leading to a prolonged induction. In these patients, intravenous induction of anaesthesia is quicker because a pulmonary transit is not necessary. A left-to-right shunt has a negligible effect on the uptake of anaesthetics as long as cardiac capacity and perfusion pressure are preserved.

Because venous return can be reduced by central regional anaesthesia, this method should be used cautiously and monitored carefully in patients in whom cardiac output is likely to be sensitive to reductions in preload. Intravenous fluid administration must be monitored carefully to avoid volume expansion or volume depletion. In contrast, peripheral nerve blocks are recommended whenever possible.

Conditions to be avoided perioperatively include:

- sympathetic stimulation/pain
- hypo-/hypervolaemia
- hypo-/hypercarbia
- acidaemia/alkalaemia
- hypoxia
- hypothermia
- atelectasis.

Postoperative considerations

Adult patients with congenital heart disease require close observation in the PACU. Patients with good haemodynamic results after minor non-cardiac surgery can be treated as any other. Patients with cyanotic congenital cardiac lesions are to be referred to an ICU or minimal medium care unit because of their intricate physiology and its sequelae, which need a close clinical and laboratory follow up.

Pregnancy and congenital heart disease

As a result of successful cardiac surgery in girls with congenital heart disease, women who had previously been unable to bear children or who would not have reached reproductive age are now presenting for obstetric and attending cardiological care. Nevertheless, one must keep in mind that the normal alterations in circulatory and respiratory physiology during pregnancy can still have deleterious effects on the mother with congenital heart disease and on her developing fetus. Especially the pregnancy-induced reduction in SVR will affect flow across right-to-left shunts.

Except for a potential increased risk of infective endocarditis, the management of labour and delivery in women with functionally mild unrepaired congenital heart disease and in women who have undergone successful cardiac surgery is the same as for normal pregnant women. The instant there are concerns about the functional adequacy of the heart and circulation, labour should be induced under controlled conditions if there are no obstetric contraindications to vaginal delivery.

Regardless of whether or not there has been surgical repair, the anticipation and management of labour delivery and the puerperium are crucial if risk is to be minimized in pregnant women with a functionally significant congenital cardiac malformation.

Caesarean delivery should be reserved as far as possible for obstetrical indications such as cephalopelvic disproportion, placenta praevia and preterm labour in a pregnant patient on oral anticoagulants. Regional anaesthesia has been used successfully, and especially segmental regional anaesthesia may attenuate haemodynamic stress during labour.

Bibliography

Baum VC, Perloff JK. Anesthetic implications of adults with congenital heart disease. *Anesth Analg* 1993; **76**: 1342–58.

Cannesson M, Collange V, Lehot JJ. Anesthesia in adult patients with congenital heart disease. *Curr Opin Anaesthesiol* 2009; **22**: 88–94.

Engelfriet P, Boersma E, Oechslin E, *et al.* The spectrum of adult congenital heart disease in Europe: morbidity and mortality in a 5 year follow-up period: the Euro Heart Survey on adult congenital heart disease. *Eur Heart J* 2005; **26**: 2325–33.

Warnes CA, Williams RG, Bashore TM, *et al.* ACC/AHA 2008 Guidelines for the Management of Adults with Congenital Heart Disease: a report of the American College of Cardiology/American Heart Association Task Force on Practice Guidelines (writing committee to develop guidelines on the management of adults with congenital heart disease). *Circulation* 2008; **118**: e714–833.

Wilson W, Taubert KA, Gewitz M, *et al.* Prevention of infective endocarditis: guidelines from the American Heart Association: a guideline from the American Heart Association Rheumatic Fever, Endocarditis, and Kawasaki Disease Committee, Council on Cardiovascular Disease in the Young, and the Council on Clinical Cardiology, Council on Cardiovascular Surgery and Anesthesia, and the Quality of Care and Outcomes Research Interdisciplinary Working Group. *Circulation* 2007; **116**: 1736–54.

Cross-references

Atrial septal defect, 129
Cardiac conduction defects, 132
Medical problems and obstetric anaesthesia, 474
Patients with heart failure, 159
Patients with pacemakers and implantable defibrillators, 161
Pulmonary hypertension, 164
Tetralogy of Fallot, 169

Coronary artery disease

Quanhong Zhou and Stefan De Hert

Cardiac complications are a major cause of perioperative morbidity and mortality. It is estimated that up to 1.4% of the general population and up to 3.9% of patients with cardiac disease suffer from major perioperative cardiac events. Especially vascular surgery patients are at increased risk with reported cardiac mortality rates of 1.5–2% for endovascular and 3–5% for open procedures. Mortality is mainly caused by the occurrence of perioperative myocardial infarction, which accounts for 10–40% of postoperative deaths.

Perioperative cardiac complications are caused either by myocardial ischaemia or by acute coronary thrombosis. Myocardial ischaemia may result from an increase in myocardial oxygen demand (tachycardia, hypertension, pain) and/or a decreased myocardial oxygen supply (hypotension, vasospasm, tachycardia, hypoxia, anaemia). Coronary plaque rupture may be caused by all factors that increase intracoronary wall stress. In addition, the presence of a hypercoagulable state, leukocyte activation and activation of the inflammatory response may greatly contribute to the pathophysiology of coronary artery occlusion.

The preoperative assessment and perioperative management of patients with coronary artery disease have been addressed recently both in the USA and in Europe, and published guidelines are now available.

Preoperative assessment

Prediction of cardiac risk

Risk stratification evaluates the risk of each particular patient suffering an adverse perioperative cardiac event. This may help to guide medical decisions and to determine optimal therapy for these patients.

The *Revised Cardiac Risk Index* allows identification of patients with an increased cardiac risk and has become one of the most widely used risk indices. It assigns 1 point for the presence of one of the following six risk factors: high-risk surgical procedure, history of ischaemic heart disease, history of congestive heart failure, history of cerebrovascular accident, preoperative treatment with insulin or a serum creatinine greater than 2.0 mg dL^{-1}. The estimated risk of major cardiac complications for indices 0, 1, 2 and 3 or higher are 0.4% (range 0.1–0.8%), 1.0% (range 0.5–1.4%), 2.4% (range 1.3–3.5%) and 5.4% (range 2.8–7.9%), respectively.

Preoperative assessment of the cardiac patient

The recent guidelines have proposed a stepwise approach for the perioperative cardiac assessment and management of cardiac patients scheduled for non-cardiac surgery.

The first step determines the urgency of surgery. In cases of urgent surgery, one should proceed immediately to surgery and take adequate measures for perioperative surveillance and treatment if indicated. Further risk stratification and risk factor management can then be planned during the immediate postoperative period.

If there is no need for emergency surgery, patients are screened for the presence of active cardiac conditions (Box 4.1). If one of these conditions is present, they should be further evaluated and, when necessary,

Box 4.1 Active cardiac conditions

- Unstable coronary syndromes:
  - unstable or severe angina
  - recent myocardial infarction (within 30 days)
- Decompensated heart failure
- Significant arrhythmias:
  - high-grade atrioventricular block
  - symptomatic ventricular arrhythmias
  - supraventricular arrhythmias with uncontrolled ventricular rate (>100 beats per minute at rest)
  - symptomatic bradycardia
  - newly recognized ventricular tachycardia
- Severe valvular disease:
  - severe aortic stenosis (mean pressure gradient >40 mmHg, area <1 cm^2 or symptomatic)
  - symptomatic mitral stenosis

treated. For all these conditions, the potential benefits of delaying surgery for further evaluation and/or to optimize treatment must be weighed against the risk of delaying the surgical procedure. With respect to a previous recent myocardial infarction, it is recommended to wait for 4–6 weeks before performing elective surgery.

If no active cardiac conditions are present, the next step is to assess the risk of surgery (Box 4.2). Many surgical procedures are associated with a low risk of perioperative complications even in high-risk patients. In such cases, it is recommended to proceed with planned surgery. In the case of intermediate- or high-risk surgery, further assessment of the patient's physical status is indicated.

Box 4.2 Surgical risk stratification

- High risk (cardiac risk >5%):
  - aortic surgery
  - major vascular surgery
  - peripheral vascular surgery
- Intermediate risk (cardiac risk 1–5%)
  - intraperitoneal and intrathoracic surgery
  - carotid endarterectomy
  - head and neck surgery
  - orthopaedic surgery
  - prostate surgery
- Low risk (cardiac risk <1%)
  - endoscopic procedures
  - superficial procedures
  - cataract surgery
  - breast surgery
  - ambulatory surgery

Subsequently, the patient's functional capacity is evaluated. When a patient is capable of performing an activity equal to or greater than 4 metabolic equivalents (METs) without symptoms, the recommendation is to proceed with surgery. If, however, the patient is symptomatic or the functional capacity of the patient is unknown, further assessment is indicated.

Which preoperative tests?

The ultimate aim of additional preoperative testing is to provide an objective measure of functional capacity, and to identify the importance of possible preoperative myocardial ischaemia and rhythm disturbances. Several non-invasive tests have been suggested to answer these questions.

Resting 12-lead electrocardiogram

The value of a preoperative resting 12-lead ECG is controversial. The guidelines still recommend it for patients with at least one clinical risk factor who will undergo vascular surgical procedures and for those patients with known coronary heart disease, peripheral arterial disease or cerebrovascular disease who are undergoing intermediate-risk surgical procedures.

Non-invasive evaluation of left ventricular function

Preoperative resting left ventricular function can be evaluated by echocardiography, radionuclide angiography and contrast ventriculography. While routine perioperative evaluation of left ventricular function is not recommended, it is considered useful in patients with dyspnoea of unknown origin, in those with current or prior heart failure and in those with worsening dyspnoea or other change in clinical status.

Stress testing

Preoperative stress testing is recommended in patients with active cardiac conditions in whom non-cardiac surgery is planned and who should be evaluated and treated before surgery and in patients with three or more clinical risk factors and a poor functional capacity (<4 METs) who require vascular surgery. It is important to note that such testing should only be performed if it will change management.

In patients who cannot exercise, two alternative techniques can be used to assess the importance of the coronary artery disease. One technique is to increase myocardial oxygen demand mainly by increasing heart rate (by pacing or dobutamine); the other is to induce a hyperaemic response by pharmacological vasodilators, such as dipyridamole or adenosine.

The most commonly used imaging techniques include echocardiography and radionuclide myocardial perfusion imaging methods. Although most currently applied tests have a satisfying sensitivity and specificity, dobutamine stress echocardiography seems to have a better diagnostic performance, especially in situations of valvular or left ventricular dysfunction.

Preoperative treatment

Revascularization

The potential benefits of preoperative coronary revascularization remain a point of debate. Basically, the indications for preoperative coronary revascularization are identical to those in the non-operative setting. This means that revascularization should be considered in patients with stable angina who have significant left main coronary artery disease, three-vessel disease, and two-vessel disease with a significant stenosis of the proximal left anterior descending coronary artery and either an ejection fraction less than 50% or demonstrable ischaemia on non-invasive testing. Also patients with unstable angina, those with non-ST-segment elevation myocardial infarction and those with acute ST-segment elevation myocardial infarction may benefit from preoperative revascularization. Finally, in patients with stable coronary artery disease, prophylactic coronary revascularization is not considered useful.

Recent evidence has indicated that prophylactic surgical revascularization is associated with a lower incidence of postoperative myocardial infarction after the subsequent non-cardiac surgery than percutaneous coronary interventions. This difference was attributed to a more complete revascularization.

Percutaneous coronary revascularization necessitates postprocedural administration of antiplatelet therapy, the duration of which depends on the type of stent used. Since antiplatelet therapy may increase the risk of perioperative bleeding, these drugs are usually discontinued at the time of surgery. It has been recognized for some time that such action may have disastrous consequences for the surgical patient and therefore specific guidelines have been developed for the management of such patients.

With respect to potential preoperative revascularization by percutaneous coronary angioplasty, a strategy of balloon angioplasty or bare-metal stent placement followed by 4–6 weeks of dual antiplatelet therapy is recommended. In patients who have received drug-eluting coronary stents and who need an urgent surgical procedure, necessitating the discontinuation of thienopyridine therapy, it is suggested that aspirin therapy should be continued and thienopyridine should be restarted as soon as possible. Elective non-cardiac surgery is not recommended within 4–6 weeks of bare-metal coronary stent implantation or within 12 months of drug-eluting coronary stent implantation in patients in whom thienopyridine therapy, or the dual therapy aspirin–thienopyridine, will need to be discontinued perioperatively. Finally, after balloon angioplasty, elective non-cardiac surgery should also be postponed for at least 4 weeks.

Medical treatment

β-Blockers

The safety of perioperative β-blockade has recently been questioned with the publication of the results of the POISE trial. This study showed a beneficial effect of a high-dose metoprolol controlled-release therapy on the risk of perioperative myocardial infarction, but this was at the cost of an increased risk of stroke and overall mortality. It was indicated, however, that, in particular, the initiation time and dose of β-blocker therapy, tight dose adjustments for heart rate control and a correct estimation of the underlying cardiac risk of the individual patient are important factors that may determine the effectiveness of the therapy.

Currently, it is recommended to continue β-blocking therapy in patients who are already on β-blocking medication. Patients at high cardiac risk undergoing vascular surgery are also believed to benefit from perioperative β-blocking therapy.

Statins

Statins were initially prescribed because their lipid-lowering properties seem highly effective in the secondary prevention of cardiac events. Different trials in patients undergoing coronary artery surgery have shown a beneficial effect of statin therapy on outcome. More recently, these positive effects have also been observed in major non-cardiac surgery with a significant reduction in postoperative cardiovascular morbidity and mortality.

It is recommended that statins should be continued for all patients scheduled for non-cardiac surgery and currently taking this medication. For patients with or without clinical risk factors undergoing vascular surgery, statins are considered reasonable. For patients with at least one clinical risk factor and scheduled for intermediate-risk surgery, statin therapy can be considered.

Others

Acetylsalicylic acid has a key role in the primary and secondary prevention of cardiovascular disease and it is commonly used, in association with clopidogrel, for the prevention of coronary stent thrombosis. Its potential beneficial effect in the perioperative period of non-cardiac surgery is less well established.

Concerns with regard to perioperative bleeding complications have been a frequent reason to interrupt this therapy. It was suggested that acetylsalicylic acid should only be discontinued if it may cause bleeding risks with increased mortality or if sequelae are similar to the expected cardiovascular risks of acetylsalicylic acid withdrawal. Acetylsalicylic acid non-adherence or withdrawal was reported to be associated with a threefold higher risk of major cardiac events.

The potential beneficial effects of perioperative α_2-agonists and calcium channel blocker remain to be definitively established. Nitrates may be considered for the prevention of myocardial ischaemia, although really strong evidence is missing about the potential effects on outcome. The strategy with regard to ACEs is controversial. Severe hypotension has been described with induction of anaesthesia, especially in the presence of concomitant ACE-inhibitor use. The severity of the hypotension seems related to the dosage of the daily therapy. Therefore, withdrawal on the day of surgery may be considered when they are prescribed for hypertension, but they should be resumed after surgery as soon as the haemodynamic status is stable. In stable patients with left ventricular dysfunction it is recommended that ACE therapy should be continued.

Intraoperative strategies

ST-segment monitoring

The occurrence of perioperative ST-segment changes has been associated with cardiac morbidity and mortality in patients undergoing non-cardiac surgery. Intra- and postoperative ST-segment monitoring with computerized ST-segment analysis is considered useful for patients with known coronary artery disease or those undergoing vascular surgery.

Pulmonary artery catheter

Perioperative use of a pulmonary artery catheter remains a controversial issue. While significant information can be obtained from its use, no differences have been observed in survival or cardiovascular morbidity compared with standard care in patients who underwent major non-cardiac surgery.

Transoesophageal echocardiography

The use of transoesophageal echocardiography has gained wide acceptance in the setting of cardiac surgery. However, to date there is not sufficient evidence to support its routine use as a diagnostic monitor or to guide therapy during non-cardiac surgery.

Blood glucose concentration

The impact of a tight blood glucose concentration on perioperative morbidity and mortality has been the subject of several recent studies. It was suggested that control of blood glucose concentrations to less than 150 mg dL^{-1} in the perioperative period may improve outcome and minimize the risk of severe hypoglycaemia in anaesthetized patients. The American College of Endocrinology recommends that preprandial glucose should be less than 110 mg dL^{-1}, maximal glucose should not exceed 180 mg dL^{-1} and, in the ICU, blood glucose concentration should be controlled to less than 110 mg dL^{-1}.

Anaesthetic management

Neuraxial techniques can result in sympathetic blockade and cause a decrease in preload and afterload. Although initially some randomized controlled trials have suggested that the use of neuraxial techniques might have beneficial effects on outcome, these data have not been unequivocally confirmed in more recent studies on larger patient populations.

A comparison of the effects on outcome of general anaesthesia with opioid analgesia to combined general-epidural anaesthesia and analgesia in intra-abdominal aortic, gastric, biliary and colon surgery revealed no overall differences in death or major complications. It seems that, to date, there is insufficient evidence to confirm (or deny) that postoperative analgesic techniques affect major postoperative morbidity and mortality.

In recent years, increasing evidence has indicated that volatile anaesthetic agents may have cardioprotective properties. In the setting of coronary artery surgery, the use of these drugs was shown to be associated with a better preservation of postoperative myocardial function and less evidence of postoperative myocardial damage. In non-cardiac surgery, however, there is at the moment no such evidence.

Other measures to be taken in the perioperative period that may help to improve outcome include maintenance of normothermia and adequate perioperative pain management.

Postoperative strategies

Pain management

Postoperative pain may increase sympathetic drive and therefore constitute a risk factor for the development of postoperative cardiac complications. However, the potential benefits of invasive analgesic techniques should be weighed against the potential dangers of their application. This is especially a concern in patients on antithrombotic or anticoagulant drugs.

Patient-controlled analgesia may be an alternative for postoperative pain relief. Non-steroidal anti-inflammatory drugs and cyclo-oxygenase 2 inhibitors may promote heart and renal failure as well as thromboembolic events and should therefore be avoided in patients with myocardial ischaemia.

Postoperative myocardial infarction

A perioperative myocardial infarction has been associated with a 30–50% perioperative mortality and reduced long-term survival. Therefore, accurate diagnosis and prompt treatment is essential.

Perioperative myocardial infarction can be documented by assessing clinical symptoms, serial ECGs, cardiac-specific biomarkers, comparative ventriculographic studies, and radioisotopic or magnetic resonance studies.

Measurements of troponin T or I have been shown to indicate myocardial damage with smaller amounts of injury. Currently, there seem to be no clear-cut standard criteria for the diagnosis of perioperative myocardial infarction in patients undergoing non-cardiac surgery. Postoperative troponin measurement is recommended in patients with electrocardiographic changes or chest pain typical of the acute coronary syndrome. Recently, assessment of pro-B-type natriuretic peptide has been gaining interest as a predictor of adverse events and outcome after non-cardiac surgery.

Bibliography

De Hert SG. Preoperative cardiovascular assessment in noncardiac surgery: an update. *Eur J Anaesthesiol* 2009; **26**: 449–57.

Devereaux PJ, Goldman L, Cook DJ, *et al.* Perioperative cardiac events in patients undergoing noncardiac surgery: a review of the magnitude of the problem, the pathophysiology of the events and methods to estimate and communicate risks. *CMAJ* 2005; **173**: 627–34.

Fleisher LA, Beckman JA, Brown KA, *et al.* ACC/AHA 2007 guidelines on perioperative cardiovascular evaluation and care for noncardiac surgery: a report of the American College of Cardiology/American Heart Association Task Force on Practice Guidelines (writing committee to revise the 2002 guidelines on perioperative cardiovascular evaluation for noncardiac surgery). *Circulation* 2007; **116**: e418–e500.

Fleisher LA, Beckman JA, Brown KA, *et al.* 2009 ACCF/AHA focused update on perioperative beta blockade incorporated into the ACC/AHA 2007 guidelines on perioperative cardiovascular evaluation and care for noncardiac surgery. *J Am Coll Cardiol* 2009; **54**: e13–e118.

Poldermans D, Bax JJ, Boersma E, *et al.* Task Force for Preoperative Cardiac Risk Assessment and Perioperative Cardiac Management in Non-cardiac Surgery of European Society of Cardiology (ESC); European Society of Anaesthesiology (ESA). Guidelines for pre-operative cardiac risk assessment and perioperative cardiac management in non-cardiac surgery: the Task Force for Preoperative Cardiac Risk Assessment and Perioperative Cardiac Management in Non-cardiac Surgery of the European Society of Cardiology (ESC) and endorsed by the European Society of Anaesthesiology (ESA). *Eur J Anaesthesiol* 2010; **27**: 92–137.

Cross-references

Cardiopulmonary exercise testing, 600
Coronary artery bypass grafting, 580
Preoperative assessment of cardiovascular risk in non-cardiac surgery, 621

Hypertension

Peter Meijer

Hypertension is a common disease and, when untreated, is associated with increased risk of mortality by stroke and congestive heart disease in the non-surgical setting. The perioperative evaluation is a unique opportunity to identify patients with hypertension and initiate appropriate therapy.

As a universally measured variable with a recognized association with coronary artery disease, hypertension serves as a useful marker for potential coronary artery disease. Untreated hypertension can result in exaggerated intraoperative blood pressure fluctuation with associated electrocardiographic evidence of myocardial ischaemia.

Perioperative risks

Pre-existing hypertension can induce a variety of cardiovascular responses that potentially increase the risk of surgery. These include diastolic dysfunction from left ventricular hypertrophy and systolic dysfunction leading to congestive heart failure, renal impairment, and cerebrovascular and coronary occlusive disease. The level of risk is dependent upon the severity of hypertension. Much of the evidence for the impact of preoperative hypertension comes from uncontrolled studies performed before more effective management was available. Furthermore, it is still unclear whether postponing surgery to achieve blood pressure control will lead to reduced cardiac risk.

The American College of Cardiology/American Heart Association (ACC/AHA) guidelines list uncontrolled hypertension as a 'minor' risk factor for perioperative cardiovascular events. However, when hypertension has caused end-organ disease, such as congestive heart failure and renal insufficiency, the probability of adverse cardiac outcome in the perioperative period increases significantly.

Preoperative screening

Because intraoperative ischaemia correlates with postoperative cardiac morbidity, it follows that control of blood pressure preoperatively may help to reduce the risk for perioperative ischaemia. Although an elevated blood pressure on an initial recording in a patient with previously undiagnosed or untreated hypertension has been shown to correlate with blood pressure lability under anaesthesia, the definition of the severity of hypertension rests with subsequent recordings in a non-stressful environment. In patients undergoing therapy for hypertension, a thorough review of current medications and dosages, along with awareness of known intolerance to previously prescribed drugs, is essential.

The physical examination should include a search for target-organ damage and evidence of associated cardiovascular pathology. A fundoscopic eye examination may provide useful data regarding the severity and chronicity of the hypertension. The physical examination and simple laboratory tests can eliminate some of the rare causes of hypertension. Further evaluation to exclude secondary hypertension is rarely warranted before surgery. If phaeochromocytoma is a serious possibility, surgery should be delayed to permit its exclusion because operative mortality may be as high as 80% in unsuspected cases. A loud abdominal bruit may suggest renal artery stenosis. A radial to femoral artery pulse delay suggests coarctation of the aorta, whereas hypokalaemia in the absence of diuretic therapy raises the possibility of hyperaldosteronism.

Management of chronic antihypertensive medication

Oral antihypertensive medications should be continued up to the time of surgery. With few exceptions, continuing antihypertensive medications is relatively safe. Furthermore, abruptly discontinuing some medications (β-blockers and clonidine) may be associated with a significant rebound hypertension. Most antihypertensive agents can be continued until the time of surgery, taken with small sips of water on the morning of surgery.

β-Blockers

β-Blockers reduce intraoperative myocardial ischaemia. In addition to a rise in blood pressure, withdrawal in patients with underlying coronary disease can lead to accelerated angina, myocardial infarction or sudden death. Atenolol or bisoprolol given before surgery to patients with, or at high risk of, coronary heart disease has been shown to decrease mortality. However, more recently, the POISE study demonstrated that the protective effect on the perioperative myocardial infarction rate of routine administration of perioperative β-blocking therapy was at the expense of a higher incidence of stroke and increased mortality. Therefore, routine administration of β-blockers in the absence of dose titration is not recommended in patients not currently taking β-blockers who are undergoing non-cardiac surgery. Given the association between hypotension or bradycardia and morbidity or mortality from the POISE trial, the haemodynamic effects of perioperative β-blockade must be incorporated and considered in any β-blocker protocol, with the goal of avoidance of bradycardia and hypotension.

Diuretics

Patients in whom chronic diuretic therapy has caused hypokalaemia may have potentiation of the effects of muscle relaxants used during anaesthesia, as well as predisposition to cardiac arrhythmias and paralytic ileus. Physicians should be aware of the potential perioperative risks associated with diuretics and pay close attention to volume and potassium replacement.

Angiotensin-converting enzyme inhibitors and angiotensin II receptor blockers

Angiotensin-converting enzyme (ACE) inhibitors and angiotensin II receptor blockers can theoretically blunt the compensatory activation of the renin–angiotensin system during surgery and result in prolonged hypotension. One study of 150 vascular surgery patients found that the incidence of hypotension during anaesthetic induction was significantly lower in patients who stopped taking captopril or enalapril the evening before surgery than in those who took the medication on the morning of surgery. A high incidence of severe hypotension in patients on an angiotensin II receptor blocker who underwent general anaesthesia has also been reported.

Although there are insufficient data upon which recommendations can be based, it seems reasonable to continue these drugs in patients who are taking them for the management of hypertension. On the other hand, it is also reasonable to withhold them on the morning of surgery in patients who are taking them for congestive heart failure in whom the baseline blood pressure is low, to avoid significant hypotension during the induction of anaesthesia.

Calcium channel blockers

Patients receiving calcium channel blockers may have an increased incidence of postoperative bleeding, probably because of inhibition of platelet aggregation. The multiple benefits of these drugs probably outweigh the small risk of continued therapy.

Postoperative hypertension

A history of hypertension preoperatively is the most important risk factor for postoperative hypertension. Other factors contributing to the development of hypertension are pain (35%), excitement on emergence from anaesthesia (16%) and hypercarbia (15%).

Postoperative hypertension usually begins within 30 minutes of the completion of surgery and lasts approximately 2 hours. On the other hand, some patients with pre-existing hypertension may experience normalization of blood pressure as a non-specific response to surgery. This response can persist for months, usually followed by a gradual return to preoperative levels.

Indications for therapy

Any patient who experiences a marked rise in blood pressure following surgery should be treated immediately. First, common causes of hypertension, such as pain, agitation, hypercarbia, hypoxia, hypervolaemia and bladder distension, should be excluded or treated.

Patients on chronic antihypertensive therapy should resume their usual medications postoperatively as needed. Those who cannot take oral medications should be given a comparable alternative. A number of parenteral antihypertensive medications are available for patients who are unable to take oral medications postoperatively. Most useful are sodium nitroprusside, nicardipine, labetalol and esmolol.

β-Blockers and clonidine should be continued because of the risk of a withdrawal syndrome resulting in excessive hypertension. For others, a comparable parenteral alternative is available. Patients taking diuretics may be given parenteral furosemide or bumetanide. Parenteral propranolol, labetalol or esmolol is available for patients taking β-blockers. Special attention is needed to restart ACE inhibitors in the postoperative period. These should only be restarted after the patient is normovolaemic, to avoid renal dysfunction.

Therapy should be considered for patients with a sustained systolic blood pressure above 180 mmHg or diastolic blood pressure greater than 110 mmHg, once common causes have been excluded or treated.

Bibliography

Casadei B, Abuzeid H. Is there a strong rationale for deferring elective surgery in patients with poorly controlled hypertension? *J Hypertens* 2005; **23**: 19–22.

Chobanian AV, Bakris GL, Black HR, *et al.* The Seventh Report of the Joint National Committee on Prevention, Detection, Evaluation, and Treatment of High Blood Pressure: the JNC 7 report. *J Am Med Assoc* 2003; **289**: 2560–72.

Fleisher LA, Beckman JA, Brown KA, *et al.* 2009 ACCF/AHA focused update on perioperative beta blockade incorporated into the ACC/AHA 2007 guidelines on perioperative cardiovascular evaluation and care for noncardiac surgery. *J Am Coll Cardiol* 2009; **54**: e13–e118.

Poldermans D, Bax JJ, Boersma E, *et al.* Task Force for Preoperative Cardiac Risk Assessment and Perioperative Cardiac Management in Non-cardiac Surgery of European Society of Cardiology (ESC); European Society of Anaesthesiology (ESA). Guidelines for pre-operative cardiac risk assessment and perioperative cardiac management in non-cardiac surgery: the Task Force for Preoperative Cardiac Risk Assessment and Perioperative Cardiac Management in Non-cardiac Surgery of the European Society of Cardiology (ESC) and endorsed by the European Society of Anaesthesiology (ESA). *Eur J Anaesthesiol* 2010; **27**: 92–137.

Cross-references

Patients with heart failure, 159

Preoperative assessment of cardiovascular risk in non-cardiac surgery, 621

Ischaemia–reperfusion injury

Stefan De Hert and Benedikt Preckel

Interruption of blood flow through the coronary circulation will induce myocardial ischaemia. Early restoration of blood flow is necessary to prevent myocardial cell death. However, reperfusion of the myocardium may itself result in tissue damage. This phenomenon is called reperfusion injury and it may manifest as arrhythmias, reversible contractile dysfunction (myocardial stunning), endothelial dysfunction and ultimately irreversible reperfusion injury with myocardial cell death. This lethal reperfusion injury may result from two mechanisms, which are necrosis and apoptosis.

Myocardial stunning

Myocardial stunning refers to the occurrence of a transient contractile dysfunction despite restoration of blood flow to the previously ischaemic myocardium. The pathogenesis of reperfusion injury still is not fully elucidated but several mechanisms are involved. Although the major consistent metabolic abnormality in the stunned myocardium is a reduction of the adenosine triphosphate (ATP) concentration in the cells, ATP depletion as such does not seem to play a major causal role in the development of reperfusion injury. Instead, release of reactive oxygen species and the disruption of the normal intracellular calcium homeostasis seem to be the major mechanisms involved in the pathogenesis of reperfusion injury. Mitochondrial dysfunction has a pivotal role in this and the key component in the development of ischaemia–reperfusion injury is the opening of a non-specific pore in the inner mitochondrial membrane, which is the mitochondrial permeability transition pore (MPTP). Normally this pore is closed, but in conditions of stress such as reperfusion of the heart after a period of ischaemia, the MPTP opens. This opening causes the mitochondriae to become uncoupled, resulting in a loss of their ATP-generating capacity, loss of the ionic homeostasis and ultimately necrotic cell death. In addition, transient opening and subsequent closure of the MPTP may occur and lead to the release of cytochrome C and other proapoptotic molecules that initiate the apoptotic cascade. Apoptosis is a controlled cellular response to moderate cell injury.

Myocardial preconditioning

The heart has the ability to protect itself against the consequences of ischaemia. Indeed, short episodes of ischaemia and reperfusion before a sustained ischaemic event, known as ischaemic preconditioning, reduce myocardial infarct size. Preconditioning represents a potent and consistently reproducible method of protection against ischaemia. In addition to a reduction in infarct size it also diminishes post-ischaemic cardiac dysfunction and arrhythmias. Ischaemic preconditioning typically consists of two windows of cardioprotection: an *early phase* that occurs immediately and produces a strong protection but has a limited duration of about 2 hours, and a *late phase* or second window which occurs about 24 hours after the initial stimulus, induces less protection but lasts for as long as 3 days.

Although the mechanisms involved in myocardial preconditioning still remain to be fully elucidated, several steps have been identified. Signalling substances trigger several intracellular signalling pathways. These pathways mainly involve a post-translational modification of proteins (translocation and phosphorylation). Protein kinase C plays a central role as intracellular mediator, but tyrosine kinase and mitogen-activated protein kinases are also involved. During the early phase of preconditioning, the cellular memory is believed to be related to translocation of protein kinase C from cytosol to the different cellular membranes, which results in a more rapid activation of protein kinase C during the prolonged ischaemic period. Several structures have been involved as end-effectors. However, the majority of experimental findings now indicate that preservation of mitochondrial function, which occurs as a consequence of mitochondrial K_{ATP} channel activation (opening), is of pivotal importance for the cardioprotective effect against ischaemia. Prevention of MPTP opening is believed to have a key role in the protection offered by the preconditioning stimulus. This results in preservation of mitochondrial function during reperfusion, thereby preventing the activation of necrotic and/or apoptotic pathways. During the late phase of preconditioning, cellular memory is thought to be related to the synthesis or activation of proteins that have a cytoprotective effect, such as the induction of several antioxidant enzymes, or the synthesis of heat-shock proteins that are involved in the stabilization of the cytoskeleton.

Ischaemic preconditioning also occurs in humans, but the clinical application of an ischaemic preconditioning protocol carries the risk of further worsening function and cell survival in an already jeopardized myocardium.

Protection against myocardial ischaemia–reperfusion injury by preconditioning can also be obtained with anaesthetic agents. Apart from the volatile anaesthetic agents, opioids and noble gases have also been shown to exhibit a preconditioning effect. The mechanisms involved in anaesthetic preconditioning strongly resemble those involved in ischaemic preconditioning.

In contrast to the experimental setting, where anaesthetic preconditioning consistently resulted in a protective action against post-ischaemic myocardial dysfunction and damage, the results of clinical studies using a preconditioning protocol are less straightforward. Although some of these studies showed either biochemical or functional signs of myocardial protection with various preconditioning protocols, others failed to observe such protective actions. The possible reasons for these variable responses seem to be related to the actual preconditioning protocol used. It was indeed recently demonstrated that protective actions (lower postoperative troponin release and/or better preservation of myocardial function) were only apparent when an intermittent administration protocol was applied instead of a continuous administration.

A more consistent cardioprotection was observed when the volatile anaesthetic was administered throughout the entire period of cardiac surgery. These observations were primarily obtained in coronary surgery patients. Outside this setting, data are less obvious. Volatile anaesthetics have been shown to exhibit protective properties in aortic valve surgery but not in mitral valve surgery. Also, during percutaneous coronary interventions no protective effects have been observed. To date, there is no evidence that such anaesthetic-induced protective effects are present in non-cardiac surgery.

Organ protection can also be achieved by an ischaemic trigger to a tissue distant from the organ intended to be protected. This phenomenon is termed *remote preconditioning*. Several studies have indicated that an ischaemic trigger to a limb (transient occlusion of blood flow to the arm or the leg) was associated with less myocardial damage in the setting of cardiac surgery.

Modulation of inflammatory markers

Volatile anaesthetic agents but also large doses of propofol have been shown to decrease the release of proinflammatory cytokines during ischaemia, thereby decreasing the extent of reperfusion injury. To date, it is unclear whether such a mechanism has an important role in clinical cardioprotection.

Myocardial postconditioning

Ischaemic postconditioning involves a cycle of brief interruptions of reperfusion applied at the onset of reperfusion and seems also to confer protective effects against myocardial ischaemia–reperfusion injury. Postconditioning involves similar pathways to those involved in preconditioning, although it still remains to be definitively elucidated through which mechanisms these pathways exert their protective effect. Ultimately, postconditioning also mediates cardioprotection through delayed or transient MPTP opening.

From a clinical point of view, just as for preconditioning, it remains hazardous to apply an ischaemic insult to an already jeopardized tissue. However, volatile anaesthetics also have a postconditioning effect.

Bibliography

Crisostomo PR, Wairiuko GM, Wang M, *et al.* Preconditioning versus postconditioning: mechanisms and therapeutic potentials. *J Am Coll Surg* 2006; **202**: 797–812.

De Hert S. Myocardial protection from ischemia and reperfusion injury. In: Mebazaa A, Gheorgiade M, Zannad FM, Parrillo JE (eds) *Acute Heart Failure*. London: Springer-Verlag, 2008, pp. 70–86.

Fräβdorf J, De Hert S, Schlack W. Anaesthesia and myocardial ischaemia/reperfusion injury. *Br J Anaesth* 2009; **103**: 89–98.

Halestrap AP, Clarke SJ, Javadov SA. Mitochondrial permeability transition pore opening during myocardial reperfusion: a target for cardioprotection. *Cardiovasc Res* 2004; **61**: 372–85.

Pagel PS. Postconditioning by volatile anesthetics: salvaging ischemic myocardium at reperfusion by activation of prosurvival signalling. *J Cardiothorac Vasc Anesth* 2008; **22**: 753–65.

Zaugg M, Lucchinetti E, Garcia C, *et al.* Anaesthetics and cardiac preconditioning. Part 1: signalling and cytoprotective mechanisms. *Br J Anaesth* 2003; **91**: 551–65.

Mitral valve disease

Jan Fräßdorf

Mitral stenosis

Epidemiology

Worldwide, rheumatic fever still is the main cause of mitral stenosis. In developing countries patients with mitral stenosis are mostly young, whereas in developed countries patients are mostly elderly and have many comorbidities. In these patients, degenerative causes are common (calcification of the mitral annulus in the elderly or in patients on dialysis). Other rare conditions are mucopolysaccharidosis, systemic lupus erythematosus, rheumatoid arthritis or abnormal serotonin metabolism (e.g. carcinoid, methysergide treatment). Prevalence in developed countries is between 0.02 and 0.2%. In rheumatic fever, women seem to be more affected, and mitral stenosis is the most common lesion in pregnancy.

Pathophysiology

The normal mitral valve area is 4–6 cm^2. If the orifice decreases to under 2 cm^2 the pressure gradient between the left atrium and left ventricle has to increase to maintain adequate filling of the left ventricle. High left atrial pressure may lead to high pulmonary pressure and, over time, to right ventricular failure.

Tachycardia is associated with a shorter diastole and therefore shorter filling time for the left ventricle. Physiological changes during pregnancy, such as tachycardia and an increase in blood volume and cardiac output, may add to the increase in left atrial pressure in pregnant women with mitral stenosis.

The atrial contribution to the filling of the left ventricle is more important in patients with mitral stenosis and loss of sinus rhythm may cause haemodynamic instability.

When mitral stenosis progresses, left atrial dilatation occurs and many of these patients present with chronic atrial fibrillation. In patients with mitral stenosis hypercoagulation is a common feature. This, in combination with left atrial dilatation, relatively low flow within the left atria and atrial fibrillation, explains the high incidence of thromboembolic events in patients with mitral stenosis.

Anaesthesia

Preassessment

Most of the patients with mitral stenosis are asymptomatic. The first symptom that occurs is, usually, atrial fibrillation or acute decompensation due to physiological changes related to pregnancy. Asymptomatic patients with a good exercise tolerance are usually not at higher risk for perioperative adverse cardiac events. Patients with severe mitral stenosis or those with pulmonary hypertension do have an increased risk of perioperative morbidity.

At physical examination special attention should be given to symptoms such as atrial fibrillation, reduced pulse pressure and weak pulse, diastolic murmur, signs of pulmonary oedema and neck vein distension. The exercise tolerance should be carefully assessed according to the AHA/ACC guidelines.

Patients who are able to manage their own life without help (cleaning, shopping) are normally not at increased risk if the heart rate is controlled. In contrast, patients with severe mitral stenosis (mitral valve orifice less than 1 cm^2) do have a significantly increased perioperative risk of cardiac adverse events. Therefore, elective surgery should be postponed in these patients and cardiological work-up should be carried out. This should include echocardiography to assess left and right ventricular function, the pressure gradient over the mitral valve, the dimensions of the heart, left atrial thrombus formation, and an estimation of left atrial and pulmonary artery pressure. Dobutamine or exercise stress echocardiography may be useful to evaluate the response to increased working conditions (increased cardiac output and heart rate). If pulmonary artery hypertension is present, its reversibility should be tested preoperatively. All this information will help arrive at a decision about potential preoperative treatment of the stenotic disease (ballon commissurotomy, mitral valve surgery).

Intraoperative management

Adequate anxiolysis is recommended to prevent tachycardia related to the patient's anxiety. However, hypercarbia must be avoided as this worsens pulmonary artery hypertension, and blood pressure has to be monitored carefully because hypotension is not well tolerated in patients with mitral stenosis.

Sinus rhythm should, if possible, be maintained, as the atrial contribution to left ventricular filling is increased. To maximize the diastolic filling time of the left ventricle, a low heart rate is recommended. As cardiac output is almost fixed through the mitral stenosis, afterload should be kept high to maintain perfusion pressure.

There is no clear advantage of a specific anaesthetic technique as long as haemodynamics are kept stable and decreases in SVR are prevented. Invasive monitoring (arterial catheter prior to induction, central venous catheter) are justified.

Although there is no evidence that the use of a pulmonary artery catheter has a positive influence on morbidity or mortality, its use can give valuable information, especially in patients with pulmonary artery hypertension. However, the use of transoesophageal echocardiography may yield more information.

Postoperative management

Dependent on the type of surgery, the patient's condition and the severity of mitral stenosis, the patient should be monitored in an adequate postoperative care unit (postanaesthesia care unit (PACU) or ICU).

Mitral regurgitation

Epidemiology

Mitral regurgitation is the most common valvular disease and occurs when normal cooptation of the mitral leaflets is lost. The prevalence of moderate to severe mitral regurgitation is estimated at 2.5% and is age-dependent (18–44 years old, 0.7%; 75 years and older, 13.3%). There are two major entities of mitral regurgitation: disturbance of the complex interaction of the different subunits of the mitral valve (functional mitral regurgitation) or structural changes of the valve apparatus (structural mitral regurgitation). The same cause (i.e. ischaemia) can lead to different mechanisms of mitral regurgitation (i.e. rupture of the papillary muscle versus ventricular remodelling and subsequently dilatation of the mitral annulus). Mitral regurgitation due to structural changes of the mitral valve apparatus is mostly caused by myxomatous degeneration, deficiency of the fibroelastic tissue and senile calcification of the valvular apparatus. Rheumatic fever causes mitral stenosis and almost always a variable degree of mitral regurgitation. Infective endocarditis can cause mitral regurgitation because of impairment of cooptation, leaflet perforation and rupture of the chordae tendineae. Diseases associated with connective tissue disorders such as Marfan or Ehlers-Danlos syndrome, cardiomyopathies or trauma are more infrequent causes of mitral regurgitation.

Pathophysiology

Mitral regurgitation imposes a large volume load on the left atrium and left ventricle. In the acute setting (i.e. rupture of the chordae tendineae) this volume overload leads to an increase in left atrial pressures, as the atrium is not able to distend acutely. The increased left atrial pressure increases pulmonary artery pressure and subsequent pulmonary oedema may occur.

In chronic mitral regurgitation, hypertrophy of the left ventricle and dilation of the left atrium occurs. Initially, left ventricular function is preserved, but, with the increase in severity, left ventricular dysfunction will develop. The ejection fraction tends to underestimate the functional consequence of the mitral valve disease since part of the ejection fraction is not pumped forward but back into the left atrium. Owing to increased left ventricular filling pressures and decreased compliance of the left ventricle, diastolic dysfunction will present in the evolution of mitral regurgitation.

Anaesthesia

Preassessment

Typical symptoms of advanced mitral valve regurgitation include fatigue, shortness of breath and decreased exercise tolerance. These are often elicited by new-onset atrial fibrillation and are typical symptoms of forward heart failure. A history of patients should be taken with special attention to these symptoms of forward failure. As chronic mitral regurgitation progresses slowly, patients tend to adapt their lifestyle and decreases in exercise tolerance may remain undetected. Auscultation of the heart reveals a pansystolic murmur and heart rhythm may be irregular owing to atrial fibrillation. The severity of mitral regurgitation is usually assessed by echocardiography. Cardiac catheterization can be useful, especially in cases of ischaemia-induced functional mitral regurgitation.

Usually, asymptomatic patients tolerate non-cardiac surgery well. Symptomatic patients who are planned for more than minor surgery should be evaluated and treatment should be optimized, especially if coronary artery disease is also present. Special attention should be paid to the use of anticoagulation if atrial fibrillation is present. Coumarin should be discontinued and replaced with heparin preoperatively. Previous medication should be continued. However, perioperative haemodynamic instability related to chronic ACE inhibitor treatment should be taken into account.

Acute mitral regurgitation is a medical emergency and elective non-cardiac surgery is contraindicated. Usually, these patients are treated with diuretics and afterload reduction. Inotropic support is frequently necessary prior to emergency cardiac surgery.

Intraoperative management

Premedication is usually well tolerated. The main haemodynamic goals are a high normal heart rate and a low SVR to promote forward flow. General, regional and neuraxial anaesthesia are well tolerated. However, if neuraxial anaesthesia is chosen, special attention should be paid to the anticoagulation therapy.

In asymptomatic patients with mild regurgitation undergoing minor surgery, no additional monitoring is warranted. Transoesophageal echocardiography may yield useful information on the morphology, volume status and function of the heart.

Postoperative management

Moderate to severe mitral regurgitation is a risk factor for major postoperative morbidity and mortality even in low-risk procedures. Postoperatively, severe complications, such as pulmonary oedema and the necessity for prolonged ventilation frequently occur with a reported morbidity of up to 27% and a mortality rate of 12%. Especially the presence of atrial fibrillation is an independent predictor of morbidity and mortality. Therefore, these patients should be monitored intensively to detect any early signs of myocardial or pulmonary decompensation.

Bibliography

Lai HC, Lai HC, Lee WL, *et al.* Mitral regurgitation complicates postoperative outcome of noncardiac surgery. *Am Heart J* 2007; **153**: 712–17.

Ling LH, Enriquez-Sarano M, Seward JB, *et al.* Clinical outcome of mitral regurgitation due to flail leaflet. *N Engl J Med* 1996; **335**: 1417–23.

Nkomo VT, Gardin JM, Skelton TN, *et al.* Burden of valvular heart diseases: a population-based study. *Lancet* 2006; **368**: 1005–11.

Silversides CK, Colman JM, Sermer M, *et al.* Cardiac risk in pregnant women with rheumatic mitral stenosis. *Am J Cardiol* 2003; **91**: 1382–5.

Cross-references

Mitral valve surgery, 583
Patients with heart failure, 159
Preoperative assessment of cardiovascular risk in non-cardiac surgery, 621

Patients with heart failure

Quanhong Zhou and Stefan De Hert

Definition and classification of heart failure

The ACC/AHA classify heart failure in four stages, based on the presence of risk factors, underlying heart diseases and symptoms. Stage A refers to the presence of risk factors for heart failure but without any structural heart disease present. Stage B refers to the presence of structural heart disease but still without symptoms. Stage C is the presence of structural heart disease with symptoms of heart failure, and stage D refers to the presence of refractory heart failure.

From a pathophysiological point of view, heart failure is usually classified in systolic and diastolic left ventricular dysfunction. Systolic heart failure is defined as a decrease in contractility of the left ventricle such that it is no longer capable of providing an adequate blood supply to the body. Usually, this occurs when left ventricular ejection fraction drops below 40%. Between 30 and 50% of patients present with heart failure in the presence of a preserved left ventricular ejection fraction. If signs and symptoms of congestive heart failure (exercise intolerance, fatigue, dyspnoea and pulmonary oedema) develop in a patient with normal or near normal systolic function, then diastolic heart failure is present. The pathophysiological basis of diastolic heart failure is related to an impairment of the normal filling pattern of the ventricle and may range from impaired myocardial relaxation to restrictive filling.

Preoperative evaluation

The presence of decompensated heart failure is one of the active cardiac conditions that necessitates prompt treatment before any elective surgery is planned. It is suggested that these patients should be stabilized for at least 1 week before undergoing elective surgery.

History and physical examination may suggest the presence of heart failure. The ACC/AHA guidelines for diagnosis and management of heart failure in adults suggest that laboratory evaluation of patients presenting with a new or suspected diagnosis of heart failure should include complete blood count, urinalysis, serum electrolytes, blood urea nitrogen, creatinine, fasting blood glucose, lipid profile, liver profile and thyroid-stimulating hormone. Pregnancy testing is advisable for patients of child-bearing age.

A 12-lead ECG is recommended for patients with heart failure to check for arrhythmias, and a chest X-ray may show the evidence of cardiomegaly, pleural effusions, prominent upper lobe veins, engorged lymphatics and alveolar oedema.

Echocardiography with Doppler flow analysis is the single most useful diagnostic test in the evaluation of patients with heart failure. It can diagnose systolic and diastolic heart failure, delineate chamber involvement and quantify ejection fraction. In addition, study of the filling patterns of the left ventricle will allow assessment of the degree of diastolic dysfunction.

Non-invasive stress testing is recommended in the following patient cohorts: (1) patients who present for major non-cardiac surgery with new symptoms of heart failure, no symptoms of ischaemia and poor functional capacity (defined as <4 METs); (2) patients with compensated heart failure and poor functional capacity presenting for major non-cardiac surgery should have non-invasive stress testing if it will change their perioperative management; and (3) non-invasive stress testing should be considered in patients with heart failure and good functional capacity who are undergoing vascular surgery. In contrast, patients who have heart failure but with good functional capacity and no history of ischaemic heart disease, cerebrovascular disease, diabetes mellitus or renal insufficiency do not need non-invasive stress testing before major non-cardiac surgery.

Preoperative treatment

For elective surgery, patients with diagnosed heart failure (both systolic and diastolic) should be aggressively and adequately treated to optimize cardiac function before surgery.

Current guidelines recommend the use of ACE inhibitors (or angiotensin receptor blockers in patients intolerant of those agents) and β-blockers as primary treatment in patients with chronic heart failure. Diuretics and digoxin are recommended in patients with heart failure who have signs or symptoms of congestive failure. The perioperative use of ACE inhibitors, β-blockers, statins and aspirin seems to be associated with a reduced incidence of in-hospital mortality in patients with left ventricular dysfunction who are undergoing major non-cardiac vascular surgery. Therefore, it is recommended that such therapies in patients with stable heart failure be continued up until surgery and that they be reinstated postoperatively, as soon as possible.

Elective surgery should be postponed until medical management has been optimized and risk assessed thoroughly against benefit. High-risk patients undergoing elective or emergency surgery may benefit from preoperative optimization in the ICU.

Intraoperative management

For patients undergoing minor interventions, local or regional anaesthesia can be considered. For more major surgery there is no evidence of the benefits of general compared with regional anaesthesia. The perioperative mortality rate appears to be more dependent on the patient's condition at the time of surgery than on the anaesthetic technique or agent used. Provided careful titration and maintenance of stable haemodynamic conditions are maintained, all modern anaesthetic agents can be safely used in these patients.

Preserving cardiac output and minimizing myocardial work are of prime importance in this patient population. Therefore, tachycardia should be avoided and arrhythmias should be aggressively treated. In addition, reduction of afterload may substantially reduce myocardial work. Cardiac contractile function must be preserved, if necessary with the use of inotropes, such as dobutamine and phosphodiesterase inhibitors. Calcium-sensitizing agents may also be considered.

In patients with high-risk heart failure and for all major surgery, invasive monitoring can guide clinical treatment. The use of a pulmonary artery catheter is recommended for surgical procedures with a high likelihood of haemodynamic disturbance. Although the use of intraoperative transoesophageal echography is not routinely recommended, it can assist haemodynamic management.

Postoperative care

Adequate oxygenation is mandatory in patients with heart failure. Careful fluid balance management is required and good pain management can avoid an excessive stress response. Most patients with heart failure who have undergone major non-cardiac surgery should be admitted to a high care unit for careful monitoring and treatment.

Perioperative management of acute exacerbations of chronic heart failure

In the perioperative period, patients with chronic heart failure may develop acute decompensation owing to the withdrawal of medication and the occurrence of perioperative haemodynamic disturbances.

The primary target of the treatment of acute heart failure is to restore proper tissue perfusion and to correct the causes of the exacerbations, such as acute rhythm disturbances, myocardial ischaemia, hypertensive crisis and hypotension.

Bibliography

Cheng JWM, Nayar M. A review of heart failure management in the elderly population. *Am J Geriatr Pharmacother* 2009; **7**: 233–49.

De Hert SG. Preoperative cardiovascular assessment in noncardiac surgery: an update. *Eur J Anaesthesiol* 2009; **26**: 449–57.

Fleisher LA, Beckman JA, Brown KA, *et al.* ACC/AHA 2007 guidelines on perioperative cardiovascular evaluation and care for noncardiac surgery: a report of the American College of Cardiology/American Heart Association Task Force on Practice Guidelines (writing committee to revise the 2002 guidelines on perioperative cardiovascular evaluation for noncardiac surgery). *Circulation* 2007; **116**: e418–e500.

Pirracchio R, Cholley B, De Hert S, *et al.* Diastolic heart failure in anaesthesia and critical care. *Br J Anaesth* 2007; **98**: 707–21.

Poldermans D, Bax JJ, Boersma E, *et al.* Task Force for Preoperative Cardiac Risk Assessment and Perioperative Cardiac Management in Non-cardiac Surgery of European Society of Cardiology (ESC); European Society of Anaesthesiology (ESA). Guidelines for pre-operative cardiac risk assessment and perioperative cardiac management in non-cardiac surgery: the Task Force for Preoperative Cardiac Risk Assessment and Perioperative Cardiac Management in Non-cardiac Surgery of the European Society of Cardiology (ESC) and endorsed by the European Society of Anaesthesiology (ESA). *Eur J Anaesthesiol* 2010; **27**: 92–137.

Toller WG, Metzler H. Acute perioperative heart failure. *Curr Opin Anaesthesiol* 2005, **18**: 129–35.

Wojciechowski P. Perioperative optimization of the heart failure patient. *Int Anesthesiol Clin* 2009; **47**: 121–35.

Cross-references

Coronary artery disease, 146
Heart transplantation, 520
Preoperative assessment of cardiovascular risk in non-cardiac surgery, 621

Patients with pacemakers and implantable defibrillators

Benedikt Preckel

The number of patients with cardiac rhythm management devices, e.g. permanent pacemakers (PMs) and/or implantable cardioverter defibrillators (ICDs), is constantly increasing.

PMs deliver a very short, low-voltage electrical current via an insulated pacing lead to the heart muscle at a preprogrammed rate. These devices also detect native electrical impulses and respond only if necessary, ensuring that there is no interference of the PM with the native rhythm of the patient. Modern PMs contain a lithium iodine battery with a battery lifespan of over 10 years. The pulse generator is surrounded by a titanium cage, removing most external electromagnetic interference (EMI), such as from microwaves, shavers or mobile phones.

Programming of the PM as well as reading information stored on the device can be by radiofrequency from an external device lying on the skin. Technical improvements and reduced size of the system have allowed implantation of these devices under local anaesthesia, probably along with additional procedural sedation. However, after implantation of an ICD, this device has to be tested, e.g. ventricular fibrillation (VF) is induced, which is subsequently recognized by the ICD and an electroshock is given by the device. These situations are uncomfortable for patients and therefore general anaesthesia is required. To ensure a successful haemodynamic response after the electroshock, an arterial line or a good plethysmography curve is needed, as electrical activity on the ECG does not necessarily mean that circulation has been restored.

Pacemaker devices

Pacing can take place in one cardiac chamber (atrium or ventricle), in two chambers (dual, atrium and ventricle) or multiple chambers (biventricular devices). Bipolar leads are mainly used in present-day systems, while older systems mostly worked with unipolar leads. Typically, pacemaker leads are placed in the right chambers of the heart (atrium, ventricle or both). The device is able to sense the electrical activity of the heart and can then trigger or inhibit pacing of the respective chamber: if no electrical activity is sensed within a preset time window, an electrical stimulation will be performed, leading to depolarization of the respective chamber. The most physiological form of pacing would be AV sequential pacing, in which atrial systole precedes ventricular systole with the same frequency.

The North American Society of Pacing and Electrophysiology/British Pacing and Electrophysiology Group (NASPE/BPEG) defined a generic code for antibradycardia, adaptive rate and multisite pacers. Usually, the programming of an individual pacemaker consists of up to five letters: pacing (atrium, A; ventricle, V; dual, D), sensing (A; V; D; none; O) and response (inhibited, I; triggered, T; D; O). Modern devices are also described by presence (R) or absence (O) for rate-adaptive mechanisms on position IV. This function allows alteration of the pacing rate to match the physiological needs of the patient (e.g. higher rates during physical activity, stress, illness). Position V indicates whether multisite pacing is present in none (O), the atria (A), the ventricle (V) or a combination of both (D).

The underlying pathophysiology in the individual patient will determine the programming of the PM: a patient with sinus bradycardia can profit from an AAI mode, whereas a patient with atrial fibrillation needs a VVI mode. In a patient with a high-degree AV block, ventricular stimulation after atrial sensing might be the mode of choice (VAT), in which sensing within the atrium triggers stimulation of the ventricle. In a DDD mode, sensing, triggering or inhibition can be performed in both the atrium and ventricle, and this is the most frequent mode used with modern devices. During operations, asynchronous modes are often used as escape modes, where a specified chamber (AOO, VOO, DOO) is paced at a fixed rate regardless of the intrinsic electrical activity.

Defibrillator devices

Modern ICDs provide a series of management strategies for episodes of ventricular tachycardia or VF, based on tachycardia zones, which depend on the individual's clinical history and electrophysiology. These strategies might be (1) observed tachycardia with no further action, (2) antitachycardia pacing, (3) low-energy synchronized shocks or (4) high-energy synchronized shocks. The coding for ICDs consist of four letters, with position I indicating which chamber is shocked (A, V, D, O), position II in which chamber antitachycardia pacing is administered (A, V, D, O), position III for antitachycardia detection (E, electrocardiogram; H, haemodynamic) and position IV indicating which chamber delivers antibradycardia pacing (A, V, D, O).

Preoperative assessment

Management of patients with a PM/ICD must take into account the underlying reason for implantation of the device, as well as functioning of the system, and must seek to avoid damage to the device, the leads or the site of lead implantation.

The most frequent indication for implantation of a PM includes sinus bradycardia of any aetiology, high-grade AV conduction block, documented episodes of asystole or after catheter ablation of the AV junction. ICDs are mostly implanted after previous VF incidents or in patients at high risk for ventricular tachycardia or VF. It is important to determine the extent to which the patient is device dependent, e.g. can the PM be set off without rhythm problems.

Preoperative assessment of patients with a PM/ICD should focus on the type of pacemaker present, its basic mode of operation, where it is sited (left, right, abdominal, to minimize the chance of iatrogenic damage) as well as the time of implantation, possible battery and/or lead replacements and whether it is currently in good working order. Recent symptoms suggesting malfunction include palpitations, syncope or dizzy spells. Mostly, this required information can be obtained from the clinic responsible for regularly following up the patient and this information should be obtained preoperatively.

It is advisable to have the unit fully checked by a PM technician before the operation, especially since a significant proportion of PM units will be sensing most of the time, and there will be little evidence on the resting ECG as to whether they are functioning or not. In addition, it is not always possible to identify the specific programme in which a unit is set (e.g. rate response) unless it is formally interrogated. There are some settings that would be better altered before general anaesthesia, but this decision is patient specific. Usually, the patient is carrying a PM card, which details the unit and programme.

Preoperative determination of urea and electrolytes is recommended, as abnormalities in potassium level can result in pacing failure. In addition, a 12-lead ECG together with a rhythm strip is advisable, although these investigations reflect only a snapshot of the current situation. However, PM spikes might be seen on the ECG and determination of baseline heart rate might be possible. If no information about the device is available (e.g. PM card), a chest X-ray can be helpful to identify the device implanted.

Intraoperative management

Standard monitoring should include ECG, blood pressure and peripheral saturation measurements. Care should be taken with EMI, which mostly comes from diathermy. Most PMs will revert to asynchronous (non-sensing mode, e.g. VOO) when exposed to continuous EMI. This may not occur with intermittent EMI, such as that generated by diathermy, and this can cause failure to pace. The major manufacturers recommend that diathermy is relatively contraindicated and that it is not used near to the generator.

Unipolar diathermy is more hazardous than bipolar, but may not always be avoided. In these cases, the grounding plate should be placed as far away from the device as possible (for head and neck surgery on the shoulder opposite to device implantation). If surgery has to be performed close to the pulse generator, an expert should be consulted as to whether the system should be set off or not, and how it can be protected against damage.

Formerly, the use of a magnet on the PM had the effect to set the system to asynchronous pacing. Nowadays, the effect of a magnet is diverse, with asynchronous pacing, timely asynchronous pacing or even no effect on the programming. Normally, in an ICD the antitachycardia programme will be set off with the antibradycardic action still working. After use of a magnet, the system should be checked for correct programming as soon as possible. The decision whether a system has to be reprogrammed or set off before an operation must be based on the anticipated amount of EMI, PM dependency, device type and rate-adaptive features. Most rate-adaptive systems should be reprogrammed to a fixed mode during the operation. This should be done by the PM technician in the operating theatre surroundings and the patient should subsequently be monitored. Reprogramming should be done immediately postoperatively in the recovery room.

If diathermy is essential, a bipolar system should be used whenever possible. Short, intermittent and irregular bursts at a low energy will lead to the least interference with the system. If system malfunction has been detected, the surgeon should be informed immediately. When an ICD has to be disabled to apply electric shocks, consideration should be given to connecting the patient to external defibrillator pads before starting surgery.

Postoperative management

If there is any doubt whether the system is functioning properly or there is a chance that damage might have occurred during the operation, the system should be checked completely immediately after the surgical procedure. In addition, reprogramming to the original settings should occur in the recovery room before the patient is discharged to the ward.

Bibliography

American Society of Anesthesiologists Task Force on Perioperative Management of Patients with Cardiac Rhythm Management Devices. Practice advisory for the perioperative management of patients with cardiac rhythm management devices. *Anesthesiology* 2005; **103**: 186–98.

Bernstein AD, Camm AJ, Fletcher RD, *et al.* The NASPE/BPEG generic pacemaker code for antibradyarrhythmia and adaptive-rate pacing and antitachyarrhythmia devices. *Pacing Clin Electrophysiol* 1987; **10**: 794–9.

Furman S, Hayes DL, Holmes DR. *A Practice of Cardiac Pacing*, 2nd edn. New York: Futura, 1989.

Hayes DL, Vlietstra RE. Pacemaker malfunction. *Ann Intern Med* 1993; **119**: 828–35.

Cross-references

Cardiac conduction defects, 132
Pacing and anaesthesia, 777

Pulmonary hypertension

Benedikt Preckel

In 2008, the Fourth World Symposium updated the clinical classification of pulmonary hypertension (PH), as follows:

Group 1 Pulmonary arterial hypertension (PAH), including idiopathic PAH, heritable PAH, drug and toxin-induced PAH, disease-associated PAH, PAH of the newborn and PAH on the basis of pulmonary veno-occlusive disease (PVOD) and/or pulmonary capillary haemangiomatosis.

Group 2 Pulmonary hypertension due to left heart disease, including systolic dysfunction, diastolic dysfunction and valvular heart disease.

Group 3 Pulmonary hypertension due to lung disease and/or hypoxia, including chronic obstructive pulmonary disease, interstitial lung disease, sleep-disordered breathing and alveolar hypoventilation as well as chronic exposure to high altitude.

Group 4 Chronic thromboembolic pulmonary hypertension.

Group 5 Pulmonary hypertension with unclear multifactorial mechanisms (e.g. haematological, systemic or metabolic disorders).

The World Symposium defined PH as a mean pulmonary artery pressure (mPAP) greater than 25 mmHg at rest (normal mPAP 14 ± 3 mmHg, range 8–20 mmHg). To define PAH, one has to additionally measure a pulmonary capillary wedge pressure of 15 mmHg or less and pulmonary vascular resistance (PVR) of at least 3 Wood units (1 Wood unit = 1 mmHg min^{-1} L^{-1} = 80 dynes s^{-1} cm^{-5}).

Pathogenesis and pathophysiology

Excessive pulmonary vascular cell proliferation, reduced cell apoptosis, excessive vasoconstriction, reduced vasodilatory effects and thrombosis play a significant role in the development of PH. This includes reduced expression and activity of endothelial nitric oxide synthase (nitric oxide is a potent vasodilator), increased production and diminished clearance of endothelin 1 (a potent vasoconstrictor), decreased prostacyclin synthase expression (prostacyclin is a potent vasodilator), as well as endothelial injuries triggering thrombotic events.

In PH, the right ventricle must adjust to an increased afterload, and, when the compensation limit is reached, right heart failure will occur. This includes right ventricular dilatation, which can also have an impact on the left heart, leading to left ventricular compression further compromising cardiac output. Reduced left ventricular outflow will also result in reduced perfusion of the right ventricle via the right coronary artery.

Preoperative assessment of patients with pulmonary hypertension

The majority of patients with PH presenting before surgery have PH on the basis of cardiac, pulmonary or thromboembolic disease.

Patients with clinical features for PH should have echocardiography to assess a cardiac cause of PH (left heart disease, congenital heart disease, valvular heart disease) and to assess right ventricular function and systolic pressure, as well as right atrial and right ventricular diameters. The work-up for other causes of PH includes pulmonary function test, sleep studies, a ventilation–perfusion scan and serology markers (e.g. HIV, connective tissue disease markers). If no cause is found, right heart catheterization should be performed to confirm the diagnosis of PAH.

Mild pulmonary hypertension has few anaesthetic consequences, whereas pulmonary artery pressures approaching systemic levels represent a significant anaesthetic risk and can lead to right heart failure and cardiogenic shock. The response of patients with pulmonary hypertension to anaesthesia depends on the aetiology of the disease, disease progression and the degree of decompensation. In many patients, the underlying cause will bear greater relevance to anaesthesia than the pulmonary hypertension itself.

Clinical findings

Right ventricular heave, loud P2 heart sound, exertional dyspnoea and finger clubbing may be present. Raised jugular venous pressure, central cyanosis (may occur early), oedema, hepatomegaly and later ascites may be present.

ECG and chest X-ray

Right ventricular hypertrophy, usually right axis deviation, P pulmonale (P >2 mm tall in lead 2) and bilaterally enlarged pulmonary arteries.

Strategies to manage pulmonary hypertension

Haemodynamic goals include minimizing and managing rises in PVR, maintaining adequate cardiac perfusion and monitoring and rapidly treating right ventricular decompensation to avoid cardiac arrest.

Oxygen is a pulmonary vasodilator and oxygen therapy should be initiated. Avoid hypoxia, hypercarbia and hypothermia, which all will lead to vasoconstriction. Avoid high intrapulmonary pressures, e.g. high tidal volumes and high positive end-expiratory pressures, as this will increase PVR and reduce right ventricular preload. An adequate preload is mandatory, and fluid boluses might be applied to optimize central venous pressure. Inotropic agents might be required to increase right ventricular contractility. β_1-Adrenergic stimulation with dobutamine (2–5 μg kg^{-1} min^{-1}) increases contractility and simultaneously decreases PVR. Systemic vasodilatation might require a peripheral vasoconstrictor, e.g. norepinephrine (0.01–0.1 μg kg^{-1} min^{-1}), that has little effect on PVR in this context. Phosphodiesterase inhibitors such as milrinone increase contractility and reduce PVR and systemic vascular resistance (SVR). As SVR will decrease, concomitant vasoconstrictive therapy will frequently be necessary. It is essential to keep the coronary perfusion pressure sufficiently high to prevent right ventricular ischaemia, which would further worsen the already compromised right ventricular function.

Pulmonary vasodilatation is a cornerstone in the therapy of PH. Inhalation of nitric oxide (NO, 20–40 p.p.m.) stimulates the guanylate cyclase to increase cyclic guanine monophosphate, a second messenger that causes vasodilatation. Because NO is rapidly inactivated within the blood, inhalational NO has virtually no systemic side-effects, allowing reduction of PVR while maintaining SVR.

Prostacyclin stimulates cyclic adenosine monophosphate, thereby acting as a vasodilator. Inhaled prostacyclin and the prostacyclin analogue iloprost can be used to reduce PH and are applied via a jet nebulizer system (30–40 ng kg^{-1} min^{-1} of prostacyclin). There is also an injectable form, epoprostenol, but systemic hypotension might limit its systemic use in PH patients. Epoprostenol has to be given continuously and interruption of therapy can cause severe rebound increases of PVR. Caution should be applied to bleeding complications, as prostacyclins inhibit platelet aggregation.

Preoperatively, application of an endothelin 1 receptor antagonist is another option to treat PH. Bosentan has been shown to improve functional capacity and to delay cardiopulmonary decompensation. Side-effects of bosentan include teratogenicity, anaemia, bleeding disorders and hepatotoxicity, as well as induction of several liver enzymes, which might lead to altered breakdown of other substances used during anaesthesia.

Next to endothelin inhibitors, phosphodiesterase 5 (PDE-5) inhibitors reduce breakdown of PDE-5, thereby increasing the amount of cyclic guanine monophosphate, producing vasodilation. A selective inhibitor of PDE-5 which can be used to treat PH is sildenafil.

Monitoring of patients with pulmonary hypertension during anaesthesia

Next to standard monitoring (ECG, oxygen saturation, capnography), intra-arterial blood pressure monitoring is suggested to promptly determine changes in systemic pressures. In addition, blood gas analysis can be performed, allowing early diagnosis of hypoxia or hypercapnia. Introducing a pulmonary artery catheter enables pulmonary artery pressures, PVR and SVR to be measured. However, introducing the catheter might lead to severe arrhythmias, and loss of sinus rhythm followed by decreased left ventricular output is detrimental in patients with PH. A central venous line is suggested to allow infusion of vasoactive substances. Transoesophageal echocardiography is very helpful to assess right and left ventricular function as well as diameters of the atria and ventricles. Valvular heart diseases can be determined and pressure gradients as well as flow velocity can be estimated.

Effect of anaesthetics on pulmonary hypertension

There is little evidence about which anaesthetic technique is best in patients with PH. The choice of anaesthetic technique has to take into account the underlying cause of PH, the severity of illness as well as surgical needs. A balanced technique with high-dose opioids and volatile anaesthetics has been shown to blunt cardiovascular responses to painful stimuli, with minimal effects on PH. Neuraxial block techniques might also be useful; however, one has to take into account that pulmonary function is essential in these patients, so high levels of blockade should be avoided. Epidural anaesthesia with slow titration of local anaesthetics might be more helpful than spinal anaesthesia, as a decrease in SVR and cardiac output can be better controlled. Peripheral nerve blocks are also helpful to avoid increases of PVR. Maintaining body temperature as well as correction of anaemia is an additional key factor in the treatment of patients with PH.

Bibliography

Archer SL, Weir EK, Wilkins MR, *et al.* Basic science of pulmonary arterial hypertension for clinicians. New concepts and experimental therapies. *Circulation* 2010; **121**: 2045–66.

Badesch DB, Champion HC, Sanchez MA, *et al.* Diagnosis and assessment of pulmonary arterial hypertension. *J Am Coll Cardiol* 2009; **54**: S55–S66.

Simonneau G, Robbins IM, Beghetti M, *et al.* Updated clinical classification of pulmonary hypertension. *J Am Coll Cardiol* 2009; **54**: S43–54.

Cross-references

Congenital heart disease in adult life, 141

Patients with heart failure, 159

Surgery after heart transplantation

Stefan De Hert

Thanks to improving surgical and perioperative care and the advances made in the prevention and treatment of graft rejection, mortality after heart transplantation has decreased substantially over the years. One year survival is now above 90% and is around 50% at 10 years. This implies that an increasing number of post-heart transplant patients will present for non-cardiac surgery. In addition, about 20–40% of these patients will require a general surgical intervention as a consequence of the complications of the transplantation and the immunosuppressive therapy. While the transplant team will be available to provide information on the allograft function and advice on the immunosuppressive therapy, these patients are mostly taken care of by general anaesthetists. All anaesthetists therefore need to be familiar with the pathophysiology of the transplanted heart and the clinical presentation of the heart transplant recipient scheduled for non-cardiac surgery.

Pathophysiology of the transplanted heart

There are several concerns for anaesthetists taking care of a patient undergoing non-cardiac surgery after previous cardiac transplantation. These include the denervation of the heart, the impact of the typical complications after cardiac transplantation and the consequences of the chronic immunosuppressive therapy.

The denervated heart

The transplanted heart is a denervated organ. Since the vagal tone is lost, the resting heart rate is relatively high in these patients and is typically between 90 and 100 b.p.m. However, tachycardia in response to physiological stress is blunted and will occur only later since it will solely depend on the effects of circulating hormones. This means that the use of drugs that may be associated with bradycardia (neostigmine) should be avoided or only administered with great care. Atropine and glycopyrrolate do not have their usual effect and, if bradycardia is to be treated, isoprenaline is the drug of choice. The absence of the reflex tachycardia response also implies that the increase in cardiac output, necessary to respond to stress, will entirely depend on the Frank–Starling mechanism. This preload dependency implies that clinical situations associated with vasodilatation should be avoided and that the choice for a central neuraxial technique should be considered only very cautiously. Similarly, vasodilating drugs should be administered very carefully.

Although with time some recovery of functional neural control may occur, these patients mostly have a higher incidence of cardiac arrhythmias owing to the absence of the vagal tone and the presence of conduction abnormalities. About 5% of heart transplant patients will need a permanent pacemaker.

Complications after cardiac transplantation

Up to 40% of heart transplant patients will develop an episode of acute rejection during the first year after transplantation. Rhythm disturbances, fever, oedema and unexplained weight gain are possible signs of rejection and should constitute a trigger to perform an endomyocardial biopsy to confirm the diagnosis.

Immunosuppression is the key approach both in the prevention and in the treatment of acute rejection. Maintenance immunosuppressive regimens are based on the administration of prednisolone, calcineurin inhibitors to suppress the production of interleukin 2 (ciclosporin or tacrolimus) and antiproliferative agents (azathioprine or mycophenolate mofetil). Additional treatments are available and the transplant team will advise on how the treatment should be continued in the perioperative phase.

Immunosuppression may interfere with wound healing and increases the susceptibility for postoperative infections. Therefore, strict aseptic techniques are essential. The number of catheters should be kept to a minimum and they should be removed as soon as possible. Treatment of infection should always be based on analysis of sensitivity to antibiotics with the use of microbiological cultures. Immunosuppressed patients are also particularly susceptible to opportunistic infections.

Cardiac allograft vasculopathy is a common complication and is, even more than malignant disease, the major cause of mortality late after heart transplantation. Both immunological and non-immunological causes, such as hyperlipidaemia and hypertension, are responsible for the development of this complication. The lesions are diffuse and may be located very distal, making complete revascularization difficult. As these patients are at risk of developing perioperative myocardial ischaemic complications it is mandatory to keep coronary perfusion pressure adequate and to prevent imbalances of the myocardial oxygen balance during anaesthesia and surgery.

Other organ systems may also be affected specifically by the immunosuppressive therapy. Ciclosporin may induce renal impairment, and about 30% of patients will develop renal dysfunction, eventually leading to renal replacement therapy in 5–8% of heart transplant patients. Proliferation signal inhibitors may further enhance the nephrotoxicity of the calcineurin inhibitors.

Ciclosporin interacts with many drugs, especially with agents that affect the cytochrome P450 system. It also interferes with bile metabolism, which may explain the high incidence of cholelithiasis and cholecystectomy in these patients. Finally, there is also a higher incidence of diabetes, pancreatitis, epilepsy and hypertension than in the normal population.

Perioperative management

Preoperative assessment

These patients are mostly under strict control of the transplant team and consequently their actual cardiac and global physical status is well documented. Because of the potential involvement of other organ systems, particular attention should be paid to liver and kidney function. Patients with a pacemaker will need the same perioperative care as non-heart transplant patients.

Intraoperative management

There is no *a priori* contraindication for a particular anaesthetic technique as long as particular care is given to maintain adequate preload. Since kidney and liver function may be compromised, care should be taken with drugs with renal and/or hepatic clearance and dose adjustments may be necessary. Effects of neuromuscular drugs may be altered: ciclosporin enhances the effect of non-depolarizing muscle relaxants, whereas azathioprine decreases the effects. Cisatracurium may be an alternative in such patients since its elimination is not affected by renal or hepatic dysfunction.

There are no specific recommendations with regard to airway management. In general, all devices can be used, remembering that, owing to the immunosuppressive therapy, there is a greater risk of bleeding. Nasal intubation is to be avoided because of the higher risk of infection.

The choice of haemodynamic monitoring is generally similar to that in the general population and will depend on the expected impact of the procedure on the cardiovascular system. Unless rejection is present, cardiac function is mostly good. Haemodynamic support should be obtained with drugs with direct cardiac effects, such as isoprenaline, epinephrine or metaraminol. Caution should be applied when administering vasodilating agents and β-blockers should be avoided. In case of tachyarrhythmias, amiodarone or verapamil may be useful.

Because of the long-lasting immunosuppressive therapies, these patients may have a frail musculoskeletal and skin structure. Therefore, particular care should be taken with positioning. As patients are frequently on steroids, the need for, and nature of, a perioperative substitution scheme should be discussed with the transplant team.

Postoperative management

Generally speaking, postoperative care is similar to that in the non-transplanted patient population. However, particular care should be taken with respect to maintenance of adequate preload, support of renal function and prevention of infection and coagulation disorders. As these patients are at increased risk for developing thromboembolic events, adequate thromboprophylaxis is a must.

Bibliography

Al-khaldi A, Robbins RC. New directions in cardiac transplantation. *Annu Rev Med* 2006; **57**: 455–71.

Blasco LM, Parameshwar J, Vuylsteke A. Anaesthesia for noncardiac surgery in the heart transplant recipient. *Curr Opin Anaesthesiol* 2009; **22**: 109–13.

Cheng DCH, Ong DD. Anaesthesia for noncardiac surgery in heart-transplanted patients. *Can J Anaesth* 1993; **40**: 981–6.

Fazel S, Everson A, Stitt LW, *et al.* Predictors of general surgical complications after heart transplantations. *J Am Coll Surg* 2001; **193**: 52–9.

Kostopanagiotou G, Smyrniotis V, Arkadopoulos N, *et al.* Anesthetic and perioperative management of adult transplant recipient in nontransplant surgery. *Anesth Analg* 1999; **89**: 613–22.

Saeed I, Rogers C, Munday A. Steering group of the UK Cardiothoracic Transplant Audit. Health-related quality of life after cardiac transplantation: results of a UK national survey with norm-based comparisons. *J Heart Lung Transplant* 2008; **27**: 675–81.

Shaw IH, Kirk AJB, Conacher ID. Anaesthesia for patients with transplanted hearts and lungs undergoing non-cardiac surgery. *Br J Anaesth* 1991; **67**: 218–20.

Taylor DO, Edwards LB, Boucek MM, *et al.* Registry of the international society for heart and lung transplantation: twenty-third official adult heart transplantation report 2006. *J Heart Lung Transplant* 2006; **25**: 869–79.

Tetralogy of Fallot

Veronika Evers

The tetralogy of Fallot (TOF) assembles a range of heart defects that include large conoventricular septal defects and variable degrees of RVOT obstruction.

The set of malformations include:

1 intraventricular communication
2 stenosis of the pulmonary artery
3 overriding aorta
4 right ventricular hypertrophy.

This constellation of findings, published in 1888 by Fallot in the first series with anatomic and pathological descriptions, is one of the most common congenital heart lesions requiring intervention in the first year of life.

TOF accounts for 10% of congenital heart diseases. Early surgical correction (<6 months) is now generally favoured, although a palliative aortopulmonary shunt followed by later definitive correction is acceptable in children who have difficult anatomy or who are subject to severe hypercyanotic spells. Only 5% of untreated patients survive beyond 25 years old. The clinical course varies and depends on the degree of obstruction.

Pathophysiology

TOF ranks among cyanotic heart defects, because the combination of RVOT obstruction and VSD usually causes an intracardiac right-to-left shunting. The physiological consequences are largely dependent upon the degree of RVOT.

The VSD is almost always large and unrestrictive, ensuring a pressure adjustment in both ventricles. As a result, the direction and magnitude of blood flow through the defect will be determined by the severity of the obstruction of the RVOT and not by the size of the VSD.

Additional sources of pulmonary blood flow, such as patent ductus arteriosus, aortopulmonary collateral vessels and surgically created aortopulmonary shunts contribute to and affect the systemic arterial saturation as well.

Owing to a missing pulmonary valve, pulmonary blood flow may derive either exclusively from a patent ductus arteriosus or, in patients with hypoplastic central pulmonary arteries, from major aortopulmonary collateral arteries. This may include an aneurysmal dilatation of the pulmonary and parenchymal arteries, which compresses the main stem and peripheral bronchi, resulting in tracheobronchomalacia, bronchospasm and air trapping.

The degree of systemic arterial desaturation depends on the SVR. When resistance of the systemic circulation is higher than the resistance to blood flow across the obstructed RVOT, blood will naturally shunt from the left ventricle to the right ventricle and into the pulmonary bed. In this situation, there is predominantly a left-to-right shunt and the patient will be acyanotic. Conversely, if systemic peripheral resistance is low, a right-to-left shunt will be present and the patient will be cyanotic.

Progressive narrowing of the RVOT heralds the potential for right ventricular failure. Chronic hypoxaemia triggers polycythaemia, causing an elevation in blood viscosity and thereby decreased perfusion with resulting decreased total oxygen delivery and an increased risk of veno-occlusive/hyperviscosity syndrome. For this reason, older untreated patients with TOF are at reasonable risk of having an embolic stroke owing to the open VSD and resultant bypass of the filtering effect of the pulmonary circulation. Infected material can thereby cause brain abscesses.

Tetralogy 'spells'

One of the physiological characteristics of TOF is that the RVOT obstruction can vary. This fluctuation can be initiated by crying, feeding or defaecation, causing 'spells' or episodes of paroxysmal cyanosis and hyperpnoea in untreated patients. These spells can generate a dynamic increase in RVOT obstruction with a subsequent increase in right-to-left shunting and the development or aggravation of cyanosis. Episodes usually resolve spontaneously but can be terminated by comforting a child or administration of intravenous β-blockers.

Diagnostic features

History and physical examination

The clinical presentation of patients with TOF is dependent upon the degree of RVOT obstruction:

- Severe obstruction and inadequate pulmonary flow typically cause a profound cyanosis in the immediate newborn period:
  - during hypercyanotic spells – hyperpnoeic, agitated, cyanotic

- blue nail beds and lips
- prominent right ventricular impulse
- occasionally a systolic thrill
- presence of prominent pulses may point to a significant patent ductus arteriosus or aortopulmonary collaterals.

- Murmur caused by a moderate obstruction and balanced pulmonary and systemic flow:
  - peripheral pulses are usually normal.
- Minimal obstruction may result in pulmonary overcirculation and heart failure.

Electrocardiogram, chest X-ray and echocardiography

- Electrocardiogram:
  - right atrial enlargement and right ventricular hypertrophy
  - right axis deviation
  - prominent R waves anteriorly and S waves posteriorly, an upright T wave in V1
  - a qR pattern in the right-sided chest leads.
- Chest X-ray:
  - 'boot-shaped' heart
  - upturned apex
  - concave main pulmonary artery segment
  - heart size is often normal
  - pulmonary flow will appear normal or decreased.
- Echocardiography:
  - location and number of VSDs
  - anatomy and severity of RVOT obstruction
  - coronary artery and aortic arch anatomy
  - presence of any associated anomalies.

Diagnostic and interventional cardiac catheterization

- Levels of RVOT obstruction.
- Coronary artery anatomy.
- Presence of aortopulmonary collaterals.
- Presence of accessory ventricular septal defects.
- Filling pressures.
- Multiple levels of right ventricular obstruction.
- Anatomy of the branch pulmonary arteries.
- Anatomy of the infundibular and pulmonary valve anatomy.
- Balloon valvuloplasty of the pulmonary valve.

Surgical procedures

Usually, surgery is performed electively in the first year or even in the first 3 months of life, if necessary.

Palliative surgical procedures

The first reported successful surgical palliation of TOF was conducted by Blalock and Taussig in 1945. They used a subclavian artery to create an aorta-to-pulmonary artery connection. Nowadays, the technique has been modified and is usually performed by using a Gortex tube to create the shunt. The Blalock–Taussig shunt remains an important palliative procedure for infants who may not be acceptable candidates for intracardiac repair because of prematurity, hypoplastic pulmonary arteries or coronary artery anatomy. But disadvantages of staged approaches such as the Blalock-Taussig shunt include long-lasting pressure overload of the right ventricle and persistent hypoxaemia with all its sequelae. Other methods for deferring corrective operations are balloon dilatation or placement of a stent in the RVOT in neonates and young infants.

Definitive surgery

Intracardiac repair of TOF consists of patch closure of the VSD and enlargement of the RVOT by resecting infundibular and subinfundibular muscle bundles and occasionally by a transannular patch. A transannular patch of the RVOT renders the pulmonary valve incompetent, which may have significant long-term haemodynamic and electrophysiological consequences, especially if severe.

Currently, a 'valve-sparing approach' is favoured whenever possible, maintaining the pulmonary valve competence, and is easily applied to patients with sufficient pulmonary annulus size. In patients with marginal pulmonary valve annulus sizes, a modest residual RVOT obstruction needs to be traded off against the obligate insufficiency that is associated with a transannular patch. A valved conduit from the right ventricle to the distal main pulmonary artery is an alternative method of surgical repair.

Anaesthetic management

Anaesthetic considerations for initial interventions

- The preoperative review should address the following questions:
  - To what extent and how is the pulmonary blood flow impaired (anatomic side and degree of RVOT obstruction)? Children with severe obstruction and inadequate pulmonary flow typically present in the immediate newborn period with profound cyanosis. Children with minimal obstruction may present with pulmonary overcirculation and heart failure.
  - Are there hypercyanotic spells?
  - Are there other pathophysiological findings that will influence the haemodynamic management (factors influencing shunt flow)?
- Select agents that maintain or increase SVR relative to PVR. Momentary increasing SVR can be facilitated by administration of phenylephrine, abdominal compression or flexion of the legs. PVR

can temporarily be lowered by hyperventilation with 100% oxygen and/or NO inhalation.

- Consider volume loading after a prolonged fasting status or in patients with diuretic therapy.
- Preoperative sedation especially in children with a history of hypercyanotic spells.
- Minimize catecholamine release by ample analgesia and cautious use of ketamine and pancuronium.
- Tracheobronchomalacia, bronchospasm and air trapping due to an aneurysmal dilation of the pulmonary and parenchymal arteries, which compress the main stem and peripheral bronchi, should be kept in mind.

Anaesthetic considerations for interventions in later life

The TOF is an example of a lesion that is 'fixed but not cured'.

- Define risk factors for and degree of cardiac dysfunction:
  - Is there a history of clinically decreased exercise tolerance and signs of right-sided congestion?
  - Assess right ventricular function.
  - Are there residual septal defects?
  - Is there presence of significant tricuspid regurgitation as a likely surrogate for the presence of substantial right ventricular dysfunction.
  - The incidence of ventricular arrhythmias on ambulatory Holter or exercise testing is significant and increases with age.
- Optimize and maintain right ventricular function (Tables 4.2 and 4.3):
  - Maintain spontaneous breathing as long or as soon as possible, because positive pressure ventilation can decrease cardiac output. It mechanically increases right ventricular afterload and decreases right ventricular filling by increasing intrathoracic pressure.
  - Adequate right ventricle filling should be maintained.
  - Drugs that significantly diminish right ventricular contractility should be avoided if contractile dysfunction is a prominent feature.
  - Sustain myocardial oxygen supply specifically in patients with restrictive physiology, as their stiff, non-compliant right ventricles may be particularly susceptible to reductions in subendocardial oxygen delivery.
  - Maintain contractility, blood pressure and oxygen-carrying capacity and keep heart rate within normal limits.
  - Avoid the combination of tachycardia, hypotension, acidosis and anaemia.

Postoperative considerations and complications

Pulmonary dysfunction was regarded as a minor postoperative residual problem but, during the last decade, it has become evident that pulmonary

Table 4.2 Factors affecting pulmonary vascular resistance (PVR)

Decrease PVR	Increase PVR
$F_iO_2 = 1$	$F_iO_2 = 0.21–0.3$
Hyperventilate to $P_aCO_2 = 3.5$ kPa	Hypoventilate to $P_aCO_2 > 7$ kPa
Short inspiratory time; no PEEP	Long inspiratory time; moderate PEEP levels
Prostacyclins	
Iloprost inhalation solution 2.5 μg 6–9 times daily to start, increased to 5.0 μg 6–9 times daily if well tolerated	
Flolan (epoprostenol sodium) for injection	
Continuously infused, 2 ng kg^{-1} min^{-1} to start, increased by 2 ng kg^{-1} min^{-1} every 15 minutes or longer until suitable efficacy/tolerability balance is achieved	
Inhaled nitric oxide (suggest 2–40 p.p.m.)	

Table 4.3 Factors affecting systemic vascular resistance (SVR)

Decrease SVR	Increase SVR
Sodium nitroprusside (infusion)	Phenylephrine (0.25–0.5 μg kg^{-1}) Norepinephrine (0.01–0.20 μg kg^{-1} min^{-1} infusion)

regurgitation is related to the most severe adverse outcomes. Right ventricular pressure and volume loading is poorly tolerated over time and is likely to result in progressive cardiac incapacity, right heart failure, ventricular arrhythmia and sudden death. Progressive systolic right ventricular dysfunction is a predictor of late morbidity and mortality.

Bibliography

Airan B, Choudhary SK, Kumar HV, *et al.* Total transatrial correction of tetralogy of Fallot: no outflow patch technique. *Ann Thorac Surg* 2006; **82**: 1316–21.

Apitz C, Webb GD, Redington AN. Tetralogy of Fallot. *Lancet* 2009; **374**: 1462–71.

Davlouros PA, Kilner PJ, Hornung TS, *et al.* Right ventricular function in adults with repaired tetralogy of Fallot assessed with cardiovascular magnetic resonance imaging: detrimental role of right ventricular outflow aneurysms or akinesia and adverse right-to-left ventricular interaction. *J Am Coll Cardiol* 2002; **40**: 2044–52.

Geva T, Sandweiss BM, Gauvreau K, *et al.* Factors associated with impaired clinical status in long-term survivors of tetralogy of Fallot repair evaluated by magnetic resonance imaging. *J Am Coll Cardiol* 2004; **43**: 1068–74.

Karamlou T, McCrindle BW, Williams WG. Surgery insight: late complications following repair of tetralogy of Fallot and related surgical strategies for management. *Nat Clin Pract Cardiovasc Med* 2006; **3**: 611–22.

Kothari SS. Mechanism of cyanotic spells in tetralogy of Fallot: the missing link? *Int J Cardiol* 1992; **37**: 1–5.

Stewart RD, Backer CL, Young L, Mavroudis C. Tetralogy of Fallot: results of a pulmonary valve-sparing strategy. *Ann Thorac Surg* 2005; **80**: 1431–8.

Cross-references

Cardiac conduction defects, 132
Congenital heart disease in adult life, 141
Patients with heart failure, 159
Patients with pacemakers and implantable defibrillators, 161
Pulmonary hypertension, 164

5

Gastrointestinal tract

Brian J Pollard

Chronic liver disease

Brian J Pollard

Cirrhosis is the most common cause of chronic liver disease and its incidence is increasing. These patients present a significant risk for surgery. Cirrhosis is the end-stage of a number of conditions, including excess alcohol intake, chronic viral hepatitis, haemochromatosis and primary biliary cirrhosis. There is severe fibrosis and nodular regeneration of the liver tissue. Patients may have had a liver biopsy and CT or MRI scan. They may be jaundiced.

Pathophysiology

Gastrointestinal tract

- Portal hypertension and associated oesophageal varices.
- Ascites, causing increased intra-abdominal pressure.
- Delayed gastric emptying and hyperacidity.
- Poor hepatocellular function with decreased drug clearance and increased free drug concentration.
- Gastrointestinal haemorrhage.

Cardiovascular system

- Vascular shunts: arteriovenous, intrapulmonary, pleural, portosystemic.
- Hyperdynamic circulation with decreased peripheral vascular resistance and increased cardiac output.
- Increased circulating volume.
- Left ventricular function may be impaired.

Respiratory

Patients with cirrhosis, particularly end-stage disease, have arterial hypoxaemia, due to:

- intrapulmonary shunts (not corrected with supplementary oxygen)
- ventilation/perfusion mismatch (correctable with supplementary oxygen)
- restrictive defects due to pleural effusions and ascites
- smoking (chronic obstructive pulmonary disease (COPD)).

Nervous system

- Encephalopathy, aggravated by sedatives and diuretics.
- Peripheral neuropathy particularly in alcoholic cirrhosis.

Renal and metabolic

- Increased sodium and water retention.
- Metabolic alkalosis with potassium loss.
- Susceptible to renal failure; acute tubular necrosis and hepatorenal failure.

Bleeding and clotting

The numerous causes of coagulopathy in patients with end-stage liver disease include:

- decreased production of vitamin K-dependent factors
- decreased production of non-vitamin K-dependent factors
- thrombocytopenia
- abnormal platelet function
- hyperfibrinolysis.

Preoperative assessment

History and examination

- Associated disease (cardiomyopathy, COPD).
- Degree of ascites (pleural effusions may coexist).
- Degree of encephalopathy (caution with sedatives).
- Bleeding from varices or elsewhere in the gastrointestinal (GI) tract.
- Neomycin (may prolong neuromuscular blockade).
- Cimetidine (may prolong action of drugs, e.g. fentanyl).
- Peripheral oedema.
- Nutritional status.
- Alcohol intake.

Investigations

- ECG.
- Arterial blood gases (ABGs):
  - P_aO_2 (if low, see if corrected with oxygen)
  - acid–base status.
- Renal function: urea, creatinine, creatinine clearance.
- Echocardiogram if left ventricular function may be impaired.
- Cardiopulmonary exercise testing may be helpful.
- Full blood count:
  - haemoglobin (Hb)
  - white cell count; look for infection
  - platelet count.

- Chest X-ray: pleural effusions, heart size.
- Lung function: restrictive or obstructive defects.
- Biochemistry: low sodium (dilutional hyponatraemia), low potassium, low albumen, raised liver enzymes.
- Coagulopathy:
  - prothrombin time (PT)
  - partial thromboplastin time (PTT)
  - bleeding time.
- Assess infection risk: hepatitis B, C antigens.

Preoperative preparation

- Ascites should be controlled in consultation with a hepatologist.
- Improve poor nutritional status and optimize coexisting disease.
- Have adequate blood cross-matched, especially for abdominal surgery. The need for fresh-frozen plasma (FFP) and cryoprecipitate should be anticipated.
- Give vitamin K for several days prior to surgery if possible.
- Start an intravenous infusion from the point of starvation.
- The patient may be receiving an infusion of octreotide to lower portal venous pressure.

Premedication

Opioids are not well tolerated. Avoid intramuscular premedication if there is a coagulopathy, and avoid drugs relying on phase I liver metabolism. Oral lorazepam is an effective anxiolytic. Anticholinergic drugs can be prescribed if necessary. Acid aspiration prophylaxis should be given.

Perioperative management

Monitoring

Routine

- ECG.
- Pulse oximeter.
- Temperature.
- Urinary catheter (hourly urine output).
- BP – non-invasive/direct.
- Capnography.
- Neuromuscular monitoring.

All but minor surgery

- Arterial line:
  - hourly ABGs
  - Hb
  - sodium and potassium
  - glucose
  - calcium
  - clotting studies.
- Central venous pressure (CVP) may be useful.
- Oesophageal Doppler may be useful.

Induction

Appropriate prophylactic antibiotics should be given before surgery. The pharmacokinetics of many drugs are altered in severe liver disease to a variable, and often unpredictable, degree. Thiopentone, etomidate or propofol are all satisfactory for induction. The action of succinylcholine may be prolonged in severe disease, but avoidance must be weighed against the increased risk of aspiration in these patients. Use it if necessary.

Maintenance

Intubation and controlled ventilation for all but minor procedures, avoiding hypocapnia. A technique based around an inhalational agent (desflurane, isoflurane or enflurane) is satisfactory. Supplement cautiously with fentanyl or alfentanil, unless postoperative ventilation is contemplated. Remifentanil may be useful. Nitrous oxide is not contraindicated but may be best avoided during abdominal surgery as bowel distension can make surgery more difficult. Atracurium is the ideal muscle relaxant. No muscle relaxants are contraindicated but their duration of action may be prolonged. Avoid hypotension and hypoxaemia as these may compromise liver function.

Urine output

- Maintenance of urine output is of paramount importance and this can be helped by meticulous attention to fluid balance.
- Aim to maintain output at above 50 mL h^{-1} in adults.
- Crystalloid infusion during surgery (dextrose 5% or dextrose/saline). Avoid excessive volumes of saline solutions.
- 100 mL boluses of 20% mannitol.
- Dopamine infusion at 3–5 μg kg^{-1} min^{-1} throughout the perioperative period has been recommended.
- Loop diuretics should be used with caution.

Coagulopathy

During major surgery with marked blood loss, regular assessment of clotting should guide replacement therapy. Laboratory tests such as PT, PTT and platelet count may be used, but thromboelastography has also been found to be a reliable and effective guide to blood product requirements.

Table 5.1 Pugh's modification of Child's classification of risks for cirrhotic patients undergoing surgery: low risk, <6 points; moderate risk, 7–9 points; high risk, >10 points

Clinical and biochemical measurements	Points scored for increasing abnormality		
	1	2	3
Encephalopathy (grade)	None	1 or 2	3 or 4
Ascites	Absent	Controlled	Not controlled
Albumin (g L^{-1})	>35	28–35	<28
Prothrombin time (seconds prolonged)	1–4	4–6	>6
Bilirubin (μmol L^{-1})	<25	25–40	>40

Temperature

Avoid hypothermia. Wrap patient in reflective blanketing. The use of a warming mattress, warm air overblanket and the warming of all fluids is vital.

Postoperative management

- Analgesia: opiates are best administered intravenously either by infusion or via a patient-controlled system. Regional analgesia is worth considering, provided there is no coagulopathy. Non-steroidal analgesics are not recommended.
- Elective ventilation should be considered for:
  - prolonged surgery
  - severe blood loss
  - continuing haemorrhage
  - hypothermia.

Careful monitoring of urine output, coagulation, and the administration of analgesia and supplementary oxygen is best carried out in a high-dependency unit (HDU).

Outcome

The leading causes of death in the surgical patient are:

- infection
- liver failure
- renal failure
- haemorrhage.

There have been few studies on survival not involving surgery for portosystemic shunts or bleeding oesophageal varices. The Pugh score divides patients into three groups, classifying them as good, moderate and poor surgical risks (Table 5.1). Open surgical operations to create portosystemic shunts have now been largely replaced by the radiological procedure of transjugular intrahepatic portosystemic shunt (TIPS).

Other factors associated with high mortality include:

- respiratory failure
- cardiac failure
- infection, particularly intra-abdominal
- emergency surgery.

Bibliography

Albers I, Hartmann H, Birsher J, Creutzfeld W. Superiority of the Child-Pugh classification to quantitative liver function tests for assessing prognosis of liver cirrhosis. *Scand J Gastroenterol* 1989; **24**: 269–76.

Mallett S, Cox D. Thromboelastography. *Br J Anaesth* 1992; **69**: 307–13.

Pugh RNH, Murray-Lyon IM, Dawson JL, *et al.* Transection of the oesophagus for bleeding oesophageal varices. *Br J Surg* 1973; **60**: 646–9.

Cross-references

Anaesthesia and chronic obstructive pulmonary disease, 91
The full stomach, 179
The jaundiced patient, 183

Disorders of the oesophagus and of swallowing

Brian J Pollard

Disorders of the oesophagus and the swallowing mechanism present hazards to the patient undergoing anaesthesia because mechanisms to clear the pharynx of foreign material and keep it clear may be compromised.

Pathophysiology

Anatomical

- Hiatus hernia results in compromise to the functional integrity of the lower oesophageal sphincter.
- Pharyngeal pouch and other diverticulas in the oesophagus may contain solid food particles or fluid for many hours after ingestion. They may also contain partially putrefied food. Discharge of the contents of the pouch may occur with changes in posture, or unexpectedly, and present an aspiration risk.
- Tracheo-oesophageal fistula, a direct communication between the trachea and oesophagus.
- Tumours of the oesophagus usually present with dysphagia, which may be partial or complete at the time of surgery. Residual food particles may remain in the oesophagus, as may liquid in the case of complete aphagia. Where obstruction is complete the patient will not be able to clear saliva.
- Achalasia of the cardia is characterized by a hypertrophy of the muscular layer at the lower end of the oesophagus resulting in increasing obstruction to the passage of material into the stomach. Although the risk of regurgitation is very low in these patients, the oesophagus may be greatly dilated above the obstruction and may contain significant volumes of swallowed material. This may be demonstrated on a preoperative barium swallow. The dilated oesophagus does not contain stomach acid.

Physiological

- Oesophageal motility is reduced in scleroderma. The lower oesophageal sphincter is functionally incompetent in these patients and this may result in reflux of gastric contents into the oesophagus. A history of heartburn can often be elicited, but is absent in patients taking omeprazole.
- Neurogenic cerebrovascular accident.

Preoperative assessment

The history should determine whether or not obstruction of the oesophagus is present and whether the patient can swallow liquid without regurgitation. A history of regurgitation of solid material hours after food suggests the presence of either a diverticulum or a dilatation above an obstruction. In the case of a pharyngeal pouch the patient may be able to prevent filling of the pouch or empty it by pressure on the neck. Prolonged avoidance of solid food allowing free fluids may help to clear solid material. A nasogastric tube placed in the oesophagus may be useful in achalasia of the cardia. A CT or MRI scan of the chest may be available.

Premedication

- Antacids are of no value in oesophageal obstruction. However, where surgery relieves an obstruction, reflux of stomach acid may occur postoperatively.
- Drying agents are beneficial if the patient is unable to swallow saliva.

Anaesthetic management

- Rapid sequence induction of anaesthesia is required when the oesophagus may not be empty at the time of induction.
- In the case of pharyngeal pouches the source of the risk is above the cricoid cartilage and cricoid pressure is of no value. Induction of anaesthesia in the lateral position should be considered with the pouch dependent.
- Intubation of the trachea with a cuffed tube is required for protection of the airway. For oesophageal tumour resections a double-lumen tube may be required.
- If the patient is unable to swallow saliva, induction in the lateral position should be considered.

Postoperative management

- Extubate the trachea with the patient awake and in the lateral position, since the risk to the airway may persist into the postoperative period.
- After intubation of an oesophageal tumour, reflux of stomach acid may occur through the tube.
- Surgery for achalasia of the cardia may render the lower oesophageal sphincter incompetent and be followed by acid reflux in the postoperative period.
- Full competence of the protective laryngeal reflexes may take several hours to return.

Cross-references

Airway and aspiration risk, 640
The full stomach, 179

The full stomach

Brian J Pollard

The avoidance of aspiration of gastric contents into the airway is of paramount importance during the administration of anaesthesia. Aspiration of solid material may cause obstruction of the airway, leading to asphyxia, lobar pneumonia or lung abscess formation. Irritation of the vocal cords during light anaesthesia by regurgitated material may cause laryngeal spasm, while aspiration of as little as 25 mL of liquid of pH less than 2.5 may cause bronchospasm, pneumonitis, bronchopneumonia and acute (adult) respiratory distress syndrome.

Pathophysiology

Both the active process of vomiting and the passive process of regurgitation of gastric contents present a hazard in a patient with a full stomach. Vomiting is a hazard at induction, during recovery, and if anaesthesia is light. Regurgitation is a hazard immediately following induction and throughout maintenance, and may occur silently. Regurgitation is predisposed to by a full stomach and any reduction in the functional integrity of the lower oesophageal sphincter (LOS).

The rate of emptying of the stomach after oral intake is variable. No patient can ever be assumed to have a completely empty stomach. In general, for a normal healthy patient, stomach emptying is complete within 6 hours after food, 4 hours after most liquids and 2 hours after water.

Delayed gastric emptying

- Obstruction of the gastrointestinal tract:
  - pyloric stenosis
  - tumours.
- Ileus:
  - postoperative
  - metabolic.
- Peritonitis.
- Pain.
- Fear/anxiety.
- Pregnancy (third trimester).
- Drugs
  - opiates
  - alcohol.

Reflux of material from the bowel

In prolonged intestinal obstruction, faeculent material may enter the stomach retrogradely.

The lower oesophageal sphincter

- Increased pressure zone (not anatomically distinct).
- Pinch-cock action of the diaphragm.
- Mucosal one-way valve.

Preoperative assessment

History

- Last oral intake of food/drink, especially alcohol.
- Possibility of swallowed blood.
- Factors known to delay gastric emptying.
- History of reflux, heartburn or hiatus hernia.
- Drugs known to reduce LOS tone:
  - alcohol, opiates
  - anticholinergics
  - tricyclics
  - dopamine
  - β-agonists.

Preparation

Delay surgery when possible to allow time for the stomach to empty. Induction of vomiting is not normally practical, and residual emetic tendency at the time of induction is dangerous. Passing a nasogastric tube and aspirating gastric contents may not be fully effective, but in the case of liquid contents will reduce intragastric pressure and thus the tendency to regurgitation. At the time of induction the presence of the tube may compromise the function of the LOS and gastric contents may leak past it and enter the oesophagus. Administration of a non-particulate acid-neutralizing drug (e.g. sodium citrate) offers protection from the effects of acid aspiration, but does not protect against regurgitation. Administration of an H_2 blocking drug or a proton pump inhibitor may only offer protection if the acid in the stomach has already been neutralized. Administration of prokinetic drugs, such as metoclopramide, may increase the rate of gastric emptying. Metoclopramide also increases the LOS tone. Anticholinergic drugs do not reliably increase gastric pH.

Perioperative management

Premedication

Avoid opiates and anticholinergics – both reduce LOS tone and delay gastric emptying.

Anaesthetic management

Management of the induction of anaesthesia depends on the cause of the full stomach and clinical circumstances. Intubation of the trachea with a cuffed tube in order to both secure and protect the airway is required.

In most cases, a rapid sequence induction with full preoxygenation and cricoid pressure is preferred. In the case of blood in the stomach, when bleeding into the airway is responsible (e.g. post-tonsillectomy bleeding), an inhalation induction with the patient in the lateral position and tilted head-down has been recommended. Although succinylcholine increases intragastric pressure it also increases LOS tone. Head-up tilt may reduce the incidence of regurgitation, but predisposes to aspiration of any material in the pharynx into the lungs. Emptying of the stomach during anaesthesia with a suitably wide-bore gastric tube should be considered. Emergence from anaesthesia carries the same potential hazards as induction and the patient should be placed in the lateral position before anaesthesia is terminated. The trachea should be extubated only on return of protective airway reflexes.

Postoperative management

- Risk continues until larynx is competent.
- Gastric emptying is delayed by pain and opiates.
- Maintain lateral position.
- Avoid sedative agents.

Bibliography

Benington S, Severn A. Preventing aspiration and regurgitation. *Anaesth Intensive Care Med* 2007; **8**: 368–72.

Maltby JR. Preoperative fasting. *Curr Anaesth Crit Care* 1996; **7**: 276–80.

Cross-reference

Airway and aspiration risk, 640

Hiatus hernia

Brian J Pollard

Hiatus hernia is a condition caused by migration of a portion of the stomach through the oesophageal hiatus in the diaphragm. It is common, particularly in later life.

Two forms are usually described, the sliding type (85% of cases) in which the gastro-oesophageal junction passes into the thorax, and the rolling type, in which the stomach itself migrates into the thorax, the gastro-oesophageal junction remaining in the abdomen.

A higher incidence of hiatus hernia is associated with the following:

- increasing age
- obesity
- pregnancy.

Although often associated with symptoms of reflux oesophagitis, a hiatus hernia may be symptomless; equally, reflux oesophagitis may occur in the absence of hiatus hernia. Reflux is associated with decreased pressure in the LOS.

The lower oesophageal sphincter

An anatomically indistinct area of the oesophagus found around the diaphragmatic hiatus, 3–5 cm long, detectable as a high-pressure zone by manometry. It is usually closed at rest. The important variable is not LOS tone, but barrier pressure (LOS pressure minus gastric pressure). Reflux is unlikely to occur if barrier pressure is greater than 13 cmH_2O, although there is wide variation between individuals.

The normal response to an increase in gastric pressure is an increase in LOS pressure, but this adaptation is lost in those who develop reflux. The response is decreased by atropine, vagotomy and in symptomatic pregnant women at term. Drugs affecting LOS pressure are shown in Table 5.2. Of more anaesthetic relevance is symptomatic evidence of gastric reflux rather than the presence of a hiatus hernia.

Preoperative assessment

History

- Epigastric or retrosternal pain and heartburn, promoted by bending or lying down, pregnancy or obesity, relieved by antacids (sliding type).
- Discomfort or 'crushing' chest pain due to distension of the stomach with food (rolling type – symptoms of reflux are unusual).
- Waterbrash and reflux of bitter fluid into the pharynx and mouth.
- Dysphagia – rare, and usually denotes oesophageal stenosis; may prevent further regurgitation and, therefore, produce a reduction in symptoms.
- Nocturnal cough – suggesting regurgitation and aspiration; may lead to aspiration pneumonitis.

Table 5.2 Drugs affecting lower oesophageal sphincter (LOS) pressure

Increase LOS pressure	Decrease LOS pressure
Antiemetics	Anticholinergics
Metoclopramide	Atropine
Prochlorperazine	Glycopyrrolate
Domperidone	Thiopentone
Anticholinesterases	Opioids
Neostigmine	Alcohol
Edrophonium	Nicotine
α-Receptor agonists	Dopamine
Histamine	α-Receptor antagonists
Succinylcholine	β-Receptor agonists
	Tricyclic antidepressants
	Ganglion blockers

Investigations

- Full blood count: chronic blood loss is common, resulting in iron-deficiency anaemia.
- Chest X-ray: to exclude aspiration pneumonia.
- Barium studies.
- CT or MRI scan.

Perioperative management

Premedication

Consideration should be given to the preoperative use of antacids, proton pump inhibitors or H_2 receptor antagonists, if not already prescribed. If the patient is symptomatic, opioids should be used with caution. Since anticholinergic drugs cause a reduction in LOS pressure, which may make regurgitation more likely, careful consideration must be given to their use as part of premedication. Metoclopramide or domperidone will increase LOS pressure, and negate the effects of anticholinergic drugs.

Airway

If the patient is asymptomatic, there are no factors present likely to increase the risk of regurgitation, and the surgery itself is short and does not require tracheal intubation, then spontaneous ventilation using a laryngeal mask following antacid premedication may be considered.

However, if there is any doubt about the patient's safety, then full precautions to prevent regurgitation and aspiration of stomach contents must be employed, i.e. preoxygenation, rapid sequence induction with cricoid pressure and tracheal intubation. This is mandatory if the hiatus hernia is symptomatic.

Emergence

Ensure emergence/extubation with the patient in the lateral position.

Postoperative management

Semirecumbent or sitting position, when practical.

Bibliography

Cotton B, Smith G. The lower oesophageal sphincter. In: Kaufman L (ed.) *Anaesthesia Review*. London: Churchill Livingstone, 1982, vol. 1.

Pollard BJ, Lipscomb GR. Gastrointestinal disorders. In: Vickers MD, Power I (eds) *Medicine for Anaesthetists*, 4th edn. Oxford: Blackwell, 1999, pp. 175–91.

Stoelting RK, Dierdof SF. *Anaesthesia and Co-existing Disease*, 4th edn. New York: Churchill Livingstone, 2002, pp. 325–41.

Cross-references

Airway and aspiration risk, 640
Obesity, 189

The jaundiced patient

Brian J Pollard

In the jaundiced patient presenting for surgery, liver disease may be divided into:

- hepatocellular
- cholestatic (obstructive).

Hepatocellular jaundice may be caused by toxins, viruses and drugs. Surgery in this group carries a poor prognosis and should be avoided, being limited to emergency procedures only. Cholestasis may be extrahepatic or intrahepatic. Causes of the former include obstruction caused by calculus, stricture and cancer. Causes of the latter include viral hepatitis and adverse drug reactions. Such drugs cause a hypersensitivity response (e.g. chlorpromazine, carbemazepine, erythromycin, imipramine, azathiaprine) or present a pure intrahepatic cholestatic picture (e.g. synthetic oestrogens). Presentation for surgery is not uncommon. Aetiology is often difficult to ascertain clinically.

Complications of surgery increase with:

- haematocrit <30% on presentation
- plasma bilirubin >200 mmol L^{-1}
- presence of malignancy
- duration of jaundice (secondary biliary cirrhosis develops).

Associated problems

Acute oliguric renal failure

Occurs in up to 17% of all jaundiced patients undergoing surgery, with a mortality of up to 50%; 75% will have a fall in glomerular filtration rate postoperatively. Factors implicated include:

- hypovolaemia and hypotension
- the presence of bile salts
- bilirubin
- endotoxins.

Glomerular and peritubular fibrin deposition has been demonstrated in affected kidneys. Hepatorenal syndrome may occur associated with deterioration of hepatic function.

Coagulopathy

The vitamin K-dependent coagulation factors (2, 7, 9 and 10) are reduced and this is manifest as a prolonged PT (>4 seconds above control is abnormal). Hepatocellular coagulopathy is often refractory to vitamin K administration. Disseminated intravascular coagulation (DIC) is associated with secondary biliary tract infection (and possibly endotoxaemia), and increases mortality.

Altered drug handling

Drugs excreted via the biliary system have prolonged elimination half-life in cholestasis. Increased volume of distribution and reduced clearance produces initial pancuronium resistance. Repeated dosing is associated with prolongation of action. Atracurium is the drug of choice for muscular relaxation. Narcotics may produce spasm in the sphincter of Oddi (biliary colic, and difficulty with cholangiography).

Pseudocholinesterase has a very long half-life, and succinylcholine apnoea is not a feature, even in fulminant liver failure, although the duration of a dose of succinylcholine may be longer than expected.

Gastrointestinal tract

Stress ulceration occurs, with gastrointestinal haemorrhage demonstrated in 16% of cases.

Wound healing

This is significantly reduced, and correlates closely with degree of malnutrition, and the presence of sepsis and malignancy.

Preoperative assessment

History and clinical examination

Look for malnutrition, malignancy, anaemia, dehydration, jaundice, pyrexia, signs of drug abuse, concomitant diseases.

Investigations

- Haemoglobin: at presentation and current.
- White cell count: cholangitis, isolates and sensitivities.
- Platelet count: reduced with severe infection and DIC.
- Clotting screen: note effect of vitamin K administration.
- Urea, electrolytes, creatinine, glucose: creatinine clearance if poor or deteriorating renal function.

- Serum bilirubin (beware if >200 mmol L^{-1}).
- Serum albumin, calcium and magnesium.
- Serum transaminases: raised in hepatocellular dysfunction.
- Blood gases: respiratory alkalosis and hypoxaemia.
- Serology: consider infective risks to staff.
- Biopsy: pattern and degree of damage.
- Ultrasound, CT scan or MRI scan to visualize the biliary and pancreatic ducts.

Preoperative preparation

Depends on severity of disease. Commonly required preparation involves:

- rehydration
- appropriate cross-match and preoperative transfusion
- perioperative antibiotic administration
- administer vitamin K
- if PT remains abnormal, arrange clotting factors
- H_2 antagonist drugs
- urinary catheter early
- optimization of concurrent disease
- percutaneous drainage (symptoms improve, prognosis unaltered).

Administration of taurocholate and selective gut decontamination is controversial.

Premedication

- Anxiolysis is useful; if there is coagulopathy avoid the intramuscular route.
- With hepatocellular disease, consider duration of action of drugs.
- Avoid sedatives in encephalopathy.
- Continue H_2 antagonist and vitamin K.

Perioperative management

Poor prognosis may relate to a reduction in hepatic blood flow associated with general anaesthetics and total hepatic necrosis can occur. Renal insult must be avoided. Therefore, stable anaesthesia avoiding hypotension is essential. Preserve cardiac output with fluid loading. Adequate circulating volume and haematocrit are essential. Isoflurane does not have a major deleterious effect in animal models of hepatic circulation. Hypercarbia produces sympathetic activation, intermittent positive pressure ventilation to P_aco_2 35–40 mmHg would be advisable. Altered drug metabolism depends upon the high and low extraction ratio and is therefore difficult to predict. Acid–base disturbance may occur; alterations in electrolytes may contribute to encephalopathy and should be monitored.

Preservation of urine output with mannitol (0.5 g kg^{-1}) and diuretics has been advocated. This should not be at the expense of circulating volume. Replace massive diuresis. Aggressive replacement of blood loss is essential. Hypoglycaemia may occur (with severe injury); monitor and treat.

In all cases, a low threshold for invasive monitoring is to be recommended. In the presence of hepatocellular disease it is essential. An oesophageal Doppler may be of value. Dopamine may be beneficial in preservation of renal function perioperatively.

Hypothermia worsens coagulopathy. Therefore, warm fluids, humidify respiratory gases, use a warming blanket and/or warm air overblanket and reduce body surface heat losses.

Postoperative management

Transfer to a high-dependency area is advisable at least for the first 24–48 hours. Hypoxaemia is common. Drain losses should be aggressively replaced; hepatocellular disease may require additional clotting factors. Monitoring with thromboelastography is helpful. Replace urine losses appropriately. Continue dopamine until cardiovascularly stable. Catecholamines may reduce hepatic and renal blood flow. Epidural analgesia can be considered in the absence of coagulopathy. Intramuscular opiate administration is inappropriate in all but minor cases.

Outcome

Relates to severity of disease. Minor worsening of liver function tests is not uncommon; morphological change is. The following may worsen jaundice postoperatively:

- blood transfusion
- haemolysis
- hepatocellular damage:
  - postoperative cholestasis
  - circulatory failure
  - drug induced
  - exacerbated chronic disease
- extrahepatic obstruction:
  - duct stone
  - bile duct injury
  - postoperative pancreatitis.

Laparotomy in the presence of hepatocellular disease has been associated with perioperative mortality of 9.5% and morbidity of 12%. Approximately 25% of jaundiced patients undergoing surgery for relief of biliary obstruction have subsequently been demonstrated to have hepatocellular disease. A combination of anaemia at presentation, serum bilirubin >200 mmol L^{-1} and presence of malignancy carries a mortality of 60%.

Bibliography

Dixon JM, Armstrong CP, Duffy SW, Davies GC. Factors affecting morbidity and mortality after surgery for obstructive jaundice a review of 373 patients. *Gut* 1983; **24**: 845–52.

Haville DD, Dummerskill WHJ. Surgery in acute hepatitis. Causes and effects. *JAMA* 1963; **184**: 257.

Wilkinson SP, Moodie H, Stamatakis JD, *et al.* Endotoxaemia and renal failure in cirrhosis and obstructive jaundice. *Br Med J* 1976; **2**: 1415–18.

Cross-references

Assessment of renal function, 199
Open and laparoscopic cholecystectomy, 451

Malnutrition

Brian J Pollard

Malnutrition occurs when protein/calorie supplies are inadequate to meet requirements and is found in approximately 50% of surgical patients, resulting in an increased incidence of postoperative complications (Box 5.1).

Pathophysiology

General effects

These include: rapid weight loss; muscle wasting and fatigue; delayed ambulation following surgery, with an increased incidence of postoperative respiratory complications; bed sores and wound infections.

Pulmonary function

- Diaphragmatic muscle mass falls in a linear fashion with body weight. There is a fall in vital capacity and maximal ventilatory volume, an increased incidence of postoperative respiratory failure and difficulty in weaning from mechanical ventilation.
- Decreased surfactant production and emphysematous changes in the lung causes alveolar atelectasis.
- Increased incidence of chest infection results from a depressed immune response, alveolar atelectasis and an ineffective cough.
- The ventilatory response to hypoxia is markedly depressed.
- The work of breathing is increased.

Visceral protein deficiency

- Depletion of serum proteins, enzymes, immunoglobulins and vital organs.
- Reduced cardiac output, stroke volume, contractility and reserve.
- Hypoalbuminaemia results in interstitial and pulmonary oedema and reduced binding of metabolites, drugs and toxins.
- Anaemia (folate or iron deficiency or mixed).
- Low serum transferrin.
- Low T-lymphocyte count and function.
- Impaired antibody response.
- Low serum IgA.
- Pseudocholinesterase deficiency in severe malnutrition (serum albumin <2 g dL^{-1}).

Preoperative assessment

Nutritional assessment

Many of the indices of malnutrition (Table 5.3) lack specificity and are poor predictors of perioperative morbidity and mortality. Immunological changes and loss of hand grip power, however, do predict those patients likely to have an increased risk of perioperative problems. Patients who demonstrate anergy at 48 hours to the intradermal injection of several antigens (*Candida*, mumps, *Trychophyton*) have a marked increase in postoperative morbidity and mortality and may benefit from preoperative nutritional support.

Clinical assessment

- Evidence of fat and muscle wasting, e.g. weight loss, fatigue, hypothermia.
- Symptoms of vitamin deficiency, e.g. anaemia (vitamin E), bleeding tendency (vitamin K).
- Reduced pulmonary function, e.g. shortness of breath.
- Heart failure, e.g. peripheral oedema, orthopnoea.
- Arrhythmias.
- Increased frequency of infection.

Investigations

- ECG: AV block, prolonged Q–T interval.
- Echocardiogram: reduced myocardial contractility.
- Pulmonary function tests: forced vital capacity (FVC) 50 mL kg^{-1} in the absence of obvious lung disease; reduced maximal ventilatory volume.

Box 5.1 Definition of malnutrition and calculation of ideal body weight

Malnutrition is defined as:

- Moderate: 15% loss of ideal body weight
- Severe: 30% loss of ideal body weight

Calculation of ideal body weight (IBW) (Broca's index):

- For men: IBW (kg) = Height (cm) – 100
- For women: IBW (kg) = Height (cm) – 105

Table 5.3 Nutritional evaluation

Value measured	Degree of malnutrition				
	Normal value	Mild	Moderate	Severe	Causes of error
Weight (%)	100	80–90	70–79	<70	
Weight loss (%)	<0	10	10–20	>20	Dehydration
Fat reserves					
Triceps skin fold (%)	100	80–90	60–79	<60	Oedema
Somatic protein					
Arm muscle circumference (%)	100	80–90	60–79	<40	Oedema
Weight (% of ideal)	100	80–90	70–79	<70	Dehydration
Weight (% of usual)	100	90–95	80–89	<80	Dehydration
Creatine/height index (%)	100	60–80	40–59	<40	Renal disease
Visceral protein					
Serum albumin (g dL^{-1})	3.5–5.0	2.8–3.4	2.1–2.7	<2.1	Liver disease
Serum transferrin (mg dL^{-1})	175–300	150–175	100–150	<100	Trauma, surgery
Retinol binding protein (mg dL^{-1})	3–6	2.7–3.0	2.4–2.7	<2.4	State of hydration
Prealbumin (mg dL^{-1})	15.7–29.6	10–15	5–9.9	<5	Increased protein loss or demand, e.g. trauma
Total lymphocytes (mm^{-3})	1500–5000	1200–1500	800–1200	<800	Abnormal white cell count
Cell-mediated immunity		Reactive	Relative anergy	Non-reactive	Steroids, immune deficiency

Preoperative management

Preoperative nutrition should be discussed with surgeons and dieticians. Enteral and total parenteral nutrition (TPN) are equally beneficial.

Examine patient for the complications associated with TPN (Box 5.2) and correct serum electrolytes and blood glucose abnormalities. TPN must not be stopped suddenly, as rebound hypoglycaemia may occur. It should be:

- continued at the same rate, controlling hyperglycaemia perioperatively as in the diabetic patient
- weaned to half the maintenance rate over 12 hours preoperatively
- replaced by 10% glucose infused at the same rate (in unstable patients).

Blood transfusion for anaemia and correction of clotting abnormalities may be required. The impact of a low plasma albumin and its correction with albumin solutions on postoperative outcome in the malnourished patient has yet to be shown. Endogenous albumin production should be encouraged with nutritional support. Exogenous albumin actually reduces the amount of albumin production by the liver. The effect of preoperative albumin infusions to increase plasma oncotic pressure is ill defined, although they may play an important role as a result of increasing the

Box 5.2 Complications of TPN

- Catheter related
- Improper central line placement
- Infection
- Fluid overload
- Especially in the elderly and patients with heart failure
- Metabolic
- Hyperglycaemia
- Hypercarbia
- Hypokalaemia
- Hypomagnesaemia
- Hypophosphataemia

binding of metabolites, drugs and toxins. Controversy exists over the routine use of albumen solutions.

Perioperative management

Monitoring includes measurement of:

- CVP
- blood sugar
- end-tidal CO_2.

Careful positioning of the patient and aseptic line placement reduces the incidence of sepsis and injury.

Mechanical ventilation is indicated by preoperative pulmonary function tests. Ability to sustain head raise, FVC greater than 15 mL kg^{-1} and maximum inspiratory force greater than −25 cmH_2O indicate adequate muscle strength prior to extubation. The malnourished heart functions at the peak of the Starling curve, and so cardiac output may fall with increased diastolic filling, precipitating cardiac failure. Judicious fluid management with CVP monitoring may be required.

There is an increased sensitivity to:

- intravenous induction agents
- succinylcholine in severe malnutrition (albumin <2.0 g dL^{-1}), since pseudocholinesterase deficiency may exist
- non-depolarizing neuromuscular blockers in the presence of hypocalcaemia, hypophosphataemia and hypomagnesaemia
- drugs bound to albumin, e.g. diazepam
- drugs bound to skeletal muscle, e.g. digoxin.

Postoperative management

- Transfer to ICU/HDU for patients with severely reduced cardiorespiratory reserve.
- Mechanical ventilation in the case of:
  - fatigue
  - increased CO_2 production due to glucose feed
  - impaired response to hypoxaemia.
- Supplemental oxygen on the ward.
- Physiotherapy.
- Analgesia to allow an effective cough.
- Restart nutritional support slowly over 12–24 hours postoperatively.
- Monitor blood glucose and serum potassium and avoid hypophosphataemia.

Outcome

Several studies have shown an increased incidence of postoperative complications in the malnourished patient, e.g. respiratory complications, wound infections and bed sores. The role of pre- and postoperative nutritional support in the malnourished patient is poorly defined. Both reduce postoperative complications and improve pulmonary function in patients with fistulas, short bowel syndrome, burns and acute renal failure, and may have a place in patients who have lost more than 20% of their usual body weight. For the maximum nutritional benefit, feeding (whether enteral or parenteral) should be started 1 week to 10 days preoperatively.

Bibliography

Hill GL, Pickford I, Young GA, *et al.* Malnutrition in surgical patients: an unrecognised problem. *Lancet* 1977; **i**: 689–92.

Meakins JL, Pietsch JB, Bubenick D, *et al.* Delayed hypersensitivity: indicator of aquired failure to host defences in sepsis and trauma. *Ann Surg* 1977; **186**: 241–50.

Meguid MM, Campos AC, Hammond WG. Nutritional support in surgical practice. *Am J Surg* 1990; **159**: 345–58.

Rochester DF, Arora NS. Respiratory muscle failure. *Med Clin North Am* 1983; **67**: 573–97.

Obesity

Brian J Pollard

Obesity is a chronic nutritional disorder characterized by hypertension, cardiovascular and respiratory disease, diabetes, cirrhosis and hiatus hernia (Box 5.3). Although medical morbidity is correlated with weight, few prospective studies have been performed relating obesity and anaesthetic outcome (Fig. 5.1). Its incidence is rising.

Pathophysiology

Cardiovascular system

In the absence of ischaemic heart disease, obesity raises end-diastolic ventricular volume, increases stroke volume, and thereby increases cardiac output. Left ventricular work rises, in part due to the increased systemic vascular resistance, and is compensated for by biventricular hypertrophy. Filling pressure and cardiac output rise promptly with exercise, which includes moving body position in the morbidly obese.

> **Box 5.3 Definition of obesity and body mass index**
>
> Obesity may be defined in a number of ways:
> - Simple: Weight greater than 30% of ideal
> - Morbid: Weight greater than 100% of ideal
>
> Calculation of body mass index (BMI)
> - BMI = Weight (kg)/(height in metres)^2
>
> Patients with a BMI greater than 25 are regarded as overweight
> Patients with a BMI greater than 30 are regarded as obese
> Patients with a BMI greater than 39 are morbidly obese

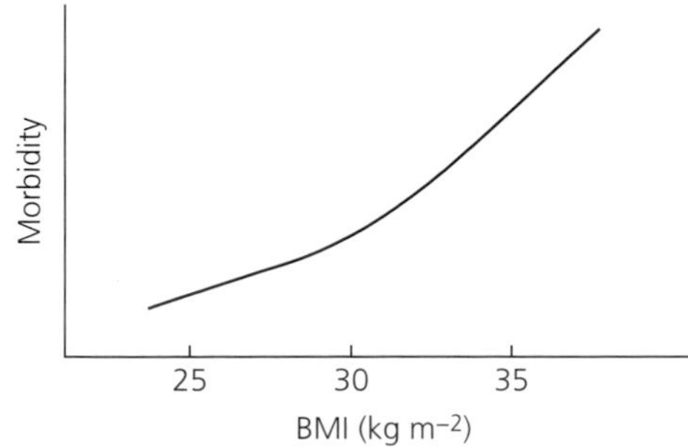

Figure 5.1 Relationship between body mass index (BMI) and morbidity.

Respiratory system

Obesity acts to impose a load on the chest wall, such that the work of breathing is raised, although lung compliance, in the absence of coexisting disease, is normal. Lung volume is reduced, and falls further with recumbency. In the morbidly obese, tidal breathing falls within the closing volume range. Arterial hypoxaemia is common, and increases pulmonary vascular resistance. In some morbidly obese patients (8%) the response to carbon dioxide is diminished – the obesity hypoventilation syndrome.

Gut

Both gastric acid and fasting gastric volume are raised in the obese. Abdominal pressure increases linearly with weight gain, and the incidence of hiatus hernia is high.

Endocrine system

Glucose tolerance in the obese is impaired and diabetes is common.

Coagulation

Laboratory evidence of hypercoagulability is slight, although some clinical reports suggest that the incidence of DVT is raised.

Preoperative assessment

Morphological

- Assessment of veins/arteries.
- Airway: mouth/jaw/dentition/neck.
- Posture for epidural, if appropriate.
- Transportation to theatre.

History

- Systematic review of associated cardiovascular and respiratory disease.
- Obesity hypoventilation syndrome:
  - day-time somnolence, poor concentration
  - night-time respiratory obstruction, nightmares and restlessness.
- Right ventricular failure.
- Smoking history.

Investigations

See Table 5.4.

Previous liver transplant

Brian J Pollard

The first human orthotopic liver transplant (OLT) was performed in 1963. This has become recognized as a therapeutic procedure for end-stage liver disease. Improvements in organ preservation, surgical and anaesthetic techniques and immunosuppression (ciclosporin initially) has led to an increase in the number of centres and in the number of cases performed. In 1993 over 3500 OLTs were performed in the USA and 700 in the UK. Today, there are many thousands of patients alive who have had a successful OLT. One year survival is 75–85% and the 5 year survival approaches 65–70%.

Patient characteristics

- Age: from infants to 70 years and over; majority are 30–60 years old.
- Medical status is generally good:
  - reversal of cardiovascular and pulmonary effects of chronic liver disease (hyperdynamic circulation and shunting) reported within 3 months of OLT
  - increased incidence of renal insufficiency in OLT patients (pre- and intraoperative factors and ciclosporin)
  - high incidence of hypertension reported after OLT.
- Normal liver function unless there is rejection, sepsis or recurrence of original disease.
- Immunosuppression increases susceptibility to infection.

Specific complications of OLT

- Early: vascular occlusion, bleeding and primary non-functional graft.
- Late: biliary leak and duct stenosis requiring reconstruction.

These will usually be dealt with at a primary transplant centre and are not further considered here.

Preoperative assessment and investigations

- Full systemic review for intercurrent or chronic problems and any evidence of infection.
- Consider the underlying pathology that led to the transplant – there may be residual effects from that pathological process.
- Formal clinical and biochemical assessment of liver function (chronic rejection, recurrent disease, biliary obstruction).
- Arrange conversion of immunosuppression from oral to intravenous administration if necessary.
- Liaise with transplant centre.

Investigations

- Full blood count: Hb, white blood cells (may be low with azathioprine).
- Liver function tests.
- Chest X-ray.
- Urea and electrolytes, plasma creatinine and creatinine clearance.
- Coagulation: PT, activate PTT, platelets with/without bleeding time.
- ECG.

Perioperative management: laparotomy

The aim is to avoid any deterioration or compromise in:

- Liver function, by optimizing hepatic oxygenation and blood flow. Maintain P_ao_2 above 15 kPa, normal P_ao_2 and pH and normovolaemia at all times. CVP and direct arterial monitoring are therefore desirable.
- Renal function, by optimizing volume status and using low-dose dopamine (1–3 μg kg^{-1} min^{-1}) and, if patient jaundiced, mannitol infusion.
- Be aware of increased infection risk. All invasive monitoring must be inserted with 'no touch' aseptic technique.

Anaesthesia

- Isoflurane or desflurane are the agents of choice: minimal metabolism and best preservation of hepatic arterial and mesenteric flow.
- Avoid halothane.
- Atracurium for neuromuscular relaxation.
- Maintain normocapnia and normal acid–base status to minimize effects on liver blood flow.

- Analgesia: epidural ideal for postoperative analgesia (NB check coagulation). If liver function is deranged, fentanyl is the safest choice intraoperatively.

Bleeding risk

May be increased because:

- previous surgery with the possibility of vascular adhesions
- abnormal liver function:
  - deranged coagulation
  - obstructive jaundice (vitamin K-dependent factors)
  - decreased synthesis of clotting proteins.

Management

- Correct prolonged PT with fresh-frozen plasma prior to surgery and invasive procedures.
- If platelet count <80 000, have platelets available for surgery.
- Drugs such as DDAVP and aprotinin (Trasylol) are useful in reducing blood loss resulting from platelet dysfunction and fibrinolysis; Trasylol also decreases 'ooze' from vascular adhesions.
- Coagulation monitoring: thrombelastography and/or serial clotting screens.

Postoperative management

For major procedures, these patients will require HDU care for a minimum of 24 hours.

- Postoperative analgesia:
  - epidural opiates/low-dose bupivacaine infusion
  - intravenous opiate infusion/patient-controlled analgesia pumps.
- Continue to ensure good oxygenation and optimize haemodynamics and volume status.
- Renal-dose dopamine for 24 hours postoperatively.
- Antibiotic prophylaxis.
- Continue immunosuppression and steroid cover.

Outcome

Increasing numbers of patients have successful liver transplants and may present months to years later with unrelated surgical problems. Careful preoperative assessment is essential, especially in relation to liver and kidney function. Perioperative management is directed to avoiding any factors that might compromise hepatic and renal function and minimizing the infection risk with antibiotic prophylaxis and careful aseptic techniques.

Bibliography

Bellamy MC. Therapeutic issues in transplant patients. *Anaesth Intensive Care Med* 2009; **5**: 248–51.

Cottam S, Jenkins S. Anaesthetic principles in liver transplantation. *Curr Anaesth Crit Care* 1999; **10**: 291–8.

Hawker F. Liver transplantation. In: Park G (ed.) *The Liver.* Philadelphia: WB Saunders, 1993, ch. 5, pp. 196–249.

Mallett SV, Cox DJA. The monitoring and treatment of coagulopathy during major surgery. *Br J Anaesth* 1992; **69**: 307–13.

Stock PG, Payne WD. Liver transplantation. Critical care of the transplant patient. *Crit Care Clin* 1990; **6**: 911–26.

Cross-reference

Liver transplantation, 527

Acute kidney injury

Denise McCarthy and George Shorten

Acute kidney injury (AKI), previously termed acute renal failure, is an acute decline in renal filtration function sufficient to result in the retention of nitrogenous end-products of metabolism, and is usually marked by an increase in serum creatinine concentration or azotaemia (an increase in blood urea nitrogen (BUN) concentration). Patients are not necessarily oliguric.

In 2004, the Acute Dialysis Quality Initiative Work Group published a consensus definition and classification system for acute kidney injury (the RIFLE classification: *r*isk of renal dysfunction, *i*njury to the kidney, *f*ailure or *l*oss of kidney function, and *e*nd-stage kidney disease). It defines three grades of severity of AKI (risk, injury and failure), based on changes to serum creatinine concentration and urine output and on two clinical outcomes (loss and end-stage). Subsequently adapted by the Acute Kidney Injury Network, the RIFLE classification has been validated in 550 000 patients. In general, the RIFLE criteria have clinical relevance for the diagnosis, classification and monitoring of progression of AKI, with modest predictive value for mortality (Fig. 6.1).

Causes

- Pre-renal – inadequate perfusion: 40–70%.
- Renal – intrinsic renal disease: 10–50%.
- Post-renal – obstructive uropathy: 10%.

The most common situation is the development of 'acute tubular necrosis' (ATN), due to ischaemia, or, occasionally, renal toxins. Necrosis is not the only form of cell death in AKI – tubular cell apoptosis (principally in the distal nephron) is an important factor in sepsis-related AKI. GFR is commonly estimated using the Cockcroft–Gault and Modification of Diet in Renal Disease study equations.

Acute tubular necrosis

Causes

- Hypoperfusion, i.e. decreased intravascular volume, sepsis, cardiogenic shock, cardiac tamponade.
- Embolic occlusion of the renal arteries.
- Severe hypoxia.

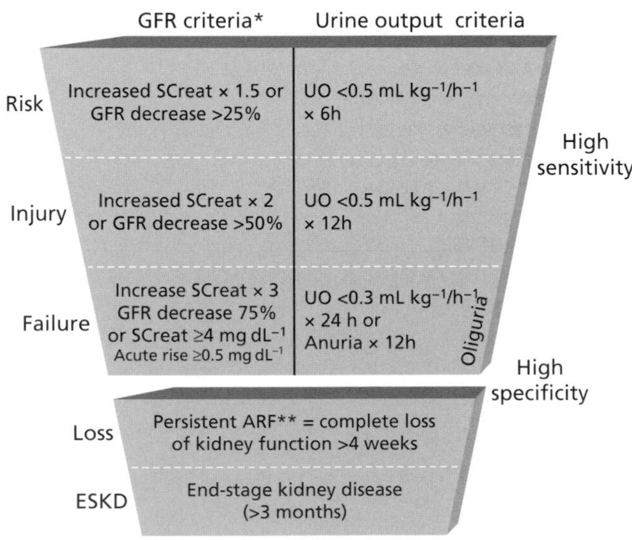

Figure 6.1 RIFLE classification of acute kidney injury. The classification system includes separate criteria for creatinine and urine output (UO). A patient can fulfil the criteria through changes in serum creatinine (SCreat) or changes in UO, or both. *GFR, glomerular filtration rate; **ARF, acute renal failure. Reproduced with permission. Bellomo *et al.* (2004) *Crit Care* 2004; 8(4): R204–R212. © BioMed Central Ltd.

- Drugs:
  - aminoglycosides
  - amphotericin B
  - radiocontrast agents
  - non-steroidal anti-inflammatory drugs (NSAIDs)
  - furosemide.
- Endogenous toxins:
  - free haemoglobin (Hb) after a transfusion reaction
  - myoglobin from rhabdomyolysis
  - abnormal reaction to succinylcholine
  - myeloma renal damage
  - crystals (urate, oxalate)
  - hypercalcaemia.

Prevention of pre-renal causes of ATN

Preoperative assessment

Detailed information should be elicited on patient factors known to be associated with increased risk for AKI (Box 6.1) and modifiable factors identified.

Box 6.1 Conditions associated with increased risk of perioperative acute kidney injury

- Preoperative renal disease
- Diabetes mellitus
- Hypertension
- Preoperative 'shock' states
- Cirrhosis
- Biliary obstruction
- Sepsis
- Multiple system trauma
- Multiple organ failure
- Cardiac failure
- Extracellular fluid volume deficit
- Elderly patients
- Aortorenal vascular disease

Perioperative management

Prevention of new perioperative AKI requires maintenance of renal perfusion and tissue oxygenation, and minimizing the use of nephrotoxic drugs:

- maintain oxygenation
- maintain normocarbia
- maintain renal perfusion pressure
- optimize intravascular volume and cardiac output
- there is no definitive evidence that any pharmacological agent can prevent or treat AKI:
  - furosemide – little or no evidence to support its use as a renoprotective agent; however, it may be useful in managing volume overload in responsive patients
  - dopamine increases renal blood flow; however, it offers no beneficial effect on renal outcome
  - mannitol – may have renoprotective effect in renal transplantation but no evidence to support its role in preventing AKI in the perioperative period in other patient populations
  - atrial natriuretic peptide – may be associated with improved outcomes when used in low doses for preventing AKI and in managing postsurgery AKI.

The observation that severe ischaemia induces renal injury less frequently in women than in men has led to a promising line of investigation of oestradiol as a renoprotective agent.

Prognosis

Perioperative AKI occurs in approximately 1% of patients undergoing general surgery procedures, and the development of AKI is associated with an eightfold increase in all-cause 30 day mortality. AKI is an independent risk factor for hospital mortality (odds ratio 3.12; 95% confidence interval 1.41, 6.93).

AKI – established

Anaesthetic assessment

A full history is taken, with particular attention to previous renal disease, infection, stones or prostatism. Examination should include a thorough assessment of intravascular volume status. Patients must have a urinary catheter and consideration should be given to using central venous pressure (CVP) monitoring.

Investigations

- Serum urea, creatinine and electrolytes.
- Ratio of urine/blood osmolality: if >1.5:1, this suggests hypovolaemia.
- Urine specific gravity and urea: intrinsic renal failure leads to a fixed specific gravity (SG) of 1010 and a urea concentration of <600 mg mL^{-1}. Urinary SG >1015 and urinary urea concentration >2 g 100 mL^{-1} are consistent with intravascular hypovolaemia.

Perioperative management

- Avoid drugs that require renal function for elimination.
- Maintain renal perfusion pressure.
- Monitor any urine output.

Bibliography

Abelha FJ, Botelho M, Fernandes V, Barro H. Determinants of postoperative acute kidney injury. *Crit Care* 2009; **13**(4): 171.

Bellomo R, Ronco C, Kellum JA, *et al.* Acute renal failure – definition, outcome measures, animal models, fluid therapy and information technology needs: the Second International Consensus Conference of the Acute Dialysis Quality Initiative (ADQI) Group. *Crit Care* 2004; **8**(4): R204–12.

Byrick RJ, Rose DK. Pathophysiology and prevention of acute renal failure: the role of the anaesthetist. *Can J Anaesth* 1990; **37**: 457–67.

Fleisher LA. *Evidence-Based Practice of Anesthesiology.* Philadelphia: WB Saunders, 2009.

Gokhale YA, Marathe P, Patil RD, *et al.* Rhabdomyolysis and acute renal failure following a single dose of succinylcholine. *J Assoc Phys India* 1991; **39**: 968–70.

Ho KM, Power BM. Benefits and risks of furosemide in acute kidney injury. *Anaesthesia* 2010; **65**(3): 283–93.

Hutchens MP, Nakano T, Kosaka Y, *et al.* Estrogen is renoprotective via a nonreceptor-dependent mechanism after cardiac arrest in vivo. *Anesthesiology* 2010; **112**(2): 395–405.

Kheterpal S, Tremper K, Heung M, *et al.* Development and validation of an acute kidney injury risk index for patients undergoing general surgery: results from a national data set. *Anesthesiology* 2009; **110**(3): 505–15.

Lerolle N, Nochy D, Guerot E, *et al.* Histopathology of septic shock induced acute kidney injury: apoptosis and leukocytic infiltration. *Intensive Care Med* 2010; **36**(3): 471–8.

Lobato EB, Gravenstein N, Kirby RR. *Complications in Anaesthesiology.* Philadelphia: Lippincott, Williams & Wilkins, 2008.

Nigwekar SU, Navaneethan SD, Parikh CR, Hix JK. Atrial natriuretic peptide for preventing and treating acute kidney injury. *Cochrane Database Syst Rev* 2009; (4): CD006028.

Srisiwat N. Modern classification of acute kidney injury. *Blood Purif* 2010; **29**: 300–7.

Uchino S, Bellomo R, Goldsmith D, *et al.* An assessment of the RIFLE criteria for acute renal failure in hospitalized patients. *Crit Care Med* 2006; **34**: 1913–17.

Cross-references

Assessment of renal function, 199
Postoperative oliguria, 779

Assessment of renal function

Denise McCarthy and George Shorten

The assessment of renal function is important to those caring for patients during the perioperative period for two reasons: (1) preoperative renal dysfunction is associated with greater risk of postoperative complications and (2) certain well-defined risk factors for new AKI or deterioration in renal function are detectable preoperatively (Box 6.2).

Box 6.2 Factors affecting renal function

- Intrinsic renal disease
- Extra-renal factors
  - intra- and extravascular fluid status
  - cardiovascular function
  - neuroendocrine factors

Perioperative AKI accounts for 50% of all patients requiring dialysis and is associated with a mortality incidence of 14–19% overall and 28–69% in patients requiring renal replacement therapy. Preoperatively, it is important to identify those patients at risk, and to take measures to protect them from developing postoperative renal complications. There is no single comprehensive test of renal function; all results should be viewed together with any significant history and examination.

Basic functions of the kidney

- Glomerular.
- Tubular.
- Endocrine.

The glomeruli are responsible for filtration and subsequent excretion of nitrogenous wastes.

Tubular function involves the selective reabsorption or secretion of particles regulating the movement of water and ions to maintain fluid balance, and the excretion/reabsorption of hydrogen ions to maintain acid–base homeostasis. Endocrine activity includes the production of renin (in the afferent arteriole), which is involved in water and electrolyte homeostasis, the release of prostaglandins (PG; the tubules synthesize PGE_2, the glomeruli both PGE_2 and prostacyclin) and the activation of both erythropoietin and vitamin D.

Assessment of renal function comprises history and examination, laboratory tests, ECG and may necessitate further investigations, e.g. chest X-ray and echocardiogram. The normal values for a 70 kg male are given in Table 6.1.

Table 6.1 Normal values for 70 kg male

Variable	Normal values
Cardiac output	5000 mL min^{-1}
Renal blood flow	1250 mL min^{-1}
Renal plasma flow	750 mL min^{-1}
Glomerular filtration rate	125 mL min^{-1}
Urine flow	2 mL min^{-1}

History and examination

Symptoms

In the early stages of renal disease there may be no symptoms. The loss of function in chronic kidney disease usually takes months or years to occur and may be asymptomatic until kidney function is less than 10% of normal. When symptoms do occur, they include:

- fatigue, general malaise, headaches
- nausea, weight loss, loss of appetite
- pruritus, dry skin
- polyuria
- polydypsia
- dysuria.

Signs

- Long-standing hypertension.
- Signs of hypervolaemia (e.g. oedema, dyspnoea) or, if overdialysed, patients may show signs of hypovolaemia (e.g. decreased skin turgor, tachycardia, hypotension).

Medication

- Diuretics.
- Potassium supplements.
- Immunosuppressive agents.
- Antihypertensive therapy.
- Dialysis schedule.

Investigations

The normal reference values for plasma and urine are given in Table 6.2.

Table 6.2 Normal reference values for measured variables in plasma and urine

	Normal range
Plasma	
Sodium	135–145 mmol L^{-1}
Potassium	3.5–5.0 mmol L^{-1}
Chloride	95–105 mmol L^{-1}
Osmolality	280–295 mOsm kg^{-1}
Urea (blood urea nitrogen (BUN))	2.5–7.0 mmol L^{-1}
Creatinine	40–120 mmol L^{-1}
Bicarbonate (HCO_3^-)	21–25 mmol L^{-1}
Calcium	2.1–2.8 mmol L^{-1}
Magnesium	0.7–1.0 mmol L^{-1}
Urine	
Sodium	50–200 mmol per 24 h
Potassium	30–100 mmol per 24 h
Chloride	100–300 mmol per 24 h
Osmolality	300–1000 mOsm kg^{-1}
Specific gravity	1003–1030
Creatinine	9.0–18 mmol L^{-1}
Creatinine clearance	110–130 mL min^{-1}
Urea clearance	60–95 mL min^{-1}
H^+	60 mEq per 24 h

Urinalysis

As a sole investigation, urinalysis is sufficient for screening patients with no history of renal or systemic disease.

Appearance

- Gross: bleeding, infection.
- Microscopic: casts, bacteria, cell forms.

pH

Normally, urine is acidic. Therefore, acidification is a measure of function.

Specific gravity

SG refers to the concentration of solutes in urine; the ability to concentrate is a measure of tubular function (Box 6.3). This is, however, non-specific.

Osmolality

- Osmolality is the number of osmotically active particles per unit of solvent (units: mOsm L^{-1}).

Box 6.3 Substances/conditions affecting SG

- Protein
- Glucose
- Mannitol
- Diuretics
- Extremes of age
- Antibiotics (carbenicillin)
- Temperature
- Hormonal imbalance (pituitary, adrenal and thyroid disease)

- Osmolality is more specific than SG, and is helpful at extreme values:
  - oliguria + osmolality >500 suggests pre-renal azotaemia
  - oliguria + osmolality <350 is likely to be ATN.

Oliguria itself also affects the osmolality value. Osmolality is useful only in low urine output states, coupled with a low SG. An osmolality of <350 mOsm kg^{-1} suggests an inability to concentrate urine and excrete electrolytes.

Protein

- <150 mg per 24 h: normal excretion (exercise and standing can increase this).
- >750 mg per 24 h: specific indicator of renal parenchymal disease.
- Massive: glomerular damage.

Glucose

Freely filtered and reabsorbed. Glycosuria occurs when an abnormally heavy load is presented to the tubules (e.g. diabetes mellitus, intravenous glucose).

BUN and creatinine

Urea is produced by protein catabolism in the liver. It is filtered and reabsorbed by the kidney. The amount reabsorbed varies with the patient's state of hydration: 33% is reabsorbed when the urine flow is <2 mL min^{-1}. Creatinine is a by-product of muscle metabolism and production is related to muscle mass. It is filtered and excreted by the kidney. Serum creatinine is an insensitive indicator of renal function – the value may be normal even if GFR is reduced by 50%. This is due to a combination of increased extrarenal metabolism and secretion of creatinine by the renal tubules. It is difficult to assess renal function using serum creatinine as it overestimates GFR. The non-renal variables affecting BUN and creatinine levels are shown in Box 6.4.

> **Box 6.4 Non-renal variables affecting BUN and creatinine levels**
>
> - Increased nitrogen absorption
> - Increased nitrogen waste production, e.g. sepsis, trauma
> - Diet
> - Body mass
> - Activity
> - Hepatic disease
> - Diabetic ketoacidosis
> - Large haematoma
> - Gastrointestinal bleeding
> - Drugs (steroids, cimetidine)

Creatinine clearance

This measures the glomerular filtration of creatinine (Cr), which approximates (although overestimates) to glomerular filtration rate:

$$\text{Cr clearance} = (\text{urine Cr} \times \text{UV})/\text{plasma Cr}$$

where UV is the urine volume.

The Cockcroft-Gault formula can also be used to calculate creatinine clearance:

$$\text{Cr clearance} = [(140 - \text{age}) \times \text{lean body weight (kg)}]/72 \times \text{plasma Cr (mg dL}^{-1})$$

Note: multiply value by 0.85 for females.

This approximation overestimates GFR by 10–20% because of creatinine secretion by peritubular capillaries.

GFR is estimated from equations using serum creatinine, age, race, sex and body size. One such equation is the Modification of Diet in Renal Disease (MDRD) Study equation.

A newer equation has been described to estimate GFR by the Chronic Kidney Disease Epidemiology (CKD-EPI) Collaboration. The CKD-EPI equation is more accurate than the MDRD Study equation overall and across most subgroups.

Biomarkers

The diagnosis of AKI has to date depended on detection of a decrease in kidney function by an increase in serum creatinine concentration, which only occurs after a significant decrease in renal function. Earlier detection of AKI would be beneficial. A number of early biomarkers of AKI are currently being investigated. Neutrophil gelatinase-associated lipocalin (NGAL), a 25 kDa protein that is bound to neutrophils and expressed in injured epithelial cells in organs including the kidney, has emerged as an accurate early biomarker of acute kidney injury. Plasma and urine NGAL have proved to be sensitive, specific and highly predictive early biomarkers of AKI after cardiac surgery in children, and these results have been confirmed in adults and in transplant patients. Other promising biomarkers are cystatin C, interleukin 18 and kidney injury molecule 1 (KIM-1). Further studies are required to validate the sensitivity and specificity of these biomarkers in clinical samples from large cohorts and from multiple clinical situations. Clinically relevant urinary biomarkers are summarized in Box 6.5.

> **Box 6.5 Clinically relevant urinary biomarkers**
>
> - Cystatin C
> - *N*-acetyl-β-D-glucosaminidase
> - Interleukin 18
> - Kidney injury molecule 1
> - Neutrophil gelatinase-associated lipocalin

Plasma electrolytes

Sodium, potassium, chloride and bicarbonate remain normal until advanced disease, when one sees a hyperkalaemic, hyperchloraemic acidosis. These changes will exacerbate dysrhythmias and compromise resuscitation. Frank renal failure results in hypocalcaemia, hyperphosphataemia and hypermagnesaemia.

Haematology

- Established renal failure: Hb = 3–9 g dL^{-1}.
- The white cell count may be abnormal if the patient is immunosuppressed.
- Uraemia causes platelet dysfunction and impaired platelet-vessel wall interaction, which can lead to impairment of coagulation and increased perioperative blood loss; however, there is also evidence indicating a prothrombotic state in these patients. Thromboelastographic indices in patients with chronic kidney disease show that all aspects of coagulation are increased, including initial fibrin formation, fibrin-platelet interaction and qualitative platelet function. There is also a reduction in fibrinolysis.

Chest X-ray

It is important to look for signs of hypertensive cardiovascular disease, pericardial/pleural effusions and, rarely, uraemic pneumonitis.

ECG

This shows the:

- toxic effects of hyperkalaemia
  - tall peaked T waves
  - ST depression
  - QRS widening
  - ventricular dysrhythmias

- toxic effects of hypocalcaemia
- signs of hypertension
- signs of ischaemic heart disease.

Echocardiography

In the presence of symptoms and signs of heart failure, left ventricular dysfunction should be evaluated. Preoperative left ventricular dysfunction has been shown to be a major risk factor for postoperative renal dysfunction and mortality.

Conclusion

At present, the measurement of creatinine clearance is the most accurate method of assessing renal function available in the clinical setting. However, it is time-consuming, has an inherent delay factor and does not offer the anaesthetist a simple, single-shot assessment of renal reserve. One relies on electrolytes, BUN and creatinine levels, which are not reliable indices of either glomerular or tubular function. A practical alternative is the use of equations estimating GFR (MDRD, CKD-EPI). The identification of novel biomarkers represents a promising step towards earlier diagnosis of kidney injury.

Bibliography

Aveline C, Leroux A, Vautier P, *et al.* Risk factors for renal dysfunction after total hip arthroplasty. *Ann Fr Anesth Reanim* 2009; **28**(9): 728–34.

Katz J, Benumof J, Kadis LB (eds). *Anesthesia and Uncommon Diseases*, 4th edn. Philadelphia: WB Saunders, 1998.

Kellen M, Aronson S, Roizen MF, *et al.* Predictive and diagnostic tests of renal function: a review. *Anesth Analg* 1994; **78**: 134–42.

Lobato EB, Gravenstein N, Kirby RR. *Complications in Anaesthesiology.* Philadelphia: Lippincott, Williams & Wilkins, 2008.

Loef BG, Epema AH, Navis G, *et al.* Postoperative renal dysfunction and preoperative left ventricular dysfunction predispose patients to increased long-term mortality after coronary artery bypass graft surgery. *Br J Anaesth* 2009; **102**(6): 749–55.

Mishra J, Dent C, Tarabishi R, *et al.* Neutrophil gelatinase-associated lipocalin (NGAL) as a biomarker for acute renal injury following cardiac surgery. *Lancet* 2005; **365**: 1231–8.

Mishra J, Ma Q, Kelly C, *et al.* Kidney NGAL is a novel early marker of acute kidney injury following transplantation. *Pediatr Nephrol* 2006; **21**: 856–63.

Moore EM, Simpson JA, Tobin A, Santamaria J. Preoperative estimated glomerular filtration rate and RIFLE classified postoperative acute kidney injury predict length of stay post-coronary bypass surgery in an Australian setting. *Anaesth Intensive Care* 2010; **38**(1): 113–21.

Nguyen MT, Devarajan P. Biomarkers for the early detection of acute kidney injury. *Pediatr Nephrol* 2008; **23**: 2151–7.

Pivalizza EG, Abramson DC, Harvey A. Perioperative hypercoagulability in uremic patients: a viscoelastic study. *J Clin Anesth* 1997; **9**: 442–5.

Prough DS, Foreman AS. Anesthesia and the renal system. In: Barash PG, Cullen BF, Stoelting RK, Cahalan M (eds) *Clinical Anesthesia*, 4th edn. Philadelphia: JB Lippincott, 2000.

Stevens LA, Schmid CH, Greene T, *et al.* Comparative performance of the CKD Epidemiology Collaboration (CKD-EPI) and the Modification of Diet in Renal Disease (MDRD) Study equations for estimating GFR levels above 60 mL/min/1.73 m^2. *Am J Kidney Dis* 2010; **56**: 486–95.

Thompson FD. Modern tests of renal function and drugs affecting the kidney. In: Kaufman L (ed.) *Anaesthesia Review*, vol. 7. Edinburgh: Churchill Livingstone, 1990, ch. 4.

Wagener G, Jan M, Kim M, *et al.* Association between increases in urinary neutrophil gelatinase-associated lipocalin and acute renal dysfunction after adult cardiac surgery. *Anesthesiology* 2006; **105**: 485–91.

Cross-reference

Postoperative oliguria, 779

Chronic kidney disease

Denise McCarthy and George Shorten

Chronic kidney disease (CKD) is defined as either (1) a glomerular filtration rate of <60 mL min^{-1} 1.73 m^{-2} for 3 months or more, irrespective of cause, or (2) kidney damage leading to a decrease in GFR, present for 3 months or more. Decreased GFR is associated in a graded fashion with increased risk of death, cardiovascular events and hospitalization, demonstrating its importance as a public health problem. The damage may manifest as abnormalities in the composition of blood or urine, on radiological imaging or in histology. It is classified into five stages depending on GFR (Table 6.3). CKD results in retention of nitrogenous waste products and inability to maintain fluid, electrolyte and acid–base homeostasis.

Table 6.3 Classification of chronic kidney disease

Stage	Description
1	Normal GFR; GFR >90 mL min^{-1} 1.73 m^{-2} with other evidence of chronic kidney damage*
2	Mild impairment; GFR 60–89 mL min^{-1} 1.73 m^{-2} with other evidence of chronic kidney damage*
3	Moderate impairment; GFR 30–59 mL min^{-1} 1.73 m^{-2}
4	Severe impairment; GFR 15–29 mL min^{-1} 1.73 m^{-2}
5	Established renal failure (ERF); GFR <15 mL min^{-1} 1.73 m^{-2} or on dialysis

*Other evidence of chronic kidney damage may be one of the following: persistent microalbuminuria; persistent proteinuria; persistent haematuria (after exclusion of other causes, e.g. urological disease); structural abnormalities of the kidneys demonstrated on ultrasound scanning or other radiological tests (e.g. polycystic kidney disease, reflux nephropathy); or biopsy-proven chronic glomerulonephritis (most of these patients will have microalbuminuria or proteinuria, and/or haematuria).

Reproduced with permission from www.renal.org.

Perioperative management of a patient with CKD requires assessment of cardiovascular status, blood volume and biochemical profile. Consideration also needs to be given to associated medical conditions, such as diabetes mellitus, to concurrent medication, and to requirement of peritoneal or haemodialysis.

Aetiology

- Diabetes mellitus, 19.8%.
- Glomerulonephritis, 10.3%.
- Pyelonephritis, 8.2%.
- Renovascular disease, 7.6%.
- Polycystic kidneys, 6.1%.
- Hyertension, 4.8%.
- Uncertain aetiology (glomerulonephritis unproven), 28%.
- Other (e.g. systemic lupus erythematosus, amyloidosis, gout, analgesic nephropathy, nephrocalcinosis), 15.2%.

Pathophysiology

CKD is associated with multisystem dysfunction resulting from the primary disease process and/or the effects of uraemia.

Biochemical

- Uraemia.
- Increased serum creatinine (>180 mmol L^{-1}).
- Electrolyte disturbance: hyperkalaemia, hyponatraemia, hyperphosphataemia, hypermagnesaemia, hypocalcaemia.
- Metabolic acidosis.

Associated cardiovascular abnormalities

- Hypertension.
- Left ventricular hypertrophy.
- Accelerated atherosclerosis.
- Fluid overload (unless dialysed).
- Cardiac failure (secondary to hypertension and increased cardiac output).
- Pericarditis and/or pericardial effusion.
- Peripheral vascular disease.
- Stroke.
- Hyperhomocystinaemia.

Respiratory

- Pulmonary oedema.
- Pleural effusion.

Haematological

- Anaemia (3–9 g dL^{-1}).
- Early stages: prothrombotic tendency; end-stage disease: prothrombotic tendency and bleeding diathesis (partly due to platelet dysfunction).

Immunological

- Immunosuppression due to uraemia or drugs.

Neurological

- Drowsiness, convulsions and coma (uraemia).
- Peripheral and autonomic neuropathies, especially if diabetic.

Gastrointestinal

- Autonomic neuropathy may lead to delayed gastric emptying and risk of pulmonary aspiration of gastric contents.
- Malnutrition.
- Stress ulceration.

Skeletal

- Renal osteodystrophy.

Preoperative assessment

History

- Drug history:
  - immunosuppressives
  - antihypertensives
  - oral hypoglycaemics.
- Review of systems particularly regarding cardiovascular disease.
- Method and time of last dialysis as well as the biochemical and haemodynamic results.

Examination

- Signs of fluid overload.
- Body weight and dialysis-related fluctuation.
- Location of arteriovenous fistula site or potential sites.

Investigations

- Full blood count (normochromic, normocytic anaemia).
- Clotting studies (including bleeding time).
- Full biochemical screen.
- ECG.
- Chest X-ray.

Premedication

The effects of premedication with sedative drugs and opioids are unpredictable and potentially dangerous. Decreased tolerance to these drugs is due to abnormal levels of plasma proteins and the effect of altered blood pH on their pharmacokinetics. Consider administration of an H_2 antagonist and/or metoclopramide preoperatively. Antihypertensive agents should generally be continued in the perioperative period (with the possible exception of angiotensin-converting enzyme inhibitors). CKD (defined as a serum creatinine >200 μmol L^{-1}) is a risk factor for perioperative cardiovascular complications. The American College of Cardiology/American Heart Association (ACC/AHA) guidelines recommend that the presence of one or more clinical risk factors, in patients having vascular or intermediate risk surgery, should prompt consideration of β-blocker therapy.

Perioperative management

One should avoid cannulating arteries or veins that might be used in the future to fashion arteriovenous fistulae. Central venous access may be indicated for monitoring fluid balance.

Induction

The pharmacokinetics of propofol are unaltered by CKD. Patients with established renal failure have been shown to require greater doses of propofol to achieve hypnosis than do patients with normal renal function (1.42 (0.24) mg kg^{-1} versus 0.89 (0.2) mg kg^{-1} respectively). In patients with CKD, thiopentone demonstrates an increased volume of distribution and decreased plasma protein binding, resulting in exposure of the brain to greater free drug concentration. Therefore, it should be administered with caution and the rate of administration decreased.

Succinylcholine administration should be avoided if the serum potassium level is greater than 5 mmol L^{-1} or if the patient has a peripheral neuropathy. Atracurium, cisatracurium and mivacurium are the neuromuscular blocking agents of choice in CKD because of their rapid elimination and independence of renal metabolism and excretion. The duration of action of vecuronium and rocuronium are increased in CKD and these agents are best administered as a single dose rather than by infusion. Sugammadex, a modified γ-cyclodextrin that selectively encapsulates steroid-based non-depolarizing neuromuscular blocking agents, may be useful in preventing postoperative residual curarization (PORC). Sugammadex is excreted unchanged in the urine but its efficacy as a reversal agent does not appear to rely on renal excretion of the cyclodextrin–relaxant complex. Sugammadex administered at reappearance of T_2 rapidly and effectively reverses neuromuscular blockade induced by rocuronium in renal failure (creatinine clearance (CL_{CR}) <30 mL min^{-1}) and healthy patients. However, it is not currently recommended for use in CKD patients with creatinine clearance <30 mL min^{-1} or in those on dialysis (European Medicines Agency; www.ema.euroa.eu).

Maintenance

- CVP monitoring may be a useful guide to maintenance of blood volume and systemic blood pressure.

- Urine output, if any, should be monitored.
- Brachial plexus block is a reasonable technique to facilitate fistulae formation; however, one must balance the benefits against the risk of a bleeding tendency. Bupivacaine and lidocaine may be safely administered. Both these agents have a shorter duration of action in patients with CKD.
- Although remifentanil has an active metabolite with 1/1000th the potency of the parent compound, its accumulation is unlikely to be clinically relevant. In patients on haemodialysis, remifentanil has a decreased clearance and prolonged elimination half-life.
- Isoflurane and desflurane are ideal inhalational agents, with minimal metabolism and augmentation of muscle relaxation. The use of enflurane is controversial owing to the potential accumulation of fluoride ions, usually <15 μmol L^{-1} (nephrotoxic concentration >50 μmol L^{-1}). Sevoflurane degrades to compound A, which is nephrotoxic in rats; however, the compound A production is minimal with Amsorb as carbon dioxide absorber.

Analgesia

- The administration of paracetamol to patients with CKD in the perioperative period is safe and does not require dose adjustment. NSAIDs should be avoided.
- Morphine and pethidine should be administered with caution, as their metabolites (morphine-6-glucuronide and norpethidine, respectively) tend to accumulate and can result in delayed onset of sedation and respiratory depression.
- Oxycodone undergoes hepatic metabolism to noroxycodone and oxymorphone, which accumulate in patients with CKD. Therefore, the dose of oxycodone should be decreased and the dose interval increased.

Postoperative management

- One should consider admission to a high-dependency unit after major surgery or if significant comorbidities.
- It is necessary to re-evaluate fluid balance and hydration regularly using clinical assessment, measurement of CVP and urine output (if any).
- Oxygen therapy to maximize carrying capacity.
- Serum electrolytes should be measured.

The later postoperative period

- Although these patients are at increased risk of bleeding, thromboembolic prophylaxis is also important.
- Patients with CKD usually require further anaesthetics, including for fistula formation for dialysis.

Bibliography

Ansell D, Feest TG, Tomson C, *et al. UK Renal Registry Report 2006*. Bristol: UK Renal Registry, 2007.

Bedford RF, Ives HE. The renal safety of sevoflurane. *Anesth Analg* 2000; **90**: 505–8.

Chauvin M, Sandouk P, Scherrmann JM, *et al.* Morphine pharmacokinetics in renal failure. *Anesthesiology* 1987; **66**: 327–31.

Craig RG, Hunter JM. Recent developments in the perioperative management of adult patients with chronic kidney disease. *Br J Anaesth* 2008; **101**: 296–310.

Dahaba AA, Oettl K, Von Klobucar F, *et al.* End-stage renal failure reduces central clearance and prolongs the elimination half life of remifentanil. *Can J Anaesth* 2002; **49**: 369–74.

Dyson D. Anesthesia for patients with stable end-stage renal disease. *Vet Clin North Am Small Anim Pract* 1992; **22**: 469–71.

Fleisher LA, Beckman JA, Brown KA, *et al.* ACC/AHA 2007 guidelines on perioperative cardiovascular evaluation and care for noncardiac surgery: a report of the American College of Cardiology/American Heart Association Task Force on Practice Guidelines (writing committee to revise the 2002 guidelines on perioperative cardiovascular evaluation for noncardiac surgery). *Circulation* 2007; **116**: e418–99.

Go AS, Chertow GM, Fan D, *et al.* Chronic kidney disease and the risks of death, cardiovascular events, and hospitalization. *N Engl J Med* 2004; **351**: 1296–305.

Goyal P, Puri GD, Pandey CK, Srivastva S. Evaluation of induction doses of propofol: comparison between endstage renal disease and normal renal function patients. *Anaesth Intensive Care* 2002; **30**: 584–7.

Higuchi H, Adachi Y, Arimura S, *et al.* Compound A concentrations during low-flow sevoflurane correlate directly with the concentration of monovalent bases in carbon dioxide absorbents. *Anesth Analg* 2000; **91**: 434–9.

Joint Specialty Committee on Renal Medicine of the Royal College of Physicians of London and the Renal Association, and the Royal College of General Practitioners. *Chronic Kidney Disease in Adults: UK Guidelines for Identification, Management and Referral.* London: Royal College of Physicians, 2006.

Kirvela M, Lindgren L, Seppala T, Olkkola KT. The pharmacokinetics of oxycodone in uremic patients undergoing renal transplantation. *J Clin Anesth* 1996; **8**: 13–18.

Levey AS, Eckardt KU, Tsukamoto Y, *et al.* Definition and classification of chronic kidney disease: a position statement from Kidney Disease: Improving Global Outcomes (KDIGO). *Kidney Int* 2005; **67**: 2089–100.

McLeod GA, Burke D. Levobupivacaine. *Anaesthesia* 2001; **56**: 331–41.

Moore EW, Hunter JM. The new neuromuscular blocking agents:do they offer any advantages? *Br J Anaesth* 2001; **87**(6): 912–25.

Naguib M. Sugammadex: another milestone in clinical neuromuscular pharmacology. *Anesth Analg* 2007; **104**: 575–81.

Ninomiya T, Perkovic V, Gallagher M, *et al.* Lower blood pressure and risk of recurrent stroke in patients with chronic kidney disease: PROGRESS trial. *Kidney Int* 2008; **73**(8): 963–70.

Rice AS, Pither CE, Tucker GT. Plasma concentrations of bupivacaine after supraclavicular brachial plexus blockade in patients with chronic renal failure. *Anaesthesia* 1991; **46**: 354–7.

Schiffrin EL, Lipman ML, Mann JF. Chronic kidney disease: effects on the cardiovascular system. *Circulation* 2007; **116**: 85–97.

Sear JW. Drug handling in renal impairment. *Curr Anaesth Crit Care* 1992; **3**: 133–9.

Smith I, Nathanson M, White PF. Sevoflurane – a long-awaited volatile anaesthetic. *Br J Anaesth* 1996; **76**: 435–45.

Staals LM, Snoeck MMJ, Driessen JJ, *et al.* Multicentre, parallel-group, comparative trial evaluating the efficacy and safety of sugammadex in patients with end-stage renal failure or normal renal function. *Br J Anaesth* 2008; **101**(4): 492–7.

Cross-references

Assessment of renal function, 199
Fluid and electrolyte balance, 754
Kidney transplantation, 522
Postoperative oliguria, 779

Goodpasture syndrome

Denise McCarthy and George Shorten

Although originally described in an 18-year-old man who developed haemoptysis and died during the influenza outbreak of 1919 following an influenza-type illness, it was not until 1958 that the term 'Goodpasture syndrome' was used to describe the entity of *pulmonary haemorrhage* and *glomerulonephritis.*

Definition of the disease/ syndrome

Goodpasture disease is glomerulonephritis with pulmonary haemorrhage and the presence of circulating antiglomerular basement membrane (anti-GBM) antibodies. Goodpasture syndrome refers to the clinical condition of glomerulonephritis with diffuse pulmonary haemorrhage and, therefore, includes those diseases which are anti-GBM antibody negative as well as positive, such as:

- polyarteritis nodosa
- Wegener's granulomatosis
- primary crescentic glomerulonephritis
- following treatment with penicillamine
- systemic lupus erythematosus.

The term anti-GBM antibody disease describes patients with serum antibodies against the basement membrane and encompasses both Goodpasture syndrome and Goodpasture disease.

Anti-GBM antibodies and antineutrophil cytoplasmic autoantibodies (ANCAs) can be assayed by immunofluorescence, allowing for a more rapid and accurate diagnosis than was possible in the past.

Pathophysiology

The pathogenic mechanism involves the development of antibodies to pulmonary and glomerular basement membranes, with an ensuing autoimmune process accounting for the renal lesions (crescentic glomerulonephritis), and pulmonary alveolitis resulting in haemoptysis. Autoantibodies to the NC1 of collagen α3(IV) are instrumental in causing renal injury. Exposure to environmental factors, such as viral infections, hydrocarbons and tobacco, can precipitate the disease and worsen the pulmonary lesions.

Patients with specific human leukocyte antigen (HLA) types are more susceptible to disease and may have a worse prognosis. Patients with Goodpasture disease have an increased incidence of *HLA-DR2* compared with control populations. In addition, *HLA-B7* is found more frequently in and is associated with more severe anti-GBM nephritis.

Epidemiology

- Annual incidence estimated 0.5–1 per 1 million population.
- Bimodal distribution: more common in the third and sixth decades of life.
- Male preponderance.
- Most patients are Caucasian.
- Genetic predisposition: HLA-DRA carriers in >80% of cases.

Presenting features

- Pulmonary features appear early:
  - dyspnoea
  - haemoptysis (rusty sputum to massive bleed) occurs in 80% of patients and is the most common presenting symptom.
- Renal:
  - haematuria
  - nephrotic picture
  - oliguria/anuria
  - hypertension.

Natural history

Once respiratory symptoms develop, oliguria and anuria usually follow. The renal recovery rate at 1 year is 95% for patients with a creatinine concentration at presentation of <500 µmol L^{-1}. Risk factors for renal non-recovery are early oligo/anuria and requirement for haemodialysis: only 5% of patients who are dialysis dependent at the start of treatment recover renal function. Renal transplantation can be performed in patients requiring chronic haemodialysis after disappearance of the circulating anti-GBM antibodies.

Patients are treated with steroids, renal support, the administration of cytotoxic drugs (e.g. cyclophosphamide) and plasmapheresis.

Pulmonary signs and symptoms are improved by decreasing anti-GBM titres with plasmapheresis and immunosuppression. Clinical lapses during treatment are characterized by fever and decreased pulmonary and renal function. Patient survival is 77% at 1 year.

Mortality is usually due to overwhelming sepsis or pulmonary haemorrhage.

Perioperative management

Elective surgery should be carried out during quiescent periods (low diffusing lung capacity for carbon monoxide (DLco)). Preoperative blood transfusion and dialysis may be necessary to optimize fluid, electrolyte and haemodynamic status.

Investigations

- Full blood count: microcytic hypochromic anaemia; 90–100% of patients have a haemoglobin concentration of <12 g dL^{-1}.
- Coagulation: usually normal.
- Urea and electrolytes: derangement reflects the degree of renal impairment.
- Chest X-ray: small discrete shadowing; confluent densities; bilateral alveolar infiltrates.
- Pulmonary function: restrictive picture; DLco elevated.
- ECG: may show signs of electrolyte abnormalities; systemic hypertension; pulmonary hypertension.

Premedication

- Avoid respiratory depression.
- Steroid cover.

Specific monitoring concerns

- Airway pressures and total pulmonary compliance should be monitored as changes may reflect intraoperative pulmonary haemorrhage.

Specific problems

- If using positive pressure ventilation, a ventilatory strategy aimed at maintaining normocapnia while minimizing the risk of volutrauma and barotrauma is recommended.
- Pulmonary haemorrhage leads to airway/endotracheal tube obstruction. Therefore, use of the largest appropriately sized endotracheal tube is advisable and endotracheal suctioning may be necessary.
- Avoid renally excreted neuromuscular blockers.
- Aseptic techniques for immunosuppressed patients.

Postoperative management

- Pulmonary physiotherapy.
- Monitor renal function.
- Increased steroid dosage.

Bibliography

Ball JA, Young Jr KR. Pulmonary manifestations of Goodpasture's syndrome: antiglomerular basement membrane disease and related disorders. *Clin Chest Med* 1998; **19**: 777–9.

Droz D. Hemorragies pulmonaires et glomerulo nephrites rapidement progressives (syndromes pneumo-renaux). *Semin Hop Paris* 1990; **66**: 407–12.

Goodpasture EW. The significance of certain pulmonary lesions in relation to the etiology of influenza. *Am J Med Sci* 1919; **158**: 863–70.

Katz J, Benumof J, Kadis LB (eds). *Anesthesia and Uncommon Diseases*, 4th edn. Philadelphia: WB Saunders, 1998.

Kelly PT, Haponik EF. Goodpasture syndrome: molecular and clinical advances. *Medicine (Baltimore)* 1994; **73**: 171–85.

Levy JB, Turner AN, Rees AJ, *et al.* Long term outcomes of anti-glomerular basement membrane antibody disease treated with plasma exchange and immunosuppression. *Ann Intern Med* 2001; **134**: 1033–42.

Plaisier E, Rossert J. Syndrome de Goodpasture. In: Kahn M-F, Peltier A-P, Meyer O, Piette J-C (eds) *Maladies et Syndromes Systemiques*. Paris: Médecine-Sciences Flammarion, 2000, pp. 763–76.

Prough DS, Foreman AS. Anesthesia and the renal system. In: Barash PG, Cullen BF, Stoelting RK, Cahalan M (eds) *Clinical Anesthesia*, 4th edn. Philadelphia: JB Lippincott, 2000.

Shah MK, Hugghins SY. Characteristics and outcomes of patients with Goodpasture's syndrome. *South Med J* 2002; **95**(12): 1411–18.

Stanton MC, Tange JD. Goodpasture's syndrome: pulmonary haemorrhage associated with glomerulonephritis. *Aust Ann Med* **1958**; 7: 132–44.

Stoelting RK, Dierdorf SF (eds). *Renal Disease in Anesthesia and Coexisting Disease*, 4th edn. Edinburgh: Churchill Livingstone, 2002.

Salama AD, Levy JB, Lightstone L, Pusey CD. Goodpasture's disease. *Lancet* 2001; **358**: 917–20.

Yang R, Cui Z, Zhao J, *et al.* The role of HLA-DRB1 alleles on susceptibility of Chinese patients with anti-GBM disease. *Clin Immunol* 2009; **133**: 245–50.

Zhao J, Cui Z, Yang R, *et al.* Anti-glomerular basement membrane autoantibodies against different target antigens are associated with disease severity. *Kidney Int* 2009; **76**: 1108–15.

Haemolytic uraemic syndrome

Denise McCarthy and George Shorten

The haemolytic uraemic syndrome (HUS) is the triad of *renal failure, haemolytic anaemia* and *thrombocytopenia* and is the most common cause of renal failure in infancy and childhood.

There are two predominant types of HUS: D+ HUS, which is associated with a prodromal diarrhoeal illness, and D– HUS, which is not. D+ HUS accounts for 90–95% of cases in children. This form is preceded by 4–6 days of diarrhoeal illness, most commonly caused by infection with Shiga toxin-producing *Escherichia coli. E. coli* serotype 0157:H7 has been associated with more than 60% of infections leading to HUS.

Of D– HUS cases, 30–50% can be attributed to dysregulation of the alternative complement pathway. This involves mutations in factor H, factor I, CD46/ membrane cofactor protein, factor B and C3 components. The aetiology of the remainder of cases is unknown. HUS patients present for anaesthesia most commonly for the creation of arteriovenous fistulae and shunts.

Pathophysiology

This is a multisystem disease affecting not only the kidneys, erythrocytes and platelets, but also the gastrointestinal tract, liver, heart and central nervous system (CNS). It is classed as a thrombotic microangiopathy.

Cardiovascular system

- Myocarditis, congestive heart failure and severe systemic hypertension.

Respiratory system

- Severe respiratory insufficiency may occur, unrelated to volume overload, pulmonary oedema or congestive heart failure.

Central nervous system

- Drowsiness, seizures, hemiparesis and coma.

Biochemical

- Evidence of acute renal failure, including acid–base and electrolyte disturbances.
- Abnormal liver function tests associated with hepatitis.

Haematological

- Haemolysis rapidly appears; haemoglobin falls to as low as 4 g L^{-1}
- Thrombocytopenia (lasting 7–14 days).
- Hepatosplenomegaly.

Renal system

- Proteinuria, haematuria and oliguria, leading to anuria.

Gastrointestinal tract

- Haemorrhagic gastritis.

Immunological

- Severe infections are common, e.g. peritonitis, meningitis and osteomyelitis.

Natural history

- In D+ HUS, the mortality rate is 3–5%. Older children and adults have poorer prognoses. Death is nearly always associated with severe extrarenal disease, including severe CNS involvement. Approximately two-thirds of children with D+ HUS require dialysis during the illness; 85% of patients regain normal renal function.
- D– HUS has a relatively poor prognosis, with a mortality rate of up to 25% in the acute phase; 50% of patients require renal replacement therapy at some point in the illness.

Management

- Fluid resuscitation may be necessary.
- Hyperkalaemia may occur and should be treated.
- Dialysis may be necessary if acute kidney injury occurs.
- Hypertension should be controlled with standard antihypertensive agents.
- Plasma exchange (plasmapheresis in combination with fresh-frozen plasma replacement) may be necessary. Plasma exchange is performed daily until remission is obtained. However, because 85% of children with haemolytic uraemic syndrome recover after supportive therapy alone, plasma exchange is generally reserved for the most severe cases.

Preoperative assessment

Examination

- Full neurological and cardiovascular examination.
- Evidence of hepatic dysfunction.
- Evidence of clotting disorders.

Investigations

- Full blood count.
- Urea and electrolytes, and creatinine.
- Liver function tests.
- Glucose.
- Clotting studies.
- Arterial blood gases.
- Chest X-ray.
- ECG.

Preoperative management

Premedication is unnecessary as patients in the acute phase tend to be lethargic and drowsy. Correction of acid–base status and electrolyte and coagulation disorders should be arranged prior to surgery. Preoperative transfusion may be necessary, and any anticonvulsant therapy should be continued perioperatively.

Perioperative management

General anaesthesia is preferred owing to the presence of coagulation disorders in an uncooperative and severely ill child. A reduction in the dose of thiopentone (less protein binding in hepatic disease) is usual. Rapid sequence induction should be performed. Isoflurane and atracurium are the ideal agents for maintenance, although administration of desflurane or mivacurium is also appropriate. In most surgery, continual monitoring of acid–base and electrolyte status, temperature and urine output will be required.

Postoperative management

Postoperative ventilation may be required in patients with severe cerebral involvement. Sepsis is a common postoperative complication.

The later postoperative period

Repeated procedures are common. A haemolytic crisis may last more than 2 weeks and the anaemia can persist for months. Renal function may recover completely, or the child may require permanent haemodialysis.

Bibliography

Caprioli J, Noris M, Brioschi S, *et al.* Genetics of HUS: the impact of MCP, CFH, and IF mutations on clinical presentation, response to treatment, and outcome. *Blood* 2006; **108**: 1267–79.

Johnson GD, Rosales JK. The haemolytic uraemic syndrome and anaesthesia. *Can J Anaesth* 1987; **34**: 196–9.

Scheiring J, Andreoli SP, Zimmerhackl LB. Treatment and outcome of Shiga-toxin-associated hemolytic uremic syndrome (HUS). *Pediatr Nephrol* 2008; **23**(10): 1749–6.

Zheng XL, Sadler JE. Pathogenesis of thrombotic microangiopathies. *Annu Rev Pathol* 2008; **3**: 249–77.

Cross-references

Anaemia, 216
Assessment of renal function, 199
Fluid and electrolyte balance, 754
Patients with heart failure, 159

Nephrotic syndrome

Denise McCarthy and George Shorten

Eighty per cent of nephrotic syndrome cases are secondary to glomerulonephritis.

Presenting features

- Proteinuria (>3 g per 24 h).
- Hypoalbuminaemia.
- Hypercholesterolaemia.
- Thromboembolic episodes.

Aetiology

Classification

Nephrotic syndrome can be primary, being a disease specific to the kidneys, or it can be secondary to a systemic condition. Injury to glomeruli is an essential feature.

Primary causes

- Minimal change nephropathy.
- Focal glomerulosclerosis.
- Membranous nephropathy.
- Hereditary nephropathies.

Secondary causes

- Diabetes mellitus.
- Lupus erythematosus.
- Amyloidosis and paraproteinaemias.
- Viral infections (e.g. hepatitis B, hepatitis C, human immunodeficiency virus).
- Pre-eclampsia.

Pathophysiology

A defect in the glomerular barrier leads to an increase in glomerular permeability, which results in proteinuria/albuminuria.

Hypoalbinaemia leads to a decrease in plasma oncotic pressure, retention of sodium and water with the accumulation of peripheral oedema, ascites, pleural effusions and hypovolaemia (Fig. 6.2). This physiologically deranged state puts the patient at risk of thromboembolism, commonly venous (deep venous thrombosis, renal vein thrombosis) but also arterial. Venous thromboembolism occurs in 10% of patients within 6 months of presentation.

Diagnosis

The definitive diagnosis is made based on renal biopsy.

Natural history

Most cases spontaneously remit without treatment; hypertension occurs commonly, although renal failure is rare.

The interval between initiating steroid therapy and disease remission is a prognostic indicator for children with idiopathic nephrotic syndrome. Patients who respond to steroid treatment within 7 days do not relapse, or relapse infrequently.

Patients may develop renal failure as well as secondary complications including thrombotic episodes and infection (which may be associated with immunosuppressive treatment).

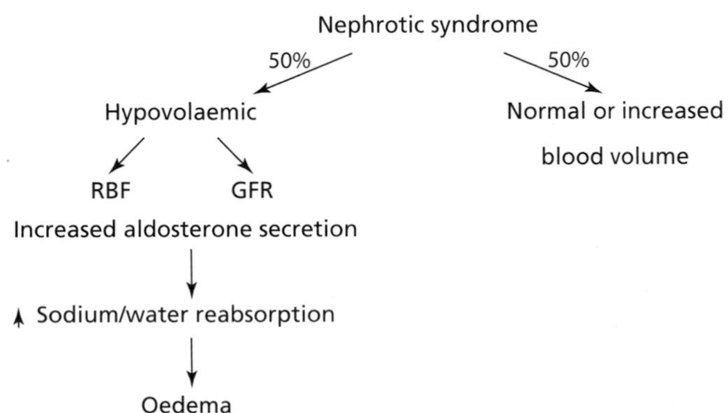

Figure 6.2 Effects of nephrotic syndrome on body fluid homeostasis. RBF, renal blood flow; GFR, glomerular filtration rate.

In patients with secondary nephrotic syndrome, morbidity and mortality are related to the primary disease process, such as diabetes mellitus or lupus. In diabetic nephropathy, the magnitude of proteinuria relates directly to mortality.

Treatment

- Diuretics.
- Angiotensin-converting enzyme inhibitors and angiotensin receptor blockers are used alone or in combination.
- Prednisolone.
- Cyclophosphamide.
- Mycophenolate.
- Ciclosporin.

Specific treatment of nephrotic syndrome depends on the aetiology. Thus, glucocorticosteroids, such as prednisone, are used for minimal change nephropathy. Prednisone and cyclophosphamide are useful in some forms of lupus nephritis. Secondary amyloidosis with nephrotic syndrome may respond to anti-inflammatory treatment of the primary disease. Patients with membranous nephropathy and a low risk for progression should be managed expectantly for the first 6 months.

Preoperative management

- Drug history: diuretics, steroids, antihypertensives.
- Clinical signs of oedema.
- CVP monitoring (to assess volume status, as these patients are likely to have depleted intravascular volume).
- Assess renal function.
- Potassium supplementation may be required; any deficiency may be due to the disease itself, or induced by diuretics/steroids.

Anaesthetic considerations

- Precautions and care, as for any patient with renal impairment/failure.
- Low plasma protein concentrations can influence the pharmacodynamics of drugs which are highly protein bound. Therefore, reduce the dose of induction agents, especially thiopentone and monitor neuromuscular blockade.

Postoperative management

- Thromboembolic prophylaxis.

Polycystic disease

- Autosomal dominant inheritance.
- The disease progresses slowly leading to end-stage kidney disease in middle age.

Pathophysiology

- Hypertension.
- Proteinuria.
- Decrease in urine-concentrating ability early in the disease.

Associated cysts

- Liver.
- CNS (intracranial aneurysms).

Treatment

- Renal replacement therapy.
- Renal transplantation.

Anaesthetic considerations

- As for end-stage kidney disease, if present.

Bibliography

du Buf-Vereijken PW, Branten AJ, Wetzels JF. Idiopathic membranous nephropathy: outline and rationale of a treatment strategy. *Am J Kidney Dis* 2005; **46**(6): 1012–29.

Jude EB, Anderson SG, Cruickshank JK, *et al.* Natural history and prognostic factors of diabetic nephropathy in type 2 diabetes. *Q J Med* 2002; **95**: 371–7.

Mahmoodi BK, ten Kate MK, Waanders F, *et al.* High absolute risks and predictors of venous and arterial thromboembolic events in patients with nephrotic syndrome: results from a large retrospective cohort study. *Circulation* 2008; **117**(2): 224–30.

Vivarelli M, Moscaritolo E, Tsalkidis A, *et al.* Time for initial response to steroids is a major prognostic factor in idiopathic nephrotic syndrome. *J Pediatr* 2010; **156**: 965–71.

Cross-references

Assessment of renal function, 199
Chronic kidney disease, 203
Fluid and electrolyte balance, 754
Serious complications of pregnancy, 482

Patient with a transplant

Denise McCarthy and George Shorten

In the UK, approximately 1500 cadaveric and 1000 living donor renal transplantations (RTs) are performed each year. Long-term transplant outcome is excellent even in older, high-risk recipients. Ethnicity and increased sensitization should not be a contraindication to RT in the elderly. The perioperative mortality is <1%, and 88–94% of the transplanted kidneys are functioning 1 year later (Box 6.6). These recipients may present for any surgery, and it is imperative that no damage occurs to the organ. Most elective surgical procedures performed on renal transplant recipients are well tolerated; in general, the renal handling of drugs is adequate, although renal function is rarely normal.

Box 6.6 Causes of death in transplant recipients

- Sepsis
- Cardiovascular disease
- Suicide
- Gastrointestinal perforation

Underlying diseases leading to need for renal transplantation

- Diabetes mellitus.
- Glomerulonephritis.
- Polycystic disease.
- Hypertension.

Problems after renal transplantation

- Opportunistic infection.
- Hepatitis B (<5% due to vaccine).
- Cancer risk (increased 30–100 times).
- Complications arising from associated medical conditions.
- Large cell lymphoma (Epstein–Barr virus infection).

Preoperative preparation

A formal assessment of renal function, coupled with a careful history and examination based on concurrent medical conditions should be undertaken. Particular note should be taken of medications including immunosuppressives and antihypertensives.

Cardiovascular factors

- Hypertension:
  - essential
  - secondary to end-stage renal failure.
- Left ventricular failure:
  - secondary to hypertension
  - secondary to a chronic increase in cardiac output (shunts, atrioventricular fistulae and anaemia).
- Ischaemic heart disease: accelerated atherosclerosis.
- Peripheral vascular disease.
- Autonomic neuropathy: postural hypotension, delayed gastric emptying.

Main anaesthetic considerations

- Continue immunosuppressive regimen perioperatively. Ciclosporin A decreases renal blood flow and glomerular filtration rate by preglomerular afferent arteriolar vasoconstriction.
- Risk of pulmonary aspiration.
- Infection risk.
- Potential for injury to existing arteriovenous fistulae.
- Gastrointestinal bleeding.
- Steroid therapy.
- Stress of surgery/anaesthesia.
- Osteoporosis (care in moving and handling of patients).
- Potential for altered drug handling.

Premedication

- Prophylactic antibiotics.
- Supplementary steroid administration.
- H_2 antagonist/metoclopramide/proton pump inhibitors.
- Benzodiazepines (avoid diazepam owing to its long half-life).
- Atropine/glycopyrrolate (20–50% renal excretion).
- Opioids are not contraindicated.
- Continue immunosuppression – if enteral administration is not possible then intravenous administration with dose adjustment will be required.

Anaesthetic technique

Local, general and regional techniques are well tolerated. General anaesthesia tends to decrease renal blood flow; this can be minimized by avoiding hyperventilation and excessive concentrations of volatile agents. Adequate graft perfusion should be ensured by maintenance of intravascular volume and avoidance of systemic hypotension.

Enflurane and sevoflurane are metabolized to produce fluoride ions (usually <15 μmol L^{-1}; nephrotoxicity at >50 μmol L^{-1}). Isoflurane and desflurane undergo minimal metabolism and augment muscle relaxation, and are therefore recommended.

If the graft is functioning, all muscle relaxants and anticholinesterases eliminated as normal. Cisatracurium and mivacuronium are probably the muscle relaxants of choice.

Opioids may be administered safely although accumulation of morphine-6-glucuronide or norpethidine are associated with a risk of convulsion.

If one is considering a regional technique then coagulation studies, including bleeding time, are indicated.

Postoperative management

Most surgery is performed without any specific complications. However, one should monitor renal function closely, especially if undertaking major procedures. Immunosuppression should be continued, with antibiotics if indicated, and any infection appropriately dealt with.

If there is any doubt concerning graft function, opioid infusions are best avoided.

Bibliography

Castaneda MA, Garvin PJ. General surgical procedures in renal allograft recipients. *Am J Surg* 1986; **152**: 717–21.

Karachristos A, Herrera A, Sifontis NM, *et al.* Outcomes of renal transplantation in older high risk recipients: is there an age effect? *J Surg Res* 2010; **161**: 173–8.

Katz J, Benumof J, Kadis LB (eds). *Anesthesia and Uncommon Diseases*, 4th edn. Philadelphia: WB Saunders, 1998.

Kaufmann L. Anaesthesia for renal transplantation. In: Kaufmann L (ed.) *Anaesthesia Review*, vol. 8. Edinburgh: Churchill Livingstone, 1991, ch. 8.

Miller RD. Anesthesia and the renal and genitourinary systems. In: Miller RD (ed.) *Anesthesia*, 5th edn. Edinburgh: Churchill Livingstone, 2000.

NHS Blood and Transplant. *Transplant Activity in the UK: 2008–2009*. Watford: NHS Blood and Transplant, 2009.

Stoelting RK, Dierdorf SF (eds). *Anesthesia and Coexisting Disease*, 4th edn. Edinburgh: Churchill Livingstone, 2002.

Cross-references

Diabetes mellitus, 60
Hypertension, 151
Kidney transplantation, 522

7
The blood

Charles Marc Samama

■ Anaemia	*Charles Marc Samama and Jean-François Schved*
■ Disseminated intravascular coagulation	*Charles Marc Samama and Jean-François Schved*
■ Glucose-6-phosphate dehydrogenase deficiency	*Charles Marc Samama and Jean-François Schved*
■ Idiopathic thrombocytopenic purpura	*Charles Marc Samama and Jean-François Schved*
■ Inherited coagulopathies	*Charles Marc Samama and Jean-François Schved*
■ Massive transfusion, microvascular haemorrhage and thrombocytopenia	*Charles Marc Samama and Jean-François Schved*
■ Mastocytosis	*Charles Marc Samama and Jean-François Schved*
■ Multiple myeloma	*Charles Marc Samama and Jean-François Schved*
■ Polycythaemia	*Charles Marc Samama and Jean-François Schved*
■ Sickle cell syndrome	*Charles Marc Samama and Jean-François Schved*
■ Thalassaemia	*Charles Marc Samama and Jean-François Schved*

Anaemia

Charles Marc Samama and Jean-François Schved

- A common condition that rarely puts fit patients at increased risk.
- There is no universally accepted minimum haemoglobin concentration.
- The management of anaemia must depend upon the cause, the patient's overall medical status and the surgery being contemplated.

Definition

The World Health Organization defines anaemia as a haemoglobin (Hb) concentration of less than:

- 13 g dL^{-1} in adult men
- 12 g dL^{-1} in adult women
- 11 g dL^{-1} in children aged 6 months to 6 years
- 12 g dL^{-1} in children aged 6–14 years.

Causes

The causes of anaemia may be divided into three categories:

- defective red cell production
- haemolysis
- haemorrhage.

Pathophysiology

The essential feature of all forms of anaemia is a decrease in the Hb content of the blood.

Since

$$\text{Arterial oxygen content} = \text{Arterial oxygen saturation} \times \text{Hb concentration}$$

and

$$\text{Oxygen delivery} = \text{Arterial oxygen content} \times \text{Cardiac output}$$

it follows that a decrease in Hb concentration will, in the absence of compensatory mechanisms, be followed by a decrease in oxygen supply to the tissues.

Compensatory mechanisms

In acute normovolaemic anaemia in otherwise healthy individuals, two mechanisms compensate for the decrease in oxygen-carrying capacity:

- an increase in cardiac output
- a decrease in blood viscosity.

In chronic anaemia a third mechanism comes into play:

- increased 2,3-diphosphoglycerate (2,3-DPG) concentration in the red cells, which shifts the oxygen dissociation curve to the right and promotes the release of oxygen to the tissues.

Clinical features

The symptoms and signs of anaemia include dyspnoea on exertion, tachycardia, palpitations, angina, increased arterial pulse pressure and capillary pulsation. However, in mild chronic anaemia which is well compensated, there may be no symptoms or signs. Anaemia is poorly tolerated by patients with coronary artery disease or pre-existing myocardial dysfunction. Such patients, who are often elderly, may present with cardiac failure.

Preoperative assessment

In some patients, anaemia is to be anticipated as a feature of the disease for which surgery is indicated. In other surgical patients, anaemia is an unexpected and unrelated finding revealed only by routine preoperative haematological testing.

Routine blood count and blood film examination will disclose:

- the severity of the anaemia
- the type of anaemia, thus suggesting its cause (Table 7.1).

Further investigations

It is always desirable to know the exact cause of any patient's anaemia. If surgery cannot be postponed, blood should be taken preoperatively so that investigations may be performed on a specimen that is undiluted by transfused blood. Renal failure is a common and often unsuspected cause of anaemia. The serum creatinine level should always be checked.

Table 7.1 Classification of causes of anaemia according to red cell morphology

Type	Cause
Hypochromic microcytic (decreased mean corpuscular volume (MCV) and mean corpuscular haemoglobin concentration)	Iron deficiency, thalassaemia, chronic disease if long-lasting anemia
Normochromic microcytic (increased MCV)	Vitamin B_{12} or folate deficiency, alcohol
Polychromatic microcytic (increased MCV)	Haemolysis
Normocytic normochromic	Chronic disease, renal failure, haemorrhage, hypothyroidism, hypopituitarism, marrow aplasia or infiltration

Correction of anaemia

What preoperative Hb level is acceptable?

There is no Hb concentration that must be met by all patients in all circumstances. Although the figure of 10 g dL^{-1} was generally accepted for many years, it has been shown that acute normovolaemic haemodilution to an Hb level of 5 g dL^{-1} is tolerated in healthy, resting volunteers, and there is evidence suggesting that Hb levels of the order of 8 g dL^{-1} are safe for many patients undergoing orthopaedic surgery or treatment in ICUs. The degree of anaemia that is acceptable depends on the cardiac reserves of the patient. A frail elderly patient with severe coronary artery disease may develop cardiac failure even at an Hb concentration of 10 g dL^{-1}.

How may the patient's Hb level be increased?

By treating the cause of anaemia

Treating the cause is the ideal solution, but many cases of anaemia are not amenable to treatment or the treatment is surgery.

By giving specific haematinics

Appropriate in specific deficiency states (iron, vitamin B_{12} or folic acid) only. Blind, haematinic treatment is useless and expensive. However, observational studies carried out to date suggest a significant role of intravenous iron in blood conservation in orthopaedic surgery. Both preoperative and postoperative iron administration are likely to reduce the need for perioperative transfusions in this group of patients.

By giving erythropoietin

This should be administered to reduce the need for allogeneic blood in certain selected patient populations (e.g. renal insufficiency, anaemia of chronic disease, rare blood groups, refusal of transfusion).

By red cell transfusion

Transfusion has only a limited place because:

- a moderate degree of anaemia is well tolerated in otherwise fit patients (see above)
- transfusion has many hazards; in particular, it is easy to overload the circulation of a normovolaemic anaemic patient.

The only patients in whom preoperative transfusion is certainly indicated are some patients with sickle cell anaemia and severely anaemic patients with cardiac decompensation in whom surgery is urgent. To minimize the risks of circulatory overload, red cell concentrates should be transfused under strict haemodynamic control (clinical surveillance, blood pressure and heart rate monitoring).

Perioperative and postoperative management

The anaesthetist's aim is to maintain oxygen delivery. To this end:

- an adequate supply of blood must be cross-matched, and blood that is lost at operation should be promptly replaced
- the decision of whether intermediate haemoglobin concentrations (i.e. 6–10 g dL^{-1}) lead to red blood cell (RBC) transfusion should be based on any ongoing indication of organ ischaemia, ongoing bleeding, and the patient's risk factors for complications of inadequate oxygenation
- particular care should be taken to ensure that:
  - hypoxaemia never develops
  - the cardiac output is not decreased.

Within this framework, there is a wide choice of anaesthetic techniques at the anaesthetist's disposal.

Bibliography

American Society of Anesthesiologists Task Force on Perioperative Blood Transfusion and Adjuvant Therapies. Practice guidelines for perioperative blood transfusion and adjuvant therapies: an updated report. *Anesthesiology* 2006; **105**: 198–208.

Auerbach M, Goodnough LT, Picard D, Maniatis A. The role of intravenous iron in anemia management and transfusion avoidance. *Transfusion* 2008; **48**: 988–1000.

Carson JL, Duff A, Berlin JA, *et al.* Perioperative blood transfusion and postoperative mortality. *JAMA* 1998; **279**: 199–205.

Hébert PC, Wells G, Blajchnian MA, *et al.* A multi-center randomised, controlled trial of transfusion requirements in critical care. *N Engl J Med* 1999; **360**: 409–17.

Nunn JF, Freeman J. Problems of oxygenation and oxygen transport during anaesthesia. *Anaesthesia* 1964; **19**: 206–16.

Weiskopf RB, Viele MK, Feiner J, *et al.* Human cardiovascular and metabolic response to acute, severe, isovolaemic anemia. *JAMA* 1998; **279**: 217–21.

Cross-references

Blood transfusion, 735

Preoperative assessment of cardiovascular risk in non-cardiac surgery, 621

Disseminated intravascular coagulation

Charles Marc Samama and Jean-François Schved

- Associated with life-threatening conditions.
- Variable presentation, with bleeding and/or thrombosis.
- Aim to correct both the underlying cause and coagulopathy.
- Involve a haematologist early.

Definition

Disseminated intravascular coagulation (DIC) involves widespread activation of those haemostatic mechanisms that normally operate locally to halt bleeding from injured vessels. The diagnosis of DIC requires the identification of a bleeding disorder with evidence of fibrinolysis and consumption of platelets and clotting factors. Microvascular thrombosis occurs and may be associated with multiple organ failure.

Pathophysiology

The normal physiological response to vascular endothelial damage involves generation of a fibrin clot at the site of injury. Thrombus formation is controlled by physiological anticoagulants such as protein C and antithrombin, and by the fibrinolytic system. DIC involves widespread activation of coagulation with microvascular thrombosis and depletion of coagulation factors. The fibrinolytic system is activated, resulting in generation of fibrin degradation products (FDPs), which themselves have anticoagulant properties. Thus, a diagnosis of DIC requires the demonstration of a consumptive coagulopathy (thrombocytopenia, hypofibrinogenaemia, disordered clotting function tests) with evidence of excessive fibrinolysis (increased levels of FDPs such as D-dimer).

Coagulation and inflammatory pathways are closely linked. In cases of systemic sepsis, release of cytokines from monocytes and macrophages results in a generalized inflammatory response and upregulation of the host's immune responses. Cytokines also produce widespread activation of coagulation and suppression of fibrinolysis, partly by stimulating expression of tissue factor on monocytes and endothelial cells. Formation of multiple fibrin clots in the microvasculature contributes to the organ dysfunction characteristic of severe sepsis. Antithrombin, protein C and protein S, which act as inhibitors of both coagulation and inflammation, are depleted in severe sepsis and DIC, raising the possibility that they might have a therapeutic role.

The trigger for DIC may be vascular damage, resulting in exposure of the blood to subendothelial collagen and activation of factor XII. The process of coagulation may also be initiated by tissue damage, releasing thromboplastins into the circulation. Box 7.1 lists the common causes of DIC.

Box 7.1 Causes of disseminated intravascular coagulation

- Infection
  - Septicaemia
  - Viraemia
  - Fungaemia
  - Protozoal, e.g. malaria
- Obstetric
  - Pre-eclampsia
  - Placental abruption
  - Amniotic fluid embolism
  - Retained products of conception
  - Placenta praevia
- Malignancy
  - Acute promyelocytic leukaemia
  - Metastatic carcinoma
- Traumatic
  - Multiple trauma, especially with shock
  - Surgery: cardiopulmonary bypass, neurosurgery
  - Burns
  - Fat embolism
- Intravascular haemolysis
  - ABO transfusion reaction
  - Snake venom
- Other
  - Shock of any cause
  - Aortic dissection
  - Extensive haemangioma
  - Severe liver disease

Clinical features

Typically, acute DIC involves depletion of clotting factors and platelets. Laboratory findings include thrombocytopenia, anaemia, prolonged prothrombin time (PT) and activated partial thromboplastin time (APTT), hypofibrinogenaemia and elevated FDPs (D-dimer).

In many cases, features of the condition are limited to laboratory abnormalities. In others, there may be widespread bruising or bleeding from the gastrointestinal tract, genitourinary tract, sites of vascular access and surgical incisions. Microvascular thrombosis may cause tissue ischaemia and necrosis, resulting in organ dysfunction that typically affects the kidneys, lungs and liver. The clinical presentation of DIC varies depending upon the aetiology, so that retained products of conception typically cause uterine haemorrhage, while carcinoma is associated with chronic vascular thrombosis.

Preoperative preparation

The underlying cause is often of greater clinical significance than the DIC itself. Antibiotics should be given for infection, and hypovolaemia must be corrected. Fluids and blood products should be warmed, as hypothermia will further impair clotting.

Surgery intended to remove the cause of the DIC, such as evacuation of retained products of conception, should be delayed no longer than is necessary to correct the coagulopathy to an acceptable level and to ensure cardiovascular stability.

Administration of blood products should be guided by the clinical condition of the patient and the results of laboratory investigations and it is important that a haematologist is involved. Correction of coagulopathy may require platelet concentrate and fresh-frozen plasma (FFP) infusion. Severe depletion of fibrinogen (blood level $<1\ g\ L^{-1}$) is an indication for giving cryoprecipitate or fibrinogen concentrate. Anaemia, due to haemorrhage or microangiopathic haemolysis, will require blood transfusion. An adequate supply of blood and blood components must be available before surgery starts.

Low-dose heparin has been used to interrupt the vicious cycle of intravascular coagulation and consumptive coagulopathy, particularly in conditions such as acute promyelocytic leukaemia. However, control is difficult, bleeding may be exacerbated and heparin is best avoided before surgery.

Antithrombin therapy has shown promise in animal studies of sepsis and DIC, but the results of human studies have been inconclusive. Recombinant activated protein C administration to patients with severe sepsis showed a decrease in the procoagulant state, a decrease in inflammatory markers and a significant decrease in mortality. In post hoc analyses, both agents have shown some kind of efficacy in the treatment of patients with DIC.

Premedication is usually unnecessary or inadvisable in the critically ill patient. Intramuscular injections are best avoided.

Perioperative management

Coagulopathy is a contraindication to regional anaesthesia, so general anaesthesia is usually used. The choice of anaesthetic agents and monitoring is dictated by the patient's clinical condition and the nature of the surgery. DIC is usually a disease of the critically ill, so controlled ventilation and invasive cardiovascular monitoring are usually appropriate. Large-bore intravenous lines are necessary to allow the rapid transfusion of blood and blood products, and all intravenous fluids should be warmed. Nasotracheal intubation should be avoided if coagulopathy is significant and care should be exercised during the insertion of nasogastric tubes.

Blood loss should be measured and promptly replaced. Platelet concentrate, FFP and cryoprecipitate or fibrinogen are given according to clinical need and laboratory results. Prothrombin complex concentrates are contraindicated as activated recombinant factor VII. When blood loss is excessive, platelet count and clotting function (including plasma fibrinogen) should be measured regularly.

Postoperative management

Patients with clinically significant DIC are best managed in an ICU and often require continued mechanical ventilation and intensive cardiovascular monitoring and support. Frequent measurement of haematological parameters should continue, with judicious administration of blood and blood products after consultation with a haematologist. Surgery, particularly in obstetric cases, may remove the cause of DIC and result in rapid resolution.

Bibliography

Bernard GR, Vincent JL, Laterre PF, *et al.* Efficacy and safety of recombinant human APC for severe sepsis. *N Engl J Med* 2001; **344**: 699–709.

Dhainaut J-F, Yan SB, Joyce DE, *et al.* Treatment effects of drotrecogin alfa (activated) in patients with severe sepsis with or without overt disseminated intravascular coagulation. *J Thromb Haemost* 2004; **2**: 1924–33.

Kitchens CS. Thrombocytopenia and thrombosis in disseminated intravascular coagulation (DIC). *Hematology Am Soc Hematol Educ Program* 2009; 240–6.

Levi M. Disseminated intravascular coagulation. *Crit Care Med* 2007; **35**: 2191–5.

Parmet JC, Horrow JC. Hematologic diseases. In: Benumof JL (ed.) *Anesthesia and Uncommon Diseases*, 4th edn. Philadelphia: WB Saunders, 1998, p. 302.

Toh CH, Hoots WK. SSC on Disseminated Intravascular Coagulation of the ISTH. The scoring system of the Scientific and Standardisation Committee on Disseminated Intravascular Coagulation of the International Society on Thrombosis and Haemostasis: a 5-year overview. *J Thromb Haemost* 2007; **5**: 604–6.

Cross-reference

Serious complications of pregnancy, 482

Glucose-6-phosphate dehydrogenase deficiency

Charles Marc Samama and Jean-François Schved

- An inherited condition.
- Haemolysis, which may be severe, can be triggered by certain agents.
- Few triggering agents are in routine anaesthetic usage.

Glucose-6-phosphate dehydrogenase (G6PD) deficiency is the most common inherited metabolic disorder of RBCs, affecting over 400 million people worldwide with varying degrees of severity. The enzyme G6PD governs the rate at which RBCs consume, utilize and detoxify oxygen. Its deficiency makes RBCs vulnerable to haemolysis. G6PD deficiency will not usually result in complications during or after anaesthesia, provided oxidant agents known to trigger haemolysis are avoided. It may confer malarial resistance.

Pathophysiology

Low levels of G6PD result in failure to generate NADPH, which is needed to maintain red cell glutathione in a reduced state. Low levels of reduced glutathione render red cell proteins susceptible to oxygenation, resulting in the formation of masses of denatured globin (Heinz bodies), which are attached to the red cell membrane. Heinz bodies are extracted from the red cells by macrophages during passage through the spleen. The inclusion-free red cells have damaged membranes and are haemolysed. Box 7.2 lists oxidant drugs that may cause haemolysis in patients with G6PD deficiency, although the response is somewhat idiosyncratic. The haemolytic episode begins 2–5 days after drug administration.

Box 7.2 Some oxidant drugs capable of triggering haemolysis in patients with glucose-6-phosphate dehydrogenase deficiency

- Analgesics
  - Aspirin in high dose
  - Phenacetin
  - Acetanilide
- Sulphonamides
- Antibiotics
  - Penicillin
  - Isoniazid
  - Ciprofloxacin
  - Chloramphenicol
- Antimalarials
  - Primaquine
  - Chloroquine
  - Quinine
- Miscellaneous drugs
  - Methylene blue
  - Vitamin K
  - Nalidixic acid
  - Naphthalene
  - Quinidine
  - Probenecid
  - Phenylhydrazine
  - Nitrates
  - Nitrofurantoin
  - Ascorbic acid in high dose

Clinical manifestations

The structural gene for G6PD resides on the X chromosome and is therefore inherited as a sex-linked characteristic. G6PD deficiency is most common in hemizygous males but is also seen in homozygous females. Heterozygous females may occasionally show clinical manifestations. There are more than 200 variants of G6PD and the clinical manifestations range from negligible to severe, depending upon the activity of the abnormal G6PD and whether the patient is a heterozygote or a homozygote/hemizygote. Two distinct clinical syndromes may result:

- In the African variant (the gene in this variant is termed A$^-$) the patient is asymptomatic until exposed to oxidant drugs or a severe infection; 11% of African Americans have the A$^-$ gene.
- In the Mediterranean and Oriental groups of variants, the G6PD deficiency is generally more severe and may be a cause of neonatal jaundice. Nevertheless, the patient is usually asymptomatic until a drug or infection precipitates haemolysis. Some individuals can also develop a fulminant haemolytic anaemia after exposure to the fava bean (favism).

Anaesthetic management

These patients should be informed of risks along with the signs and symptoms of an acute haemolytic crisis. Elective surgery should not be performed during a haemolytic crisis. The classical features of such a crisis include abdominal pain, jaundice, a decrease in haemoglobin concentration, an increasing reticulocyte count and the presence of Heinz bodies in the peripheral blood film.

When providing anaesthetic care for patients with G6PD deficiency, it is important to avoid oxidant agents associated with the triggering of haemolysis. These are listed in Box 7.2. In addition to these, it has been recommended that nitroprusside, and prilocaine in large amounts, be avoided.

Bibliography

Elyassi AR, Rowshan HH. Perioperative management of the glucose-6-phosphate dehydrogenase deficient patient: a review of literature. *Anesth Prog* 2009; **56**: 86–91.

Jandl JH. Heinz body hemolytic anemias. In: Jandl JH (ed.) *Blood: Textbook of Hematology*. Boston, MA: Little, Brown & Co., 1987, pp. 338–41.

Smith CL, Snowdon SL. Anaesthesia and glucose-6-phosphate dehydrogenase deficiency. *Anaesthesia* 1987; **42**: 281–8.

Idiopathic thrombocytopenic purpura

Charles Marc Samama and Jean-François Schved

- Thrombocytopenia can lead to severe haemorrhage.
- Platelet count should be increased to above 50×10^9 L^{-1}, if possible (higher for neurosurgery).
- Patients may be taking drugs, e.g. steroids, with significant side-effects.
- Platelet transfusions may increase the platelet count for no more than 1 hour.

Pathophysiology

Idiopathic thrombocytopenic purpura (ITP) is a destructive thrombocytopenia caused by the presence of an antibody (usually IgG) against platelet membrane glycoproteins IIb/IIIa. The binding of antibody to platelets leads to their phagocytosis by cells of the reticuloendothelial system (mainly in the spleen but also in the liver) and, therefore, to a decreased platelet lifespan.

ITP may be acute or chronic. The acute form occurs most commonly in children (of both sexes). It is usually preceded by a viral infection and leads to spontaneous remission in the vast majority of patients. The chronic form of the disease affects mainly young women and is a relatively common haematological disorder.

Clinical features

- Petechial haemorrhage.
- Easy bruising.
- Skin purpura.
- Menorrhagia.
- Mucosal bleeding.
- Rarely, intracranial haemorrhage.

Diagnosis

- Decreased platelet count (usually 10–50 $\times 10^9$ L^{-1}).
- Increased or normal megakaryocytes in an otherwise normal marrow.
- Splenomegaly is unusual and suggests another diagnosis.
- Increased platelet-associated IgG (PAIgG) in most patients (this test is not sufficiently sensitive or specific to justify its routine use in uncomplicated ITP).
- There is no specific test.

The diagnosis of ITP is made after the exclusion of other causes of thrombocytopenia based on the history, physical examination, blood count and blood film. Many feel that additional investigations, such as bone marrow and platelet antibodies, are unnecessary except in patients aged >65 years, those with atypical findings or those refractory to treatment.

Treatment

There is a lack of randomized clinical trials comparing the different treatment options, and treatment should therefore be tailored to the individual patient.

High-dose oral corticosteroids can lead to a rapid increase in platelet numbers and long-term remission, but continued low-dose therapy is often required to produce adequate platelet counts. As the side-effects of long-term steroid therapy are not inconsiderable, the aim of therapy should be to provide adequate platelet numbers for haemostasis rather than to achieve a normal platelet count.

In general, patients with platelet counts $>30 \times 10^9$ L^{-1} do not need treatment unless they require surgery, dental procedures or are shortly to give birth.

Recommendations for 'safe' platelet counts in adults:

- surgery: $\geq 50 \times 10^9$ L^{-1}
- neurosurgery: $\geq 80 \times 10^9$ L^{-1}
- pregnancy: see later.

Splenectomy is often recommended if steroid therapy fails. The operation carries a low mortality in experienced hands and the response, if it occurs, is usually rapid, with normalization of platelet count within 2 weeks. Unfortunately, relapse is common. Patients should be given prophylactic polyvalent pneumococcal vaccine, *Haemophilus influenzae* B vaccine and meningococcal C conjugate vaccination at least 2 weeks before splenectomy. The efficacy of lifelong antibiotics is unproven.

Around 70–85% of patients achieve remission with steroid therapy and/or splenectomy. For patients refractory to these treatments, the options are many; but, even if therapy is successful, relapse is common.

Intravenous immunoglobulins are of special interest in children, especially during the preoperative period. Their efficacy is generally transient.

Anti-CD20 therapy (rituximab) is an effective agent, as well as the least toxic, when splenectomy fails: the short-term response rate is 50% and the sustained response rate more than 30%.

The remaining treatment options include vinca alkaloids, cyclophosphamide, azathioprine, danazol, colchicines, intravenous anti-D and dapson. They should be reserved for patients with severe disease refractory to both splenectomy and rituximab.

ITP in pregnancy

ITP may occur *de novo* in a pregnant patient or pregnancy may occur in a patient with pre-existing ITP. ITP must be distinguished from gestational thrombocytopenia (platelet count rarely <80 × 10^9 L^{-1}), which is a benign self-limiting condition not associated with a bleeding risk to mother or child.

Intrapartum and postpartum haemorrhage may prove life-threatening to the mother. As PAIgG can cross the placenta, the fetus may become thrombocytopenic and is at risk of haemorrhage, particularly in the central nervous system. There has been debate on whether vaginal delivery or caesarean section is the safer option for the baby. It is now generally agreed that the mode of delivery should be determined by obstetric considerations alone. In the neonate, the platelet count may be low and continue to decrease in the first week of life.

The asymptomatic mother with ITP does not need therapy until delivery is imminent if the platelet count is >20 × 10^9 L^{-1}, but should be monitored closely both clinically and haematologically. If the platelet count falls below this level, low-dose steroid therapy or immunoglobulin may be given. The neonate may also receive steroids and immunoglobulin if necessary.

- Platelet counts >50 × 10^9 L^{-1} should be considered safe for vaginal delivery in patients with otherwise normal coagulation.
- Platelet counts >80 × 10^9 L^{-1} should be considered safe for caesarean section and spinal or epidural anaesthesia in patients with otherwise normal coagulation.

Anaesthetic management

Advice should be sought from a haematologist. If the procedure is elective, steroid and immunoglobulin administration may increase platelet count sufficiently for surgery to be undertaken safely. A platelet count of >80 × 10^9 L^{-1} is an acceptable target. Platelet transfusion is rarely indicated, as platelet survival is usually <1 hour. However, it may be the only option in acute life-threatening haemorrhage.

The side-effects of drug therapy should be looked for and managed appropriately if present. For steroids, these include hyperglycaemia, hypokalaemia and hypertension.

During splenectomy, platelets should be given once the splenic artery is clamped – this is logical but is based only on relatively poor published evidence. Regional anaesthetic techniques should usually be avoided if the platelet count is <80 × 10^9 L^{-1}. Each case should be considered individually and both the benefits and risks of regional anaesthesia considered.

Bibliography

British Committee for Standards in Haematology. Guidelines for the investigation and management of idiopathic thrombocytopenic purpura in adults, children and in pregnancy. *Br J Haematol* 2003; **120**: 574–96.

Bussel JB. Traditional and new approaches to the management of immune thrombocytopenia: issues of when and who to treat. *Hematol Oncol Clin North Am* 2009; **23**: 1329–41.

Michel M. Immune thrombocytopenic purpura: epidemiology and implications for patients. *Eur J Haematol Suppl* 2009; **71**: 3–7.

Cross-reference

Serious complications of pregnancy, 482

Inherited coagulopathies

Charles Marc Samama and Jean-François Schved

- Rare.
- Most patients presenting for anaesthesia are already aware of their disease.
- Specific concentrates are available for all the commoner types.

The following are the more common ones and may be encountered by the anaesthetist:

- factor VIII deficiency (haemophilia A or classical haemophilia)
- factor IX deficiency (haemophilia B or Christmas disease)
- von Willebrand's disease
- factor XI deficiency
- factor VII deficiency.

Haemophilia

There are about 5500 patients with haemophilia A in the UK, of whom 34% are HIV positive. There are about 1100 patients with haemophilia B in the UK, of whom 5% are HIV positive.

The genes for factor VIII and factor IX production are carried on the X chromosome, and consequently haemophiliacs are usually male. The severity of haemophilia A is determined by the level of functional factor VIII (Table 7.2).

Clinical manifestations

The mild form (factor VIII levels 25–50 units 100 mL^{-1}) is asymptomatic, and the diagnosis may not be made until the patient has surgery. Any family history of abnormal bleeding, however vague, should be taken seriously and the patient's haemostatic mechanisms thoroughly investigated. In the severe form, spontaneous bleeding into joints, muscles and other organs occurs and can give rise to long-term dysfunction of the sites of bleeding. The clinical manifestations of haemophilia B are similar and depend on the level of factor IX.

The APTT is prolonged in haemophilia and can be corrected by the addition of normal plasma. Quantitative assays of factor VIII or IX will identify the type and severity of the disease.

Management

A haematological opinion should be sought if possible. For minor surgery, factor VIII or IX levels should be ≥50% of normal. For major surgery, the levels should be as near normal as possible before surgery and should be maintained at >50% of normal for several days after surgery.

FFP should only be given to patients with haemophilia A in extreme emergencies. FFP does not work in patients with haemophilia B.

Most hospitals have adequate supplies of factor VIII and factor IX concentrates, all of which have been subject to some form of virucidal treatment. Most of them are recombinant factors. Some are plasmatic. Hospitals which do not stock these concentrates can usually obtain supplies within 24 hours.

Older patients who received factor concentrates before 1985, when heat treatment was introduced, may be infected with some or all of the following viruses:

- hepatitis B
- hepatitis C
- human immunodeficiency virus (HIV).

Haemophiliacs may develop anti-VIII or anti-IX antibodies, requiring the use of activated prothombin complex concentrates (FEIBA) or activated recombinant factor VII (NovoSeven) for several days before and after the surgical procedure.

Table 7.2 Relationship between plasma factor VIIIc levels and severity of bleeding in classical haemophilia*

Factor VIIIc level (units 100 mL^{-1})	Bleeding symptoms
50	None
25–50	Excess bleeding after major surgery or accident
5–25	Excess bleeding after minor surgery
1–5	Severe bleeding after minor surgery and some spontaneous haemorrhage
<1	Spontaneous haemorrhage

*Adapted from Rizza CR. Clinical management of haemophilia. *Br Med Bull* 1997; **33**: 225–30.

von Willebrand's disease

von Willebrand's disease (vWD) is an autosomal dominant disease and is therefore seen in both sexes. Severe forms of the disease are probably about as common as factor IX deficiency. It is caused by a deficiency of von Willebrand's factor (vWF), which has a complex molecular biology. It can be associated with gene deletion, point mutations or intragenic replications. Although the frequency of abnormal genes may be as high as 1:2000 in the UK population, relatively few affected people have a haemostatic abnormality. Most of the patients with vWD have an inherited type 1 (quantitative defect). Type 2 (qualitative defect in vWF) and type 3 (homozygous deficiency) are much less frequent. Basically, patients with blood groups A, B and AB have a normal plasma level of vWF, as compared with patients with group O, in whom vWF is generally decreased (50% could be normal for such a patient).

vWF is a multifunctional plasma glycoprotein that is secreted by endothelial cells and binds to factor VIII, collagen, heparin and to platelet membrane glycoproteins. In severe vWD, platelets do not adhere to endothelium, and the factor VIII level is low owing to lack of carrier protein.

Clinical manifestations

The severity of the disease depends upon the vWF levels. Problems range from frequent nose bleeds, heavy periods and marked bleeding after dental extraction to more serious problems such as mucosal bleeds and haemarthroses. Diagnosis is by the demonstration of a prolonged Platelet Function Analyzer 100 test, a non-constant decrease in factor VIII activity, a decrease in von Willebrand antigen (vWF-Ag, for type I and III only) and a decrease in ristocetin-cofactor activity (vWF-RCo).

Management

DDAVP treatment (0.3 $\mu g\ kg^{-1}$ intravenous infusion) works only for type I vWF disease. It can increase vWF levels for a few days, but does so at the expense of body stores. For severe forms of the disease, replacement therapy can be given using either some recombinant or plasmatic factor VIII concentrates that contain vWF multimers or directly vWF concentrates.

Factor XI deficiency

There are about 250 patients with factor XI deficiency in the UK, of whom around half are Ashkenazi Jews. It is an autosomally inherited condition. Specific factor XI concentrates are available. In mild and moderate deficits, tranexamic acid may be of value.

Factor VII deficiency

Factor VII deficiency is the most frequent among rare congenital bleeding disorders and, in the UK, is usually seen in Muslims of Indian origin, probably as a result of consanguinity. It is autosomally inherited. Recombinant activated factor VII can be used (15–30 $\mu g\ kg^{-1}$).

Bibliography

Budde U. Diagnosis of von Willebrand disease subtypes: implications for treatment. *Haemophilia* 2008; **14** (Suppl. 5): 27–38.

Choi S, Brull R. Neuraxial techniques in obstetric and non-obstetric patients with common bleeding diatheses. *Anesth Analg* 2009; **109**: 648–60.

Hermans C, Altisent C, Batorova A, *et al.*; European Haemophilia Therapy Standardisation Board. Replacement therapy for invasive procedures in patients with haemophilia: literature review, European survey and recommendations. *Haemophilia* 2009; **15**: 639–58.

Iorio A, Matino D, D'Amico R, Makris M. Recombinant factor VIIa concentrate versus plasma derived concentrates for the treatment of acute bleeding episodes in people with haemophilia and inhibitors. *Cochrane Database Syst Rev* 2010; (8): CD004449.

Lapecorella M, Mariani G; International Registry on Congenital Factor VII Deficiency. Factor VII deficiency: defining the clinical picture and optimizing therapeutic options. *Haemophilia* 2008; **14**: 1170–5.

Martín-Salces M, Jimenez-Yuste V, Alvarez MT, *et al.* Review: Factor XI deficiency: review and management in pregnant women. *Clin Appl Thromb Hemost* 2010; **16**: 209–13.

Cross-reference

Blood transfusion, 735

Massive transfusion, microvascular haemorrhage and thrombocytopenia

Charles Marc Samama and Jean-François Schved

- Restore and maintain adequate circulating blood volume.
- Maintain sufficient oxygen-carrying capacity.
- Coagulopathy is unlikely to occur until at least one blood volume has been transfused.
- Secure haemostasis:
  - give FFP if PT ratio and APTT ratio (PTR, APTTR) >1.5
  - give platelet concentrate concomitantly if platelet count $<50 \times 10^9$ L^{-1}, or $<75 \times 10^9$ L^{-1} if bleeding is still ongoing, or $<100 \times 10^9$ L^{-1} if there is a risk of intracranial haemorrhage
  - give cryoprecipitate or fibrinogen concentrate if fibrinogen level <100 mg dL^{-1}.

Definition

Massive transfusion can be defined as the loss of one circulating blood volume in a 24 hour period (70 mL × body weight). This equates to a blood loss of 5 litres in a 70 kg man, and represents the transfusion of only six units of RBCs to an adult patient with a target haematocrit of 27%. More practical definitions have been developed to allow earlier recognition of major haemorrhage, and because the rate of blood loss has important haemostatic consequences. Massive transfusion can, therefore, also be defined as a >50% loss of circulating blood volume in 3 hours, or a rate of blood loss greater than 150 mL min^{-1}.

Pathophysiology

Massive blood loss leads to a decrease in circulating blood volume, and the effects of hypovolaemia must be separated from those of anaemia. The clinical manifestations of hypovolaemia related to percentage blood loss are given in Table 7.3.

Massive transfusion is associated with microvascular haemorrhage in 30% of patients. In the absence of inherited disorders of haemostasis, the main causes

Table 7.3 Classification of hypovolaemic shock according to blood loss

	Class I	Class II	Class III	Class IV
Blood loss:				
Percentage	<15%	15–30%	30–40%	>40%
Volume (mL)	750	800–1500	1500	>2000
Blood pressure:				
Systolic	Unchanged	Normal	Reduced	Very low
Diastolic	Unchanged	Raised	Reduced	Very low, unrecordable
Heart rate (min^{-1})	Slight tachycardia	100–120	120 (thready)	>120 (very thready)
Capillary refill	Normal	Slow (>2 s)	Slow (>2 s)	Undetectable
Respiratory rate	Normal	Normal	Tachypnoea	Tachypnoea
Urinary flow rate (mL h^{-1})	>30	20–30	10–20	0–10
Extremities	Normal colour	Pale	Pale	Pale and cold
Complexion	Normal	Pale	Pale	Ashen
Mental state	Alert	Anxious or aggressive	Anxious, aggressive or drowsy	Drowsy, confused or unconscious

are a dilutional deficiency of clotting factors and DIC. The development of component therapy and the use of plasma-poor red cells (SAGM blood; Box 7.3) has changed the usual cause of the dilutional coagulopathy from low platelet count to clotting factor deficiency. DIC is a feared complication of major haemorrhage and is more likely to develop in conjunction with prolonged shock, hypothermia and extensive muscle or cerebral damage. It causes bleeding, tissue necrosis and microthrombosis, which can lead to irreversible organ damage.

Box 7.3 Contents of blood components

- Red cells in additive (stored at 4 ± 2°C, use within 4 hours at room temperature)
  - SAGM (saline, adenine, glucose, mannitol) units = 350 + 70 mL
- Platelet concentrates (stored at 22 ± 2°C, continuously agitated, use within 2 hours)
  - Single unit = 50 ± 10 mL fresh plasma, contains 55×10^9 platelets
  - Pooled platelet pack = 320 ± 26 mL fresh plasma, contains 250×10^9 platelets
- FFP (30 minutes to thaw, use within 2 hours)
  - Single unit = 150–200 mL, dose is 12–15 mL kg^{-1}

Management

Mortality and morbidity associated with major haemorrhage are high, and the institution of locally agreed major haemorrhage protocols is essential to ensure effective management (Fig. 7.1). Initial management of the patient requires a full clinical assessment, insertion of large-bore intravenous lines and invasive monitoring. The clinical priority is rapid restoration of circulating blood volume with simultaneous surgical, medical or radiological intervention to stop bleeding. It is essential to prevent prolonged hypotension, as this leads to a progressive acidosis and tissue and organ damage that both predispose to the development of DIC. Mortality increases with the duration and severity of shock. Hypothermia increases bleeding by interfering with haemostasis. Patient temperature should always be kept above 35.5°C. Active rewarming is mandatory.

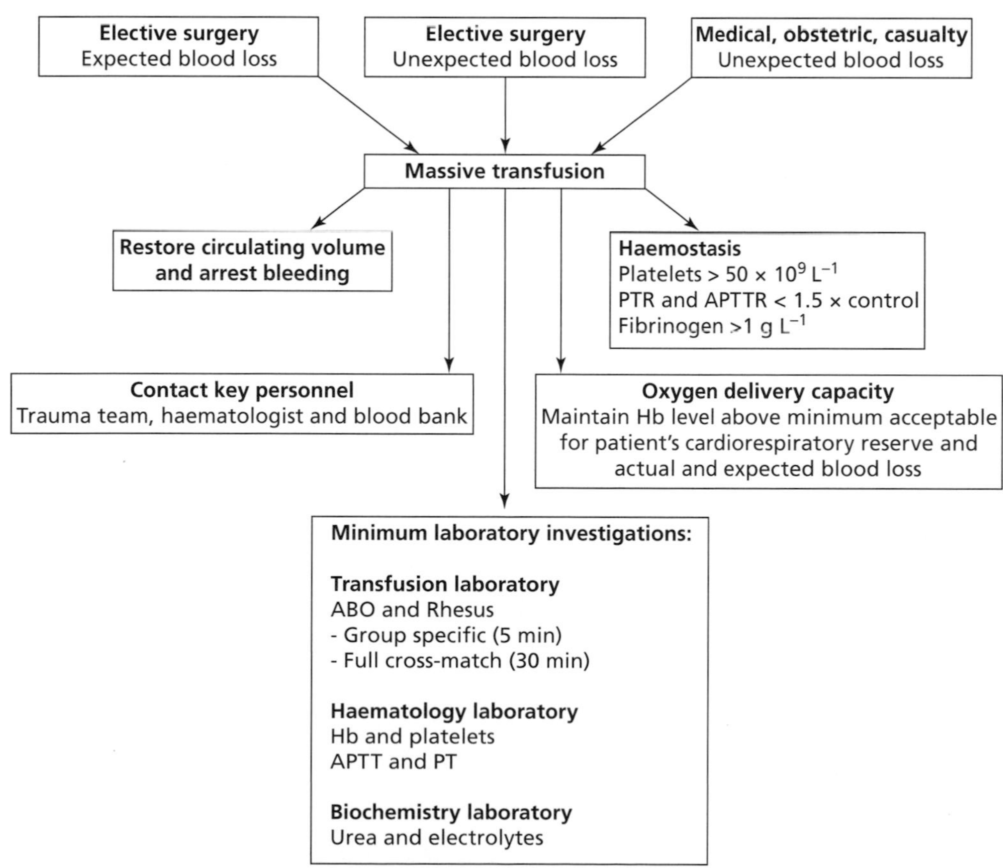

Figure 7.1 Key issues of massive blood loss and transfusion.

Debate continues as to the preferred choice of initial resuscitation fluid: crystalloid or colloid. About 50–75% less colloid than crystalloid is needed to achieve the same volume expansion, but at increased cost, risk of allergic reactions and, in large volumes, altered haemostasis. Pragmatically, it seems reasonable to use a combination of both crystalloids and colloids, but to restrict the total amount of these solutions in order to keep haemostasis under control.

The critical level of oxygen delivery (Do_2) is an unknown value, but recent evidence suggests that an Hb concentration of 7–8 g dL^{-1} may be sufficient for the majority of patients. On the other hand, RBCs play a major role in haemostasis (platelet adhesion, aggregation, thrombin generation) and some authors recommend to target 10 g dL^{-1} Hb in the bleeding patient. A blood transfusion is likely to be required when 30% of total blood volume is lost. This decision must always be guided by laboratory investigations and the clinical picture, including an evaluation of the patient's cardiorespiratory reserve and the rate of blood loss, together with the extent of anticipated further blood loss.

Formulaic replacement therapy, i.e. the automatic administration of a unit of FFP and/or platelets for each set number of units of blood transfused, has not been shown to be effective in preventing microvascular haemorrhage. However, recent data show that plasma to RBC units ratios should increase and that plasma and platelet concentrate should be given earlier. A moderate deficiency of coagulation factors is common in massively transfused patients, but does not contribute to microvascular haemorrhage until levels fall to <50% of normal. The APTT and PT should be monitored regularly, but interpretation must always be related to the clinical picture. These tests are not predictive for the bleeding risk. Supplementation with fibrinogen concentrate has been shown to be effective in some retrospective studies.

A dilutional thrombocytopenia is unlikely unless more than two blood volumes are lost or the patient's platelets are functionally abnormal. Extracorporeal circulatory techniques used in cardiac surgery, renal insufficiency or treatments with antiplatelet agents can cause an acquired functional defect, leading to an increase in the bleeding risk.

DIC can be caused by a variety of triggers that include shock. The coagulation defect occurs as a result of consumption of coagulation factors and platelets, and increased fibrinolytic activity. Laboratory investigations show a mixed picture of low platelets, low fibrinogen, prolonged PT and APTT, and increased FDPs or D-dimer. Senior haematological advice, platelets, FFP and cryoprecipitate or fibrinogen will all be required. Up to now, no benefit of prothombin complex concentrate has been shown.

Protocols for accurate identification of transfusion specimens and of designated units of blood, platelets and FFP must be adhered to even in the stress of an emergency situation, as clinical errors at this time account for most transfusion-related error morbidity.

Bibliography

American Society of Anesthesiologists Task Force on Perioperative Blood Transfusion and Adjuvant Therapies. Practice guidelines for perioperative blood transfusion and adjuvant therapies: an updated report. *Anesthesiology* 2006; **105**: 198–208.

British Committee for Standards in Haematology, Stainsby D, Maclennan S, Thomas D, *et al.* Guidelines on the management of massive blood loss. *Br J Haematol* 2006; **135**: 634–41.

Fenger-Eriksen C, Lindberg-Larsen M, Christensen A, *et al.* Fibrinogen concentrate substitution therapy in patients with massive haemorrhage and low plasma fibrinogen concentrations. *Br J Anaesth* 2008; **101**: 769–73.

Hardy JF, De Moerloose P, Samama CM; Members of the Groupe d'Intereret en Hemostase Perioperatoire. Massive transfusion and coagulopathy: pathophysiology and implications for clinical management. *Can J Anaesth* 2006; **53**(Suppl.): S40–58.

Hiippala S. Replacement of massive blood loss. *Vox Sang* 1998; **74**(Suppl. 2): 399–407.

Nascimento B, Callum J, Rubenfeld G, *et al.* Clinical review: fresh frozen plasma in massive bleedings – more questions than answers. *Crit Care* 2010; **14**: 202.

Rossaint R, Bouillon B, Cerny V, *et al.* Management of bleeding following major trauma: an updated European guideline. *Crit Care* 2010; **14**: R52.

Sihler KC, Napolitano LM. Complications of massive transfusion. *Chest* 2010; **137**: 209–20.

Cross-references

Blood transfusion, 735

Serious complications of pregnancy, 482

Mastocytosis

Charles Marc Samama and Jean-François Schved

- Rare but potentially fatal.
- Multidisciplinary care of the patient.
- Premedicate with antihistamines and cromoglycate.
- Avoid histamine-releasing agents.
- Be prepared for cardiovascular instability.

Definition

Mastocytosis is a rare disorder (1–4:10 000) of mast cell proliferation that occurs in both cutaneous (urticaria pigmentosa) and, in about 10% of cases, systemic forms (particularly affecting the reticuloendothelial system). Two thirds of patients develop the disease in childhood, with an equal distribution between the sexes, and the condition has been reported in all races. Familial cases have been documented, although most patients have no familial association. Symptoms and signs result from immune and non-immune stimulation of mast cells, resulting in the local and systemic release of a variety of biologically active mediators.

Pathophysiology

Currently, the only established pathological mechanism appears to be the presence of a somatic mutation in codon 816 of the c-*kit* proto-oncogene, leading to constitutive activation of the KIT receptor (a type III tyrosine kinase receptor), which drives mast cell proliferation and survival.

Stimulation of the mast cells results in the release of preformed mediators (including histamine, heparin, chemotactic factors and cytokines) and newly formed mediators (including prostaglandin D_2 (PGD_2) leukotrienes and platelet-activating factor). Clinically, the most important of these are histamine and PGD_2, their physiological effects being widespread:

- Cardiovascular:
  - venous dilatation resulting in increased vascular capacity
  - arteriolar dilatation resulting in decreased arterial pressure
  - increased capillary permeability with rapid loss of fluid into the tissue spaces.
- Respiratory:
  - bronchospasm and increased production of airway secretions.
- Cutaneous:
  - increased blood flow to the skin with erythema and flushing
  - pruritus.
- Gastrointestinal:
  - increased gastric secretions
  - increased gut motility.
- Other:
  - increased uterine contraction.

Symptoms

The diverse nature of the disease, with both acute 'attacks' and chronic organ involvement, results in symptoms that are variable in terms of severity and duration. Symptoms range from pruritus and flushing to dyspnoea, abdominal pain and even syncope, and are attributable to the wide-ranging physiological effects of the secreted mast cell mediators (Box 7.4). Episodes of syncope and hypotension are rare, as are deaths associated with mast cell mediator release.

Precipitating factors

Mast cell stimulation results from both immune and non-immune mechanisms. Perioperatively, the latter are of greater significance and may be classified into non-pharmacological or pharmacological triggers.

Non-pharmacological triggers

Mechanical irritation of the lesions, temperature changes, exercise, vomiting, pain and psychological stress.

Pharmacological triggers

A multitude of drugs have been implicated, including alcohol, opiates (morphine, tramadol, pethidine, codeine), thiopenthal, atracurium, rocuronium, mivacurium, succinylcholine, non-steroidal anti-inflammatory drugs, nefopam, vancomycin, aspirin, radiocontrast media, β-receptor antagonists, α-receptor agonists and drug preservatives, including sodium metabisulphate and parabens. Gelatin solutions (plasma expanders) are also contraindicated.

Box 7.4 Symptoms and signs of mastocytosis

- Cardiopulmonary:
  - chest pain
  - dizziness
  - dyspnoea
  - palpitations
  - syncope
- Gastrointestinal:
  - abdominal cramps
  - diarrhoea
  - epigastric pain
  - nausea and vomiting
  - hepatosplenomegaly
- Skin
  - bullae
  - urticaria and oedema
  - flushing and pruritis
- Neurological
  - cognitive disorganization
  - headaches
- Skeletal
  - bone pain
  - pathological fractures
- Constitutional
  - fatigue
  - fever
  - malaise
  - weight loss
- Haematological
  - anaemia and thrombocytopenia
  - bleeding diathesis

Preoperative assessment

A detailed history may suggest organ involvement and may highlight any known trigger agents. All patients with suspected systemic involvement should have a full blood count and a peripheral smear to exclude an associated haematological disorder. Abnormal findings should prompt a bone marrow biopsy. Although liver function tests are usually normal, an abdominal ultrasound scan should be performed to rule out hepatic or splenic involvement.

Serum α-tryptase is elevated in patients with systemic mastocytosis regardless of whether or not they are experiencing acute symptoms, and it can be used to assess the total-body mast cell burden. A plasma level >20 $\mu g\ L^{-1}$ should be considered as a cut-off. Urinary methylimidazole acetic acid (a histamine metabolite) levels have been shown to correlate closely with the extent of mast cell disease, being highest in patients with widespread systemic involvement. Beyond these tests, any additional work-up should be tailored to individual specific symptoms and may include gastrointestinal tract endoscopy, bone scans and lymph node biopsy.

Preoperative preparation

Epinephrine and other resuscitation drugs and equipment must be immediately available. Premedication with H_1 and H_2 histamine receptor antagonists and non-steroidal anti-inflammatory agents is recommended, although the latter can act as trigger agents. Sodium cromoglycate may help stabilize mast cells, although prophylactic steroids have not been shown to be of any benefit. There are several reports of preoperative intradermal skin tests being used to identify drugs that may be safely administered during anaesthesia. However, the specificity of these tests is uncertain.

Perioperative management

Premedication

Anxiolysis and sedation may be achieved using benzodiazepines. Anticholinergic drugs such as hyoscine should be avoided.

Monitoring

In addition to standard monitoring, invasive blood pressure, temperature and urine output should be measured. Central venous access and pressure measurement should be considered, depending upon the type of surgery.

Induction and maintenance of anaesthesia

Haemodynamic instability should be anticipated, and resuscitation drugs and equipment must be immediately available at all times. Large-bore intravenous cannulae should be inserted and monitoring instituted before induction of anaesthesia. Drugs known to cause histamine release should be avoided. Drugs that have been safely administered include hydroxyzine, propofol, ketamine, etomidate, fentanyl, sufentanil, remifentanil, vecuronium, volatile anaesthetic agents (ether-linked anaesthetic agents inhibit mast cell degranulation), nitrous oxide, benzodiazepines, paracetamol and preservative-free amide local anaesthetics. If an anticholinergic drug is required, glycopyrrolate is preferred. The number of pharmacological agents used should be kept to a minimum. Regional anaesthetic techniques may be used, although these have still been associated with acute reactions.

Environment

A warm, calm environment should be maintained throughout the perioperative period. Hypothermia should be prevented by both active and passive means. Local tissue trauma should be minimized by careful patient handling, positioning and padding of all pressure points. Tourniquets should be used with caution if they are deemed necessary.

Postoperative management

A calm environment, adequate analgesia and normothermia should be maintained after surgery. Skin irritation and trauma should continue to be minimized, and resuscitation drugs and equipment should remain immediately available.

Bibliography

Chaar CI, Bell RL, Duffy TP, Duffy AJ. Guidelines for safe surgery in patients with systemic mastocytosis. *Am Surg* 2009; **75**: 74–80.

Konrad FM, Schroeder TH. Anaesthesia in patients with mastocytosis. *Acta Anaesthesiol Scand* 2009; **53**: 270–1.

Lerno G, Slaats G, Coenen E, *et al.* Anaesthetic management of systemic mastocytosis. *Br J Anaesth* 1990; **65**: 254–7.

Tharp MD, Longley Jr BJ. Mastocytosis (review). *Med Dermatol* 2001; **19**: 679–96.

Cross-reference

Urticaria and angio-oedema, 293

Multiple myeloma

Charles Marc Samama and Jean-François Schved

Myeloma can cause:

- severe bone pain and spontaneous fractures
- renal failure
- hypercalcaemia.

Definition

Multiple myeloma is a diffuse proliferation of B lymphocytes and plasma cells largely confined to bone marrow. It is characterized by the production of a monoclonal immunoglobulin and the occurrence of osteolytic bone lesions. The diagnosis is made by the coexistence of at least two of the following:

- excess plasma cells in the marrow
- monoclonal immunoglobulin concentration of >1 g dL^{-1} (IgG or IgA) or excess light chains in the urine
- X-ray evidence of lytic lesions.

It is a disease of the elderly, with a mean age at diagnosis of 60 years.

Pathophysiology

Bone lesions

Lytic lesions, through which pathological fractures occur, result from the secretion of an osteoclast-stimulating cytokine by the abnormal plasma cells. Bones fracture either spontaneously or after trivial injuries; vertebral collapse is particularly common. Patients often suffer from severe bone pain.

Hypercalcaemia

In general, this occurs only in those patients with extensive osteolysis. It is exacerbated by dehydration secondary to vomiting and the inability to retain salt and water owing to renal involvement. It may also be precipitated by bed rest and infection. Hypercalcaemia can cause vomiting, constipation, anorexia, depression, confusion, drowsiness and even coma.

Renal impairment

Renal impairment is due to a combination of dehydration, hypercalcaemia, pyelonephritis, deposition of myeloma protein in the kidney, and in some cases, renal amyloidosis. In acute renal failure secondary to myeloma, the most important measure is correction of dehydration and treatment of any precipitating renal infection. This has to be considered as a major issue in these patients.

Haematological abnormalities

Normochromic, normocytic anaemia is common and may be severe because of marrow failure or renal failure. Haemostatic abnormalities may be due to interference with clotting and platelet function by monoclonal immunoglobulin, hyperviscosity, renal failure or, rarely, thrombocytopenia as a result of marrow infiltration or chemotherapy.

Hyperviscosity

This is a rare complication associated with high plasma levels of monoclonal immunoglobulin. It is more likely to occur in IgA myelomatosis, in which there is polymerization of monoclonal immunoglobulin molecules. It can cause a variety of neurological, ocular, haematological and cardiac problems, including cardiac failure. It may also result in spurious hyponatraemia and predispose to venous thrombosis.

Immune system

Synthesis of all immunoglobulins apart from the monoclonal immunoglobulin is depressed, leading to increased susceptibility to infection, especially by staphylococci and Gram-negative organisms.

Nervous system

The most important neurological manifestations are peripheral neuropathy, paraplegia secondary to an epidural plasmacytoma, and spinal root compression due to paravertebral masses or collapsed vertebrae.

Anaesthetic management

There has been little research into the anaesthetic management of patients with multiple myeloma and, therefore, all recommendations have to be based purely on an understanding of the abnormalities associated with the disease.

Preoperative

Management should be directed towards the detection and correction of abnormalities associated with myeloma, with particular attention to fluid balance, hypercalcaemia, haemostatic abnormalities and renal impairment. Patients with symptomatic hyperviscosity should be treated with plasmapheresis preoperatively.

Intraoperative

Regional anaesthesia

This may be absolutely contraindicated for medical reasons (haemostatic abnormalities) or relatively contraindicated for medicolegal reasons (active neurological disease).

General anaesthesia

Attention to the positioning of the patient is essential in view of the increased susceptibility to fractures. Strict asepsis is important in view of the impairment of immune function that may be further impaired by general anaesthesia. In theory, adjustment of doses of intravenous agents may be necessary in view of changes in plasma proteins.

Postoperative

Duration of immobility should be minimized to decrease the risk of precipitating hypercalcaemia and of developing venous thromboses.

Bibliography

Dewhirst WE, Glass DD. Haematological diseases. In: Katz J, Benumof JL, Kadis LB (eds) *Anaesthesia and Uncommon Diseases*. Philadelphia: WB Saunders, 1990, pp. 406–8.

Raab MS, Podar K, Breitkreutz I, *et al.* Multiple myeloma. *Lancet* 2009; **374**: 324–39.

Polycythaemia

Charles Marc Samama and Jean-François Schved

- Chronic myeloproliferative disease with a clinical course that is characterized by a low rate of transformation into acute myeloid leukaemia and myelofibrosis.
- Can be associated with abnormal bleeding during and after surgery.
- Postoperative thromboembolic events are common.
- Poses a greater risk to the patient than anaemia.

Definition

Polycythaemia may be defined as an increase in RBC mass such that Hb concentration and haematocrit exceed the values shown in Table 7.4.

Table 7.4 Definition of polycythaemia

	Male	Female
Haemoglobin (g dL^{-1})	17.5	15.0
Haematocrit (%)	51	48

Causes

- Primary polycythaemia (increased red cell mass).
- Secondary polycythaemia (increased red cell mass).
- Apparent polycythaemia (normal red cell mass).

Primary polycythaemia

Also known as *polycythaemia rubra vera*, this is a non-malignant stem cell disease of clonal origin. In 2005, a somatic activating mutation in the *JAK2* non-receptor tyrosine kinase (*JAK2V617F*) was identified in most patients (95%) with polycythaemia, bringing many hopes for the understanding and the treatment of polycythaemia. The same mutation was also found in a large proportion of patients with essential thrombocytosis and primary myelofibrosis. Polycythaemia gives rise to an increase in granulocyte and platelet count in addition to an increase in RBC mass. Hb can exceed 20 g dL^{-1}, platelet count is often in the range 450–800 × 10^9 L^{-1} and can exceed 1000 × 10^9 L^{-1}. It is a disease of older adults (median age 55–60 years) and of both sexes. To assert the diagnosis, the global RBC mass should exceed 36 mL kg^{-1} in men and 32 mL kg^{-1} in women. Less than 5% of cases present before the age of 40 years. Splenomegaly and hepatomegaly are common. High blood viscosity resulting from the high haematocrit can lead to episodes of thrombosis with resulting ischaemic damage. Primary polycythaemia may be an incidental finding, but is classically associated with digital ischaemia, stroke, headache, mental clouding, facial plethora, myocardial infarction, pruritus, bleeding and gout. Although thrombosis is more common in patients with a high platelet count, it can also occur in those with normal platelet numbers. Paradoxically, patients with primary polycythaemia can also suffer from abnormal bleeding as platelet function is sometimes abnormal. Rarely, patients with primary polycythaemia may present with anaemia as a result of chronic gastrointestinal haemorrhage. Without treatment, the median survival of patients is about 2 years after diagnosis. The mainstay of treatment is repeated venesection to maintain the haematocrit <45%. Hydroxyurea is given to control the platelet count. Small molecule inhibitors of JAK2 are currently being tested in clinical trials.

Secondary polycythaemia

The majority of secondary polycythaemias are caused by a compensatory increase in erythropoietin production in response to hypoxia. Common causes include chronic obstructive pulmonary disease, high altitude and congenital cyanotic heart disease. A smaller number of patients have abnormal excess secretion of erythropoietin. Causes include hypernephroma, hepatoma, cerebellar haemangioblastoma and phaeochromocytoma. Polycystic and transplanted kidneys can secrete inappropriately large amounts of erythropoietin.

Apparent polycythaemia

This term is applied to patients who have an increased haematocrit but normal RBC mass. The mechanism is unclear but smoking, hypertension, obesity, diuretics and high alcohol intake have all been associated with apparent polycythaemia. Management is aimed at reversing any potential cause, e.g. stopping smoking, and treatment by venesection is recommended in patients with a haematocrit >54% or in those with an increased risk of vascular occlusion. In addition, there are clinical situations in which the normal ranges for haemoglobin and haematocrit are exceeded with a normal RBC mass if the plasma volume is substantially reduced, e.g. plasma loss in burns and severe fluid loss suffered as a result of gross dehydration or prolonged bowel obstruction.

Anaesthesia and polycythaemia

Polycythaemia probably presents a much greater risk to the patient undergoing surgery than anaemia. It is not surprising that controlled, randomized studies of patients who have undergone surgery with or without treatment of their polycythaemia are not available. Two retrospective, uncontrolled and non-randomized studies suggested some important points about the anaesthetic and surgical management of patients with primary polycythaemia:

- Patients with untreated primary polycythaemia experience substantially greater morbidity and mortality after surgery than those who are adequately treated.
- Patients with adequately treated primary polycythaemia may have a similar morbidity and mortality to unaffected patients.
- The commonest complications in patients with untreated primary polycythaemia are haemorrhage and thrombosis. The risk of deep vein thrombosis after major surgery is at least fivefold increased.
- The decrease in postoperative morbidity and mortality seen in patients whose primary polycythaemia has been treated is proportional to the duration of haematological control.

Preoperative management

Polycythaemia most often comes to light during the investigation of some other disorder or at routine preoperative testing. It should be considered if small vessel occlusive disease is the indication for surgery, or if the patient has plethoric facies, a history of ischaemic heart disease or abnormal bleeding.

If a high Hb concentration or haematocrit is identified preoperatively, acute plasma volume reduction as a cause can usually be excluded on history and clinical grounds. If true polycythaemia is identified, hypoxaemia as a cause can be readily excluded by performing arterial blood gas measurement. If the surgical procedure is elective, the patient should then be referred to a haematologist for investigation and treatment. It has been suggested that the peripheral blood count and the blood volume should be normalized before surgery.

If the surgery is urgent and blood volume is clinically normal, isovolaemic haemodilution can be performed by venesecting the patient and replacing the withdrawn volume with colloid. It is logical to retain the withdrawn blood for administration to the patient should surgical blood loss be excessive. Subcutaneous low-molecular-weight heparin administration should be considered.

Perioperative management

If the polycythaemia is secondary, then steps must be taken to account for the primary disease process, e.g. chronic obstructive pulmonary disease and congenital cyanotic heart disease. Venous stasis and hypotension, both of which can cause thrombosis, should be avoided. Regional anaesthesia offers advantages to the polycythaemic patient in that the incidence of postoperative thromboembolic events may be decreased. The anaesthetist should take care to ensure that the results of clotting and platelet function tests are normal before embarking on neuraxial blocks.

Cyanosis occurs when the concentration of reduced (deoxygenated) haemoglobin exceeds a value of about 5 g dL^{-1}. This will occur at higher oxygen saturations in patients with a high Hb concentration. If the Hb concentration exceeds 20 g dL^{-1}, cyanosis may occur at saturations equal to the normal mixed venous oxygen saturation, i.e. 75%. Figure 7.2 shows the oxygen saturation at which cyanosis may occur for a range of Hb concentrations.

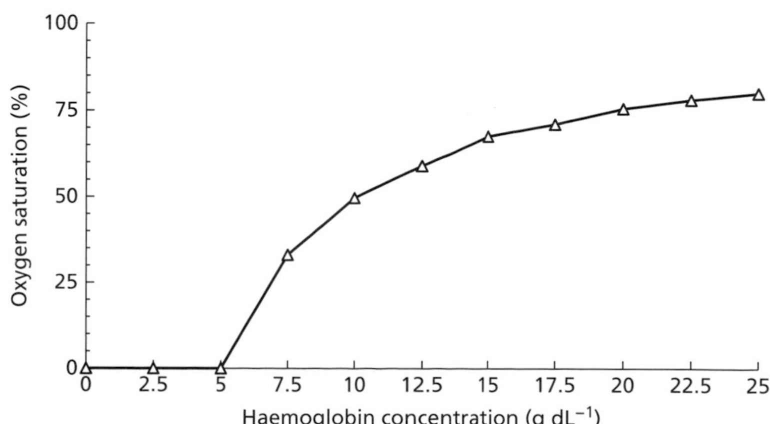

Figure 7.2 Oxygen saturation at which cyanosis may occur over a range of haemoglobin concentrations.

Bibliography

Barabas AP. Surgical problems associated with polycythaemia. *Br J Hosp Med* 1980; **23**: 289–90.

Levine RL, Gilliland DG. Myeloproliferative disorders. *Blood* 2008; **112**: 2190–8.

Messinezy M, Pearson TC. ABC of clinical haematology. Polycythaemia, primary (essential) thrombocythaemia and myelofibrosis. *Br Med J* 1997; **314**: 587–90.

Provan D, Weatherall D. Red cells II: acquired anaemias and polycythaemia. *Lancet* 2000; **355**: 1260–68.

Ruggeri M, Rodeghiero F, Tosetto A, *et al.*; Gruppo Italiano Malattie Ematologiche dell'Adulto (GIMEMA) Chronic Myeloproliferative Diseases Working Party. Postsurgery outcomes in patients with polycythemia vera and essential thrombocythemia: a retrospective survey. *Blood* 2008; **111**: 666–71.

Wasserman LR, Gilbert HS. Surgical bleeding in polycythemia vera. *Ann N Y Acad Sci* 1964; **115**: 122–38.

Sickle cell syndrome

Charles Marc Samama and Jean-François Schved

- Includes HbSS, HbSC and HbSThal.
- Life-threatening sickle crises can occur.
- Finding compatible blood can be difficult as a result of RBC antibodies.

Definition

Sickle cell syndromes are inherited haemoglobinopathies in which the dominant Hb is the unstable haemoglobin S. They include sickle cell anaemia (HbSS) and the double heterozygote conditions sickle C (HbSC) and sickle thalassaemia (HbSThal).

Pathophysiology

The sickle gene causes a single amino acid substitution on the β chain of the Hb molecule. There is some evidence that haemoglobin S confers a limited resistance to infection with malaria, a fact that may explain the greater incidence of the sickle gene in equatorial Africa.

When haemoglobin S is deoxygenated, the molecules polymerize into long chains called 'tactoids' and become insoluble. This results in deformation of the red cell membrane into the characteristic sickle shape. Although the process is often reversible with oxygenation, haemolysis will occur if the cell membrane is damaged. During prolonged periods of deoxygenation, irreversible sickling may occur. In this situation, the cells aggregate and occlude small blood vessels, which leads to tissue infarction and further hypoxia. Hypoxia is aggravated by lung infarction, which is a common cause of death. The major features of sickle cell disease are, therefore, a chronic anaemia and the occurrence of sickle cell 'crises' in which multiple episodes of tissue infarction occur.

Sickling occurs in individuals who are homozygous for the sickle gene (HbSS) and also in those in whom the sickle gene is inherited along with another variant such as HbC or β-thalassaemia. Tactoid formation is enhanced in the presence of HbC compared with the normal HbA. Patients with HbSC may have an Hb concentration towards the lower end of the normal range, but are liable to sickle and have a high incidence of venous thrombosis. Inheritance of the β-thalassaemia gene results in greatly reduced β-chain synthesis.

Individuals with sickle cell trait (HbAS) are usually asymptomatic, although sickling may occur under conditions of severe hypoxaemia. Patients with sickle cell trait are not at increased risk during a properly conducted anaesthetic, although the use of a tourniquet may be hazardous.

Preoperative assessment

Patients from susceptible populations should be screened for haemoglobin S with a quick solubility test, e.g. Sickledex. This will not distinguish between HbAS and the more dangerous phenotypes, but other abnormalities in the full blood count, and examination of the blood film, should alert the laboratory to the presence of an important haemoglobinopathy. Haemoglobin electrophoresis is necessary to confirm the diagnosis.

The history and examination should identify the frequency, pattern and severity of recent sickle crisis, and the presence of organ damage.

Patients with HbSS are usually well adapted to their low haemoglobin concentration, and increases in the haematocrit will increase the risk of a vaso-occlusive crisis. Patients who have received multiple transfusions in the past may have many red cell antibodies. Consequently, compatible blood may be difficult to find and transfusion reactions are relatively common. The optimum haemoglobin concentration and the acceptable proportion of HbS are both debatable and are determined in part by the proposed surgical procedure. In general, blood transfusion is usually unnecessary for patients undergoing minor surgery. For major surgery, simple red cell transfusion to increase the haemoglobin concentration to 10 g dL^{-1} seems to be as effective in preventing complications as more complex transfusion regimens to reduce the HbS concentration. However, a haematologist must be involved in this aspect of the patient's management.

See also Table 7.5.

Perioperative management

No specific anaesthetic technique is recommended. The principal objectives are to avoid any factors that may promote sickling. In particular, care should be taken to maintain good oxygenation, hydration, normothermia and normal acid–base balance. Limb

Table 7.5 Points to note in the preoperative assessment of patients with sickle cell disease

System	Point to note
Cardiovascular system	Cardiomegaly Increased cardiac output at rest Blood pressure typically low
Respiratory system	Pulmonary infarctions common – chest pain Consider measuring arterial blood gases
Blood	Oxyhaemoglobin dissociation curve shifted to left Low arterial oxygen saturation Increased blood viscosity
Abdomen	Abdominal crises may mimic a surgical emergency
Renal	Impaired concentration ability causes polyuria Chronic renal failure common
Neurological	Cerebral infarction may result in focal deficits Proliferative sickle retinopathy

tourniquets are best avoided, although there are reports of their uncomplicated use. If a tourniquet is essential, it should be applied as distally as possible, the limb should be thoroughly exsanguinated and the ischaemic time should be minimized.

The high standard of care delivered in the operating theatre must continue into the postoperative period. This may require advanced planning to ensure that a bed on a high-dependency unit is available.

Pain management presents a number of problems. Opioids may cause respiratory depression with consequent acidosis and hypoxia. Some patients may have developed a tolerance to opioids if they have required frequent treatment for sickle cell crises. In theory, regional pain techniques seem preferable, although there is little evidence to support this. Careful patient monitoring is essential.

Painful sickle crises may present in the postoperative period; these need to be distinguished from the surgical pain and treated appropriately. The acute chest syndrome is an acute pain crisis presenting as pleuritic chest pain, fever, hypoxaemia and lung infiltrates on the chest X-ray. It has a high mortality and requires urgent treatment with oxygen therapy and exchange transfusion to decrease the HbS concentration.

Bibliography

Firth PG. Anaesthesia for peculiar cells: a century of sickle cell disease. *Br J Anaesth* 2005; **95**: 287–99.

Firth PG. Anesthesia and hemoglobinopathies. *Anesthesiol Clin* 2009; **2**: 321–36.

Stenberg MH. Management of sickle cell disease. *N Engl J Med* 1999; **340**: 1021–30.

Vijay V, Cavenagh JD, Yate P. The anaesthetist's role in acute sickle cell crisis. *Br J Anaesth* 1998; **80**: 820–8.

Cross-references

Anaemia, 216

Thalassaemia, 241

Thalassaemia

Charles Marc Samama and Jean-François Schved

- β-Thalassaemia major, a transfusion-dependent anaemia, is the form most likely to present problems.
- The major problems are:
  - cardiomyopathy and liver disease as a result of haemosiderosis
  - difficult airway management
  - difficulty in finding compatible blood.

Definition

The thalassaemias are an inherited group of haematological diseases in which there is deficient synthesis of α- or β-globin chains. They are the most common monogenic blood diseases and are more frequently found in people originating in the Mediterranean, Central Africa, China and Southeast Asia.

In normal adults, the majority of haemoglobin is HbA, which has two α and two β chains, i.e. α2β2. There are four genes controlling α-chain production (two on each chromosome 16) and two controlling β-chain production (one on each chromosome 11).

α-Thalassaemia

The classification of α-thalassaemia into α0 and α+ has replaced the older nomenclature of type 1 (severe) and type 2 (mild).

α0-Thalassaemia results from elimination of α1 and α2 genes and /or regulatory sequences. α+-thalassaemia results from a single gene deletion or point mutation that prevents normal α-chain production. Deletion of only one gene controlling α-chain production produces haematological indices which overlap with those of the normal population. The α-thalassaemia trait is caused by the interaction of the normal haplotype with α0- or α+-thalassaemia determinant or homozygosity for two α+ haplotypes. The resulting anaemia is mild and of little anaesthetic significance.

Haemoglobin H disease is caused by the interaction of α0 and α+ determinants (loss of three genes). The clinical picture is of chronic haemolytic anaemia with Hb levels of 8–10 g dL^{-1}.This stimulates erythropoietin production and results in excess production of large amounts of β chains that form insoluble tetramers (HbH). The anaemia is characterized by jaundice, hepatosplenomegaly, leg ulcers, gallstones and folic acid deficiency. Haemolysis may be increased by oxidant drugs. Inability to produce any α chains results in hydrops fetalis in which death occurs *in utero* or soon after birth.

β-Thalassaemia

Usually inherited as a recessive disorder (some cases in which unstable β chains are produced are dominantly inherited), they present as a quantitative reduction in β-chain production. Underproduction of β chains results in an excess of α chains, which are unstable and precipitate in red cell precursors, which are destroyed in the bone marrow.

β-Thalassaemia trait results from the inheritance of a single abnormal gene (βo or β+) and is associated with mild iron-resistant hypochromic anaemia but with little or no other disability.

β-Thalassaemia major results from the presence of two abnormal genes, and sufferers are unable to produce any β chains. Production of fetal haemoglobin (α2γ2) leads to a haemoglobin concentration of 30–50% of the normal adult levels. This condition is associated with a severe anaemia that requires blood transfusion from the first year of life. Patients almost invariably develop antibodies making cross-matching of blood difficult. Patients must be treated with desferrioxamine (an iron-chelating agent) to decrease iron overload and haemosiderosis. Patients may be treated with bone marrow transplantation early in life before iron overload occurs.

Clinical features of thalassaemia

Clinically significant forms of thalassaemia are associated with bone marrow hyperplasia because of excessive erythropoietin production. This can lead to skeletal abnormalities including head bossing, prominent maxillae and a sunken nose, which may make tracheal intubation difficult.

There may be gross hepatosplenomegaly with hypersplenism. Repeated transfusion puts the patients at risk of blood-borne infections and haemosiderosis. The latter may give rise to cardiomyopathy, left ventricular dysfunction and clinically significant heart failure. In addition, haemosiderosis can also cause hepatic failure, diabetes, hypothyroidism, hypoparathyroidism and adrenal insufficiency. Individuals who have undergone bone marrow transplantation may be taking immunosuppressant drugs.

Preoperative assessment

Careful assessment of the patient's airway is essential. Ease of venous access should be assessed as repeated transfusions may have damaged peripheral veins. Skeletal abnormalities should be assessed as the patient may be kyphoscoliotic, which may have implications for lung function and positioning on the operating table. Symptoms and signs of cardiac, hepatic or endocrine disorders should be sought.

Investigations should include a full blood count, urea and electrolytes, blood glucose estimation, liver function tests and ECG (and echocardiogram if cardiac dysfunction is suspected). Allow extra time for blood cross-matching.

Perioperative management

Appropriate steps should be taken for any abnormalities identified preoperatively. Transfusion to normal haemoglobin levels is not indicated unless it is necessary to improve cardiorespiratory function. If the patient has an associated cardiomyopathy, intensive preoperative chelation therapy may improve cardiac function. Individuals who have had a splenectomy (for hypersplenism) should have had pneumococcal vaccine and should receive antibiotic prophylaxis.

Bibliography

Aldouri MA , Wonke B, Hoffbrand AU. High incidence of cardiomyopathy in β thalassaemia patients receiving regular transfusion and iron chelation. *Acta Haematol* 1990; **84**: 113–17.

Firth PG. Anesthesia and hemoglobinopathies. *Anesthesiol Clin* 2009; **2**: 321–36.

Modell B, Letskey EA Flynn DM. Survival and desferrioxamine in thalassaemia major. *Br Med J* 1986; **284**: 2031–9.

Orr B. Difficult intubation: a hazard in thalassaemia. *Br J Anaesth* 1967; **39**: 585.

Rodgers GP. Pharmacological therapy. *Baillière's Clin Haematol* 1998; **II**(1): 239–55.

Schrier SL. Pathophysiology of thalassaemia. *Curr Opin Haematol* 2002; **9**: 123–6.

Weatherall DJ. Fortnightly review: the thalassaemias. *Br Med J* 1997; **314**: 1675.

Zurlos MG, de Stefans P, Borgna-Pignatti C, *et al.* Survival and causes of death in thalassaemia major. *Lancet* 1989; **ii**: 27–30.

Cross-reference

Anaemia, 216

8 Bones and joints

Alain Borgeat

- Ankylosing spondylitis — *Alain Borgeat and José A Aguirre*
- Dwarfism — *José A Aguirre and Alain Borgeat*
- Marfan syndrome — *José A Aguirre and Alain Borgeat*
- Metabolic and degenerative bone disease — *José A Aguirre and Alain Borgeat*
- Rheumatoid disease — *José A Aguirre and Alain Borgeat*
- Scoliosis — *Alain Borgeat and José A Aguirre*

Ankylosing spondylitis

Alain Borgeat and José A Aguirre

Ankylosing spondylitis (AS) is a disease that affects young people and presents at around 26 years of age. Men are more often affected than are women (2:1). About 80% of patients develop the first symptoms before 30 years and less than 5% present at older than 45 years. There is a rough correlation between the prevalence of human leukocyte antigen (HLA) B27 and the incidence and prevalence of this disease: 90–95% of patients are positive for HLA B27 and the risk of this disease developing is about 5% in HLA B27-positive individuals and higher in HLA B27-positive relatives. However, most HLA B27-positive individuals remain healthy. Overall, the prevalence of AS is between 0.1 and 1.4%, and in mid-Europe it is 0.3–0.5% (similar to that for rheumatoid arthritis).The incidence of AS is between 0.5 and 14 per 100 000 population per year. These differences are due to selection of the target populations, screening criteria such as back pain, the choice of diagnostic criteria (Box 8.1) to confirm the diagnosis and the prevalence of HLA B27 and the distribution of its subtypes.

Box 8.1 Modified New York criteria for ankylosing spondylitis (AS)

Diagnosis of AS requires one radiological criterion with at least one clinical criterion. AS is the probable diagnosis if >3 clinical criteria and/or radiological criteria are present.

- Clinical criteria
  - Low back pain >3 months' duration, improves with exercise and is not relieved by rest
  - Limitation of motion of the lumbar spine in sagittal and coronal planes
  - Limitation of chest expansion relative to normal values corrected for age and sex
- Radiological criteria
  - Bilateral sacroiliitis – grade 2 (sclerosis with some erosions) or higher
  - Unilateral sacroiliitis – grade 3 (severe erosions, pseudodilatation of joint space and partial ankylosis) or grade 4 (complete ankylosis)

Functional restrictions in patients with AS are greater in those with a history of physically demanding jobs, more comorbid conditions and in smokers than in those with higher levels of education and a family history of this disease. Young age at the onset of symptoms is associated with worse functional outcome. In juvenile patients with spondyloarthritides, clinical symptoms can be different and include severe tarsitis. Male patients have more structural changes, including bamboo spine, than do female patients.

Pathophysiology

Musculoskeletal disease

Characteristic symptoms of AS are spinal stiffness and loss of spinal mobility, which are explained by spinal inflammation, structural damage or both. Spinal inflammation can arise as spondylitis, spondylodiscitis or spondylarthritis. Structural changes are mainly caused by osteoproliferation rather than by osteodestruction. Syndesmophytes and ankylosis are the most characteristic features of this disease, which are visible on conventional X-rays after some months to many years. Low bone density, osteoporosis and an increased rate of fractures may add to the hyperkyphosis predominantly seen in male patients. Decreased movement of the lumbar spine results with a proportion progressing to ankylosis and complete rigidity with a classical X-ray picture of 'bamboo spine'.

Complications of severe spinal disease include fractures with little or no history of trauma, collapse of vertebral end-plates (spondylodiscitis) and spinal nerve root compression. Cervical fractures, which occur commonly at C5–6, are often overlooked because they occur with minimal trauma or hyperextension. Clinically significant atlantoaxial subluxation occurs in 21% of patients with AS. About 47% of AS patients with vertebral compression fractures have a neurological complication ranging from paraesthesia to loss of muscle strength.

The most common joints affected are the hips and shoulders. End-stage hip disease requiring hip replacements occurs in 20% of patients with juvenile-onset AS, in about 10% of patients with onset in late teens, and is rare when the onset is in the twenties to thirties. Peripheral joint involvement occurs in 50% of patients and is more common in patients with concomitant psoriasis. Temporomandibular joint involvement causes limited mouth opening in 10% of patients, rising to 30–40% in those with long-standing disease. The disease rarely causes arthritis of the cricoarytenoid joint, but can lead to dyspnoea, hoarseness and vocal cord fixation. AS often affects costovertebral and costotransverse joints, causing local tenderness and pain on coughing or sneezing. Other features include plantar fasciitis and Achilles tendonitis.

Respiratory system

Upper lobe pulmonary fibrosis is a recognized complication of long-standing AS. Along with costovertebral involvement this may significantly impair the respiratory reserve of the patient. Chest X-rays may show apical fibrosis while pulmonary function testing may reveal a restrictive lung defect.

Cardiovascular system

Cardiovascular involvement occurs in up to 10% of patients with severe spondylitis. Fibrous proliferation of the intima of the aorta can result in aortitis and aortic insufficiency, occasionally affecting the mitral valve. Involvement of the Purkinje fibres may cause conduction defects, increasing the risk of myocardial infarction. Long-term disease is associated with a greatly increased cardiovascular mortality.

Neurological system

Neurological effects include spinal cord compression, cauda equina syndrome, cervical spine fracture, focal epilepsy, vertebrobasilar insufficiency and peripheral nerve lesions. Spinal fractures can lead to acute epidural haematoma and neurological deficits.

Other

Anterior uveitis (iridocyclitis) occurs in 20–40%, psoriasis in 9% and inflammatory bowel disease in up to 6%. Anterior uveitis classically presents with sudden onset of blurred vision associated with eye pain, redness and photophobia. Some can progress to become chronic uveitis with permanent visual impairment.

Preoperative assessment

A thorough preoperative assessment is essential to evaluate the severity of the disease, in particular airway involvement and the extra-articular manifestations of the disease. Preoperative neurological deficits must be documented. The range of movement of all joints should be assessed to plan optimal positioning of the patient. The extent of preoperative investigations mainly depends on the severity of the disease, and these include echocardiography, lung function tests, imaging of the cervical spine and arterial blood gas analysis. Owing to the potential for conduction defects, a preoperative electrocardiogram (ECG) is mandatory. An echocardiogram is required to assess the severity of valvular disease (Table 8.1).

There is no clear consensus regarding the management of anti-tumour necrosis factor α (TNF-α) blockers in the perioperative period. There is a significant association between infectious complications following orthopaedic surgery and treatment with anti TNF α agents, although the perioperative continuation of anti-TNF-α agents is not a significant risk factor for surgical wound infections and infection risk appears not to be a reason to withhold therapy.

Perioperative management

Premedication

If fibreoptic intubation is to be performed or difficulty with intubation is anticipated then an antisialagogue should be prescribed with or without an antacid.

Planning anaesthesia

If general anaesthesia is the only possibility, careful airway management of the patient is paramount. Difficult intubation is associated with AS involving the

Table 8.1 Preoperative investigations for patients with AS and rheumatoid arthritis

Investigations	Result
Full blood count	Anaemia normochromic, normocytic (severe, hypochromic; gastrointestinal bleed)
Urea and electrolytes	Abnormal (iatrogenic – gold, ciclosporin)
ECG	Heart block
	Ischaemic (arteritis)
	Left ventricular hypertrophy (valvular heart disease)
Chest X-ray	Rheumatoid nodules
Cervical spine X-ray	Atlantoaxial subluxation (lateral subatlantoaxial subluxation and odontoid views)
Spirometry	Restrictive flow pattern
Indirect laryngoscopy	Degree of cricoarytenoid involvement

cervical spine and can be compounded further when the temporomandibular joint is involved. There is significant risk of neurological injury with any excessive neck extension in patients with chronic cervical kyphosis. Neck extension can cause vertebrobasilar insufficiency as a result of bony encroachment on the vertebral artery. Injuries to the cervical spine and spinal cord, such as dislocation of C6 vertebra and quadriparesis after an emergency intubation, have been reported. Fixed cervical flexion deformities limit access to the trachea and tracheostomy may be impossible. Neck supports should be used during anaesthesia and forcible movements of the neck in the presence of neuromuscular blockade avoided. Awake fibreoptic intubation is the safest option, especially in those patients in whom it is not possible to visualize the larynx on indirect laryngoscopy or in those with severe chin on chest deformity. It also allows for constant neurological monitoring during placement of the tracheal tube. Retrograde intubation may also be considered.

The laryngeal mask is more appropriate in patients with restricted mouth opening of <2 cm or in patients who do not require intubation. It may not be possible to place a laryngeal mask in patients with AS when the mouth opening is <1.2 cm and if a fixed extension deformity and large cervical osteophytes are present.

The 'intubate at all costs' approach is not appropriate for elective surgery, and if maintaining the airway is reasonably easy a laryngeal mask is useful. If airway maintenance is extremely difficult or impossible, then allowing the patient to wake up and postponing surgery is prudent.

In the emergency situation there may be insufficient skill/equipment available to perform fibreoptic intubation and emergency tracheostomy/cricothyrotomy may be necessary. (However, with a severe flexion deformity these may be impossible!)

Central neuraxial blocks are frequently difficult in these patients because of ankylosis of the intervertebral joints, or are ill advised because of neurological complications of the disease. AS has been reported as an independent risk factor for spinal haematoma after epidural anaesthesia. This may be due to technical difficulties and repeated trauma or perhaps non-steroidal anti-inflammatory drug (NSAID) therapy. Continuous peripheral nerve blocks should be applied whenever possible. The peripheral catheter is very useful for postoperative analgesia and will reduce the need of opioids.

Respiratory system

Preoperative assessment should indicate whether any degree of respiratory compromise exists and if consideration should be given to postoperative ventilation.

Cardiovascular system

Aortic or mitral incompetence should be treated as in primary cardiac disease, with caution in the use of vasodilating drugs. Antibiotic cover may be appropriate and preoperative pacing may be necessary.

Conduct of anaesthesia

Peripheral nerve blocks should be used whenever possible. Central neuraxial blocks are technically difficult. The paramedian approach may be used and the number of attempts limited to three because of the risk of bleeding.

For general anaesthesia there are no specific contraindications to the use of any anaesthetic agent. Care should be taken with regard to patient transfer and positioning in order to avoid vertebral or neurological damage and minimize backache postoperatively. Ensuring that patients have full control of their airway prior to extubation is essential, as reintubation may prove very difficult.

Postoperative management

The use of continuous peripheral nerve block analgesia is the ideal option whenever possible. High doses of opioids must be balanced against the risk of oversedation and compromising the airway. Patient-controlled analgesia (PCA) may be helpful in these circumstances.

Re-establishment of regular NSAID therapy will help to relieve pain due to AS, which may be greater than the surgical pain.

Physiotherapy, breathing exercises and early mobilization should be instituted early because patients are at increased risk of respiratory complications. The effects of fluid shifts and the effects of medications on perioperative fluid balance should be monitored.

Long-term management

Patients with AS may present for any type of surgery, but as the duration of the disease lengthens so does the likelihood of the surgery relating to the disease or complications of its treatment. Previous anaesthetic notes are essential, with particular reference to intubation/airway difficulties.

Bibliography

Akkoc N, Khan MA. Overestimation of the prevalence of ankylosing spondylitis in the Berlin study: comment on the article by Braun *et al. Arthritis Rheum* 2005; **52**: 4048–9; author reply 4049–50.

Bakland G, Nossent HC, Gran JT. Incidence and prevalence of ankylosing spondylitis in Northern Norway. *Arthritis Rheum* 2005; **53**: 850–5.

Branten AJ. Risk of infectious complications during anti-TNFalpha therapy. *Neth J Med* 2008; **66**: 50–2.

Braun J, Bollow M, Remlinger G, *et al.* Prevalence of spondylarthropathies in HLA-B27 positive and negative blood donors. *Arthritis Rheum* 1998; **41**: 58–67.

Brewerton DA, Hart FD, Nicholls A, *et al.* Ankylosing spondylitis and HL-A 27. *Lancet* 1973; **1**: 904–7.

Brophy S, Pavy S, Lewis P, *et al.* Inflammatory eye, skin, and bowel disease in spondyloarthritis: genetic, phenotypic, and environmental factors. *J Rheumatol* 2001; **28**: 2667–73.

Burgos-Vargas R, Vazquez-Mellado J. The early clinical recognition of juvenile-onset ankylosing spondylitis and its differentiation from juvenile rheumatoid arthritis. *Arthritis Rheum* 1995; **38**: 835–44.

Cooper C, Carbone L, Michet CJ, *et al.* Fracture risk in patients with ankylosing spondylitis: a population based study. *J Rheumatol* 1994; **21**: 1877–82.

den Broeder AA, Creemers MC, Fransen J, *et al.* Risk factors for surgical site infections and other complications in elective surgery in patients with rheumatoid arthritis with special attention for anti-tumor necrosis factor: a large retrospective study. *J Rheumatol* 2007; **34**: 689–95.

Feldtkeller E, Khan MA, van der Heijde D, *et al.* Age at disease onset and diagnosis delay in HLA-B27 negative vs. positive patients with ankylosing spondylitis. *Rheumatol Int* 2003; **23**: 61–6.

Giles JT, Bartlett SJ, Gelber AC, *et al.* Tumor necrosis factor inhibitor therapy and risk of serious postoperative orthopedic infection in rheumatoid arthritis. *Arthritis Rheum* 2006; **55**: 333–7.

Hyderally HA. Epidural hematoma unrelated to combined spinal-epidural anesthesia in a patient with ankylosing spondylitis receiving aspirin after total hip replacement. *Anesth Analg* 2005; **100**: 882–3.

Jacobs WB, Fehlings MG. Ankylosing spondylitis and spinal cord injury: origin, incidence, management, and avoidance. *Neurosurg Focus* 2008; **24**: E12.

Jimenez-Balderas FJ, Mintz G. Ankylosing spondylitis: clinical course in women and men. *J Rheumatol* 1993; **20**: 2069–72.

Karberg K, Zochling J, Sieper J, *et al.* Bone loss is detected more frequently in patients with ankylosing spondylitis with syndesmophytes. *J Rheumatol* 2005; **32**: 1290–8.

Khan MA. Epidemiology of HLA-B27 and arthritis. *Clin Rheumatol* 1996; **15**(Suppl. 1): 10–12.

Kumar CM, Mehta M. Ankylosing spondylitis: lateral approach to spinal anaesthesia for lower limb surgery. Can *J Anaesth* 1995; **42**: 73–6.

Lu PP, Brimacombe J, Ho AC, *et al.* The intubating laryngeal mask airway in severe ankylosing spondylitis. *Can J Anaesth* 2001; **48**: 1015–19.

Nederlandse Vereniging voor Reumatologie. Medicijnen: Het toepassen van TNF blockade in de behandeling van reumatoide arteritis. Dutch Society for Rhematology, 2008.

Peters MJ, van der Horst-Bruinsma IE, Dijkmans BA, Nurmohamed MT. Cardiovascular risk profile of patients with spondylarthropathies, particularly ankylosing spondylitis and psoriatic arthritis. *Semin Arthritis Rheum* 2004; **34**: 585–92.

Saraux A, Guedes C, Allain J, *et al.* Prevalence of rheumatoid arthritis and spondyloarthropathy in Brittany, France. Societe de Rhumatologie de l'Ouest. *J Rheumatol* 1999; **26**: 2622–7.

Shaikh SA. Ankylosing spondylitis: recent breakthroughs in diagnosis and treatment. *J Can Chiropr Assoc* 2007; **51**: 249–60.

Stone M, Warren RW, Bruckel J, *et al.* Juvenile-onset ankylosing spondylitis is associated with worse functional outcomes than adult-onset ankylosing spondylitis. *Arthritis Rheum* 2005; **53**: 445–51.

van der Linden SM, Valkenburg HA, de Jongh BM, Cats A. The risk of developing ankylosing spondylitis in HLA-B27 positive individuals. A comparison of relatives of spondylitis patients with the general population. *Arthritis Rheum* 1984; **27**: 241–9.

Vosse D, van der Heijde D, Landewe R, *et al.* Determinants of hyperkyphosis in patients with ankylosing spondylitis. *Ann Rheum Dis* 2006; **65**: 770–4.

Wanders A, Landewe R, Dougados M, *et al.* Association between radiographic damage of the spine and spinal mobility for individual patients with ankylosing spondylitis: can assessment of spinal mobility be a proxy for radiographic evaluation? *Ann Rheum Dis* 2005; **64**: 988–94.

Ward MM, Weisman MH, Davis Jr JC, Reveille JD. Risk factors for functional limitations in patients with long-standing ankylosing spondylitis. *Arthritis Rheum* 2005; **53**: 710–17.

Wulf H. Epidural anaesthesia and spinal haematoma. *Can J Anaesth* 1996; **43**: 1260–71.

Cross-references

Aortic valve disease, 126
Cardiac conduction defects, 132
Difficult airway: management, 651
Mitral valve disease, 156
Regional anaesthesia techniques, 719
Restrictive lung disease, 114

Dwarfism

José A Aguirre and Alain Borgeat

People with short stature conventionally are divided into two categories: those with proportionate growth and those with disproportionate growth, and it is the latter group that are classified as dwarfs. Patients with dwarfism are often considered as having a single disease entity, but this is an oversimplification. There exist over 100 different types of dwarfism, many of which pose specific anaesthetic problems.

Although each particular type of dwarfism is relatively rare, the large number of types means that any practising anaesthetist is likely to meet dwarfs. Achondroplasia, the commonest cause of dwarfism, has an incidence of 1:10000 to 1:40000. There is a defect in the fibroblast growth factor receptor. This affects endochondral bone formation, i.e. long-bone growth, while membranous and periosteal bones are unaffected. Achondroplasia is congenital and hereditary (autosomal dominant); 80–90% of cases are probably new mutations.

Anaesthetic problems

These patients may have multiple problems. Monitoring and anaesthetic techniques need to be considered in relation to both the underlying diagnosis and the planned surgical procedure.

Traditionally, general anaesthesia has been the technique of choice. This is despite the risks of airway obstruction with some syndromes. This is in part because of the difficulties encountered in performance of spinal and epidural blockade, such as poor landmarks, spinal deformities including lumbar lordosis and spinal stenosis with a narrow epidural space. Nevertheless, there are numerous reports of successful spinal and epidural anaesthesia for caesarean section. Decreased volumes of local anaesthetic are needed and epidural may be preferable to spinal as the dose can be titrated according to the height of the block. Continuous peripheral nerve blocks may be challenging, but in many cases can be successfully performed and should be used whenever possible.

Preoperative assessment

Respiratory system

- Clinical assessment of airway: narrow nose passage, intraorally anatomical changes.
- Obstructive airway lesions, especially in patients with mucopolysaccharidoses.
- Previous problems with airway maintenance or intubation.
- Positioning problems owing to reduced mobility of the atlanto-occipital joint. Risk of atlanto-occipital luxation.
- Restrictive defects secondary to rib hypoplasia and kyphoscoliosis.
- Sleep apnoea.

Cardiovascular system

- Pulmonary hypertension.
- Congenital heart disease.
- Coronary artery disease.
- Valvular heart disease.
- Cardiomyopathy.

Neurological system

- Macrocephaly and hydrocephaly.
- Cervical spine instability.
- Spinal cord compression.
- Nerve root compression.
- Temperature regulation problems.

Others

- Endocrinopathy (hyperglycaemia).
- Prone to infections.
- Bleeding problems.
- Renal function.
- Positioning damage due to deformities.

Premedication

Midazolam can be given in the majority of the patients and provides good anxiolysis. Anticholinergic agents can be considered in patients with marked secretions, and in those in whom problems with the airway or intubation are anticipated. Avoid sedatives in patients with potential upper airway obstruction (sleep apnoea syndrome). Consider also sodium citrate or H_2-receptor blocker.

Intraoperative management

Venous access

Peripheral and central access are often challenging. These patients are frequently obese and, in addition, may possess subcutaneous infiltrates with lax skin. Cervical abnormalities, including very short necks and, frequently, stabilization devices, may make access to the jugular vein extremely difficult. In these circumstances there may be no option but to use either a femoral or subclavian approach.

Monitoring

Because of the different proportions, non-invasive blood pressure cuffs may lead to wrong measurements. In the case of hydrocephalus, a possible rise in intracranial pressure must be anticipated.

Induction

Awake intubation with conscious sedation (propofol and remifentanil) or inhalational induction with maintenance by spontaneous respiration are thought to be relatively safe techniques in patients in whom difficulties with airway maintenance or intubation are predicted. Nasal intubation should be avoided. Restrictive lung disease, if present, will prolong an inhalational induction. Muscle relaxants should be avoided until it is certain that the patient can be ventilated by mask.

Intubation

This can prove to be extremely difficult and exposure of the larynx may prove impossible with a conventional laryngoscope in some patients with very short necks. In these circumstances, a short-handled laryngoscope may enable visualization of the glottis, but if this fails then fibreoptic-guided intubation either awake or under general anaesthesia will be required. In patients with foramen magnum stenosis or atlantoaxial instability it is important to avoid neck movements during attempts at intubation, and under these circumstances fibreoptic control of the airway may be preferable.

There is some controversy as to the selection of the correct size of tracheal tube. For patients with achondroplasia the formula

$$(Age/4) + 4$$

usually correctly predicts the internal diameter. In extreme circumstances, a tracheostomy may be necessary, but in patients with mucopolysaccharidoses this may not completely relieve the tracheal obstruction due to distal tracheal distortion.

Respiratory support

The low functional residual capacity (FRC) and high closing volume frequently found in patients with respiratory involvement predisposes these patients to atelectasis and ventilation/perfusion (V/Q) mismatching. This may cause severe problems with oxygenation. For all but the shortest and simplest surgical procedures, arterial cannulation for intra- and postoperative blood gas estimation is strongly recommended for any patient with respiratory dysfunction. Postoperative ventilation, which can be prolonged, may be required, especially in patients with thoracic dystrophy.

Cardiovascular problems

Cardiology opinion may be required to delineate the extent of cardiac compromise. Pulmonary hypertension is the most frequent cardiovascular complication seen. Clinical suspicion may be raised by the presence of a parasternal heave, a loud widely split second heart sound and a pulmonary systolic ejection murmur. Right ventricular enlargement can best be confirmed by echocardiography. In patients with pulmonary hypertension, the anaesthetic has to be planned to avoid pulmonary arterial vasoconstriction while still maintaining an adequate cardiac output. Care must be taken to avoid hypoxia, hypercapnia and respiratory or metabolic acidosis, which can cause profound rises in pulmonary artery pressures. In mildly affected individuals, oxygen and inhalational anaesthetics are often used. In patients with right ventricular failure, high-dose narcotic techniques are preferred. In children, ketamine has been safely used, even in cases with right ventricular failure, although this is not recommended in adults. In patients with congenital heart lesions, or corrected lesions, endocarditis prophylaxis is mandatory.

Neurological problems

Most of these problems revolve around the stability of the cervical spine, especially at the atlantoaxial and craniocervical junctions, and problems with raised intracranial pressure (ICP). In patients with spinal cord compression, an autonomic hyper-reflexic state may develop. Document any pre-existing neurological deficit if central blockade is considered.

The problems of anaesthetizing a patient with raised ICP are formidable: an inhalational induction can be associated with hypercapnia and a rise in ICP, whereas an intravenous induction can be associated with apnoea in a patient who cannot be intubated or ventilated. These patients thus require consideration on a case-by-case basis.

Rarely, hyperthermia, usually without the clinical features of malignant hyperthermia (MH), develops. Therapy consists of simple cooling measures alone. A few cases that are clinically indistinguishable from MH have been observed in patients with osteogenesis imperfecta. It was only by muscle biopsy that the diagnosis was able to be refuted. Thus, potential trigger agents do not need to be avoided unless MH is clinically suspected.

Bleeding problems

Osteogenesis imperfecta is the only chondrodystrophy associated with a coagulopathy. These patients require formal evaluation with a bleeding time preoperatively. Platelets and fresh-frozen plasma should be available.

Bibliography

Berkowitz ID, Raja SN, Bender KS, Kopits SE. Dwarfs: pathophysiology and anesthetic implications. *Anesthesiology* 1990; **73**: 739–59.

Carstoniu J, Yee I, Halpern S. Epidural anaesthesia for caesarean section in an achondroplastic dwarf. *Can J Anaesth* 1992; **39**: 708–11.

Crawford M, Dutton DA. Spinal anaesthesia for caesarean section in an achondroplastic dwarf. *Anaesthesia* 1992; **47**: 1007.

Dvorak DM, Rusnak RA, Morcos JJ. Multiple trauma in the achondroplastic dwarf: an emergency medicine physician perspective case report and literature review. *Am J Emerg Med* 1993; **11**: 390–5.

Monedero P, Garcia-Pedrajas F, Coca I, *et al.* Is management of anesthesia in achondroplastic dwarfs really a challenge? *J Clin Anesth* 1997; **9**: 208–12.

Walts LF, Finerman G, Wyatt GM. Anaesthesia for dwarfs and other patients of pathological small stature. *Can Anaesth Soc J* 1975; **22**: 703–9.

Cross-references

Cardiomyopathy, 136
Congenital heart disease in adult life, 141
Difficult airway: management, 651
Monitoring, 690
Pulmonary hypertension, 164

Marfan syndrome

José A Aguirre and Alain Borgeat

Marfan syndrome was first described in 1896 by Marfan. The incidence is 1 in 10 000 live births in the USA. There is no gender preference. The inheritance is autosomal dominant, with a 25% incidence of spontaneous mutation, and there is clinical variability with complete penetrance. The syndrome is due to mutations in gene *FBN1* encoding fibrillin 1 on chromosome 15q21.1. Clinical diagnosis requires a family history of Marfan syndrome with involvement of an organ system, but increased organ involvement is needed for the diagnosis if there is no family history.

Pathophysiology

Cardiovascular

Cardiac abnormalities are the most serious medical complication of the syndrome. Historically, the mean age of survival was 43 years for men and 46 years for women, but the average life span has now been extended to 72 years, with early deaths occurring at an average age of 41 years. Mitral valve insufficiency, aortic valve insufficiency, and both ascending and descending aortic dilatation may lead to a dissecting aneurysm, which is the most frequent cause of death. Congenital Marfan syndrome is a particularly serious variant with an 80% incidence of cardiac abnormalities and a 14% mortality rate during the first year of life.

Skeletal

The long bones are slender, with long limbs, and arm span usually exceeds the patient's total height. There is joint laxity and arachnodactyly, abnormal lengthening of the digits. The 'thumb sign' in Marfan syndrome is positive when the nail of the thumb in a clenched fist extends beyond the ulnar border of the small finger. Another sign of arachnodactyly is the 'wrist sign', in which the patient encircles the wrist with their contralateral hand and the thumb overlaps the small finger. Protrusio acetabuli is another feature of Marfan syndrome.

Significant scoliosis is common and spine deformity occurs early in life. Dural ectasia is common; 63% of patients with Marfan syndrome were reported to have scoliosis and >50% had kyphosis; 12% developed progressive scoliosis requiring surgery. Further complications may include instrumentation fixation failure, pseudarthrosis and curve decompensation.

Respiratory

Thoracic insufficiency syndrome in Marfan syndrome can be from chest wall constriction from pectus carinatum or excavatum, and scoliosis can further contribute to thoracic insufficiency syndrome volume depletion deformity of the thorax from spine rotation. There are also intrinsic lung problems. Spontaneous pneumothorax and bronchospasm may be a problem and pulmonary function is often adversely affected.

Ocular

These include lens dislocation, myopia, retinal detachment, glaucoma and cataracts.

Preoperative assessment

Particular attention should be paid to cardiopulmonary investigations. These should include chest X-ray, ECG, echocardiography, lung function tests and arterial blood gases. When aortic dilatation exceeds 5–5.5 cm in adults, prophylactic graft replacement of the aortic valve and ascending aorta may be necessary. Vital capacity and forced expiratory volume in 1 second (FEV_1) may appear to be lower than expected when compared with predicted values, owing to greater height or arm span. Before surgery, patients should be screened for platelet count, prothrombin time (PT) and partial thromboplastin time (PTT).

Perioperative management

Prophylactic antibiotics must be given because of the high risk of bacterial endocarditis. In patients undergoing spine operations for Marfan syndrome, a deep infection rate of 10%, dural tears of 8% and a mean blood loss of 2400 mL for scoliosis and 3000 mL for kyphosis has been reported. Careful handling and positioning are essential to avoid joint trauma and dislocation.

Whenever possible, a continuous peripheral nerve block should be performed in order to avoid any intervention on the airways and a good control of the surgical-induced stress reaction. Intubation may be difficult owing to the long, high arched palate. Gentle laryngoscopy should be performed to avoid cervical spine and temporomandibular joint damage.

Surges of blood pressure should be avoided, e.g. on laryngoscopy or in response to surgical stimulation. β-Blockade will reduce aortic wall tension. Blood pressure should be maintained with the diastolic pressure high enough to ensure good coronary flow, but not too high so as to risk dissection. There may be little cardiac reserve, and volatile agents may be very depressant.

Spontaneous pneumothorax may become a tension pneumothorax in a patient on positive pressure ventilation. Maintain low airway pressures and avoid overinflation of the lungs.

The risk of malignant hyperthermia may be increased; therefore, the use of intravenous agents is preferred.

Monitoring

In addition to the minimal monitoring standards produced by the Association of Anaesthetists of Great Britain and Ireland (AAGBI), capnography, airway pressures, arterial cannulation (but increased risk of morbidity because of weak arterial wall) and temperature are recommended.

Choice of anaesthetic

The choice of anaesthetic technique is broad and no one agent or technique is suggested. Following careful induction with thiopentone, propofol or etomidate while monitoring blood pressure, anaesthesia may be maintained with nitrous oxide/oxygen/narcotic/muscle relaxant/volatile agent. Blood pressure may be further controlled by β-blockade, if needed. Care must be taken to maintain intravascular volumes and filling pressure.

Bibliography

Birch JG, Herring JA. Spinal deformity in Marfan syndrome. *J Pediatr Orthop* 1987; **7**: 546–52.

De Paepe A, Devereux RB, Dietz HC, *et al.* Revised diagnostic criteria for the Marfan syndrome. *Am J Med Genet* 1996; **62**: 417–26.

Dietz HC, Cutting GR, Pyeritz RE, *et al.* Marfan syndrome caused by a recurrent de novo missense mutation in the fibrillin gene. *Nature* 1991; **352**: 337–9.

Groenink M, Rozendaal L, Naeff MS, *et al.* Marfan syndrome in children and adolescents: predictive and prognostic value of aortic root growth for screening for aortic complications. *Heart* 1998; **80**: 163–9.

Hall JR, Pyeritz RE, Dudgeon DL, Haller Jr JA. Pneumothorax in the Marfan syndrome: prevalence and therapy. *Ann Thorac Surg* 1984; **37**: 500–4.

Jones KB, Erkula G, Sponseller PD, Dormans JP. Spine deformity correction in Marfan syndrome. *Spine (Phila Pa 1976)* 2002; **27**: 2003–12.

Konig P, Boxer R, Morrison J, Pletcher B. Bronchial hyperreactivity in children with Marfan syndrome. *Pediatr Pulmonol* 1991; **11**: 29–36.

Morse RP, Rockenmacher S, Pyeritz RE, *et al.* Diagnosis and management of infantile Marfan syndrome. *Pediatrics* 1990; **86**: 888–95.

Nallamshetty L, Ahn NU, Ahn UM, *et al.* Dural ectasia and back pain: review of the literature and case report. *J Spinal Disord Tech* 2002; **15**: 326–9.

Nienaber CA, Von Kodolitsch Y. Therapeutic management of patients with Marfan syndrome: focus on cardiovascular involvement. *Cardiol Rev* 1999; **7**: 332–41.

Silverman DI, Burton KJ, Gray J, *et al.* Life expectancy in the Marfan syndrome. *Am J Cardiol* 1995; **75**: 157–60.

Sponseller PD, Hobbs W, Riley 3rd LH, Pyeritz RE. The thoracolumbar spine in Marfan syndrome. *J Bone Joint Surg Am* 1995; **77**: 867–76.

Streeten EA, Murphy EA, Pyeritz RE. Pulmonary function in the Marfan syndrome. *Chest* 1987; **91**: 408–12.

Taylor LJ. Severe spondylolisthesis and scoliosis in association with Marfan's syndrome. Case report and review of the literature. *Clin Orthop Relat Res* 1987; (221): 207–11.

Walker BA, Murdoch JL. The wrist sign. A useful physical finding in the Marfan syndrome. *Arch Intern Med* 1970; **126**: 276–7.

Cross-references

Abdominal aortic reconstruction: elective open repair, 505
Aortic valve disease, 126
Cardiac conduction defects, 132
Cataract surgery, 342
Mitral valve disease, 156
Restrictive lung disease, 114

Metabolic and degenerative bone disease

José A Aguirre and Alain Borgeat

Osteomalacia

Osteomalacia is a metabolic disease of bone in which normal bone is replaced by unmineralized osteoid. When this condition occurs in children, the disease is called rickets. Clinically, it can be extremely difficult to differentiate osteomalacia and osteoporosis. The finding of a low serum phosphate suggests osteomalacia, but the only certain diagnostic method is to take a bone biopsy.

Osteomalacia is caused by an inadequate level of 1,25-dihydrocholecalciferol (1,25-DHCC); this is an active metabolite of vitamin D. The commonest cause of osteomalacia is deficiency of vitamin D due to diet or inadequate exposure to sunlight. Rarely, malabsorption can interfere with absorption of vitamin D leading to osteomalacia. Severe renal disease is a potent cause of osteomalacia because 25-hydroxycholecalciferol is exclusively converted to the active 1,25-DHCC in the kidney. Osteomalacia may develop in patients on long-term therapy with drugs that induce hepatic mixed function oxidase, because this interferes with vitamin D metabolism. Clinical features include bone pain, pathological fractures and proximal myopathy.

Treatment of the underlying cause and replacement of vitamin D is important. This may be administered either as calciferol or the active metabolite 1-α-cholecalciferol. Replacement therapy must be closely monitored since there is a risk of hypercalcaemia developing. Calcium supplements are only used if the patient is hypocalcaemic.

Anaesthetic problems in osteomalacia

- Abnormal drug metabolism if mixed function oxidase induced.
- Potential for hypercalcaemia if on therapy with vitamin D supplements.
- Great care with positioning (fractures can easily occur).
- Deformity, if occurs before epiphyseal fusion.
- Hypocalcaemia – may increase non-depolarizing muscle relaxant duration.
- Chronic renal failure.

Osteoporosis

In osteoporosis the overall quantity of bone is reduced, whereas its shape, composition and morphology remain normal. It generally occurs in the elderly, especially women. The commonest precipitating factor is the menopausal withdrawal of oestrogens. However, endocrinopathies, long-term corticosteroid therapy, smoking, alcohol, poor nutrition/malabsorption and immobilization can also result in osteoporosis. The net effect appears to be a relative overactivity of the osteoclasts, leading to bone loss. Because of the bone loss, fractures occur far more readily, frequently after minimal trauma.

Common sites of fractures include vertebrae (usually crush or wedge fractures), neck of femur, distal radius, proximal humerus and pelvis. Multiple vertebral fractures leading to a kyphosis are not uncommon. This may be associated with marked respiratory impairment. Despite their frequency, it is unusual for vertebral fractures to be associated with serious neurological sequelae, although sciatica is common.

Patients may require surgical stabilization, but any immobilization tends to worsen the conditions. Current attempts are directed at prevention, by increasing the bone mass before the menopause with the aid of calcium supplementation and physical activity and by reducing the rate of bone resorption by using hormone replacement therapy, bisphosphonates and vitamin D.

Paget disease

Paget disease is a metabolic disease of unknown aetiology. Both environmental and genetic factors have been implicated in its pathogenesis. Several genetic loci have been linked to this disease and three genes have been identified in these loci. It is characterized by excessively rapid remodelling of bone. There is intense resorption of bone by abnormal osteoclasts. The new bone formed by osteoblasts is architecturally distorted and its mineralization is defective. The affected bones and bone marrow are initially very vascular. Eventually, the bone may become dense and hard with a reduced vascularity. It is these sclerotic areas that are weak and lead to the common complication of fractures.

The incidence of Paget disease is ~5% of over 55 year olds and tends to run in families. The most frequently affected sites are the pelvis, femur, tibia, skull and the spine. Because of the involvement of the skull and spine, spinal cord compression, atlantoaxial instability and brainstem compression may develop.

Patients may be asymptomatic, but commonly bone pain or fractures are the presenting feature. Occasionally, patients present in high-output cardiac failure owing to the increased bone vascularity; 1% of patients develop bone sarcoma.

Specific treatment is indicated for patients with symptoms or complications of the disease. Calcitonin, which acts primarily as an inhibitor of bone resorption, has been used in patients with bone pain and before orthopaedic procedures to reduce the vascularity of the bone. Increasingly, the bisphosphonates (e.g. alendronate) are being used to control bone pain, their effect often far outlasting the duration of treatment. They are adsorbed onto hydroxyapatite crystals, so slowing both their rate of growth and dissolution, and reducing the rate of bone turnover.

Anaesthetic management of Paget disease

- Careful evaluation for atlantoaxial and craniocervical instability.
- Assess lung function in patients with a kyphosis.
- Cardiac failure, if present, must be treated.
- Careful moving and positioning of the patient (fractures occur very easily).
- General or regional techniques may be used. Spinal and epidural placement can be difficult. Most dental cases are performed under general anaesthesia because extractions are difficult and the risk of postoperative bleeding is increased.
- Corticosteroid treatment may be required, depending upon previous treatment.
- Consideration should be given to the use of calcitonin before major orthopaedic procedures.

Osteoarthritis

Osteoarthritis is a common degenerative disease of the joint surface. There is damage to hyaline cartilage, with sclerosis and osteophyte formation in underlying subchondral bone. This leads to a reduced joint space. The aetiology is unclear, but may be related to joint trauma and joint overuse. Osteoarthritis is a major cause of disability and is universally evident after age 60.

Patients usually complain of pain that is worse with movement and at the end of the day and of stiffness that improves with use. Characteristically, the hip and knee joints are involved, but there may be involvement of the distal interphalangeal joints and degeneration of the spine. The middle and lower cervical spine and lower lumbar spine are the areas most likely to be involved. Spinal cord compression or nerve root compression can occur because of degenerative discs. Spinal fusion is rare.

Treatment of osteoarthritis is symptomatic, using physiotherapy and NSAIDs. Corticosteroids are not used since they are associated with a worsening of the degenerative process. Reconstructive joint surgery has much to offer these patients, but can be associated with considerable blood loss and carries a high risk of thromboembolic phenomena. The use of regional anaesthesia for these procedures, either alone or in combination with general anaesthesia, has been shown to reduce the blood loss and to decrease the incidence of deep venous thrombosis from 33% to 9%. Graduated compression stockings and thromboprophylaxis are also used in an attempt to further reduce the incidence of thromboembolism.

Bibliography

Agarwal R. Vitamin D, proteinuria, diabetic nephropathy, and progression of CKD. *Clin J Am Soc Nephrol* 2009; **4**: 1523–8.

Altman RD. Early management of osteoarthritis. *Am J Manag Care* 2010; **16**(Suppl. Management): S41–7.

Cody JD, Singer FR, Roodman GD, *et al.* Genetic linkage of Paget disease of the bone to chromosome 18q. *Am J Hum Genet* 1997; **61**: 1117–22.

Ebeling PR. Clinical practice. Osteoporosis in men. *N Engl J Med* 2008; **358**: 1474–82.

Gagnon C, Li V, Ebeling PR. Osteoporosis in men: its pathophysiology and the role of teriparatide in its treatment. *Clin Interv Aging* 2008; **3**: 635–45.

Hocking LJ, Herbert CA, Nicholls RK, *et al.* Genomewide search in familial Paget disease of bone shows evidence of genetic heterogeneity with candidate loci on chromosomes 2q36, 10p13, and 5q35. *Am J Hum Genet* 2001; **69**: 1055–61.

Holick MF. Vitamin D deficiency. *N Engl J Med* 2007; **357**: 266–81.

Poole KE, Compston JE. Osteoporosis and its management. *BMJ* 2006; **333**: 1251–6.

Scharla S. Diagnosis of disorders of vitamin D-metabolism and osteomalacia. *Clin Lab* 2008; **54**: 451–9.

Cross-references

Epidural and spinal anaesthesia, 707
Regional anaesthesia techniques, 719
Repair of fractured neck of femur, 541

Rheumatoid disease

José A Aguirre and Alain Borgeat

Rheumatoid disease (RA) is a common systemic chronic inflammatory disease affecting up to 3% of women and 1% of men in the UK with an onset typically between 30 and 50 years. It is HLA DR4 linked. It is thought to be an autoimmune condition perhaps triggered by an infectious agent. It usually affects multiple joints symmetrically, the hand and wrists most commonly, but also elbows, neck, shoulders, hips, knees and feet. Virtually every organ can be affected by the disease and compelling evidence exists to relate active and severe RA. Patients with RA may develop anaemia, systemic complications and other coexisting autoimmune disorders.

Pathophysiology

Musculoskeletal

The destructive synovitis associated with rheumatoid disease attacks the small joints of the hands, ankles, knees, temporomandibular joints, wrists, elbows and joints of the spinal column. The disease progresses until the inflammation eventually moves into a fibrotic phase, leaving characteristic fixed deformities in the joints of the hands. A number of studies have demonstrated that involvement of the cervical spine is common among patients with early or late disease and is associated with poor outcomes. Approximately 40–85% of patients with RA develop neck pain and radiographic evidence of instability (atlantoaxial subluxation, and superior migration of the odontoid process) and 50% of these patients are asymptomatic. In a prospective observational study of 100 patients with early RA (less than 1 year's duration), 12% developed atlantoaxial subluxation within the first 5 years of disease. Involvement of the temporomandibular and cricoarytenoid joints is also commonly seen.

Respiratory

Patients with RA have a decrease in vital capacity, total lung volume and arterial hypoxaemia. Pleural disease occurs in 3–12.5% of patients and more commonly in men. Ribcage stiffness and interstitial lung fibrosis combine to produce a restrictive picture. Other pulmonary manifestations include the presence of rheumatoid nodules in the lungs that may rupture or cavitate and become sites of infection, pleural effusions (typically unilateral) and, rarely, fibrosing alveolitis. Pulmonary vasculitis should be considered as a potential cause of pulmonary hypertension. Iatrogenic pulmonary disease occurs in up to 5% of patients treated with methotrexate, and appears as a progressive interstitial fibrosis. Sulphasalazine therapy may lead to the development of eosinophilic pneumonitis.

Cardiovascular

The prevalence of cardiovascular disorders has been estimated to be up to 40%, with pericardial disease being the most common. Of rheumatoid patients, 1–5% have mitral valve disease, with other valves being less commonly involved. Conduction abnormalities have been reported. When inflamed, the condition is referred to as pericarditis. Inflammation of heart muscle (myocarditis) can also develop. Rheumatoid vasculitis can range in severity from a widespread, life-threatening disease refractory to treatment. It can lead to skin ulcerations, bleeding stomach or small bowel ulcerations and neuropathies with the nerve problems causing pain, numbness or tingling.

Haemopoietic

A mild normocytic anaemia is common in rheumatoid patients and tends to correlate with disease activity. It is important that other causes of anaemia are excluded, in particular bleeding from the gastrointestinal tract secondary to either steroid or NSAID therapy. The normal responses to infection may not be present owing to concomitant immunosuppressive therapy. Methotrexate, sulphasalazine, gold, azathioprine and penicillamine may induce bone marrow suppression.

Other

Gastrointestinal symptoms are generally secondary to drug therapy: NSAIDs and steroids causing ulceration, azathioprine leading to nausea and vomiting and possibly even pancreatitis, and oral gold therapy causing irritation of the gut.

Renal and hepatic failure often occurs as the result of amyloidosis or drug therapy. Subclinical renal and hepatic dysfunction is common in patients with RA. Renal impairment may occur secondary to gold, penicillamine, ciclosporin or NSAIDs, or, rarely, amyloidosis.

Methotrexate, sulphasalazine, azathioprine, gold and ciclosporin can all cause hepatotoxicity. Methotrexate is also responsible for haematological and pulmonary side-effects, e.g. pancytopenia and irreversible pulmonary fibrosis. Treatment with leflunomide has been associated with disturbances in the gastrointestinal tract and with the development of peripheral neuropathy. Etanercept has also been suggested to have been the cause of acute lung injury and polyneuropathy owing to demyelinization of nerve fibres.

Neurological complications include peripheral neuropathy (usually mainly sensory), mononeuritis multiplex, entrapment neuropathy (e.g. carpal tunnel syndrome) and spinal cord lesions secondary to cervical disease.

Infections of all kinds are more common in rheumatoid disease, especially joint infections.

Preoperative assessment

- Neck movement/mouth opening/dentition.
- Veins/arteries/bruising.
- Presence of painful joints and limitations.
- Suitability for regional technique.
- Complete neurological, respiratory and cardiovascular history.
- Drug history.
- Previous anaesthetic problems.
- Investigations – see Table 8.1.

Perioperative management

Consideration should be given to performing the procedure under local or regional blockade if feasible, as this will avoid the need for airway manipulation. However, the involvement of the spine may make epidural or spinal anaesthesia difficult if not impossible. Peripheral blocks should be performed whenever possible. The need for sedation (propofol and remifentanil) is often necessary because of pain due to positioning on the operating table.

If general anaesthesia is to be used then the cervical spine and airway are the areas likely to cause most concern. The development of fibreoptic laryngoscopes has altered the management of rheumatoid patients when general anaesthesia with intubation is considered necessary.

Premedication

If fibreoptic intubation is to be performed or difficulty with intubation is anticipated, then an antisialagogue should be prescribed.

Cervical spine

On induction of anaesthesia the cervical spine will lose any protective tone around the unstable neck, and thus it is important to determine the range of comfortable neck movement before induction and limit it to this with the use of sandbags, etc. If tracheal intubation is necessary, it may be that with severe cervical spine involvement early consideration should be given to awake fibreoptic intubation, especially if there is posterior atlantoaxial subluxation (neck extension potentially hazardous).

When intubation is not required, then oropharyngeal or nasopharyngeal airways may reduce the amount of cervical manipulation required. The laryngeal mask is useful in longer procedures, although the larynx may be displaced in cervical spine disease, making placement difficult. Use manual in-line stabilization during airway manipulation in unconscious patients unless certain the cervical spine is stable.

Airway

Temporomandibular joint involvement may lead to difficulty in mouth opening and forward jaw protrusion, thus leading to difficulty in inserting a laryngoscope as well as viewing the larynx. Rarely, cricoarytenoid involvement can result in acute airway obstruction. Anticipated problems or previous difficulty should lead to early consideration of the fibreoptic laryngoscope.

Conduct of anaesthesia

There are no restrictions on anaesthetic agents used in rheumatoid disease, although iatrogenic, hepatic or renal disease may alter the amount of free drug available and increments should be administered with care. Great care should be taken to protect the joints during anaesthesia, with careful handling and positioning of the patient and protection of pressure points. Mechanical ventilation may be necessary in those patients with severe pulmonary disease.

Postoperative management

Analgesia is the main problem in the postoperative period, as these patients tend to be more sensitive to opioids. PCA may be difficult for the rheumatoid patient owing to hand deformities, although special modifications are available. Continuous regional analgesia may provide the optimal form of analgesia in this group of patients, if appropriate.

Early physiotherapy is indicated to prevent chest infections both in patients who have a restrictive lung defect, and thus a propensity to develop atelectasis, and in those who are more difficult to mobilize because of musculoskeletal dysfunction.

Steroid cover should be continued when indicated, and there should be close monitoring of renal function, especially if preoperative dysfunction was present.

Long-term management

These patients tend to require multiple surgical procedures because of the relentless progression of their disease. Careful attention should be paid to previous anaesthetic notes, and any problems with intubation, analgesia, etc. should be noted.

Bibliography

Bharti N, Madan R, Mohanty PR, Kaul HL. Intrathecal midazolam added to bupivacaine improves the duration and quality of spinal anaesthesia. *Acta Anaesthesiol Scand* 2003; **47**: 1101–5.

Fulling PD, Roberts JT. Fiberoptic intubation. *Int Anesthesiol Clin* 2000; **38**: 189–217.

Horlocker TT, Kopp SL, Pagnano MW, Hebl JR. Analgesia for total hip and knee arthroplasty: a multimodal pathway featuring peripheral nerve block. *J Am Acad Orthop Surg* 2006; **14**: 126–35.

Huggett MT, Armstrong R. Adalimumab-associated pulmonary fibrosis. *Rheumatology (Oxford)* 2006; **45**: 1312–13.

Kohjitani A, Miyawaki T, Kasuya K, *et al.* Anesthetic management for advanced rheumatoid arthritis patients with acquired micrognathia undergoing temporomandibular joint replacement. *J Oral Maxillofac Surg* 2002; **60**: 559–66.

Lacomis D, Zivkovic SA. Approach to vasculitic neuropathies. *J Clin Neuromuscul Dis* 2007; **9**: 265–76.

Lim AY, Gaffney K, Scott DG. Methotrexate-induced pancytopenia: serious and under-reported? Our experience of 25 cases in 5 years. *Rheumatology (Oxford)* 2005; **44**: 1051–5.

Magro CM, Crowson AN. The spectrum of cutaneous lesions in rheumatoid arthritis: a clinical and pathological study of 43 patients. *J Cutan Pathol* 2003; **30**: 1–10.

Murali Krishna T, Panda NB, Batra YK, Rajeev S. Combination of low doses of intrathecal ketamine and midazolam with bupivacaine improves postoperative analgesia in orthopaedic surgery. *Eur J Anaesthesiol* 2008; **25**: 299–306.

Oien RF, Hakansson A, Hansen BU. Leg ulcers in patients with rheumatoid arthritis: a prospective study of aetiology, wound healing and pain reduction after pinch grafting. *Rheumatology (Oxford)* 2001; **40**: 816–20.

Paimela L, Laasonen L, Kankaanpaa E, Leirisalo-Repo M. Progression of cervical spine changes in patients with early rheumatoid arthritis. *J Rheumatol* 1997; **24**: 1280–4.

Quoss A, Buurman C. [Anesthesiological considerations in rheumatic diseases]. *Anaesthesiol Reanim* 2000; **26**: 116–21.

Skues MA, Welchew EA. Anaesthesia and rheumatoid arthritis. *Anaesthesia* 1993; **48**: 989–97.

Smolen JS, Emery P. Efficacy and safety of leflunomide in active rheumatoid arthritis. *Rheumatology (Oxford)* 2000; **39**(Suppl. 1): 48–56.

Takeuchi K, Kuroda Y. [Rheumatoid vasculitis with multiple intestinal ulcerations: report of a case]. *Ryumachi* 2000; **40**: 639–43.

Cross-references

Anaemia, 216
Arthroscopy, 538
Difficult airway: management, 651
Iatrogenic adrenocortical suppression, 72
Mitral valve disease, 156

Scoliosis

Alain Borgeat and José A Aguirre

Scoliosis is a fixed, structural, lateral curvature of the spine with associated rotation of the vertebrae. The severity of the curve is evaluated on standing spinal X-rays using the Cobb angle. Scoliosis can be congenital or acquired. Congenital scoliosis, which may present at any age, is the result of either failure of vertebral segmentation (called a *bar*) or failure of formation (called a *hemivertebra*). Congenital scoliosis is often part of a generalized condition, such as Goldenhar syndrome or spina bifida, and may be associated with abnormalities in the renal, cardiac, respiratory or neurological systems. The indication for surgery is documented progression at any age. Most acquired scoliosis is idiopathic. Infantile-onset idiopathic scoliosis (scoliosis before the age of 8 years) carries the most serious prognosis and, if left unchecked, is likely to result in cardiopulmonary failure in middle age.

Aetiology

Scoliosis is a sign, not a disease. It may arise from several different causes; although presentation, complications and management may be similar, the prognosis may differ greatly for different aetiologies (Table 8.2).

Classification of scoliosis

- *Functional scoliosis*. Secondary to discordant leg length, etc. The curve disappears when the patient lies down.
- *Structural scoliosis*. There are three main groups:
  - Congenital: associated with vertebral anomalies. May have abnormalities of the heart and genitourinary tract.
  - Idiopathic: accounts for 60–80% of cases and has the best prognosis of all aetiologies. This is a diagnosis of exclusion.
  - Neuromuscular: scoliosis occurring secondary to a neuropathy (upper or lower motor neurone or other neuropathy), e.g. cerebral palsy, poliomyelitis, Friedreich's ataxia, or myopathy, e.g. Duchenne's muscular dystrophy. This group includes many of the syndromes associated with scoliosis, e.g. Prader–Willi syndrome.
- In addition:
  - Mesenchymal: abnormalities of the tissues, e.g. Marfan syndrome, Ehlers–Danlos syndrome.
  - Trauma.
  - Tumours: intraspinal or skeletal.
  - Metabolic: this category includes several miscellaneous causes, e.g. rickets, hyperphosphatasia.

The severity of scoliosis can be defined by the Cobb angle, which is measured from an anteroposterior X-ray of the spine. The first line is taken from the most tilted vertebral body above the scoliosis and extended laterally. The second line is taken from the most tilted vertebra below the scoliosis. The measured angle is at the intersection of these two lines. Although, occasionally, patients may have a scoliosis which is

Table 8.2 Aetiology of structural scoliosis (relative frequencies)

Idiopathic (70%)	
Congenital	Abnormal spinal cord/vertebral development
Neuromuscular (15%)	Neuropathic: cerebral palsy, syringomyelia, poliomyelitis
	Myopathic: muscular dystrophies, neurofibromatosis, Friedreich's ataxia
Mesenchymal disorders	Rheumatoid arthritis, Marfan syndrome, osteogenesis imperfecta
Metabolic bone disease	Osteoporosis, Paget disease
Malignancy	Primary and secondary tumours
Trauma/surgery	Fracture, radiotherapy, surgery
Infection	Tuberculosis, osteomyelitis

largely in the lumbar region, it is more often the case that the thoracic vertebrae are involved. In these circumstances, the larger the angle, the more severe is the scoliosis and the greater the likelihood of compromised respiratory and cardiovascular function. Patients with neuromuscular-type scoliosis may have significant impairment despite lesser abnormalities.

Pathophysiology

Respiratory system

Respiratory impairment usually shows a restrictive pattern, with lung volumes being related inversely to the angle of curvature. Vital capacity is the most severely affected, but total lung capacity and FRC are also reduced. The abnormalities of ribcage development cause abnormal development of the underlying lung, with alveolar volume being compressed to, or below, FRC. Rib abnormalities result in mechanical disadvantage of muscles of respiration and reduced chest wall compliance. This results in alveolar hypoventilation. The commonest arterial blood gas abnormality is a reduced P_ao_2.

Associated with the compressed alveoli is restricted development of the pulmonary vascular bed and diversion of blood into high-resistance extra-alveolar vessels. The resulting V/Q mismatch causes an increased alveolar to arterial oxygen gradient and exacerbates the alveolar hypoventilation. An increase in P_ao_2 occurs late and is a poor prognostic indicator. In addition, patients with more severe scoliosis have a decreased respiratory sensitivity to elevated P_ao_2.

Cardiovascular system

There is a relatively high incidence of congenital heart disease in patients with scoliosis. Thoracic scoliosis of any aetiology may result in right-sided cardiac problems. The V/Q mismatch causes an increased pulmonary vascular resistance. Low lung volumes, chronic hypoxia and abnormal development of the pulmonary vascular bed all contribute to these changes. Right atrial dilatation and right ventricular hypertrophy are late in appearance.

Preoperative assessment

Surgical intervention is generally warranted in cases in which the curvature is >50%, or >40% in skeletally immature patients, or in patients in whom curvature is progressing despite bracing. Patients with congenital or neuromuscular causes of scoliosis, such as muscular dystrophy or cerebral palsy, may be at risk for more aggressive progression of scoliosis, and therefore may warrant earlier surgical treatment.

Surgical correction is aimed at partial straightening of the curvature, stabilization of the spine and cessation of further progression of scoliosis. Hardware is secured segmentally to the vertebral pedicles, followed by partial straightening, termed distraction, of the spine with rigid rods that are manipulated to achieve the desired degree of lesser curvature.

Assessment involves determining the aetiology of the scoliosis and associated problems. See Table 8.3 and Boxes 8.2 and 8.3 for the different ages.

Respiratory function

- Clinical assessment of airway and intubation may be difficult in, for example, fixed flexion deformities, large meningomyelocele with or without encephalocele, 'halo' or other neck immobilizing traction.
- Exercise tolerance.

Table 8.3 Suggested preoperative investigations before major spinal surgery

	Minimum investigations	Optional investigations
Airway	Cervical spine lateral X-ray with flexion/ extension views	CT scan
Respiratory system	Plain chest radiograph	Pulmonary function tests
	Arterial blood gas analysis	Pulmonary diffusion capacity
	Spirometry (FEV_1, FVC)	
Cardiovascular system	Electrocardiograph	Dobutamine stress echocardiograph
	Echocardiography	Dipyridamole/thallium scintigraphy
Blood tests	Full blood count	Liver function tests
	Clotting profile	
	Blood cross-match	
	Urea, electrolytes	
	Albumin, calcium (neoplastic disease)	

FVC, forced vital capacity; FEV_1, forced expiratory volume in 1 second.

Box 8.2 Anaesthetic considerations for spinal surgery in children

- Preoperative considerations
  - Evaluation of all organ systems to pick up other congenital defects
  - Evaluation of the nervous system and documentation of neurological deficit
  - Evaluation for anatomical abnormalities leading to 'airway challenge'
  - Specific age-related anaesthetic considerations
  - Awareness of associated pathology (Arnold–Chiari malformation, cerebral paresis, etc.)
  - Evaluation of respiratory and cardiovascular status
  - Previous anaesthetic records
  - Awareness of potential for latex allergy
  - Psychological status
  - Premedication as appropriate
- Preoperative investigations
  - Full blood count
  - Urea and electrolytes
  - Clotting profile
  - Liver function tests
  - Chest X-ray
  - Baseline arterial blood gas analysis
  - Spirometry as appropriate, when possible
  - Cervical spine imaging as appropriate
  - ECG and echocardiogram as appropriate
- Induction of anaesthesia
  - Consider fibreoptic-aided intubation if anticipating a difficult airway or for unstable spinal injuries Consider intubation in the lateral position to protect the neuroplaque
  - Secure adequate venous access
  - Routine monitoring – include invasive blood pressure monitoring when appropriate
- Maintenance of anaesthesia
  - Airway maintenance and securing the tube well
  - Prone position and ensuring safety in the prone position
  - Use of appropriate agents for anaesthetic maintenance
  - Facilitation of spinal cord monitoring
  - Maintenance of spinal cord perfusion pressure
  - Prevention of hypothermia
  - Maintenance of volume status
  - Awareness of potential for blood loss – blood/products organized
  - Blood conservation techniques where appropriate
  - Antibiotic prophylaxis after discussion with the surgical team
- Monitoring
  - Oximetry, capnography and gas monitoring
  - ECG, blood pressure (usually invasive) and core temperature
  - Monitoring of neuromuscular block
- Postoperative considerations
  - High-dependency/intensive care nursing where appropriate
  - Postoperative analgesia

- Chest expansion and ability to cough.
- Formal lung function tests – if the scoliosis is <65° or lung function tests are greater than 30% of the predicted value, ventilation problems are rare. If vital capacity <30% the patient is more likely to need postoperative mechanical ventilation.
- Arterial blood gas measurements – if the patient is unable to perform lung function tests or has scoliosis >65°.

Cardiac function

- Clinical examination – right ventricular enlargement, loud pulmonic second sound, murmur of pulmonary insufficiency.
- ECG – P wave >2.5 mm and R>S in V_1 and V_2. These changes are rare and occur late.
- Echocardiography – a more sensitive detector of cardiac abnormalities secondary to pulmonary hypertension.

Box 8.3 Anaesthetic concerns for spinal surgery in neonates

- Peculiarities of the neonatal respiratory control and mechanics
  - Hypercarbia stimulates respiration to a lesser extent than in adults
  - Hypoxia leads to sustained respiratory depression
  - Tendency to periodic breathing and increased risk of postoperative apnoea up to 60 weeks after conceptual age
  - Neonates are at increased risk of atelectasis
  - Diaphragm is susceptible to fatigue
  - Increased risk of airway obstruction and thoracoabdominal asynchrony under anaesthesia
- Characteristics of neonatal circulation and myocardial function
  - Limited functional reserve
  - Myocardium less able to generate force
  - Myocardium more dependent on extracellular calcium
  - Balance in favour of the parasympathetic system
- Immature hepatic function
  - Require adjustment of drug dosing intervals and maintenance dosing
- Immature renal function
  - Tolerate fluid restriction and fasting poorly
- Higher incidence of intraoperative complications
  - Dislodgement of the tracheal tube
  - Tracheal tube obstruction
  - Bronchial intubation
  - Pneumothorax
  - Failure of anaesthetic equipment
  - Hypothermia

Perioperative management

Premedication

A benzodiazepine, e.g. midazolam, is adequate to control preoperative anxiety. Consider preoperative physiotherapy in those with poor respiratory function.

Monitoring

- AAGBI minimal monitoring standards.
- Arterial cannulation is useful both for measuring blood pressure and for postoperative measuring of arterial blood gasses and is mandatory for patients with neuromuscular scoliosis.
- Core temperature – there is a higher incidence of malignant hyperthermia in patients with scoliosis.
- Nasogastric tube – decompression of the stomach assists ventilation, and distraction of the spine may be associated with the development of paralytic ileus.
- Consider central venous pressure and urine output monitoring, particularly for surgery associated with high blood loss.

Anaesthesia

- Intravenous anaesthesia without the use of succinylcholine is a safe practice since it avoids triggering malignant hyperthermia in susceptible patients.
- Hyperkalaemia may occur following the use of succinylcholine in patients with neuromuscular problems.
- Rhabdomyolysis and myoglobinuria may occur following the use of succinylcholine and halothane in patients with myopathies.
- Consider the prone position and its complications (Box 8.4).

Box 8.4 Complications of the prone position

- Unintentional extubation
- Eye complications
  - Corneal abrasions
  - Conjunctival and periorbital oedema of the dependent eye
  - Retinal ischaemia
  - Postoperative visual loss because of ischaemic optic neuropathy
- Entangling of cables
- Accidental dislodgement of access and monitoring lines
- Abdominal compression leading to impaired ventilation, increased bleeding from epidural plexus and decreased cardiac output
- Improper head and neck positioning leading to venous and lymphatic obstruction
- Macroglossia
- Possibility of venous air embolus

Surgery

Evidence of pulmonary hypertension or right ventricular hypertrophy carries a poor prognosis. Right ventricular failure must be treated before surgery. There is no specific contraindication to local or regional anaesthesia. Placement of one or two epidural catheters by the surgeon at the end of surgery is a very efficient way to control postoperative pain. Most patients who undergo scoliosis surgery are children or young adults.

The aims of surgery are:

- correction of curve
- prevention of progression of curve
- relief or prevention of back pain

- prevention of neurological compromise
- prevention of respiratory compromise
- cosmetic.

Patients usually present for corrective surgery before the onset of pulmonary hypertension. Surgery may be via an anterior approach, posterior approach or both (carried out as two separate procedures several days apart or during a single session). The anterior approach requires access to the vertebrae on the convex side of the curve. This is achieved via thoracotomy and costectomy and usually precedes posterior fusion. The posterior approach requires the patient to be placed prone.

Anaesthetic – specific considerations

- Blood loss may be considerable and rapid. Hypotensive techniques have been associated with spinal cord ischaemia and paresis. Consider methods of blood preservation, such as cell salvage and haemodilution. Attempt to maintain temperature with fluid warmers and a warming blanket. Patients with Duchenne's muscular dystrophy and central paresis appear to bleed more.
- Postoperative pain, hypoventilation and atelectasis are severe following thoracotomy. Thoracic epidural analgesia provides good operating conditions and excellent pain relief and may be continued for several days postoperatively.
- Anaesthesia must facilitate spinal cord monitoring ('wake-up' test, sensory or motor-evoked potentials). Total intravenous anaesthesia using an infusion of propofol with remifentanil is a suitable technique.
- Prone position is used for the posterior approach. Careful positioning is required, including abdominal decompression (decreases blood loss). Complications of the prone position include retinal artery thrombosis, brachial plexus injury and suprascapular nerve injury.

Neurological risks associated with scoliosis surgery

Neurological impairment, particularly paraparesis or paraplegia, is an infrequent but potentially devastating complication of scoliosis surgery. As with other types of spine surgery, the spinal cord and nerve roots are at risk for mechanical injury as hardware is affixed to the vertebral pedicles. The likelihood of misdirection of hardware is probably higher in scoliosis surgery because of the abnormal curvature and rotation of the vertebrae, and the risk of spinal cord injury is probably higher because the spinal cord is often situated very close to the concave wall in the scoliotic spine. In addition, certain techniques require passing of sublaminar hardware through the epidural space, further exposing the spinal cord to potential trauma.

The greatest risk of spinal cord injury during scoliosis surgery occurs during distraction of the spine. Injury may result from stretching or compression of the cord or of the anterior spinal artery or its feeding radicular vessels, causing spinal cord ischaemia and infarction. The anterior spinal circulation supplies the descending corticospinal tracts and the anterior horn, and infarction in this territory may result in paraparesis or paraplegia. Among those undergoing scoliosis surgery, a higher rate of neurological complications is seen in patients with hyperkyphosis, in those with a high degree of rigid curvature, in those with congenital scoliosis, neuromuscular scoliosis or cerebral palsy, and in those undergoing combined anterior and posterior approaches.

Neurophysiological intraoperative monitoring including somatosensory-evoked potentials, motor-evoked potentials, spontaneous electromyography and triggered electromyography is standard for scoliosis surgery (Fig. 8.1).

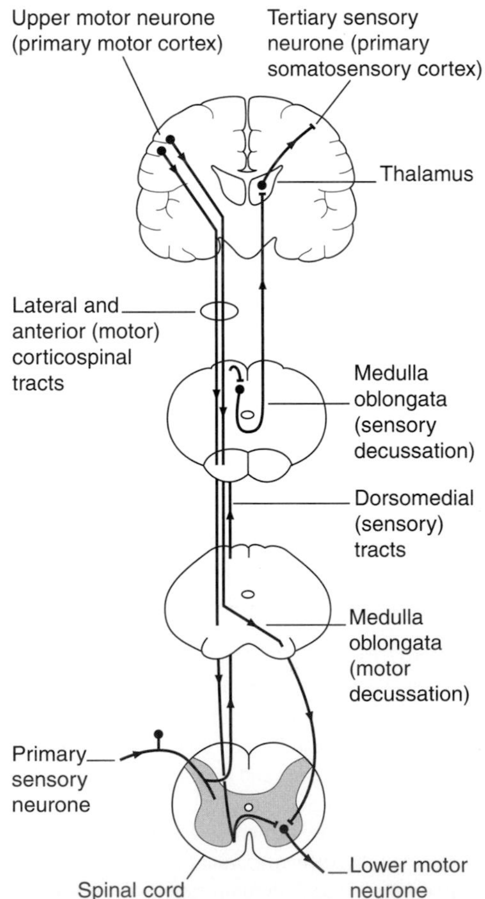

Figure 8.1 Diagrammatic representation of motor and sensory pathways of the spinal cord.

Postoperative care

- ICU or postanaesthesia care unit following corrective scoliosis surgery, major general surgery and minor surgery under general anaesthesia if there is significant respiratory or cardiovascular compromise.
- Postoperative intermittent positive pressure ventilation may be required.
- Continuous oxygen therapy.
- Regular physiotherapy.
- Multimodal analgesia.

Bibliography

American Electroencephalographic Society. Guidelines for intraoperative monitoring of sensory evoked potentials. *J Clin Neurophysiol* 1987; **4**: 397–416.

Berven S, Bradford DS. Neuromuscular scoliosis: causes of deformity and principles for evaluation and management. *Semin Neurol* 2002; **22**: 167–78.

Blumenthal S, Min K, Nadig M, Borgeat A. Double epidural catheter with ropivacaine versus intravenous morphine: a comparison for postoperative analgesia after scoliosis correction surgery. *Anesthesiology* 2005; **102**: 175–80.

Blumenthal S, Borgeat A, Nadig M, Min K. Postoperative analgesia after anterior correction of thoracic scoliosis: a prospective randomized study comparing continuous double epidural catheter technique with intravenous morphine. *Spine (Phila Pa 1976)* 2006; **31**: 1646–51.

Borgeat A, Blumenthal S. Postoperative pain management following scoliosis surgery. *Curr Opin Anaesthesiol* 2008; **21**: 313–16.

Bridwell KH. Surgical treatment of idiopathic adolescent scoliosis. *Spine* (*Phila Pa 1976*) 1999; **24**: 2607–16.

Coe JD, Arlet V, Donaldson W, *et al.* Complications in spinal fusion for adolescent idiopathic scoliosis in the new millennium. A report of the Scoliosis Research Society Morbidity and Mortality Committee. *Spine* (*Phila Pa 1976*) 2006; **31**: 345–9.

Colomina MJ, Godet C. [Anesthesia for scoliosis surgery: preoperative assessment and risk screening of patients undergoing surgery to correct spinal deformity]. *Rev Esp Anestesiol Reanim* 2005; **52**: 24–42; quiz 3, 7.

Gonzalez AA, Jeyanandarajan D, Hansen C, *et al.* Intraoperative neurophysiological monitoring during spine surgery: a review. *Neurosurg Focus* 2009; **27**: E6.

Guigui P, Blamoutier A. [Complications of surgical treatment of spinal deformities: a prospective multicentric study of 3311 patients]. *Rev Chir Orthop Reparatrice Appar Mot* 2005; **91**: 314–27.

Hod-Feins R, Abu-Kishk I, Eshel G, *et al.* Risk factors affecting the immediate postoperative course in pediatric scoliosis surgery. *Spine* (*Phila Pa 1976*) 2007; **32**: 2355–60.

Kinnear WJ, Johnston ID. Does Harrington instrumentation improve pulmonary function in adolescents with idiopathic scoliosis? A meta-analysis. *Spine* (*Phila Pa 1976*) 1993; **18**: 1556–9.

Koumbourlis AC. Scoliosis and the respiratory system. *Paediatr Respir Rev* 2006; **7**: 152–60.

Malfair D, Flemming AK, Dvorak MF, *et al.* Radiographic evaluation of scoliosis: review. *AJR Am J Roentgenol* 2010; **194**: S8–22.

Qiu Y, Wang S, Wang B, *et al.* Incidence and risk factors of neurological deficits of surgical correction for scoliosis: analysis of 1373 cases at one Chinese institution. *Spine* (*Phila Pa 1976*) 2008; **33**: 519–26.

Roach JW. Adolescent idiopathic scoliosis. *Orthop Clin North Am* 1999; **30**: 353–65.

Cross-references

Marfan syndrome, 251
Muscular dystrophies, 74
Restrictive lung disease, 114

9
Connective tissue

Brian J Pollard

- Bullous and vesicular skin disorders *Brian J Pollard*
- Disorders of epidermal cell kinetics and differentiation *Brian J Pollard*
- Ehlers–Danlos syndrome *Brian J Pollard*
- Epidermolysis bullosa *Brian J Pollard*
- Glycogen storage disease *Brian J Pollard*
- Mucopolysaccharidoses *Brian J Pollard*
- Polyarteritis nodosa *Brian J Pollard*
- Polymyositis and dermatomyositis *Brian J Pollard*
- Pseudoxanthoma elasticum *Brian J Pollard*
- Scleroderma *Brian J Pollard*
- Systemic lupus erythematosus *Brian J Pollard*
- Urticaria and angio-oedema *Brian J Pollard*

Bullous and vesicular skin disorders

Brian J Pollard

This chapter considers bullous and vesicular skin disorders with the exception of epidermolysis bullosa, which is the subject of a separate entry.

Pemphigus and pemphigoid

These rare autoimmune conditions are characterized by a bullous eruption of the skin and mucous membranes. There are several variants of each disease. In pemphigus, blisters form intradermally; in pemphigoid, lesions occur at the dermal–epidermal junction.

Pemphigus vulgaris is the most common form of pemphigus and occurs predominantly in patients of Mediterranean or Jewish origin, with a peak incidence between 30 and 50 years old. It was uniformly fatal before the advent of steroid therapy. There is a familial tendency and an increased incidence of human leukocyte antigen 13 (HLA-13) among affected individuals. There may be an association with other autoimmune diseases, such as thymoma, myasthenia gravis and systemic lupus erythematosus. Large, superficial, flaccid blisters occur spontaneously or in response to trauma and are found in the groins, axillae and over the trunk. Oral lesions may pre-date cutaneous bullae by several months. Pressure with torsion may result in blister formation in normal-looking skin (Nikolsky's sign). The bullae are fragile, rupturing easily with coincident loss of large areas of skin; healing occurs without scarring. Lesions may occur on the lips and in the mouth, nose, pharynx and larynx, causing difficulty in eating and hoarseness. In some variants of pemphigus, e.g. pemphigus erythematosus and pemphigus foliaceus, bulla formation occurs more superficially within the epidermis. These forms tend to be less severe.

Pemphigoid includes both bullous and cicatricial types. Bullous pemphigoid is clinically similar to pemphigus, but occurs predominantly in patients over 50 years old. If untreated, it follows a chronic relapsing course and the mortality is low. It tends to be self-limiting and the patient's health remains good. The characteristic feature of the condition is large, tense bullae, often occurring on the inner aspects of the thighs, on the flexor surfaces of the forearms, axillae and groins, and over the lower abdomen. The oral cavity may be affected but, unlike pemphigus, is rarely the initial manifestation. Blister formation is thought to result from the activation of complement in association with neutrophil and eosinophil migration. Cicatricial pemphigoid is rare and primarily affects the mucous membranes. Skin is involved in 10–30% of cases, but rarely in the absence of mucosal lesions. It is a chronic condition and the lesions usually heal with scarring. This may lead to nasal obstruction, dysphagia and laryngeal stenosis. Blindness may complicate ocular involvement.

Treatment in both pemphigus and pemphigoid is with steroids and, occasionally, other immunosuppressant drugs, e.g. methotrexate, azathioprine or cyclophosphamide. Lower doses of corticosteroids are used in pemphigoid. Gold injections and plasmapheresis may also be used in pemphigus.

Erythema multiforme

Erythema multiforme (EM) is more common and is an acute, self-limiting eruption of the skin and mucous membranes. It is characterized by distinctive target or iris lesions. Fifty per cent of cases have no identifiable cause but, for the rest, a wide variety of triggers, including infective agents, drugs and neoplasms, has been described. Those of particular importance to the anaesthetist include barbiturates, antibiotics, anticonvulsants, antipyretics and cimetidine. The pathogenesis of EM is not fully understood, but there is evidence that it may be a hypersensitivity reaction. It may present in various forms (hence its name), ranging from a mild, self-limited, skin eruption through to the Stevens–Johnson syndrome (SJS) with its systemic involvement and high mortality (5–15%) if untreated. EM may present as symmetrical target lesions (dull red macules up to 2 cm in diameter with a clear centre) on the extensor surfaces of the extremities, as a series of urticarial plaques or with vesicle or bullae formation.

SJS is a more severe form of EM, with involvement of mucosal surfaces and viscera in association with marked constitutional symptoms. There is a prodrome lasting up to 14 days consisting of fever, malaise, myalgia, arthralgia, respiratory and gastrointestinal symptoms. It is followed by the explosive eruption of bullous lesions of the mouth, lips and conjunctivae, and variable skin involvement. In severe cases, the oesophagus and respiratory tract are involved. Pneumonitis, pleural effusions and bullae of the visceral pleura are seen, the last occasionally leading to pneumothorax or even bronchopleural fistula. Myocarditis, atrial fibrillation and renal failure are recognized complications. There may also be anaemia and fluid and electrolyte imbalance. Treatment in SJS is supportive, although steroids have also been used for SJS and in severe cases of EM.

Preoperative assessment

History and examination

- Fully assess the disease together with its extent and the duration of the illness. In particular, assess the distribution and severity of lesions, especially those involving the airway.
- Assess nutritional state.
- Note drug therapy and dose, especially systemic corticosteroids and immunosuppressants.
- Consider the effects of plasmapheresis on cholinesterase levels in pemphigus.

Investigations

- Full blood count:
  - anaemia may occur in SJS
  - leukopenia and thrombocytopenia may result from immunosuppressant therapy.
- Urea and electrolytes: abnormalities may exist in SJS or as a result of steroid therapy.
- Assess renal function, especially in SJS.
- Blood glucose: may be raised because of steroid therapy.
- Flow-volume loops may be of use where upper respiratory tract stenosis is suspected.
- Consider cholinesterase activity following plasma-pheresis.

Premedication

- Ensure that premedication is sufficient to prevent struggling during induction. Struggling may risk new bulla formation.
- The intramuscular route might appear unsuitable for fear of inducing new lesions; however, new bullae formation has not been reported.

Perioperative management

Induction

- Intramuscular ketamine has been used successfully.
- Suture intravenous cannulae in place.
- Avoid barbiturates.
- For children, encourage the presence of parents in the anaesthetic room in order to reduce the chances of struggling and restlessness on induction, thereby reducing chances of blister formation.

Airway considerations

A major concern in all the blistering diseases must be the potential to cause new bullae during airway manipulation or intubation. It is wise to use manoeuvres to avoid unnecessary airway manipulation.

- Use face-masks with a soft air cushion.
- Pad face-masks with Vaseline gauze.
- Place Vaseline gauze under chin to protect skin from anaesthetist's fingers.
- If possible, avoid the use of airway adjuncts, such as Guedel airways.
- An inhalational induction may be required where laryngeal stenosis is present; helium/oxygen mixtures may help.
- Consider the use of a hood for inhalational induction.
- Protect front of neck with Vaseline gauze if cricoid pressure must be used.
- Laryngoscopy and oral intubation may be difficult in all of the blistering diseases owing to pre-existing airway bullae.
- Laryngeal stenosis has been reported in SJS and cicatricial pemphigoid. The use of small uncuffed tracheal tubes may be necessary.
- The use of nasotracheal tubes has not been reported.
- Secure tracheal tubes with simple loose ties rather than with adhesive tape.

Maintenance

- Intermittent positive pressure ventilation (IPPV) may be hazardous in SJS because of the risk of pneumothoraces or bronchopleural fistulae.
- Drug disposition will be affected by hypo-albuminaemia and renal disease in SJS.
- Intravenous ketamine and diazepam infusions, in the absence of intubation, have proven useful in SJS.

Regional techniques

Spinal and epidural anaesthetic techniques appear safe. No new lesions have occurred at the sites of spinal needle insertion. Modifications should be made to the skin-cleansing routine – apply liquid skin cleanser and do not use applicator sponges; avoid rubbing the skin; avoid subcutaneous injections of local anaesthetic solutions. If using EMLA cream do not apply self-adhesive occlusive dressing.

Monitoring

- Well-padded non-invasive blood pressure (BP) cuffs do not appear to cause bullae, probably because direct pressure is less harmful than frictional or shearing forces.
- The pulse oximeter should be attached using a simple clip rather than adhesive or tape.
- Use ECG pads without adhesive; needle ECG electrodes may be an alternative.
- A weighted untaped precordial stethoscope may be useful.
- Secure intravenous lines with sutures, not tape.
- Arterial lines may be of use: secure with sutures.
- Do not use self-adhesive electrodes for monitoring neuromuscular function.

Positioning

- Keep sheets and other linen free from creases.
- Pad heels, elbows and bony prominences using foam.
- Allow patients to move themselves onto trolleys or the operating table in order to minimize skin trauma.
- Inform theatre staff of the need for special care during patient positioning.
- Take care with the positioning of a diathermy pad and do not use a self-adhesive type.

Emergence and recovery

- If pharyngeal suction is required, use a soft flexible catheter.
- Use protective Vaseline gauze under oxygen masks.
- For children, encourage the presence of parents in the recovery room in order to reduce the chances of struggling and restlessness on emergence.
- Regional techniques may allow the provision of high-quality continuous postoperative analgesia (do not secure the catheter using self-adhesive tape).

Postoperative management

- New skin lesions are a common complication.
- Continue steroid supplements.

Bibliography

Cucchiara RF, Dawson B. Anesthesia in Stevens–Johnson syndrome: report of a case. *Anesthesiology* 1971; **35**: 537–9.

Drenger B, Zidenbaum M, Reifen E, Leitersdorf E. Severe upper airway obstruction and difficult intubation in cicatricial pemphigoid. *Anaesthesia* 1986; **41**: 1029–31.

Prasad KK, Chen L. Anesthetic management of a patient with bullous pemphigoid. *Anesth Analg* 1989; **69**: 537–40.

Vatashsky E, Aronson HB. Pemphigus vulgaris: anaesthesia in the traumatised patient. *Anaesthesia* 1982; **37**: 1195–7.

Cross-references

Anaemia, 216
Assessment of renal function, 199
Iatrogenic adrenocortical suppression, 72

Disorders of epidermal cell kinetics and differentiation

Brian J Pollard

Psoriasis

Psoriasis is a chronic skin disorder, characterized by an accelerated epidermal turnover and epidermal hyperplasia. These are caused by an increased rate of epidermal protein synthesis, rapid epidermal cell growth, shortened epidermal cell cycle and an increase in the proliferative cell population. The exact aetiology of psoriasis is unknown, although both genetic and environmental factors are thought to play a part. Lesions tend to involve the extensor surfaces (elbows, knees), sacral area and scalp. They consist of loosely adherent, thickened, non-coherent, silver skin scales which have an increased vascularity. Mechanical trauma leading to removal of skin causes small blood droplets to appear on the skin (Auspitz's sign). Psoriatic lesions often follow trauma of the skin (Koebner's phenomenon). Psoriatic arthropathy occurs in 5–10% of patients and resembles seronegative rheumatoid arthritis. Psoriasis is also associated with ulcerative colitis and Crohn disease. Psoriatic lesions have a tendency to increased colonization by bacteria, especially *Staphylococcus aureus*, compared with normal skin. Severe psoriasis may be associated with hyperuricaemia, anaemia (chronic illness, folate or vitamin B_{12} deficiency), negative nitrogen balance, iron loss and hypoalbuminaemia.

Two forms of psoriasis produce marked systemic effects on the body: psoriatic erythroderma (see below) and generalized pustular psoriasis. The latter is characterized by waves of sterile pustules over the skin of the trunk and extremities, together with fever up to 40°C lasting for several days. There may be associated weight loss, muscle weakness, congestive cardiac failure and hypocalcaemia.

The treatment of psoriasis involves the use of topical steroids, coal tar or dithranol, ultraviolet light (with or without a psoralen), retinoids (vitamin A derivatives), cytotoxic agents (e.g. methotrexate, azathioprine) and ciclosporin A.

Erythroderma

Erythroderma (or exfoliative dermatitis) describes a generalized inflammatory disorder in which there is widespread scaling and erythema of the skin. The skin is hot and oedematous, and the disorder is associated with systemic effects, including disturbances of the cardiovascular, thermoregulatory and metabolic systems. In the acute stages of the disorder there may be marked hypothermia, pyrexia-related hypovolaemia and heart failure. The more common causes are psoriasis, eczema, drug reactions and the reticuloses. Normally, total skin blood flow is approximately 1 L min^{-1} at 37°C; however, in erythroderma, this may increase to 5 L min^{-1}, reaching as much as 10 L min^{-1} in the presence of pyrexia. As a result, high-output cardiac failure is a risk and may be exacerbated by hypoalbuminaemia, hypercatabolism and an iron- or folate-deficiency anaemia. Treatment of erythroderma relies on treating the cause of the disorder.

Ichthyosis

Ichthyosis describes a group of conditions which are characterized by the accumulation of large amounts of dry scales on the skin. It is a disorder of keratinization. The most common form is ichthyosis vulgaris, an autosomal dominant disease. Other common forms include X-linked ichthyosis, lamellar ichthyosis (autosomal recessive) and epidermolytic hyperkeratosis (autosomal dominant). Ichthyosis is also seen in association with neoplasia such as lymphoma, multiple myeloma and carcinomas of the lung and breast. Treatment of ichthyosis is directed at increasing the water content of the skin (urea-containing creams), causing separation of the cells using keralytic agents (salicylic acid ointment), or by affecting epidermal metabolism (lactic acid ointment). Occasionally, methotrexate and the retinoids are used.

Preoperative assessment

History and examination

- Fully assess the disease together with its extent and the duration of the illness. In particular, assess the distribution and severity of lesions.
- Assess nutritional state.
- Assess any cardiovascular dysfunction, e.g. congestive cardiac failure in erythroderma or generalized pustular psoriasis.

- Exclude hypovolaemia (owing to increased transepidermal water loss or pyrexia) in erythroderma.
- Check core temperature in erythroderma and pustular psoriasis.
- Note drug therapy and dose, especially immunosuppressants and steroids.

Investigations

- Full blood count: anaemia may be due to chronic illness or deficiencies of iron, vitamin B_{12} or folate; leucopenia and thrombocytopenia may result from immunosuppressant therapy.
- Urea and electrolytes: abnormalities may exist in erythroderma; measure calcium levels if hypoalbuminaemia exists; assess renal function in erythroderma.
- ECG and chest X-ray if there is clinical evidence of heart failure.
- Cross-match blood in erythroderma (risk of blood loss).

Premedication

Do not inject intramuscular premedication into areas of psoriasis (risk of Auspitz's phenomenon and infection due to skin colonization).

Perioperative management

Induction

- Avoid using psoriatic sites for intravenous access (risk of Auspitz's phenomenon and infection due to skin colonization).
- Suture intravenous cannulae in place. Adhesive tape is likely to denude skin (ichthyosis or psoriasis), cause bleeding (psoriasis) or the Koebner phenomenon (psoriasis).
- The hyperdynamic circulation in erythroderma may alter the speed of onset of intravenous and inhalational anaesthetic agents.
- Hypervolaemia, hypovolaemia, congestive cardiac failure, hypoalbuminaemia and a reduction in renal blood flow may affect the kinetics of drug distribution and excretion.

Maintenance

- Hypervolaemia, hypovolaemia, congestive cardiac failure, hypoalbuminaemia and a reduction in renal blood flow may affect the kinetics of drug distribution and excretion.
- The increased skin blood flow and high cardiac output in erythroderma may lead to excessive bleeding during surgery.
- Use space blankets or warm air blankets with care in erythroderma because of the risk of hyperthermia. These patients have difficulty in regulating their body temperature, have an increased metabolic rate and may not be able to sweat.

Regional techniques

- Avoid using psoriatic sites for regional techniques (risk of Auspitz's phenomenon and infection due to skin colonization).
- Modifications should be made to the skin-cleansing routine; use swabs soaked in an aqueous solution of antiseptic or pour solution over skin in ichthyosis. Alcohol-based solutions may cause intense pain. Avoid skin scrubbing.
- Secure extradural catheters using bandage, as adhesive tape may cause skin loss.

Monitoring

- Attach ECG electrodes and pulse oximeter to unaffected skin areas.
- Central venous pressure monitoring will be of use in erythroderma, in which fluid replacement must be undertaken with care.
- Use ECG pads without adhesive in ichthyosis/erythroderma.
- A weighted untaped precordial stethoscope may be useful in ichthyosis/erythroderma.
- Monitor core temperature in erythroderma.
- BP cuffs may cause the Koebner phenomenon, so pad them underneath.

Bibliography

Greaves MW, Weinstein GD. Treatment of psoriasis. *N Engl J Med* 1995; **332**: 581–8.

Love JB, Wright CA, Hooke DH, *et al.* Exfoliative dermatitis as a risk factor for epidemic spread of methicillin resistant *Staphylococcus aureus*. *Intensive Care Med* 1992; **18**: 189.

Smart G, Bradshaw EG. Extradural analgesia and ichthyosis. *Anaesthesia* 1984; **39**: 161–2.

Cross-references

Anaemia, 216
Assessment of renal function, 199

Ehlers–Danlos syndrome

Brian J Pollard

Ehlers–Danlos syndrome (EDS) consists of a group of hereditary disorders of connective tissue characterized by hypermobile joints, extensibility and fragility of skin, and easy bruising. There are nine distinct types (referred to as types I–IX) depending on biochemical studies, the severity of joint and skin manifestations and the degree of involvement of other tissues and organs.

In most forms of EDS, the condition is inherited as an autosomal trait. Specific mutations of some of the 20 collagen genes have been described in different types of EDS. Variations in the specific types of collagen involved and their distribution in different tissues result in diverse clinical manifestations (Table 9.1). Type IV (ecchymotic form) is the most severe form owing to abnormalities in type III collagen, which result in marked weaknesses in blood vessels and the possibility of spontaneous vessel rupture.

Other features of EDS include cardiac conduction defects, mitral valve prolapse, pes planus, scoliosis, hernias, bladder diverticuli, pulmonary emphysema, spontaneous pneumothorax, periodontitis and loose teeth. Clotting is usually normal, but severe bruising, due to friable vessels, is common.

Table 9.1 Clinical manifestations of different forms of Ehlers–Danlos syndrome

Form	Effects
I, III, V, VI, VII, X	Hyperextensible joints resulting in recurrent dislocations
IV	Thin skin with prominent veins Spontaneous rupture of: major vessels, uterus, bowel Aneurysmal dilatation
VI	Blue sclera Rupture of eye
Most types	Laxity of skin
I, IV, VIII	Easily torn skin that heals with 'cigarette paper' scars
V	Mitral and tricuspid valve prolapse

Preoperative assessment

History and examination

- Determine the exact form of EDS and its severity.
- Assess pre-existing cardiovascular and arterial disease with emphasis on valvular abnormalities, aneurysms and arrhythmias.
- Assess jaw opening.
- Assess cervical spine mobility (may be increased).
- Check for loose teeth and periodontitis.

Investigations

- Coagulation studies (correct any abnormalities).
- Cross-match blood (large volumes may be required).
- ECG to exclude arrhythmias and conduction defects.

Perioperative management

Premedication

- The patient should be warned of the risks of anaesthesia.
- Avoid intramuscular premedication (risk of haematoma formation).
- Prophylaxis for bacterial endocarditis if mitral valve disease is present.
- Consider cardiac pacing in the presence of conduction defects.

Induction

Cannulation of vessels may be difficult:

- lax mobile skin makes vessel fixation difficult
- there may be loss of the normal sensation when a vessel wall is pierced
- vessels may be fragile
- risk of haematoma formation with all vessel punctures, especially of arteries and central veins (avoid puncture of a vessel where direct pressure cannot be easily used to control bleeding, e.g. subclavian)
- securing cannulae may be difficult owing to mobile skin
- subcutaneous extravasation may be marked and undetected because of skin laxity.

Maintenance

- Care with insertion of nasogastric tubes (risk of haemorrhage).
- Avoid systemic hypertension (risk of haemorrhage and aneurysmal rupture).

Airway considerations

- Avoid tracheal intubation, if possible, because of the potential for local haemorrhage.
- Modify the hypertensive response to intubation to reduce the risk of aneurysm rupture.
- Special care should be taken during intubation because of the risk of cervical spine damage.
- Use the oral route for intubation in preference to nasal.
- Avoid IPPV, if possible, as there is a risk of pneumothorax if high inflation pressures are required.

Regional techniques

Regional techniques are said to be inadvisable in patients with easy bruising because of the risk of haematoma formation. However, spinal and epidural (caudal and lumbar) techniques have been used without complication.

Positioning

Lax and fragile skin demands that extra care be taken when moving and positioning the patient for surgery. Also take care with movements of joints.

Other considerations

- During surgery meticulous attention should be paid to haemostasis.
- Risk of major blood loss is significant.
- Ligaments and skin may not hold sutures – risk of wound dehiscence.

Postoperative care

- Intramuscular injections are best avoided in case of haematoma formation.
- Intravenous opiate infusions, patient-controlled analgesia or continuous regional techniques would appear to be the most suitable.

Bibliography

Abouleish E. Obstetric anaesthesia and Ehlers–Danlos syndrome. *Br J Anaesth* 1980; **62**: 1283–6.

Brighouse D, Guard B. Anaesthesia for Caesarian section in a patient with Ehlers–Danlos syndrome type IV. *Br J Anaesth* 1992; **69**: 517–19.

Dolan P, Sisko F, Riley E. Anaesthetic considerations for Ehlers–Danlos syndrome. *Anesthesiology* 1980; **52**: 266–9.

Pyeritz RE. Ehlers Danlos syndrome. *N Engl J Med* 2000; **342**: 730–2.

Cross-references

Abdominal aortic reconstruction: elective open repair, 505

Blood transfusion, 735

Epidermolysis bullosa

Brian J Pollard

Epidermolysis bullosa (EB) encompasses a group of hereditary diseases characterized by blistering of skin, either spontaneously or following minimal mechanical trauma. Direct pressure to the skin seems less likely to cause damage than frictional or shearing forces. Separation of the outer layer of the epidermis with accumulation of fluid within the space forms a large blister. Mucous membranes, particularly the mouth, pharynx and oesophagus, may also be affected. Over 20 different subtypes of EB exist, but they can be classified into three major groups – dystrophic (EBD), junctional (EBJ) and simplex (EBS) – depending on the plane within the skin where separation occurs. EBD has the greatest anaesthetic significance. Treatment may involve systemic corticosteroids or drugs with collagenase activity, e.g. phenytoin and monocycline. Patients with EB often require repeated surgery for repair of syndactyly, oesophageal dilatation, skin grafting, dental surgery, removal of skin cancer or change of dressings. Infections of bullae are common.

Dystrophic epidermolysis bullosa

EBD may be transmitted as either an autosomal dominant or recessive disorder with an incidence ranging from 1 in 50 000 to 1 in 300 000 births. It is characterized by low amounts of type VII collagen, possibly due to excessive collagenase activity. Blister formation occurs beneath the lamina densa of the epidermal basement membrane. The disease may start at birth or in early infancy, and is characterized by extensive skin bullae with subsequent scarring. The bullae are large, flaccid and may become infected or haemorrhagic. In the hand, scar formation eventually results in syndactyly. Flexural contractures also occur. Involvement of the mucous membranes of the mouth, pharynx and oesophagus may lead to feeding difficulties, microstomia, fixation of the tongue to the floor of the mouth, and oesophageal stricture. Anaemia is common and poor nutrition may lead to growth retardation.

Junctional epidermolysis bullosa

EBJ describes a group of autosomal recessive conditions leading to blister formation immediately above the basal membrane in the lamina lucida. Death usually occurs in the first 2 years of life. Patients who survive infancy often develop many of the complications of EBD.

Simplex epidermolysis bullosa

EBS may be generalized or localized. Some forms are inherited as autosomal dominant disorders, others as autosomal recessive. EBS is the least disabling form.

Preoperative assessment

History and examination

- Fully assess the form of EB, together with the extent and duration of the illness.
- Note drug therapy, especially systemic corticosteroids and phenytoin.
- Assess venous access.
- Carefully assess the airway (see below).

Investigations

- Full blood count – anaemia and thrombocytosis are common.
- Urea and electrolytes – abnormalities may exist in severe EB; assess renal function.
- Serum iron, folate and vitamin B_{12} levels – anaemia may be due to iron or folate deficiency.
- Liver function tests.
- Albumen – hypoalbuminaemia is common.
- Phenytoin levels, if receiving phenytoin.

Premedication

- Ensure that if premedication is needed it is sufficient to keep the patient calm during induction (struggling may risk new EB lesions).
- The intramuscular route tends to be avoided for fear of inducing new EB lesions; however, it seems unlikely that intramuscular injections cause such problems.
- Prophylaxis against gastric aspiration may be required if oesophageal complications exist.

Perioperative management

Induction

- Venous access may be difficult and cut-down or central vein cannulation may be necessary. Suture

intravenous cannulae in place – do not use adhesive tape.
- An inhalation induction may be needed if venous access is difficult.
- Intramuscular ketamine has proven useful.
- Succinylcholine appears to be safe – there have been no new EB lesions reported after muscle fasciculations and hyperkalaemia response is not seen, despite muscle atrophy.
- Thiopentone appears to be safe, despite fears of associated porphyria.
- For children, encourage the presence of parents in the anaesthetic room in order to reduce the chances of struggling and restlessness on induction.

Airway considerations

Concern has been expressed over the possibility of causing new EB lesions during airway manipulation or intubation. Although pharyngeal lesions do occur, the hazards of intubation appear to have been overstated, since there are no reports of laryngeal or tracheal lesions following tracheal intubation or tracheostomy. However, spontaneous EB lesions are possible in all of these sites.

- Use a face-mask with a soft air cushion and pad with Vaseline gauze.
- Place Vaseline gauze under the chin to protect the skin from the anaesthetist's fingers.
- If possible, avoid the use of airway adjuncts, such as Guedel airways.
- The use of a well-lubricated and carefully placed laryngeal mask appears to be safe.
- Consider the use of a hood for inhalational induction rather than a mask.
- Use a rapid sequence induction when there are oesophageal symptoms (regurgitation is a risk).
- Protect the front of the neck with Vaseline gauze when applying cricoid pressure.
- New head and neck lesions are often associated with difficult or failed intubation.
- Laryngoscopy and oral intubation may be difficult owing to poor dentition, limited mouth opening and adhesion of the tongue to the floor of the mouth. Consider fibreoptic intubation.
- Nasal airways or tubes should be avoided or well lubricated and used with great care.
- Lubricate the laryngoscope blade well.
- Hydrocortisone ointment has been recommended for lubrication but care must be taken with potential absorption of steroid through mucous membranes.
- Use small uncuffed tracheal tubes if possible, always taking into account the surgical field and the need to prevent airway soiling.
- Secure tracheal tubes with simple loose ties and not adhesive tape.
- Treat haemorrhage from mucous membrane lesions using sponges soaked in epinephrine (1:200 000).
- Avoid using a nasogastric tube if possible.

Maintenance

Drug disposition will be affected by decreased muscle bulk, hypoalbuminaemia and any renal disease.

Regional techniques

Although regional anaesthesia has traditionally been avoided, many blocks have been used without complication (e.g. brachial plexus, spinal, epidural (lumbar and caudal), femoral nerve, digital, wrist, lateral cutaneous nerve of thigh). For skin cleansing, apply liquid cleaning agent to skin and do not rub with applicator sponges. Avoid subcutaneous injections of local anaesthetic solutions. If using EMLA cream do not apply self-adhesive occlusive dressing.

Monitoring

- Well-padded non-invasive BP cuffs do not appear to cause bullae, probably because direct pressure is less harmful than frictional or shearing forces.
- The pulse oximeter should be attached using a simple clip rather than adhesive or tape.
- Use ECG pads without adhesive; needle ECG electrodes may be an alternative.
- A weighted untaped precordial stethoscope may be used.
- Arterial lines may be of use – if so, secure with sutures not tape.

Positioning

- Protect the eyes using bland ointment and Vaseline gauze pads, not adhesive tape (bullae may lead to corneal ulceration and globe perforation).
- Keep sheets and other linen free from creases.
- Pad heels, elbows and bony prominences using foam.
- Allow patients to move themselves onto trolleys or the operating table to minimize skin trauma.
- Inform theatre staff of the need for special care during patient positioning.
- Take care with the positioning of a diathermy pad and do not use the self-adhesive type.
- Tourniquets do not appear to be hazardous if the skin is protected by sufficient padding.

Emergence and recovery

- Pharyngeal suction must be performed extremely carefully using a soft, flexible catheter.
- Use protective Vaseline gauze under oxygen masks.
- For children, encourage the presence of parents in the recovery room in order to reduce the chances of struggling and restlessness on emergence.

Postoperative care

Common problems or complications include new skin lesions, regurgitation leading to aspiration pneumonia.

Bibliography

Ames WA, Mayou BJ, Williams K. Anaesthetic management of epidermolysis bullosa. *Br J Anaesth* 1999; **82**: 746–51.

Boughton R, Crawford MR, Vonwiller JB. Epidermolysis bullosa – a review of 15 years' experience, including experience with combined general and regional anaesthetic techniques. *Anaesth Intensive Care* 1988; **16**: 260–4.

Fine J, Bauer EA, Briggaman RA, *et al.* Revised clinical and laboratory criteria for subtypes of inherited epidermolysis bullosa. *J Am Acad Dermatol* 1991; **24**: 119–35.

Griffin RP, Mayou BJ. The anaesthetic management of patients with dystrophic epidermolysis bullosa. A review of 44 patients over a 10 year period. *Anaesthesia* 1993; **48**: 810–15.

James I, Wark H. Airway management during anaesthesia in patients with epidermolysis bullosa dystrophica. *Anesthesiology* 1982; **56**: 323–6.

Smith GB, Shribman AJ. Anaesthesia and severe skin disease. *Anaesthesia* 1984; **39**: 443–55.

Cross-references

Assessment of renal function, 199
Difficult airway: management, 651
Paediatric plastic surgery, 402
Peripheral limb surgery, 405
Rigid bronchoscopy, 423

Glycogen storage disease

Brian J Pollard

Glycogen is a polysaccharide made up of glucose units and found in virtually every tissue in the body. The principal storage sites of glycogen are the liver and muscle. Liver glycogen is concerned with maintenance of blood glucose; muscle glycogen constitutes the energy store for muscle itself and does not contribute to blood glucose homeostasis.

Glycogen consists of chains of six to 12 glucose units joined at carbon atoms 1 and 4. The chains are joined by 1:6 linkages to form branching structures. Metabolism is under the control of a variety of enzymes, which synthesize and break glycogen down to its constituent glucose units (liver glycogen) or to pyruvate and lactate in muscle. Muscle glycogen is principally used in anaerobic metabolism via the relatively inefficient glycolytic pathway. Metabolism occurs in situations where sudden bursts of activity are required and there is no time for increases in cardiac output and delivery of oxygen. Lactate diffuses into general circulation and may then be resynthesized to glucose by the liver. Muscle and blood lactate also rise in shocked states and this is stimulated by epinephrine.

Glycogen storage disease

Numerous enzymes are required in the synthesis and breakdown of glycogen. In 1952 von Gierke disease was described, in which there is a deficiency of glucose-6-phosphatase. This enzyme hydrolyses glucose-6-phosphate to glucose and phosphate immediately prior to release of glucose into the general circulation. Since then, 13 types of glycogen storage disease have been described.

Type I glycogenosis: von Gierke disease

- Diagnosis is by liver or muscle biopsy and enzyme studies.
- Deficiency of glucose-6-phosphatase in the liver, kidney and intestine, with an inability to immobilize liver glycogen to maintain blood glucose.
- Autosomal recessive disorder.
- Short stature; prominent, rounded abdomen owing to liver enlargement; kidneys also enlarge; fat deposits in cheeks and buttocks.
- Hypoglycaemic, hyperlipidaemic and a tendency to acidosis (ketoacidosis and lactic acidosis).
- Prolonged bleeding time owing to platelet glucose-6-phosphatase deficiency.
- Frequent or nasogastric feeding is needed to maintain blood glucose.
- A portacaval shunt enables absorbed glucose to bypass the liver.
- Diazoxide may be effective as it inhibits insulin release and raises blood glucose.

Type II glycogenosis: Pompe disease

- 1:4-α-Glucosidase (acid maltase).
- Lysosomal enzyme; normally breaks 1:4 linkage in glucose chains.
- Glycogen present in excessive quantities in liver, heart, muscle, tongue and central nervous system (especially anterior horn cells).
- Blood sugar, lipid and ketone concentrations and response to glucagon and epinephrine are normal, but the prognosis is poor because of muscle weakness and heart failure.

Type III glycogenosis: Cori disease

- Deficiency of amylo-1,6-glucosidase (debranching enzyme).
- Features similar to type I but milder; able to mobilize glucose from outer chains of glycogen molecule.
- Liver enlarged, growth retardation, hypoglycaemia, elevated blood lipid concentrations and increased hepatic glycogen.
- Treatment consists of frequent feeds with a high protein diet (gluconeogenic pathway intact); hypoglycaemia can cause mental retardation.

Type IV glycogenosis: Andersen disease

- Deficiency of 1,4-glucose-6-glucosyl transferase (brancher) enzyme.
- Normal at birth, but fails to thrive.
- Enlarged liver and spleen, muscles hypotonic.
- Problems are those of liver disease; death in the second year of life.

Type V glycogenosis: McArdle syndrome

- Lack of muscle phosphorylase, which normally removes glucose units from glycogen as glucose-1-phosphate for metabolism to pyruvate and lactate; therefore, unable to maintain glucose supply.
- Symptoms usually develop in the second decade of life.

- Muscle of glycogen moderately elevated; severe pain and muscle cramps at the start of exercise owing to a lack of glucose availability, but passes off (second wind) if exercise persists because of increased cardiac output, vasodilatation and availability of circulating glucose and fatty acids; advised to start exercise gradually.

Type VI glycogenosis: Hers disease

- Reduced hepatic phosphorylase.
- Clinically mild form of type I; enlarged liver and mild hypoglycaemia.

Types VII–XIII glycogenoses

- Extremely rare.

Anaesthesia

Experience is limited. With hepatic glycogenosis (type I and type III), problems are hypoglycaemia and acidosis. Both lactic acidosis in type I and ketoacidosis in type IX have been described along with hyperthermia. It is thus important to provide enteral or parenteral nutrition pre- and postoperatively and to monitor acid–base status.

With type II disease, problems are of myocardial involvement with congestive or obstructive cardiomyopathy and skeletal muscle weakness. A large tongue may cause airway problems. Successful surgery has been undertaken with ketamine and vecuronium and obsessional attention to detailed monitoring, particularly oxygenation. Also, an enlarged heart has caused bronchial obstruction.

Anaesthetic experience with type V disease is also very limited. On theoretical grounds, succinylcholine should be avoided because of the potential myoglobin release and renal damage. Atracurium and alcuronium have been used uneventfully, as has extradural spinal anaesthesia with bupivacaine. Any increased metabolic demand on, or diminution in, the blood supply to skeletal muscle is a potential problem, e.g. hypotension, hypothermia and shivering. The use of a tourniquet should be avoided.

Bibliography

Casson H. Anaesthesia for portocaval bypass in patients with metabolic disease. *Br J Anaesth* 1975; **47**: 969–75.

Coleman P. McArdle's disease. Problem of anaesthetic management of Caesarian section. *Anaesthesia* 1984; **39**: 784–7.

Cox JM. Anesthesia and glycogen storage disease. *Anesthesiology* 1968; **29**: 1221–5.

Edelstein G, Hershman CA. Hyperthermia and ketoacidosis during anaesthesia in a child with glycogen storage disease. *Anesthesiology* 1980; **52**: 90–2.

McFarlane HJ, Soni N. Pompe's disease and anaesthesia. *Anaesthesia* 1986; **41**: 1219–24.

Rajah A, Bell CF. Atracurium and McArdle's disease. *Anaesthesia* 1986; **41**: 93.

Samuels TA, Coleman P. McArdle's disease and Caesarian section. *Anaesthesia* 1988; **43**: 161–2.

Mucopolysaccharidoses

Brian J Pollard

A group of rare familial disorders caused by deficiencies of enzymes required to metabolize the mucopolysaccharide (MPS) constituents of connective tissue. MPS accumulates in skin, bone, blood vessels, brain, heart, liver, spleen, cornea and the tracheobronchial tree, causing anatomical and biochemical malfunction. All sufferers exhibit progressive joint, skeletal and craniofacial abnormalities. Survival beyond the second decade is rare, the majority of childhood deaths being attributable to recurrent pneumonia or cardiac disease. In later years, death occurs from cardiac failure or related complications.

MPS enzyme deficiencies are recessively inherited. All variants are autosomal, with the exception of the Hunter syndrome, which is X linked. Urinary excretion of connective tissue substrates assists diagnosis, but skin biopsy and biochemical enzyme analysis may also be required. Anaesthesia may be required for surgical correction of anatomical abnormalities, relief of distressing symptoms, diagnostic investigation or coincidental disease.

Cardiovascular system

The mitral and aortic valves are distorted and thickened, causing incompetence or stenosis. Myocardial and coronary vessel involvement leads to hypertrophic cardiomyopathy, congestive cardiac failure, myocardial ischaemia and infarction. Arrhythmias and conduction block may occur. Chronic respiratory disease and airway obstruction may produce cor pulmonale.

Respiratory system

Airway obstruction may occur as a result of an enlarged tongue, orofacial abnormalities, adenotonsillar hypertrophy, laryngomalacia, tracheomalacia and mucosal deposition of MPS throughout the respiratory tree. Excessive secretions may cause further compromise. Age-related anterocephalad displacement of the larynx occurs in some types. Kyphoscoliosis and obstructive lung disease increase susceptibility to pulmonary sepsis. Mitral valve disease, pulmonary hypertension and chronic right ventricular failure may further affect respiratory function.

Central nervous system

Mental function ranges from normal intellect to severe retardation. Intellectual deterioration may arise from the disease process or be secondary to hydrocephalus and raised intracranial pressure (ICP). Visual and hearing impairment may complicate assessment.

Gastrointestinal tract

Hepatosplenomegaly is routinely present, but liver and splenic function are usually unaffected. Umbilical and inguinal hernias are common owing to abdominal wall weakness.

Skeletal

Macrocephaly, hypertelorism and abnormalities of the oropharynx and temporomandibular joints occur frequently. Abnormalities of the neck and cervical spine are common, including 'silent' atlanto-occipital subluxation and delayed vertebral ossification. Joint deformities may be aggravated by muscle contractures.

Preoperative assessment

History

- Previous operations and anaesthetic problems.
- Physical and mental disability.
- Respiratory or cardiovascular history.
- Symptoms of obstructive sleep apnoea.

Examination

General

- Skeletal abnormalities (craniofacial, contractures, etc.).
- Skin and peripheral veins.

Respiratory

- Upper airway and orofacial abnormalities.
- Axial anomalies (cervical spine, kyphoscoliosis, etc.).
- Proximal and distal airways obstruction.
- Evidence of chronic lung disease.
- Secretion and sputum production.
- Active pulmonary infection.

Cardiovascular

- Cardiac valve incompetence or stenosis.
- Cardiomegaly, left ventricular hypertrophy.
- Cor pulmonale.
- Univentricular and biventricular failure.
- Arrhythmias.

Central nervous system

- Raised intracranial pressure, papilloedema.
- Visual and hearing impairment.

Investigations

See Table 9.2.

Preoperative preparation

- Treatment of active respiratory infection.
- Chest physiotherapy.
- Treatment of cardiac failure and arrhythmias.
- Full discussion with parents, and consideration of parental accompaniment to the anaesthetic room.

Premedication

- Increased sensitivity to narcotic analgesics – risk of respiratory depression/sleep apnoea.
- Antisialagogue advisable (use glycopyrrolate if tachyarrhythmias are predicted).
- Benzodiazepines effective, but unpredictable.
- Ketamine useful if difficult airway anticipated.
- Consider the need for prophylaxis against bacterial endocarditis.
- Use of EMLA cream helps maintain cooperation of the child.

Perioperative management

The mucopolysaccharidoses present a wide range of potential anaesthetic problems (Table 9.3).

Induction

- Arrange a full range of airway adjuncts.
- Tracheal tube size not predictable from age/weight; therefore, a full range of sizes must be available.
- Oral abnormalities and temporomandibular stiffness may reduce airway access.
- There is a strong case for using fibreoptic intubation in the majority of patients with mucopolysaccharidoses. Difficulties in intubation are common and cervical spine abnormalities may cause critical spinal stenosis, which may be asymptomatic. In such patients, positioning the patient for conventional laryngoscopy may produce significant cord compression. Fibreoptic intubation avoids the necessity to extend the neck and should reduce this risk. When a laryngeal mask is inserted to facilitate endoscopic intubation, neck extension should similarly be avoided.
- Nasal intubation may cause epistaxis; adenoidal tissue may obstruct the nasal tube.
- Laryngeal mask is useful, but may cause excessive secretions or laryngospasm.
- Inhalational induction with oxygen/halothane is useful if a difficult airway is likely.
- Small titrated doses of intravenous anaesthetic drug maintaining spontaneous ventilation may be used until the airway is secured.
- Ketamine is often used; avoid if ICP is raised.

Table 9.2 Investigations for mucopolysaccharidoses

Investigation	Result
Spirometry	Decreased vital capacity, FRC, TLC
Arterial blood gases	Hypoxaemia, hypercapnia
Chest X-ray	Pneumonia, atelectasis, subglottic narrowing
ECG	LVH, RVH, arrhythmias, conduction block
Echocardiogram	Decreased ejection fraction, valve lesions, dyskinesia
Cardiac catheterization	Valve pressure gradients, coronary artery occlusion
CT scan of brain	Hydrocephaly, increased ICP
Cervical spine X-rays	Decreased ossification, atlanto-occipital instability
MR scan of cervical spine	Decreased ossification, atlanto-occipital instability
Haematology profile	Increased white cell count, anaemia
Urea and electrolytes	Diuretic and digoxin effects
Liver function tests	Liver dysfunction

FRC, functional residual capacity; ICP, intracranial pressure; LVH, left ventricular hypertrophy; RVH, right ventricular hypertrophy; TLC, total lung capacity.

● **Table 9.3** Anaesthetic problems associated with various syndromes

Syndrome (type)	Major anaesthetic considerations
Hurler (I)	Macroglossia, kyphoscoliosis, odontoid hypoplasia, mitral incompetence, cardiomegaly
Scheie (I)	Macroglossia, prognathia, short neck, aortic incompetence
Hurler–Scheie (I)	Macroglossia, micrognathia, short neck, mitral and aortic incompetence
Hunter (II)	Hydrocephaly, short neck, ischaemic cardiomyopathy
San Filippo (III)	Macroglossia, vertebral abnormalities
Morquio (IV)	Kyphoscoliosis, odontoid hypoplasia, short neck, C1/C2 instability, aortic regurgitation
Maroteaux–Lamy (VI)	Macroglossia, kyphoscoliosis, odontoid hypoplasia, mitral and aortic valve lesions
Sly (VII)	Contractures, thoracic gibbus, odontoid hypoplasia, mitral and aortic valve lesions, aortic dissection

- Intravenous induction agents should be used cautiously, as they may precipitate apnoea.
- Avoid neuromuscular blockade until the trachea is intubated or ventilation can be assured.

Regional techniques

These are seldom appropriate for surgery alone owing to mental retardation of many patients.

Airway considerations

- Always consider cervical spine involvement.
- Oral airways may cause obstruction by pushing the epiglottis backwards; nasal airways less so.
- Difficult intubation is common, and becomes progressively more so with increasing age.
- Cartilaginous softening/airway distortion may make tracheostomy/cricothyrotomy difficult.

Maintenance

- Nitrous oxide/volatile agent mix as appropriate.
- Use caution with narcotic analgesics because of increased sensitivity.
- Spontaneous breathing techniques are generally inadvisable unless the procedure is of short duration or intubation proves impossible.

Monitoring

In addition to standard anaesthesia monitoring techniques, it is recommended that somatosensory-evoked potentials should be monitored in patients with a high risk of compression of the cervical spinal cord (types I, IV, VI, VII), particularly during airway manipulations. In such patients, preoperative MRI may be valuable in assessing the risk of cord compression.

Positioning

This may be difficult because of kyphoscoliosis.

Emergence and recovery

- Delayed awakening is a recognized problem.
- Extubate when awake to avoid airway obstruction; consider a nasopharyngeal airway.

Analgesia

- Titrate narcotic analgesics in reduced dosage.
- Local or regional techniques are beneficial.

Postoperative care

- Consider ITU admission for close monitoring.
- Chest physiotherapy and antibiotics.

Common problems include:

- restlessness or aggressive behaviour
- arrhythmias
- respiratory obstruction/depression
- obstructive sleep apnoea
- pulmonary infection
- reduced cough and secretion clearance.

With appropriate management, the perioperative morbidity and mortality of patients with mucopolysaccharidoses is low.

Bibliography

Diaz JH, Belani KG. Perioperative management of children with mucopolysaccharidoses. *Anesth Analg* 1993; **77**: 1261–70.

Cross-references

Aortic valve disease, 126
Cardiomyopathy, 136
Difficult airway: overview, 647
Mitral valve disease, 156
Raised intracranial pressure/cerebral blood flow control, 791

Polyarteritis nodosa

Brian J Pollard

Polyarteritis nodosa (PAN) is a rare systemic disease in which a necrotizing arteritis affects the small- and medium-sized arteries. The consequence of this vasculitis depends on the site and number of vessels involved and may range from localized lesions with clinically insignificant effects to life-threatening organ failure. Typically, there is aneurysm formation in the medium-sized arteries, and both haemorrhage and infarction in major organs. Prognosis in PAN is significantly influenced by the size of vessel affected and by the presence of renal involvement. Up to 40% of patients with PAN die within a year of diagnosis.

The histology of classical PAN is a fibrinoid necrosis of the media of affected arteries associated with infiltration of the intima and media by polymorphs. It occurs more often in women, with a peak incidence in the 40–50 year age group. Presenting symptoms often include malaise, fever and weight loss. Approximately 60% have arthralgia, 50% a rash (erythematous, purpuric or vasculitic) and 40% a peripheral neuropathy. The gastrointestinal system is involved in about 45% of cases; gut or gallbladder infarction, gastrointestinal haemorrhage and pancreatitis being the common presentations. Approximately 25% have renal impairment. Myalgia may also be a presenting symptom. It is usually treated with immunosuppressant drugs (e.g. cyclophosphamide) and systemic corticosteroids.

In some patients with PAN there is little evidence of major organ involvement, with the exception of severe renal disease (microscopic polyarteritis). Although all of the features of classical PAN can occur in microscopic polyarteritis, they are less frequent. The patient often presents with haematuria (microscopic or macroscopic), proteinuria or oliguria. Haemoptysis, frank pulmonary haemorrhage (occasionally requiring mechanical ventilation), pleurisy and asthma may also be the initial symptoms. In microscopic polyarteritis histological examination reveals a focal segmental necrotizing glomerulonephritis with fibrinoid necrosis and thrombosis of the glomerular tufts. Treatment of microscopic polyarteritis is as for PAN; azathioprine is occasionally added. Plasmapheresis may be used when cytotoxics and steroids appear to have no benefit.

Preoperative assessment

History and examination

- Assess the extent and duration of the illness. Discover whether the patient has an acute arteritis or is in remission, as this will affect perioperative risk and outcome.
- Assess systemic involvement:
  - cardiovascular (angina, heart failure, cardiomegaly, pericarditis)
  - respiratory (asthma, pneumonia, haemoptysis, pleurisy)
  - renal (renal failure, hypertension)
  - central nervous system (CNS) (peripheral neuropathy, cerebrovascular accident (CVA))
  - airway (acute pharyngeal oedema).
- Check drug history:
  - systemic corticosteroids
  - other immunosuppressant drugs
  - cardiac drugs.

Investigations

ECG

- Cardiac ischaemia, myocardial infarction.
- Arrhythmias, pericarditis.

Echocardiography

- Assess cardiac contractility, pericardial effusions.

Chest X-ray

- Pulmonary infection, haemorrhage.
- Pulmonary infiltrates (pulmonary eosinophilia).
- Pulmonary fibrosis.
- Cardiac failure.

Arterial blood gases

- Look for hypoxaemia.
- The critically ill patient is likely to have a metabolic acidosis.

Urea and electrolytes

- Usually normal until disease is very severe.
- Assess renal function (creatinine and potassium).

Full blood count

- Anaemia is common; leukocytosis is a frequent finding.
- Leukopenia may result from immunosuppressant drug therapy.

Liver function tests

- Albumin and clotting factors as indicators of liver function.
- Approximately 30% of patients with PAN carry the hepatitis B surface antigen.

Lung function tests

- Request if there is clinical evidence of lung disease.

Plasma cholinesterase levels

- Reduced by plasmapheresis.
- Action inhibited by cyclophosphamide.

Preoperative preparation

- Preoperative optimization of cardiovascular and respiratory systems:
  - chest physiotherapy
  - antibiotics
  - control of hypertension
  - treatment of angina (e.g. nitrates).
- Patients with severe cardiovascular disease may require invasive haemodynamic monitoring.
- Perioperative steroid cover will be needed for patients receiving systemic steroids.

Perioperative management

Throughout the perioperative phase there should be scrupulous anti-infection measures because of the high risk of sepsis in PAN.

An anxiolytic premedicant may be advantageous to reduce the risk of tachycardia and hypertension from catecholamines. Avoid anticholinergic premedication (risk of tachycardia).

Induction

- Avoid drugs and techniques likely to cause tachycardia, hypertension, hypotension or reduced myocardial contractility (e.g. ketamine, thiopentone).
- Use a cardiostable anaesthetic technique (e.g. high-dose opioid) to limit the hypertensive response to laryngoscopy.
- Preoxygenate prior to induction.
- Pharyngeal oedema, although rare, has been reported in PAN.

Maintenance

- Avoid drugs and techniques likely to cause tachycardia, hypertension, hypotension or reduced myocardial contractility.
- Administer high concentrations of oxygen when there is a history of cardiac or respiratory disease.
- Maintain good tissue blood and oxygen supply.
- Avoid hypotension and maintain fluid balance, especially in patients with renal involvement.
- Drug handling is altered in renal disease. Avoid drugs which are primarily excreted by the kidneys.
- Hypoalbuminaemia will affect drug distribution.
- Avoid vasoconstrictor drugs, if possible, because of the risk of vascular occlusion.
- When plasmapheresis has been recent, remember that the action of ester drugs (e.g. succinylcholine) will be prolonged.
- The action of succinylcholine may be prolonged by cyclophosphamide.

Regional techniques

- Avoid use of epinephrine-containing local anaesthetic solutions because of the risk of vascular occlusion.
- Document existing sensorimotor neuropathies prior to use of regional techniques.

Monitoring

- A CM5 lead for ECG is useful to detect myocardial ischaemia and arrhythmias.
- Radial artery cannulation may be inadvisable in the presence of aneurysmal disease because of the risk of vascular occlusion.
- Transoesophageal echocardiography may be helpful intraoperatively if there is severe cardiac disease.

Postoperative management

Common problems/complications include:

- deterioration in cardiovascular function
- respiratory failure resulting from pneumonia
- risk of systemic sepsis.

Continue systemic steroid supplements.

Cross-references

Assessment of renal function, 199
Chronic kidney disease, 203
Obstruction or perforation, 447
Preoperative assessment of cardiovascular risk in non-cardiac surgery, 621
Preoperative assessment of pulmonary risk, 625

Polymyositis and dermatomyositis

Brian J Pollard

Dermatomyositis (DM) and polymyositis (PM) are members of an uncommon group of connective tissue disorders known as idiopathic inflammatory myopathies. Other members of the group include cancer-associated myositis, connective tissue disease-associated myositis, childhood dermatomyositis, inclusion body myositis and eosinophilic myositis. Their cause is unknown but genetic factors, toxins, drugs and infectious agents may all play a part. The incidence of malignancy is increased. Both DM and PM present with muscle weakness, usually involving proximal muscle groups, and are associated with other multisystem connective tissue diseases, such as systemic lupus erythematosus, rheumatoid arthritis, Hashimoto's thyroiditis and systemic sclerosis. In DM there are characteristic violaceous skin lesions, often involving the upper eyelid. Treatment is usually with oral steroids. In some cases, other immunosuppressive drugs, such as azathioprine, cyclophosphamide, methotrexate or ciclosporin are added. Patients may present with side-effects of therapy. Plasmapheresis has also been used and may lower plasma cholinesterase levels. The potential problems associated with these diseases do not seem to hold major implications for the anaesthetist. Morbidity and mortality seem to be low and when they occur it is usually because of respiratory disease.

Pathophysiology

Muscle

Chronic inflammation leads to weakness, muscle tenderness, myalgia and, eventually, atrophy and fibrosis of skeletal muscle. Characteristically, there is a rise in serum enzymes derived from muscle, e.g. creatine phosphokinase, and their levels usually parallel disease activity. Myoglobin may be released from muscle, leading to myoglobinaemia and myoglobinuria. The risk of malignant hyperthermia is unknown, but recent *in vitro* studies have shown that muscle from some patients produces significant contracture to caffeine or halothane, but not both (i.e. malignant hyperthermia equivocal).

Respiratory

Of the patients with idiopathic inflammatory myopathies, 5–10% have associated interstitial pulmonary disease, predominantly fibrosis. Pulmonary compromise can also occur because of intercostal and diaphragmatic weakness or aspiration pneumonia. Patients with myositis who have no pulmonary symptoms and a normal chest X-ray may exhibit abnormal pulmonary function tests. Vocal cord dysfunction may exist.

Cardiac

Cardiac disease is a major cause of death. The principal cardiac manifestations are arrhythmias, conduction defects, myocarditis, cardiomyopathy and cor pulmonale. Steroid-induced hypertension may occur.

Gastrointestinal

Poor coordination of swallowing, nasal regurgitation and pooling of secretions in the vallecula and cricopharyngeal spaces may predispose to pulmonary aspiration. There may also be oesophageal reflux, delayed gastric emptying and decreased intestinal motility.

Preoperative assessment

History and examination

Review of associated cardiovascular, respiratory and gastrointestinal disease and assessment for other associated autoimmune disorders. Review of drug therapy and its possible complications. Treat any chest infection.

Investigations

- ECG – look for tachyarrhythmias, conduction abnormalities, ventricular hypertrophy, cor pulmonale.
- Chest X-ray – look for pulmonary fibrosis, ventricular dilatation.
- Spirometry – look for decreased vital capacity, decreased functional residual capacity, decreased tidal volume.
- Blood gas analysis – look for hypoxaemia, hypercapnia.
- Full blood count – look for anaemia, leukopenia.

Premedication

- Continue systemic steroid cover and avoid intramuscular injections.

Perioperative management

Induction/maintenance

- Avoid malignant hyperthermia trigger agents.
- Controlled ventilation should be used in the presence of preoperative ventilatory compromise.

Muscle relaxants

Conflicting evidence exists regarding the use of neuromuscular blocking agents. Succinylcholine has produced an abnormal muscle contraction prior to relaxation in a child with DM. The use of succinylcholine has been avoided by other workers because of the potential, yet unproven, risk of malignant hyperthermia and hyperkalaemia.

The use of non-depolarizing neuromuscular blocking agents has also resulted in conflicting evidence. Several workers have noted no problem, yet there are reports of prolonged neuromuscular paralysis following the use of both vecuronium in PM and atracurium in eosinophilic myositis. A myasthenic-like response has been reported, but this may be related more to associated malignancy than to myositis.

- Use small doses of short-acting neuromuscular blocking agents, preferably after a test dose (remember that there is reduced muscle mass).
- Avoid succinylcholine if possible (because of the potential risk of malignant hyperthermia or, in acute myositis, hyperkalaemia).

Airway considerations

- The use of a tracheal tube is strongly recommended, especially if there is risk of aspiration.
- Rapid sequence induction should be used if pharyngeal, oesophageal or gastric symptoms are present.

Intraoperative monitoring

- Neuromuscular monitoring is essential.
- Extubation and termination of assisted ventilation should follow measurement of lung volumes (e.g. tidal volume, vital capacity).

Postoperative care

- Extubate awake or in the lateral position, because of the risk of aspiration.
- Continue systemic steroid supplementation postoperatively.
- Avoid intramuscular analgesics; titrate small intravenous doses of opiates.
- Postoperative physiotherapy when necessary.
- Immediate postoperative recovery appears to be normal in most patients, yet the following complications might be expected from knowledge of the disease:
  - prolonged recovery from neuromuscular blockade, requiring IPPV
  - lung atelectasis
  - postoperative pneumonia
  - postoperative respiratory failure
  - aspiration if pharyngeal muscles are weak.

Bibliography

Flusche G, Unger-Sargon J, Lambert DH. Prolonged neuromuscular paralysis with vecuronium in a patient with polymyositis. *Anesth Analg* 1987; **66**: 188–90.

Gabta R, Campbell IT, Mostafa SM. Anaesthesia and acute dermatomyositis/polymyositis. *Br J Anaesth* 1988, **60**: 854–8.

Heytens L, Martin JJ, Van de Kleft E, Bossaert LL. In vitro contracture test in patients with various neuromuscular diseases. *Br J Anaesth* 1992; **68**: 72–5.

Johns RA, Finholt DA, Stirt JA. Anaesthetic management of a child with dermatomyositis. *Can Anaesth Soc J* 1986; **33**: 71–4.

Plotz PH, Dalakas M, Leff RL, *et al.* Current concepts in the idiopathic inflammatory myopathies: polymyositis, dermatomyositis, and other related disorders. *Ann Intern Med* 1989; **111**: 143–57.

Cross-references

Rheumatoid disease, 255
Systemic lupus erythematosus, 290

Pseudoxanthoma elasticum

Brian J Pollard

Pseudoxanthoma elasticum (PXE) is a disorder of elastic and collagen tissue in which there is progressive calcification and degeneration of elastin fibres and the supportive collagen matrix in skin and mucous membranes of affected areas. Similar processes may affect the arterial system, leading to arterial occlusion and ischaemia. Ocular and myocardial involvement may also occur. The underlying biochemical lesion is unknown, but the condition is inherited as either an autosomal dominant or recessive disorder. Diagnosis is usually confirmed by skin biopsy. It is unclear why the areas of the body most rich in elastic tissue (e.g. aorta, lungs, palms, soles) are spared, and the pattern follows more closely the distribution of collagen. The prevalence of PXE is estimated to be between 1 in 50 000 and 1 in 200 000 adults, with females being more commonly affected. Acceleration of symptoms may occur during pregnancy. The disease occurs at any age and, although average life expectancy is normal, premature death in childhood is a recognized risk. The majority of patients with PXE who undergo anaesthesia and surgery have an uncomplicated course and outcome. Those with severe cardiovascular involvement are at greater risk, as are those suffering complications such as gastrointestinal haemorrhage, requiring emergency surgery.

Skin

There is a variable tendency to loosening of the skin, particularly in the neck, face, axillae, abdomen and groin (including the genitalia). Most affected individuals show evidence of these changes by their second decade, but some may have minimal involvement even in later life. The loose skin becomes thickened and 'pebbled', sometimes being described as 'peu d'orange'. A characteristic skin deposition of yellowish lesions, mainly in the antecubital fossae, gives a xanthoma-like appearance and the disorder its name. Similar deposition and calcification may occur in mucous membranes, lower lip, rectum and vagina.

Airway and respiratory system

Laryngeal involvement with PXE has been reported. This may cause loss of elasticity of the laryngeal structures, leading to difficult tracheal intubation. Respiratory complications may occur secondary to cardiac involvement.

Vascular system

Arterial involvement may lead to a reduction or absence of peripheral pulses, often with associated medial calcification. Distal ischaemic problems are uncommon, presumably because the slow process allows time for collateral circulation to develop. Renovascular arterial occlusion may cause severe hypertension, even in young patients. Vascular aneurysms also occur in PXE.

Heart

Calcification within the endocardium may affect conduction, and predisposes to arrhythmias. Mitral valve thickening and incompetence have been reported. Coronary arterial lesions may result in severe angina, even in the young; myocardial ischaemia and infarction may result. Coronary artery bypass grafting has been necessary in teenage sufferers and a fatal myocardial infarction has been reported in a 6-week-old infant.

Eye

PXE produces well-recognized ocular manifestations in the form of retinal streaks extending radially from the optic disc over the fundus. The 'angioid streaks' are the result of reduced elasticity of Bruch's membrane, and may lead to scarring and retinal or vitreous haemorrhage.

Gastrointestinal system

Acute gastrointestinal haemorrhage is common, often presenting in children and young adults. The cause appears to be vascular involvement which prevents normal healing responses to minor abrasions of the mucosa. Peptic ulceration and oesophagitis also occur.

Central nervous system

Psychiatric disturbances are commonly associated with the condition. Cerebral ischaemia and haemorrhage are also recognized complications of PXE.

Preoperative assessment

Patients with PXE may require surgery for the ocular, cardiovascular or gastrointestinal complications of the disease. Increasingly, patients present for the surgical treatment of disfiguring cutaneous manifestations.

History and examination

- Assess the extent of the disease, taking note of the degree of involvement of the cardiovascular and respiratory systems:
  - angina, myocardial infarction
  - dyspnoea
  - syncopal attacks (arrhythmias)
  - arterial pulses
  - BP
  - heart murmurs.
- Assess venous access, both peripheral and central.

Investigations

- ECG.
- Chest X-ray.
- Urea and electrolytes (baseline test of renal function).

Preoperative preparation

Temporary cardiac pacing may be indicated in selected patients with conduction defects.

Perioperative management

Induction

- Venous access may be difficult owing to the loose and thickened skin.
- The antecubital fossae are often unsuitable for intravenous access.
- Neck involvement may prevent use of the internal jugular veins.
- Groin involvement may prevent use of the femoral veins.
- Venous cut-down may be necessary.
- An inhalation induction may be necessary.

Anaesthetic technique

There appear to be no specific contraindications to the use of any particular anaesthetic drug. However, in planning the anaesthetic technique, the following points should be borne in mind:

- risks of undiagnosed cardiac ischaemia and dysrhythmias
- risk of major haemorrhage
- risks of hypertension, e.g. subendocardial ischaemia, intracranial haemorrhage.

Airway considerations

- Tracheal intubation may be difficult because involvement of the laryngeal ligaments and cartilages may cause laryngeal rigidity.
- Rigid bronchoscopy has been necessary to assist with endotracheal intubation.

Maintenance

Care should be taken to avoid upper gastrointestinal trauma from the use of a nasogastric tube.

Regional techniques

Thickened loose skin may make regional techniques difficult.

Monitoring

- BP monitoring, although essential, may be difficult:
  - non-invasive oscillotonometric methods are likely to be unreliable in the presence of occlusive arterial disease
  - invasive BP monitoring may be difficult because of arterial occlusion or vessel calcification.
- Central venous access for central venous pressure monitoring may be difficult.
- Care should be taken to avoid upper gastrointestinal trauma from the use of an oesophageal stethoscope or oesophageal temperature probe.

Bibliography

Levitt MWD, Collison JM. Difficult endotracheal intubation in a patient with pseudoxanthoma elasticum. *Anaesth Intensive Care* 1982; **10**: 62–4.

Wilson Krechel SL, Ramirez-Inawat RC, Fabian LW. Anesthetic considerations in pseudo-xanthoma elasticum. *Anesth Analg* 1981; **60**: 344–7.

Cross-references

Cardiac conduction defects, 132
Coronary artery bypass grafting, 580
Hypertension, 151

Scleroderma

Brian J Pollard

A chronic multisystem disorder of unknown aetiology. There is fibrosis of skin, vascular damage and organ involvement. It involves many organs, in particular skin, gastrointestinal tract, lungs, heart and kidneys. There is evidence of an autoantibody response and the types of antibody present may be used to categorize different subgroups. Females are affected more than males (4–10 times). Onset is usually between the ages of 20 and 50 years. Symptoms may be exacerbated by pregnancy.

There is excessive deposition of collagen and other extracellular matrix proteins in affected tissues. Sufferers often possess certain common HLA antigens and there is evidence of both disordered cell-mediated immunity and abnormal endothelial cell function. Additionally, some chemicals (e.g. silica) induce scleroderma-like syndromes. Most cases of scleroderma fall into one of two subsets: progressive systemic sclerosis or limited cutaneous systemic sclerosis.

Clinical features (Table 9.4)

- Shiny, waxy, taut skin with loss of skin folds.
- Perioral contractures, which limit mouth opening, and poor dental hygiene.
- Oesophageal involvement (dysphagia, reflux and stricture formation) in about 80% of patients.
- The heart is involved in approximately 50–80% of patients, leading to conduction defects, cardiomyopathy, pericarditis, cardiomegaly, arrhythmias, reduced ventricular contractility and pericardial effusions.
- Pulmonary fibrosis resulting in decreased compliance and decreased vital capacity. Pulmonary hypertension may develop.
- Weakness of the intercostal muscles and diaphragm has been reported.
- The skin of the chest wall may be involved, thus limiting normal chest expansion.

Table 9.4 Clinical features and natural history of scleroderma subtypes*

Diffuse cutaneous systemic sclerosis		
Early onset of Raynaud's (<1 year)	Early (<5 years after onset)	Late (>5 years after onset)
Truncal and sacral skin involved	Rapid progression of skin thickening	Skin involvement stable or regresses
Early systemic disease (interstitial lung fibrosis, renal failure, gastrointestinal and myocardial involvement)	Increased risk of renal, cardiac, pulmonary, articular, vascular complications and digital ulcers	Progression of existing visceral disease, but reduced risk of new visceral involvement
Antitopoisomerase antibody in ≈40%		
Limited cutaneous systemic sclerosis		
Raynaud's phenomenon for years	Early (<10 years after onset)	Late (>10 years after onset)
Face, hands, feet and forearm skin affected	No progression of skin lesions	No progression of skin lesions
Late incidence of pulmonary hypertension, trigeminal neuralgia, skin calcification and telangiectasia	Raynaud's phenomenon, digital tip ulceration, oesophageal symptoms are common	Raynaud's phenomenon, digital ulceration and calcification, oesophageal stricture, malabsorption and pulmonary hypertension
Anticentromere antibody in 70–80%		

*Modified from Leroy *et al*. (1988) and Steen and Medsger (1990).

- Renal disease may lead to hypertension. Hypertensive crises may follow withdrawal of angiotensin-converting enzyme inhibitors.
- Lower gut involvement may result in malabsorption, obstruction or perforation.
- Other findings include peripheral neuropathies, Sjögren syndrome, non-pitting oedema, telangiectasia and diminished sweating.
- Raynaud disease is common.

The CREST syndrome, a variant of scleroderma, is the combination of calcinosis, Raynaud's phenomenon, oesophageal involvement, sclerodactyly and multiple telangiectasia of the skin, lips, oral mucosa and gut.

Preoperative assessment

History and examination

- Assess the extent and duration of the illness.
- Assess venous access.
- Assess mouth opening.
- Assess state of dentition (often poor).
- Look for mucosal telangiectasia in the mouth.
- Assess neck mobility.
- Assess degree of cardiac and respiratory symptoms (e.g. exertional dyspnoea or the dry cough of pulmonary fibrosis); examine for cardiac dysrhythmias, a pericardial effusion and signs of pulmonary hypertension. Cardiopulmonary exercise testing may be useful.
- Check preoperative BP.
- Ask about dysphagia and oesophageal reflux.
- Ask about symptoms of Raynaud's phenomenon.
- Check for evidence of chronic renal failure.
- Examine for peripheral neuropathies.
- Check drug history – in particular for systemic corticosteroids and immunosuppressant drugs.

Investigations

- ECG and echocardiography: 24 hour ECG recording may be indicated. The presence of a normal resting ECG does not exclude involvement of the heart in scleroderma; up to 40% of such patients may have abnormalities on 24 hour rhythm analysis. There may be diastolic dysfunction, asymmetric septal hypertrophy or pericardial effusion.
- Chest X-ray: look for signs of pulmonary fibrosis; exclude preoperative inhalation of gastric contents.
- Cervical spine X-ray: assess associated spinal disease and neck mobility.
- Arterial blood gases: look for hypoxaemia.
- Urea and electrolytes: baseline test of renal function.
- Full blood count: look for anaemia or leukocytosis due to treatment.
- Lung function tests: decreased functional vital capacity and/or impaired diffusing lung capacity for carbon monoxide (DLco) in early scleroderma is predictive of lung disease. Pulmonary fibrosis may lead to decreased lung compliance and reduced total lung capacity or vital capacity. Impaired gas transfer may occur; DLco is abnormal in 70% of patients with progressive systemic sclerosis.
- Coagulation studies: these may be abnormal because of malabsorption.
- Thyroid function tests: hypothyroidism may occur in scleroderma.

Preoperative preparation

- Xerostomia and poor dental hygiene may be helped by frequent preoperative mouthwashes.
- Steroid cover may be needed if the patient is receiving systemic corticosteroids.
- Use prophylactic H_2 blockers and prokinetic drugs (but beware of inducing arrhythmias), when oesophageal disease is present.
- Vitamin K may be required when malabsorption has led to a bleeding tendency.
- Temporary cardiac pacing may be indicated in selected patients with conduction defects.

Operative management

Induction

Venous access may be difficult owing to vasoconstriction; cut-down or central vein cannulation may be necessary. An inhalational induction or fibreoptic intubation technique may be necessary. Do not administer a muscle relaxant until it is certain that the larynx can be viewed and intubation is possible.

Airway

A rapid sequence induction may not be practicable if intubation difficulties are anticipated. Cricoid pressure may be ineffective if the oesophagus is fibrosed. Consider awake fibreoptic intubation. Intubation should be performed very gently to avoid injury to the mouth. Use oral intubation in preference to the nasal route as nasopharyngeal telangiectasia may lead to bleeding. In very severe cases, consider tracheostomy.

Maintenance

Maintain the patient's temperature at 37°C (risk of Raynaud's phenomenon). Warm all intravenous fluids; warm theatre; warming blanket. Reduced lung and chest wall compliance may make ventilation difficult. Dry eyes make eye care especially important: eyelids should be taped shut; use bland ointments or artificial tears. Use a heat and moisture exchanger in the airway. Avoid hypotension and maintain fluid balance, especially in patients with renal involvement. Drug metabolism is altered in renal failure. Avoid vasoconstrictor drugs if possible. Increased concentrations of oxygen may be required.

Regional techniques

Ischaemic effects of tourniquets make the use of intravenous regional anaesthesia unwise. Nerve blocks, including brachial plexus and sciatic nerve, have been used successfully, but may be associated with prolonged duration of block. Raynaud's phenomenon may follow wrist blocks. Avoid use of epinephrine-containing local anaesthetic solutions. Unilateral local anaesthetic stellate ganglion blocks have worsened Raynaud's phenomenon on the contralateral side.

Monitoring

Limb contractures may make BP measurement difficult. Radial artery cannulation or sampling should be avoided if possible (if it is essential then careful assessment of collateral flow (Allen's test) is necessary or use a larger artery). ECG monitoring to detect arrhythmias and conduction defects.

Positioning

Consider the risks of pressure effects on fibrotic skin during prolonged operations.

Emergence and recovery

The maintenance of a head-down position is advisable until patient is fully conscious. Patients should be nursed upright once awake, in order to prevent regurgitation. Increased oxygen requirements may result from a diffusion block in cases of lung fibrosis.

Postoperative management

Common problems/complications include postoperative chest infection, respiratory failure (due to respiratory muscle weakness or pneumonia), increased postoperative analgesic requirements (possibly due to increased numbers of sensory nerve fibres in skin). Continue systemic steroid supplements.

Bibliography

Black CM, Stephens C. Systemic sclerosis (scleroderma) and related disorders. In: Maddison PJ, Isenberg DA, Woo P, Glass DN (eds) *Oxford Textbook of Rheumatology*. New York: Oxford University Press, 1993, pp. 771–94.

Leroy EC, Black S, Eleischmajor R, *et al.* Scleroderma (systemic sclerosis): classification, subsets and pathogenesis. *J Rheumatol* 1988; **15**: 202–5.

Neill RS. Progressive systemic sclerosis. Prolonged sensory blockade following regional anaesthesia in association with a reduced response to systemic analgesics. *Br J Anaesth* 1980; **52**: 623–5.

Omote K, Kawamata M, Namiki A. Adverse effects of stellate ganglion block on Raynaud's phenomenon associated with progressive systemic sclerosis. *Anesth Analg* 1993; **77**: 1057–60.

Roberts JG, Sabar R, Gianoli JA, Kaye AD. Progressive systemic sclerosis: clinical manifestations and anesthetic considerations. *J Clin Anesth* 2002; **14**: 474–7.

Smith GB, Shribman AJ. Anaesthesia and severe skin disease. *Anaesthesia* 1984; **39**: 443–55.

Smoak LR. Anesthesia considerations for the patient with progressive systemic sclerosis (scleroderma). *J Am Assoc Nurse Anesth* 1982; **50**: 548–54.

Steen VD, Medsger TA. Epidemiology and natural history of systemic sclerosis. *Rheum Dis Clin North Am* 1990; **16**: 1–10.

Wigley FM. When is scleroderma really scleroderma? *J Rheumatol* 2001; **28**: 1471–3.

Younker D, Harrison B. Scleroderma and pregnancy. Anaesthetic considerations. *Br J Anaesth* 1985; **57**: 1136–9.

Cross-references

Difficult airway: management, 651

Disorders of the oesophagus and of swallowing, 177

Systemic lupus erythematosus

Brian J Pollard

Systemic lupus erythematosus (SLE) is a chronic inflammatory disease affecting most body systems and characterized by abnormal immune function. Increased numbers of hyperactive B lymphocytes, together with impaired T-cell regulation, lead to the production of immunoglobulin G (IgG) antibodies, which are specific for exogenous and endogenous antigens. The serum in SLE contains a variety of autoantibodies directed against nuclear material (anti-DNA antibodies in particular), and histological examination of affected tissue shows evidence of immune complex deposition. The origin of SLE appears to be multifactorial - diet, drugs, toxins, infection, stress, surgery, pregnancy, environment, hormones, genetics, etc., all seem to play a part. Drug-induced SLE may occur with isoniazid, hydralazine, anticonvulsants, procainamide, methyldopa and chlorpromazine.

SLE is more common in females than males (9:1), and the usual onset is in the third and fourth decades. It is an episodic disease with periods of prolonged remission punctuated by life-threatening exacerbations. Usually, the onset involves arthralgia, fever, weight loss, rash, anaemia and leukopenia; involvement of other organs produces a wide clinical spectrum of disease (Box 9.1). The presence of hypertension and/or nephritis indicates a poor long-term prognosis.

Of particular note to the anaesthetist is involvement of the cardiovascular, respiratory and renal systems. Myocarditis occurs in approximately 15% of cases, pericarditis in up to 60% and valvular lesions (Libman-Sach endocarditis) in almost 25%. Pleuritic pain is found in about 50% of cases, pleural effusions in 25% and interstitial fibrosis, pulmonary vasculitis and interstitial pneumonitis in 20%. Renal disease is the most common cause of death. Of those patients with renal disease, 50% have hypertension.

Up to 30% of patients have a circulating anticoagulant (lupus anticoagulant), which may prolong the activated partial thromboplastin time (aPTT) but also risks the formation of arterial and venous thromboses and predisposes to recurrent abortions. The presence of the anticardiolipin antibody is also associated with these problems.

Treatment of SLE is with a combination of non-steroidal anti-inflammatory drugs (NSAIDs), antimalarial agents, corticosteroids and immunosuppressant drugs (e.g. cyclophosphamide, azathioprine). Some centres use plasmapheresis for patients who are resistant to conventional therapy.

Box 9.1 Clinical features of SLE

- Bones/joints
  - Flitting arthralgia
  - Polyarthritis (wrists, elbows, knees)
  - Aseptic necrosis of large joints
- Skin
  - 'Butterfly' rash in malar region
  - Photosensitivity
  - Raynaud's phenomenon
- Cardiovascular system
  - Pericarditis/pericardial effusion
  - Myocarditis
  - Endocarditis
  - Leg ulcers
  - Limb gangrene
  - Necrotic finger pulp lesions
- Respiratory system
  - Pleurisy/pleural effusions
  - Pulmonary infiltration
  - Diffusion block
- Renal system
  - Proteinuria
  - Nephrotic syndrome
  - Hypertension
  - Acute and chronic renal failure
- Muscular system
  - Myalgia
  - Myositis
  - Wasting/weakness
- Nervous system
  - Seizures
  - Psychosis
  - Peripheral sensorimotor neuropathy
  - Hemiplegia
  - Cranial nerve palsies
- Gastrointestinal system
  - Peritonitis
  - Gastrointestinal haemorrhage
  - Vasculitic ischaemia
- Haematological system
  - Anaemia
  - Leukopenia
  - Thrombocytopenia
  - Bleeding diathesis (circulating anticoagulants)

Preoperative assessment

History and examination

- Assess the extent and duration of the illness. Discover whether the patient has acute disease or is in remission, as this will affect perioperative risk and outcome.
- Assess systemic involvement:
  - cardiovascular (tachycardia, heart failure, cardiomegaly, pericardial effusion, valve lesions)
  - respiratory (pleurisy, dyspnoea)
  - renal (renal failure, hypertension)
  - CNS (peripheral neuropathy, CVA)
  - Raynaud's phenomenon.
- Check drug history:
  - NSAIDs
  - antimalarials
  - systemic corticosteroids
  - other immunosuppressant drugs
  - cardiac drugs
  - use of plasmapheresis.

Investigations

- ECG: myocarditis, dysrhythmias, pericarditis.
- Echocardiography: cardiac contractility, pericardial effusions.
- Chest X-ray: pleural effusion, pulmonary fibrosis, pericardial effusion, cardiac failure.
- Arterial blood gases: look for hypoxaemia, usually with a normal or low $P_{a}CO_2$.
- Urea and electrolytes: baseline test of renal function.
- Full blood count: anaemia is common, leukopenia from immunosuppressant drug therapy or from SLE itself; thrombocytopenia may occasionally occur.
- Lung function tests: clinical signs, symptoms and chest X-ray may not reflect the degree of pulmonary involvement; pulmonary fibrosis will cause a restrictive defect; diffusing capacity may be reduced.
- Coagulation studies: prolonged aPTT or kaolin cephalin clotting time due to anticardiolipin antibody and lupus anticoagulant. Prothrombin time may be normal.
- Plasma cholinesterase levels are reduced by plasmapheresis and cyclophosphamide.

Preoperative preparation

- Preoperative optimization of cardiovascular and respiratory systems. In particular:
  - control of hypertension
  - treatment of angina (e.g. nitrates)
  - treatment of arrhythmias
  - treatment of heart failure
  - drainage of pericardial/pleural effusions
  - treatment of intercurrent pneumonia.
- Patients with severe cardiovascular disease may require perioperative invasive haemodynamic monitoring.
- Perioperative steroid cover will be needed for the patient receiving corticosteriods.
- Take antithrombotic measures perioperatively in patients with anticardiolipin antibody:
  - antiembolic stockings
  - avoid dehydration
  - subcutaneous heparin.

Patients with the anticardiolipin antibody and a history of thrombotic events require permanent anticoagulation with either warfarin or aspirin. They should receive heparin as an infusion perioperatively. Blood transfusions can exacerbate SLE.

Perioperative management

Induction

- Avoid drugs and techniques likely to cause tachycardia, hypertension, hypotension or reduced myocardial contractility (e.g. ketamine, thiopentone).
- Use a cardiostable anaesthetic (e.g. opiate induction, intravenous lidocaine) to limit the hypertensive response to laryngoscopy.
- Preoxygenate.

Airway considerations

There are rare reports of a narrowed airway due to cricoarytenoid arthritis in SLE.

Maintenance

- Avoid drugs and techniques likely to cause tachycardia, hypertension, hypotension or reduced myocardial contractility.
- When plasmapheresis has been recent, the action of ester drugs (e.g. succinylcholine) may be prolonged.
- The action of succinylcholine may be prolonged by cyclophosphamide.
- Administer high concentrations of oxygen when there is cardiorespiratory disease.
- Avoid hypotension and maintain fluid balance, especially in the patient with renal involvement.
- Drug metabolism is altered in renal disease; avoid drugs which are metabolized/excreted by the kidneys.
- Hypoalbuminaemia in nephrotic syndrome will affect drug distribution.
- Avoid vasoconstrictors in Raynaud disease.

Regional techniques

- Be absolutely sure of the patient's coagulation status before embarking upon regional anaesthetic techniques.
- Document existing sensorimotor neuropathies prior to use of regional techniques.

Monitoring

- A CM5 lead ECG is useful to detect myocardial ischaemia and arrhythmias.
- Radial artery cannulation may be inadvisable in the presence of Raynaud's phenomenon.
- Transoesophageal echocardiography is helpful intraoperatively in severe cardiac disease.
- Neuromuscular junction monitoring is essential if cyclophosphamide or plasmapheresis used.

Postoperative management

Common problems/complications include deterioration in cardiovascular function, renal failure and risk of arterial or venous thromboses. Continue systemic steroid supplements.

Bibliography

Davies SR. Systemic lupus erythematosus and the obstetrical patient: implications for the anaesthetist. *Can J Anaesth* 1991; **38**: 790–6.

Menon G, Allt-Graham J. Anaesthetic implications of the anticardiolipin antibody syndrome. *Br J Anaesth* 1993; **70**: 587–90.

Malinow AM, Rickford WJK, Mokkiski BLK, *et al.* Lupus anticoagulant. Implications for the obstetric anaesthetist. *Anaesthesia* 1987; **42**: 1291–3.

Cross-references

Aortic valve disease, 126
Chronic kidney disease, 203
Inherited coagulopathies, 226

Urticaria and angio-oedema

Brian J Pollard

Urticaria is a well demarcated, usually pruritic, skin reaction characterized by erythematous, raised, palpable lesions, often with pale centres, which blanch on pressure. Urticarial lesions result from a transient increase in capillary permeability causing focal oedema of the superficial part of the dermis. Angio-oedema describes a condition in which there is circumscribed, non-pitting subepithelial oedema, sometimes with erythema. It may involve the eyelids, lips, tongue, larynx, pharynx, respiratory tract, gastrointestinal tract, renal system and, occasionally, the central nervous system. This may result in airway obstruction, pleural effusions, abdominal pain, vomiting, diarrhoea, hemiplegia and seizures.

Urticaria and angio-oedema often accompany each other; however, in those cases of angio-oedema due to a deficiency of the C_1-esterase deficiency (see below), urticaria does not occur. Individual attacks of urticaria and angio-oedema usually last no longer than 48 h. If episodes of urticaria/angio-oedema occur for more than 2 months, the condition is termed 'chronic'.

Box 9.2 Aetiology of urticaria and angio-oedema

- Idiopathic
- Foodstuffs and additives
- Drugs:
  - Antibiotics
  - Muscle relaxants, e.g. tubocurarine
  - Opiates, e.g. morphine
  - Heparin
  - Protamine
  - Antihypertensives, e.g. ACE inhibitors
  - NSAIDs
  - Psychotropic drugs
- Insect bites and stings
- Physical:
  - Dermatographism
  - Cold/heat
  - Vibration
  - Exercise
  - Delayed pressure urticaria
- Infections
- Collagen vascular disease
- Endocrine disease
- Vasculitis
- Malignancy
- Hereditary and acquired angio-oedema
- Miscellaneous

Many common forms of urticaria and angio-oedema (Box 9.2) result from the antigen-induced release of biologically active substances from mast cells which are found in organs rich in connective tissue (e.g. skin, respiratory tract, etc.). Urticaria/angio-oedema may also be caused by drugs which cause direct mast cell degranulation or which activate the arachidonic acid or complement pathways. In all these cases, release or activation of mediators (e.g. histamine, heparin, tryptase, chymase, chemotactic factors, prostaglandins, leucotrienes, platelet activating factor (PAF), adenosine, oxygen radicals) causes altered vascular permeability, smooth muscle contraction and chemotaxis of leucocytes. This results in a spectrum of signs and symptoms ranging from simple urticaria or angio-oedema to fulminant anaphylaxis.

Some forms of angio-oedema result from a functional deficiency of the inhibitor of the first component of the complement cascade (C_1), and this is known as C_1 esterase inhibitor (C_1EI). Hereditary angio-oedema (HAO) is an autosomal dominant disorder characterized by recurrent spontaneous episodes of oedema of the skin and the mucous membranes of the respiratory tract and gut. Minor trauma, concomitant illness or perioral surgery (e.g. dentistry or tonsillectomy) may precipitate an attack. Attacks may increase during pregnancy (when C_1EI levels are low) or during menstrual bleeding. The major serious complication of an acute attack of HAO is upper airway obstruction, although oedema of the bowel wall may be mistaken for an acute abdomen and result in unnecessary, and risky, surgery. Low levels of C_1EI also occur as an acquired disorder (Box 9.3). Acquired

Box 9.3 C_1-esterase inhibitor (C_1EI) deficiency

Hereditary C_1EI deficiency

- Type 1 (85%)
  - Impaired synthesis
  - Mostly autosomal dominant
- Type 2 (15%)
  - Dysfunctional protein
  - Heterogeneous genetic groups,
  - Mostly autosomal dominant
- Aquired C_1EI deficiency
  - B-cell lymphoproliferative disorders
  - Connective tissue diseases
  - Monoclonal gammopathies
  - Antibodies to C_1EI

C_1EI deficiency can be distinguished from HAO by the absence of complement abnormalities in other family members, late age of onset and by the reduced level of C_1 seen in the acquired form.

Long-term treatment of urticaria/angio-oedema

Chronic urticaria/angio-oedema

- Identify and avoid precipitating factors
- Avoid drugs which may aggravate disease, e.g. salicylates, NSAIDs, opiates
- Treat with H_1-receptor antagonists, e.g. chlorpheniramine
- Add a β-adrenergic agonist, e.g. terbutaline
- Add an H_2-receptor antagonist, e.g. ranitidine
- Consider use of a tricyclic antidepressant, e.g. doxepin (this acts against both H_1- and H_2-receptors)
- Corticosteroids are used only in very severe disease
- Adrenaline is used for severe attacks of anaphylaxis.

C_1EI deficiency (hereditary and acquired)

- Androgens, e.g. stanozolol; stimulate hepatic synthesis of C_1EI
- Antifibrinolytic agents, e.g. tranexamic acid or epsilon aminocaproic acid (EACA); these inhibit plasmin activation (plasmin is a potent catalyst for complement activation)
- Purified C_1EI concentrate.

Preoperative assessment

History and examination

Specifically ask about:

- Atopy
- Hypersensitivity
- Drug reactions
- Family history
- Previous episodes of urticaria/angio-oedema, including frequency, duration, effect, etc.
- Drug therapy (see above).

Investigations

- C_1EI function in HAO
- Radioallergosorbent (RAST) tests.

Preoperative preparation

Skin testing may be useful, but results are often unreliable and there is a small risk of severe anaphylaxis during test. Avoid precipitating drugs or factors in chronic urticaria/angio-oedema.

Premedication

Avoid precipitating drugs or factors in chronic urticaria/angio-oedema. In all cases of urticaria/angio-oedema, suitable premedication should be used to allay anxiety.

In chronic urticaria/angio-oedema, the following agents may be useful as a part of the premedication:

- H_1 antagonist (antihistamine)
- H_2 antagonist
- β-Adrenergic agonist
- Corticosteroid.

In HAO, attempts should be made to increase C_1EI levels preoperatively using:

- Androgens
- Antifibrinolytics
- Two units of fresh frozen plasma (FFP)
- Purified C_1EI concentrate (IMMUNO AG).

If the patient is not receiving long-term therapy with androgens or antifibrinolytics, these should be administered for several days prior to surgery. Although they start to act within 24 h, they require 1–2 weeks to reach maximum effect. Alternatively, the administration of 2 units of FFP given in the immediate preoperative period will restore the C_1EI to a safe level (40% of normal) for between 1 and 4 days. These measures also seem appropriate for the acquired form of C_1EI deficiency, although there is little documentation of their use.

Perioperative management

Induction/maintenance

Venepuncture has precipitated forearm angio-oedema in a patient with HAO.

Use the most 'immunologically benign' agents, particularly in atopic patients. Avoid histamine-releasing drugs, where possible.

Avoid airway manipulation and intubation, where possible.

In cold urticaria:

- Warm intravenous fluids
- Warm the laryngoscope blade
- Use a warming blanket and warm air circulating cover
- Humidify respiratory gases.

Monitoring

Monitor core temperature, especially in cold and cholinergic (heat) urticaria.

Positioning

In pressure urticaria, use extra protection for bony prominences, tourniquets, etc.

Regional techniques

These may allow the avoidance of tracheal intubation.

Cardiopulmonary bypass

Cardiopulmonary bypass (CPB) has been undertaken successfully in patients with certain forms of urticaria/angio-oedema.

Management of acute attacks of urticaria and angio-oedema

- Always have facilities available to treat anaphylaxis or airway obstruction, e.g. intubation equipment and tracheostomy facilities.
- Treat acute attacks of chronic urticaria/angio-oedema with adrenaline, steroids and antihistamines.
- Treat attacks of angio-oedema due to C_1EI deficiency with FFP or purified C_1EI concentrate (1000–1500 plasma units).
- There is unlikely to be any response during an acute attack of HAO to adrenaline, steroids, or antihistamines.
- Monitor coagulation status in HAO.
- Remember that C_1EI levels will fall due to haemodilution if patients with C_1EI deficiency undergo CPB.
- CPB in a patient with cold urticaria has led to a rise in arterial histamine levels during rewarming.

Bibliography

Johnston WE, Moss J, Philbin DM *et al.* Management of cold urticaria during cardiopulmonary bypass. *New England Journal of Medicine* 1982; **306**: 220–221

Kharasch ED. Angiotensin-converting enzyme inhibitor-induced angioedema associated with endotracheal intubation. *Anesthesia and Analgesia* 1992; **74**: 602–604

Razis PA, Coulson IH, Gould TR *et al.* Aquired C_1 esterase inhibitor deficiency. *Anaesthesia* 1986; **41**: 838–840

Wall RT, Frank M, Hahn M. A review of 25 patients with hereditary angioedema requiring surgery. *Anesthesiology* 1989; **71**: 309–311

Cross references

Allergic reactions, 727

Intraoperative bronchospasm, 762

Intraoperative hypertension, 765

Part 2
Surgical Procedures

10

Neurosurgery

Martin Smith

- General principles of neuroanaesthesia — *Michelle Leemans*
- Anaesthesia for interventional neuroradiological procedures — *Mary Newton and Robin Kumar*
- Anaesthesia for intracranial neurovascular surgery — *Sally Wilson and Tamsin Gregory*
- Anaesthesia for magnetic resonance imaging — *Ugan Reddy and Sally Wilson*
- Anaesthesia for non-craniotomy neurosurgery — *Shulpa Reddy and Katharine Hunt*
- Anaesthesia for posterior fossa surgery — *Ugan Reddy and Katharine Hunt*
- Anaesthesia for spine surgery — *Michelle Leemans*
- Anaesthesia for supratentorial surgery — *Ian Appleby and Tamsin Gregory*
- Anaesthesia for trans-sphenoidal hypophysectomy — *Nicholas Hirsch*
- Anaesthetic and ICU management of the head-injured patient — *David Highton and Martin Smith*
- Neuromonitoring — *David Highton and Martin Smith*

General principles of neuroanaesthesia

Michelle Leemans

Neuroanaesthesia broadly concerns intracranial and spinal surgery, and interventional neuroradiology. For intracranial procedures, the conduct of anaesthesia should be based on the type of procedure, the patient's general medical condition and also on the effects of anaesthetic agents on cerebral physiology. For example, anaesthesia for an elective craniotomy is quite different from a craniotomy following a traumatic brain injury (TBI). It is particularly the case that in brain-injured patients (from any cause) special consideration must be taken of the effects of anaesthetic agents on altered cerebral physiology.

Effects of anaesthetic agents on cerebral physiology

The choice of agent is based on consideration of its effects on cerebral blood flow (CBF) and cerebral blood volume (CBV), cerebral metabolic rate ($CMRo_2$), intracranial pressure (ICP), cerebral pressure autoregulation and carbon dioxide reactivity. For intracranial surgery, a balanced anaesthetic technique using sevoflurane in an air–oxygen mix is a popular choice and allows rapid wake-up and early neurological assessment. Total intravenous anaesthesia (TIVA) with propofol is an acceptable alternative, but there is no evidence to suggest that this is superior to a volatile-based technique under most circumstances.

Intravenous agents

Agents such as thiopental and propofol cause a reduction in CBF secondary to a decrease in $CMRo_2$ because of a direct cerebral vasoconstrictive effect. Both are used to reduce ICP in patients with TBI. All intravenous agents preserve autoregulation in normal subjects but their influence in those with impaired autoregulation is variable. They also have minimal effects on the CO_2 responsiveness of cerebral vessels. Despite the potential advantages conveyed by intravenous agents there is no evidence in elective neurosurgical cases that they are superior to volatile agents. It is, however, prudent to use an intravenous technique in brain-injured patients because of the beneficial effects on ICP. Thiopental and propofol are both powerful cardiovascular depressants, and it is important to maintain systemic blood pressure to avoid a reduction in cerebral perfusion pressure (CPP).

Volatile agents

All volatile agents cause cerebral vasodilatation and a dose-dependent increase in CBF. Flow–metabolism coupling persists during volatile anaesthesia but the balance may be shifted to allow a higher flow for a given metabolic rate. Since volatile agents cause a reduction in $CMRo_2$, they also result in a coupled reduction in CBF. The overall cerebrovascular effect therefore reflects a balance between the direct vasodilatory and indirect flow–metabolism-mediated vasoconstrictive effects of a particular agent and dose.

Halothane is the most potent cerebrovasodilator and is no longer used during neuroanaesthesia. Isoflurane is the most marked metabolic depressant of the older volatile agents and therefore the least cerebrovasodilating. Desflurane and sevoflurane have similar cerebrovascular effects to isoflurane. Cerebral autoregulation is impaired by volatile agents in a dose-dependent manner, being preserved at 0.5 MAC but abolished at 1.5 MAC. Enflurane should not be used during neuroanaesthesia since it is epileptogenic in at-risk patients.

Nitrous oxide

Nitrous oxide is a potent cerebrovasodilator and causes a rise in ICP. It has minimal effects on autoregulation and CO_2 reactivity. However, most authorities consider that nitrous oxide no longer has a role in neuroanaesthesia.

Opioids

Morphine has negligible effects on cerebral haemodynamics and metabolism but may cause hypotension secondary to histamine release. Synthetic narcotics have variable cerebrovascular and metabolic effects but, with the exception of alfentanil, which in some circumstances has been reported to increase ICP, have little direct effect on ICP. However, all opioids have the potential to cause systemic hypotension and postoperative hypoventilation, which may have deleterious effects on CPP. Remifentanil has gained popularity because its favourable pharmacological profile confers many advantages over more established agents. A remifentanil infusion allows rapid titration of analgesic levels during highly stimulating periods but, because its context-sensitive half-life remains consistent at 3–5 minutes, rapid wake-up is not affected.

Muscle relaxants

Succinylcholine causes a transient rise in ICP, but this effect is not long lasting and is irrelevant under most circumstances. Non-depolarizing muscle relaxants have no effect on CBF and $CMRo_2$. The use of continuous neuromuscular blockade is determined by the surgical procedure and individual preference of the anaesthetist, although the requirement for neuromuscular blockade is limited if remifentanil is included in the anaesthetic technique.

Preoperative assessment

In addition to a routine preoperative assessment, special consideration should be given to focal neurological deficits, pupillary abnormalities and alterations in the level of consciousness. Attention should be paid to the use of antiplatelet drugs since it may be necessary to stop these preoperatively or specifically continue them in some neuroradiological procedures. The appropriate postoperative destination should be identified in advance (see below).

Airway management

- Endotracheal intubation and mechanical ventilation is recommended for intracranial neurosurgical procedures to allow control of P_aco_2 and maintenance of adequate oxygenation. Traditionally, reinforced endotracheal tubes have been used, although conventional endotracheal tubes are suitable for most procedures in the supine position. A well-seated reinforced laryngeal mask airway (LMA) or ProSeal LMA may be a suitable alternative in short extracranial surgery and during radiological procedures.
- Ventilation should be adjusted to maintain normoxia and P_aco_2 between 4.5 and 5.0 kPa during intracranial surgery.
- The head may be secured using a Mayfield three-point pin fixator during cervical spine or intracranial procedures. The airway is relatively inaccessible during surgery because of the position of the operative field.
- Neck positioning should remain as neutral as possible with slight reverse Trendelenburg positioning to facilitate venous drainage.
- Haemodynamic surges and coughing during intubation or patient positioning should be prevented by judicious use of opioids and muscle relaxation.
- Most elective patients are extubated at the end of surgery. Some neuroanaesthetists favour 'deep' extubation whereas others extubate all patients awake. Intuitively it makes sense to avoid coughing during extubation but there is no evidence to support one technique over the other.

Fluid management

- Circulating volume should be normalized during neuroanaesthesia. The choice of fluid (with the exception of dextrose) is less important than the volume given, and crystalloid or colloid can both be used for fluid replacement. Fluid flux across the blood–brain barrier is determined by osmolality rather than oncotic pressure and, therefore, hypotonic fluids should be avoided. Compound sodium lactate (CSL) is effectively hypo-osmolar because of the tendency for molecular aggregation of sodium ions, but there is no evidence that the judicious use of CSL for elective neurosurgical procedures is detrimental. It is prudent to use 0.9% saline for patients with an acute brain injury, although large volumes may cause hyperchloraemic acidosis.
- Unless hypoglycaemia is suspected, glucose-containing solutions should be avoided. First, after glucose metabolism the residual free water can worsen cerebral oedema and, second, hyperglycaemia is correlated with poor outcome after brain injury. Hypoglycaemia should always be avoided to ensure continued cerebral glucose supply. Aim for a blood sugar of 6.0–10.0 mmol L^{-1} in the perioperative period.
- Blood loss should be replaced with colloid and blood products to maintain haemoglobin ≥8 g dL^{-1}.

Monitoring

- Routine monitoring should include ECG, S_po_2, capnography and arterial cannulation for direct blood pressure measurement as well as intermittent blood gas sampling. A large-bore cannula and a temperature probe are also mandatory.
- Central venous pressure (CVP) monitoring will assist in fluid management if severe blood loss is anticipated or to manage comorbidities. Although placement of CVP lines in the internal jugular veins is unlikely to obstruct venous return in the majority of cases, head-down tilt should be avoided during insertion in patients with intracranial pathology. For this reason, some centres prefer femoral or subclavian routes. Practice, however, is varied as

these routes have increased risks of infection or pneumothoraces, respectively.

- A urinary catheter should be inserted for long cases or if mannitol is likely to be used.
- ICP monitoring, oesophageal Doppler ultrasonography and electrophysiological monitoring (somatosensory-evoked potentials (SSEPs), motor-evoked potentials (MEPs), VIIth nerve) may be indicated for specific cases.

Temperature management

Although moderate hypothermia (temperature ~34–35°C) reduces ICP, there are no data to recommend its routine use during neuroanaesthesia. However, many neuroanaesthetists do allow mild passive hypothermia during procedures in which the brain is most at risk of ischaemia. These include neurovascular procedures and surgery in which prolonged brain retraction is required. Under these circumstances, forced-air rewarming is used to restore normal temperature before the end of the procedure. A recent prospective randomized study investigating the role of hypothermia during clipping of aneurysms showed no significant benefit.

Positioning

- *Supine*: reverse Trendelenburg with 15–30° head-up tilt helps promote venous drainage and is suitable for most cases.
- *Prone*: used for posterior spinal and posterior fossa surgery. Careful positioning to avoid pressure on the eyes, face, axillae and breasts is essential. It is also important to ensure that there is no pressure on the abdominal contents to avoid excessive rises in venous pressure.
- *Lateral/park bench*: for lateral spinal operations and some posterior fossa surgery. Ensure that the head and body are well supported. Avoid jugular compression and pressure on nerves, particularly the brachial plexus (use axillary pad).
- *Sitting* (now rarely used): beware hypotension and venous air embolism.

Thromboembolic prophylaxis

Neurosurgical patients are at high risk of development of venous thromboembolism (VTE). Risk factors include age over 60 years, tumour excision, surgery over 4 hours and lower limb paresis. Because of the catastrophic risks of postoperative intracranial haemorrhage, clinicians remain reticent to routinely prescribe unfractionated or low-molecular-weight heparins (LMWHs). Mechanical methods provide a useful alternative, but there is little evidence to support either compression stockings or intermittent pneumatic compression (IPC) devices to prevent VTE. Practice in the UK remains varied between centres and even between clinicians. Generally, intraoperative compression stockings and IPC are used for all neurosurgical procedures, with the early use of LMWHs in high-risk patients and their introduction at 48 hours postoperatively in routine circumstances. Clinicians should be aware that the period of risk for VTE exists even after discharge.

Pain, nausea and vomiting

Neurosurgical procedures can be painful, and postoperative pain was historically poorly controlled. This was because of concerns that opioids may obscure the signs of neurological deterioration and cause respiratory depression, or that non-steroidal anti-inflammatory drugs (NSAIDs) may result in postoperative bleeding.

Paracetamol

This simple analgesic should be given routinely unless there are contraindications. The advent of an intravenous formulation has facilitated its routine intraoperative use. Paracetamol is unlikely to be adequate as a sole analgesic agent, but is very effective when given in combination with NSAIDs or opioids.

Opioids

Codeine phosphate has traditionally been used after neurosurgery because it was thought to cause less respiratory depression than other opioids. However, it remains mostly ineffectual at adequately controlling pain. Use of morphine, including by patient-controlled analgesia, is safe and effective after craniotomy. All patients receiving potent opioids should be monitored in the postoperative period to ensure that respiratory depression does not occur since elevated $P_{a}CO_2$ may cause brain swelling and deterioration in neurological status. However, there is no evidence to suggest that this is more likely with one opioid than another, or that it is a problem when appropriate doses are used.

Non-steroidal anti-inflammatory drugs

NSAIDs are frequently used after spinal surgery and by many neuroanaesthetists after intracranial surgery. The concern about increased bleeding tendency because of their antiplatelet action is probably unjustified, but some neuroanaesthetists prefer to wait 24 hours before introducing NSAIDs. In paediatric neuroanaesthesia, NSAIDs are routinely used postoperatively with no increased adverse effects.

Local anaesthesia

The beneficial effects of surgical infiltration along wound edges are often underestimated. A skull block will abolish sympathetic response to head pin insertion at the beginning of surgery and contribute to postoperative analgesia.

Nausea and vomiting

Nausea and vomiting are common after craniotomy despite the widespread use of dexamethasone and other antiemetics. There is no convincing evidence favouring one antiemetic agent over another and multimodal therapy is often required.

Other postoperative considerations

- Electrolyte abnormalities are common in neurosurgical patients and urine output and plasma electrolytes should be closely monitored and treatment initiated as appropriate.
- Seizures should be treated aggressively in the postoperative period to minimize the risk of secondary ischaemic brain damage. Some recommend prophylactic anticonvulsant therapy for 'at-risk' patients, but there is no evidence to support this practice.
- Postoperative destination: following a routine craniotomy, an extended recovery or high-dependency unit (HDU) bed is advocated in most instances.

Bibliography

Constantini S, Kanner A, Freidman A, *et al.* Safety of perioperative minidose heparin in patients undergoing brain tumour surgery: a prospective, randomised double blind study. *J Neurosurg* 2001; **94**: 918–21.

De Gray LC, Matta BF. Acute and chronic pain following craniotomy: a review. *Anaesthesia* 2005; **60**: 693–704.

Dinsmore J. Anaesthesia for elective neurosurgery. *Br J Anaesth* 2007; **99**: 68–74.

Duffy CM, Matta BF. Sevoflurane and anaesthesia for neurosurgery: a review. *J Neurosurg Anesthesiol* 2000; **12**: 128–40.

Goldsack C, Scuplak SM, Smith M. A double blind comparison of codeine and morphine for postoperative analgesia following intracranial surgery. *Anaesthesia* 1996; **51**: 1029–32.

Leslie K, Williams DL. Postoperative pain, nausea and vomiting in neurosurgical patients. *Curr Opin Anaesthesiol* 2005; **18**: 461–5.

Smith M. Post-operative neurosurgical care. *Curr Anaesth Crit Care* 1994; **5**: 29–35.

Sneyd JR, Andrews CJH, Tsubokawa T. Comparison of propofol/remifentanil and sevoflurane/remifentanil for maintenance of anaesthesia for elective neurosurgery. *Br J Anaesth* 2005; **94**: 778–83.

Cross-references

Complications of position, 743

Raised intracranial pressure/cerebral blood flow control, 791

Thrombosis and embolism, 793

Anaesthesia for interventional neuroradiological procedures

Mary Newton and Robin Kumar

Interventional neuroradiology is a rapidly evolving specialty in which radiologists perform increasingly complex and high-risk procedures in patients with a wide variety of intracranial and spinal pathologies. The administration of anaesthesia by an anaesthetist with expertise in the care of this group of patients, many of whom are critically ill, is mandatory.

Although the requirement for the provision of anaesthesia in this area is increasing, the working environment is often remote and poorly designed for its purpose. The development of interventional neuroradiological services should allow for the same standards of anaesthetic care afforded to the neurosurgical patient in the operating theatre. Ideally, there should be a dedicated anaesthetic room and the anaesthetist should always be assisted by appropriately trained personnel. All members of the team should be familiar with the clinical needs of the patients undergoing general anaesthesia and must communicate effectively, particularly when emergency situations arise. These aspects of care are reinforced by the World Health Organization Safe Surgery Checklist, modified to serve this patient population.

Neuroradiological procedures

The intracranial and spinal circulations can be accessed by fluoroscopically guided catheters inserted through a sheath, usually via a femoral artery. Microcatheters can be guided selectively into specific vessels and used to inject glue and particles, or to deploy coils or stents. The majority of interventional procedures require general anaesthesia because immobility is essential at critical moments.

- Diagnostic angiography is usually painless and performed in awake patients. General anaesthesia may be required for uncooperative patients or long procedures, such as spinal angiography.
- The International Subarachnoid Aneurysm Trial (ISAT), which enrolled patients between 1994 and 2002, demonstrated a significant reduction in risk of death at 5 years for aneurysms treated by endovascular coiling compared with surgical clipping; this has resulted in an increased number of aneurysms being treated by coiling. Stents are now also used to treat wide-necked or giant aneurysms previously untreatable by the endovascular route, but these are very high-risk procedures in patients with recently ruptured aneurysms.
- Angioplasty is used in symptomatic cerebral vasospasm that is unresponsive to medical therapy. A balloon is guided into the stenosed section of artery and briefly inflated, and the procedure repeated along the area of spasm. Additionally, vasospasm affecting larger areas may be achieved by the injection of nimodipine directly into the affected cerebral artery.
- Embolization of arteriovenous malformations (AVMs) may be performed as a staged procedure or prior to surgery or radiosurgery.
- Highly vascular cerebral and spinal tumours can also be embolized prior to surgery to reduce operative bleeding.
- Stenting (sometimes in combination with angioplasty) is an effective procedure for the management of occlusive cerebrovascular disease.
- Intra-arterial thrombolysis with recombinant tissue plasminogen activator and/or mechanical clot extraction can be used in patients with acute ischaemic stroke in whom intravenous thrombolysis has failed. Current evidence suggests that intra-arterial thrombolysis can be used up to 6 hours after symptom onset for anterior circulation stroke, increasing to 12 hours for posterior circulation stroke.

Some procedures in awake patients require the presence of an anaesthetist for cardiovascular monitoring/management and management of anticoagulation. These include carotid and vertebral artery stenting, and 'test' balloon occlusions.

- Carotid stenting is an alternative to carotid endarterectomy for occlusive carotid disease. The International Carotid Stenting Study (ICSS) 2010 recommended carotid endarterectomy as the treatment of choice for patients suitable for surgery because it is associated with lower rates of stroke and fatal myocardial infarction. However, the Carotid Revascularisation Endarterectomy vs. Stenting Trial (CREST) 2010 indicated that both procedures have similar long-term outcomes, with a possible benefit for stenting in younger patients. Profound bradycardia can occur with dilatation of the artery; therefore, atropine should be immediately available. Vertebral arteries can also be stented.

- Test balloon occlusion of the internal carotid and vertebral arteries is performed in awake patients to determine whether they will tolerate permanent sacrifice of the artery during surgery for tumour resection or the management of giant aneurysms. Anticoagulation is essential to prevent clot development proximal to the balloon and subsequent distal embolization when it is deflated. Urgent anaesthetic intervention may be required if the patient fails the occlusion test and loses consciousness.

Ionizing radiation and contrast medium

- Repeated imaging results in the use of high doses of ionizing radiation, and minimizing exposure of patients and staff is essential. The dose exposure of radiation declines proportionally to the square of the distance from the radiation source (inverse square law) so, in addition to wearing protective lead coats and thyroid shields, staff should position themselves as far as practically possible from the source. Female patients of child-bearing age should have the date of their last menstrual period checked.
- Considerable doses of contrast medium may be injected during neuroradiological procedures and dehydration should be avoided in all patients to minimize the risk of nephrotoxicity. Additionally, it is essential that the radiologist is aware of the patient's renal function (serum creatinine and estimated glomerular filtration rate) and adjusts the contrast medium dosage accordingly to minimize the risk of renal failure. There is no consensus on the use of *N*-acetylcysteine as a renal protectant. Patients on metformin should omit doses for 48 hours after the procedure or until renal function returns to normal.
- Contrast medium can also cause anaphylaxis and anaesthetists and radiologists must be familiar with the recognition and management of this life-threatening complication. Treatment algorithms should be readily available in all radiology departments.

Equipment

Equipment provision should meet the same requirements for patients undergoing general anaesthesia for complex procedures in an operating department. It is imperative that geographically remote areas are kept well stocked with drugs and equipment for the provision of a variety of anaesthetic techniques, including TIVA.

- Venous thromboembolic prophylaxis measures and patient warming should be a standard of care.
- Urinary catheterization is necessary because of the osmotic diuresis caused by the contrast medium and the large volumes of saline flush used to maintain vascular catheter patency.
- A naso/orogastric tube is required in patients requiring intraprocedural administration of aspirin or clopidogrel. The radiologist can confirm the correct position of the gastric tube during the procedure.
- An angiography table capable of head-up tilt is useful in patients with intracranial hypertension.
- Frequent movement of the table and imaging equipment increases the risk of accidental extubation and decannulation. Breathing system tubing and intravascular lines should be extended to compensate for this.
- Equipment for near-patient testing of anticoagulation should be available in the angiography suite.

Monitoring

- In addition to standard minimal monitoring, most patients require intra-arterial pressure monitoring to guide cardiovascular management (see below). Intra-arterial monitoring can be achieved via a dedicated arterial line or via the femoral sheath being used by the radiologist.
- Central temperature should be measured and hyperthermia should be avoided. Nasopharyngeal probes do not interfere with imaging.
- A peripheral nerve stimulator should be attached to an easily observed limb if neuromuscular blocking agents are used.

Conduct of anaesthesia

- Meticulous control of blood pressure during induction of anaesthesia and intubation is essential. Hypertension may result in aneurysmal/AVM rupture, and hypotension may exacerbate pre-existing cerebral ischaemia. Spraying the vocal cords with local anaesthetic prior to intubation may improve cardiovascular stability during patient transfer.
- Patient movement may interfere with image appearances and is potentially dangerous.

Therefore, tracheal intubation and mechanical ventilation is standard practice. Tracheal intubation provides a secure airway in situations in which the ability to move quickly and safely is required, such as emergency transfer to the operating theatre or CT scanner.

- Maintenance of anaesthesia with intravenous or volatile agents is acceptable. Remifentanil infusions are widely used and avoid the need for repeated administration of neuromuscular blocking agents. Nitrous oxide should be avoided to reduce the risk of cerebral or spinal cord infarction by air microemboli.
- It is essential to maintain cardiovascular stability throughout the procedure, including patient transfers. A stable circulation helps the radiologist estimate blood flow through the cerebral or spinal vasculature, and, in particular, helps to determine the required concentration and quantity of glue for injection. Sampling of arterial blood must not occur at critical steps of the procedure as loss of monitoring risks missing a change in blood pressure that accompanies aneurysmal rupture. The radiologist must be informed immediately of any cardiovascular instability.
- A strategy should be in place for the emergency treatment of hypertension if an aneurysm or AVM ruptures. Propofol is particularly valuable in this situation.
- ICU patients with an ICP monitor in place should have monitoring continued during the procedure. Significant rises in ICP can occur during transfers and when the patient is laid flat. A target mean arterial pressure should be set to achieve an adequate CPP.
- Similar care must be taken when transferring patients with external ventricular drains *in situ*. The drain should be opened slowly once the patient is properly positioned, to avoid sudden drainage. The height of the angiography table should not be altered before alerting the anaesthetist so that drain height can also be adjusted.
- Anticoagulation regimens vary from unit to unit. Heparin is commonly used to achieve an activated clotting time of twice normal. Many radiologists avoid reversal with protamine in aneurysmal rupture so that the procedure can be completed and the aneurysm secured. Nevertheless, protamine must be readily available and administered on the radiologist's request.
- 'Antiplatelet' medications such as aspirin are often administered during the procedure at the radiologist's request. These can be given via the naso/orogastric tube or intravenously if that formulation is available.
- Protocols should be immediately available for the preparation of infrequently used medications required in emergency situations. These include intra-arterial nimodipine for vasospasm, and intra-arterial abciximab (ReoPro) for intra-arterial thrombus formation.

Postprocedure care

- Patients must be managed in a recovery or critical care unit experienced in the care of neurosurgical and interventional neuroradiological procedures.
- Neurological status (Glasgow Coma Scale score, alertness, limb power) should be monitored carefully and compared with preprocedural status. Subtle neurological changes may indicate a significant complication such as stent occlusion or postembolization tumour swelling.
- There should be clearly defined instructions on postprocedure blood pressure management. Reperfusion injury can occur in patients with treated stenoses and any hypertension should be treated aggressively. Induced hypertension (as part of the triad of hypervolaemia, hypertension and haemodilution –'triple-H' therapy) may be required to treat cerebral vasospasm.
- Antiplatelet agents are often prescribed for 14 days to prevent thrombus formation on the surface of coils and stents. They should not be stopped without consulting an interventional radiologist.
- Most procedures are not painful, although significant analgesia may be required after interventions for dural lesions and bone tumour embolizations since they may become painful as the lesion becomes ischaemic. A severe, persistent headache following AVM treatment may indicate significant 'venous escape'. The early recognition of this and movement of the patient to a HDU may reduce morbidity.
- There is a significant risk of femoral artery haematoma following removal of the arterial sheath. This can be minimized by the use of vascular occlusion devices and reduced leg movement. However, protocols should be readily available for the management of major haemorrhage.

Bibliography

Brott T, Hobson R, Howard G, *et al.* Stenting versus endarterectomy for treatment of carotid-artery stenosis. *N Engl J Med* 2010; **363**: 11–23.

International Carotid Stenting Study Investigators. Carotid artery stenting compared with endarterectomy in patients with symptomatic carotid stenosis (International Carotid Stenting

Study): an interim analysis of a randomised controlled trial. *Lancet* 2010; **375**: 985–97.

Molyneux AJ, Kerr RSC, Birks J, *et al.* Risk of recurrent subarachnoid haemorrhage, death, or dependence and standardised mortality ratios after clipping or coiling of an intracranial aneurysm in the International Subarachnoid Aneurysm Trial (ISAT): long-term follow-up. *Lancet Neurol* 2009; **8**: 427–33.

Cross-references

Intraoperative hypertension, 765
Subarachnoid haemorrhage, 39

Anaesthesia for intracranial neurovascular surgery

Sally Wilson and Tamsin Gregory

Patients may require neurosurgery for treatment of cerebral aneurysms, arteriovenous malformations and other vascular abnormalities, or following intracranial haemorrhage.

Intracranial aneurysms

Intracranial aneurysms result from progressive degenerative changes in the vessel wall and usually occur at the junction of vessels in the circle of Willis (see Section 1, Central nervous system). Ninety per cent are found in the anterior circulation and 10% in the posterior circulation. The commonest site is the anterior communicating artery. The pathogenesis and risk factors of aneurysms are multifactorial (Box 10.1). Their incidence increases with age and they are more common in women.

Clinical features

The majority of patients present following aneurysm rupture with the signs and symptoms of subarachnoid haemorrhage (SAH). Usually the patient describes a severe, sudden onset (thunderclap) headache. Unruptured aneurysms may be an incidental finding or present following screening. Other presentations of SAH include:

- loss of consciousness due to raised intracranial pressure (ICP)
- seizures
- focal neurological deficits
- isolated cranial nerve palsies
- drowsiness, agitation and restlessness.

Neurosurgical treatment

Following the publication of the International Subarachnoid Aneurysm Trial (ISAT), neurosurgical intervention for intracranial aneurysms is increasingly uncommon. ISAT demonstrated that an endovascular technique (coiling) is preferable to an open approach (clipping) in patients with ruptured aneurysms in the anterior and posterior cerebral circulations. There are still some aneurysms that require neurosurgical intervention and these include those with a wide neck or difficult anatomy, or those that are too distal to be reached using endovascular techniques. There are also some patient groups (e.g. pregnancy, allergy to contrast) who are unsuitable for prolonged neuroradiological procedures. Surgery may also be required to place an external ventricular drain (EVD) in patients with SAH-related hydrocephalus.

Most intracranial aneurysm surgery is performed on unstable patients with the associated intracranial and systemic problems of SAH. Many present acutely following failure of an endovascular procedure. Others may be treated surgically if the aneurysm is associated with haematoma-producing mass effect or as an elective procedure if it has been found incidentally.

Box 10.1 Factors associated with intracranial aneurysms

- Familial (first-degree relatives)
- Smoking
- Hypertension
- Adult polycystic kidney disease
- Coarctation of the aorta
- Fibromuscular dysplasia
- Marfan syndrome
- Hereditary haemorrhagic telangiectasia

Anaesthesia following aneurysmal rupture

Preoperative assessment

- Patients with poor grade SAH may already be intubated and ventilated on the ITU.
- Patients with grade I or grade II SAH are usually extremely anxious and require reassurance. Routine sedative premedication is rarely used as it may impair conscious level pre- and postoperatively.
- Headache should be controlled with appropriate analgesia.
- Anticonvulsant drugs and calcium channel antagonists (nimodipine) should be continued preoperatively.
- Consider the many systemic problems associated with SAH.
- Cardiac function should be optimized and an ECG is essential since many patients with SAH have ECG abnormalities, including ST segment changes, prolonged QTc interval and arrhythmias.
- Hypertension should be treated: analgesia may be enough, but persistent hypertension should be managed with short-acting antihypertensive agents, e.g. labetalol.

- Patients may be intravascularly depleted and need fluid resuscitation.

Intraoperative management

Anaesthetic management is similar to that for any other supratentorial procedure but particular attention should be paid to:

- Careful induction to maintain cardiovascular stability and minimize changes in blood pressure. An increase in the transmural pressure in the affected cerebral artery can precipitate aneurysm rupture, while hypotension may worsen cerebral ischaemia and cause infarction. Rupture during induction of anaesthesia is rare but has a mortality of 75%.
- Standard monitoring includes ECG, S_pO_2, invasive blood pressure, end-tidal CO_2 ($ETco_2$), temperature and measurement of urinary output.
- Other monitoring, such as central venous pressure (CVP), electroencephalogram (EEG), bispectral index, evoked potentials and transcranial Doppler, is used as appropriate.
- Anaesthesia can be maintained with a volatile agent (e.g. sevoflurane) and remifentanil infusion, or total intravenous anaesthesia (TIVA) (propofol and remifentanil).
- The $ETco_2$ should be maintained between 4.5 and 5.0 mmHg.
- Normotension is the cardiovascular goal and hypotensive and pressor agents used as appropriate.
- Cardiac dysfunction and arrhythmias are common and should be managed with correction of electrolyte imbalance in the first instance.
- Normothermia should be maintained as intra-operative cooling does not improve neurological outcome.
- Patient position depends on the site of the aneurysm. Anterior circulation aneurysms are approached via a frontoparietal craniotomy with the patient supine, while posterior circulation aneurysms require the patient to be in the park bench position.

Intraoperative aneurysm rupture

Intraoperative aneurysm rupture occurs most commonly as the neck is dissected. At this stage, a temporary clip can be used to stop haemorrhage from the main vessel. However, if the aneurysm ruptures as the dura is being opened, and the circle of Willis is not dissected, the situation will be uncontrolled. Under these circumstances, acute hypotension is essential to allow surgical access and control of haemorrhage. Blood pressure should be reduced only to a level that allows the surgeon to gain control under direct vision by:

- deepening anaesthesia by increasing the remifentanil infusion
- boluses of thiopental/propofol
- labetalol in increments of 5–10 mg.

Following control of the aneurysm, hypertension should be induced to restore perfusion to the compromised area.

Postoperative management

Postoperative management is as for any craniotomy. A rapid smooth emergence prevents rises in ICP and allows early neurological assessment. The patient should be closely monitored in a critical care area and blood pressure fluctuations treated. If vasospasm is suspected, higher than normal blood pressure targets may be required. Consideration should be given to postoperative ventilation only if the patient was severely obtunded preoperatively or if there was an intraoperative catastrophe.

Anaesthesia for elective aneurysm surgery

This is increasingly uncommon and the techniques are similar to those for emergency cases. The risk of vasospasm is less and blood pressure control less critical.

Arteriovenous malformations

Arteriovenous malformations (AVMs) are congenital abnormalities of the vascular network in which abnormal connections between arteries and veins, without intervening capillary, result in a direct arterial-to-venous shunt and development of twisted dilated vessels. Approximately 5–10% of AVMs present acutely following a SAH, but the majority present with seizures, headache or progressive neurological signs.

Many AVMs are now treated by staged radiological glue embolization and/or gamma knife. For some this may be curative but, in others, surgical excision is required. This may be an elective procedure, but urgent intervention is required for an expanding haematoma causing mass effect.

Anaesthetic issues

- The anaesthetic technique is similar to that for aneurysm surgery, with particular attention to blood pressure control.
- Substantial blood loss can occur during open surgery.

Postoperative problems

- Severe postoperative headache may be a warning sign of intracranial haemorrhage and should prompt a CT scan.
- Since blood is chronically shunted through the AVM, the surrounding brain tissue becomes ischaemic

and local autoregulatory control is usually lost. However, once the AVM is removed, there is a return of normal perfusion to the previously ischaemic and non-autoregulating brain and this can result in diffuse swelling and microhaemorrhage. This is called normal perfusion pressure breakthrough.

- Hyperaemia may occur if the venous outflow is removed but arterial flow persists.
- Maintenance of normotension in the postoperative period reduces the incidence of complications.

Intracerebral haemorrhage

Intracerebral haemorrhage (ICH) has a high mortality and morbidity and is the cause of 10–15% of all strokes.

Pathology and aetiology

Risk factors for ICH are shown in Box 10.2. After the initial haemorrhage, there is expansion of the haematoma and surrounding brain oedema causing further neurological deterioration.

Presentation

The specific signs and symptoms depend on the site of the haematoma, but most patients present with a rapid onset neurological deficit associated with vomiting, headache, seizures and decreased level of consciousness, including coma.

Management

Many patients with an ICH, particular those with intraventricular extension, will require surgery for an EVD. Surgical treatment for evacuation of the haematoma is more controversial and still being tested in clinical studies. Patients with a large compressive posterior fossa haematoma definitely benefit from clot evacuation and some with a superficial lobar may also do better with surgery. Decompressive craniectomy is an option in patients with uncontrollable increases in ICP.

Specific issues related to the management of ICH include:

- mannitol may be used to reduce brain swelling while awaiting definitive treatment
- anaesthetic considerations are the same as for other forms of supratentorial lesions; many patients will already be intubated, sedated and ventilated on the ITU
- blood pressure control is vital pre- and postoperatively to minimize haematoma expansion and secondary brain injury
- patients often have cardiac and other systemic complications resulting from chronic hypertension and multiple comorbidities
- postoperative intensive care is often required and an ICP monitor should be inserted at the end of surgery if the patient will remain sedated.

Box 10.2 Risk factors of primary intracerebral haemorrhage

- Increasing age
- Male sex
- African/Asian descent
- Chronic hypertension
- Amyloid angiopathy
- Anticoagulation treatment
- Excess alcohol
- Recreational drugs, e.g. cocaine, ecstasy

Bibliography

Elliott J, Smith M. The acute management of intracerebral hemorrhage. *Anesth Analg* 2010; **110**: 1419–27.

Gross B, Bendok B, Hage Z, *et al.* Advances in open neurovascular surgery 2007. *Stroke* 2009; **40**: 324–6.

Hartmann A, Mast H, Choi J, *et al.* Treatment of arteriovenous malformations of the brain. *Curr Neurol Neurosci Rep* 2007; **7**: 28–34.

Molyneux A, Kerr R, Stratton I, *et al.* International Subarachnoid Aneurysm Trial (ISAT) of neurosurgical clipping versus endovascular coiling in patients with intracranial aneurysms. *Lancet* 2002; **360**: 1262–3.

Todd M, Hindman B, Clarke W, Torner J. Mild intraoperative hypothermia during surgery for intracranial aneurysm. *N Engl J Med* 2005; **352**: 135–45.

Cross-references

Hypertension, 151

Raised intracranial pressure/cerebral blood flow control, 791

Subarachnoid haemorrhage, 39

Anaesthesia for magnetic resonance imaging

Ugan Reddy and Sally Wilson

MRI produces excellent images of soft tissue. It is used extensively for imaging the central nervous, musculoskeletal and cardiovascular systems, as well as the pelvis and liver. MRI is now commonly used for interventional procedures and, more recently, to guide neurosurgical procedures.

Principles of MRI

Images are produced by placing patients within a strong magnetic field and applying pulses of radiofrequency (RF) energy. This results in intermittent release of RF energy from hydrogen nuclei, which is detected by a series of close-fitting receiving antennae known as coils. The RF signals are collected and interpreted by computer to produce extremely accurate images. The strength of the magnetic field used during MRI is measured in tesla (T). One tesla is equal to 10 000 gauss (G), and the magnetic field of the earth is approximately 0.5–1.5 G. The most common strengths of magnetic resonance (MR) scanners in clinical use range from 0.5 to 3 T, although the majority of scanners used for general diagnostic purposes are 1.5 T. The MR scanner is designed to place the patient in the centre of a magnetic field within the bore of a magnet and, as a result, the patient is effectively enclosed within a narrow tube to which access is extremely limited. Newer designs include open and wider bore magnets that allow improved access and are less claustrophobic for awake patients.

MR scans are produced in sequences of up to 10 minutes and any movement during that time produces profound distortion of the final images. The aim of anaesthesia for MRI is, therefore, to provide immobility to obtain the best possible images, while maintaining safety and patient comfort throughout.

Safety issues in MR units

- The strong magnetic field poses the most important hazard related to anaesthesia and care of patients requiring MRI.
- Ferromagnetic objects within the 50 G line will be subject to movement and may be rapidly accelerated into the magnetic field. They then become dangerous projectiles causing injury to anyone in their path, damage to equipment and interference with the MR image generated.
- Implanted ferromagnetic objects may move in the magnet or heat up significantly, causing local tissue damage. This includes foreign bodies in the eye that may be dislodged during scanning, with the associated risk of vitreous haemorrhage.
- Non-ferromagnetic metals may heat up in the scanner, causing burns. They will also cause image artefact if they are adjacent to the area being scanned.
- Implanted pacemakers, defibrillators and other devices may be inactivated, reprogrammed, dislodged or revert to an asynchronous mode by the magnetic field. Although implanted programmed devices are a general contraindication to MRI, some patients may be scanned under strictly controlled conditions in specialist centres.
- Pregnant patients and staff should not enter the scanner during the first trimester.
- Noise levels above the safe level of 85 decibels may be generated by the scanner and can cause potential hearing loss in those having long scans. Staff and all patients, whether awake or anaesthetized, should wear ear protection.

The most commonly used intravenous MR contrast agent is gadolinium dimeglumine (Gd-DTPA), which can cause mild side-effects including nausea, vomiting and pain on injection. It has an extremely low incidence of anaphylactoid reactions. However, Gd-DTPA has been implicated in nephrogenic systemic fibrosis in patients with impaired renal function. An assessment of renal function (e.g. estimated glomerular filtration rate) should therefore be performed if a patient's scan requires contrast.

Practical considerations

The MR unit is often isolated from the main operating theatres and must be self-sufficient in terms of anaesthesia and resuscitation equipment. Since the patient is placed inside a narrow bore tube for the duration of the scan, he or she is relatively inaccessible and may be difficult to observe. Furthermore, many MR units were not designed with anaesthesia in mind and space is often limited. Although the anaesthetic and recovery rooms should ideally be placed adjacent to the scanner, many units have these areas in distant sites. The arrangements for anaesthesia will therefore be determined by local circumstances, but the following general points always apply:

- all personnel must be trained in the local rules before entering the unit
- ferromagnetic items, such as scissors, oxygen cylinders and laryngoscopes, must never be taken into the scanning room.

Monitoring and equipment

Equipment used in the MR unit may be *MR safe*, which indicates that it can be used in the scanning room with no additional risk to patients or personnel. It is *MR unsafe* if it is known to pose hazards in all MR environments. Alternatively, equipment may be *MR conditional*, meaning that it has been demonstrated to pose no known hazard in a specified MR environment with specified conditions of use. Field conditions that define the specified MR environment include field strength, spatial gradient, rate of change of magnetic field, RF fields and specific absorption rate.

As well as conforming to the same standards as applied in the operating theatre, monitoring and equipment in the MR unit has additional and specific requirements:

- Monitoring should be established to allow the anaesthetist to view the monitor and patient from outside the scanning room.
- MR conditional monitors allow accurate monitoring within the scanning room. Previously, anaesthetists have used standard monitoring that has been modified for use in the scanner, or have placed monitors outside the scanning room and passed long cables through specially shielded holes in the scanning room wall. This practice cannot be recommended now that MR conditional equipment is readily available.

Box 10.3 Indications for general anaesthesia during MRI

- Children
- Ventilated and other ITU patients
- Patients with severe movement disorders
- Patients whose position is limited by pain
- Adults with learning disorders
- Claustrophobic patients
- Certain patients undergoing stereotactic neurosurgical procedures
- Patients receiving intraoperative MRI

- ECG cables must be shielded and special electrodes used. Furthermore, the magnetic field causes specific problems with ECG interpretation, including MR-induced changes in the ST segment and T waves similar to those seen with hyperkalaemia or pericarditis.
- Pulse oximeters must use fibreoptic cables to avoid burns.
- There may be a delay in obtaining a capnograph signal and monitoring of airway pressures and gases because the sampling tubing is longer than normal.
- Measurement of temperature is difficult in the MR scanner but the technology is now available to measure peripheral temperature.
- The anaesthetic machine may be sited outside the scanning room and long breathing circuits passed through the wall, as described above. However, an anaesthetic machine (with piped anaesthetic gases) should always be available inside the scanning room and this should ideally be MR conditional. Non-MR conditional anaesthetic machines must either be bolted onto the floor or kept outside the 50 G line. All gas cylinders must be MR safe.

Patient assessment

The types of patients who may require general anaesthesia during MR scanning are shown in Box 10.3.

Screening is essential to exclude those who cannot enter the magnetic field, and this is generally conducted by radiographers using a standard checklist. The exact make of an implantable device is required in order to assess its safety in the MR scanner. All patients with pacemakers and internal defibrillators may be excluded, as these devices may be inactivated by the magnetic field. Any metallic implants must be screened because aneurysm clips, cochlear implants and prosthetic heart valves may become dislodged, heat up or cause the induction of electric currents. Patients who are metal workers or who have known intraocular foreign bodies must also be screened with a plain X-ray prior to scanning and all female patients should have a pregnancy test. Tattoos may heat up in the magnetic field.

Anaesthetic management

An MRI scan is not painful, and the requirements of anaesthesia are therefore hypnosis, amnesia and immobility. Recovery will be rapid and most patients can be treated as day cases. The following are simple rules that facilitate anaesthesia in the MRI suite:

- The patient is anaesthetized on a tipping trolley in the anaesthetic room.

- Most patients can be anaesthetized using short-acting agents and a laryngeal mask airway (LMA). With a standard LMA, the pilot balloon must be taped away from the site to be scanned, as the small spring inside it may cause artefact. The airway should be clear as partial airway obstruction may cause increased respiratory movement and image artefact.
- Maintenance of anaesthesia is usually easier with an inhalational agent such as sevoflurane, as this avoids the need for MR compatible infusion pumps or the use of long extensions and a pump placed outside the 50 G line.
- Patients with a poor gag or reflux and pregnant women may need intubation and ventilation. A preformed endotracheal tube will allow close-fitting head coils to be applied, but the pilot balloon must again be taped away from the site to be scanned.
- Padding should be placed between the patient's skin and monitoring cables to prevent burns. Loops in cables must be avoided.
- Patients are transferred to a docking table or are taken into the scanning room on a non-ferromagnetic trolley.
- Contrast may be needed for scans to examine tumours or for MR angiography.
- In the event of a cardiac arrest or other critical incident the patient must be removed from the scanner for resuscitation.

Sedation in the MR unit

Many patients can have MRI successfully performed under sedation. There are different considerations for adults and children.

Adults

- Claustrophobic adults may often be adequately managed with oral benzodiazepines.
- Pulse oximetry should be used in all cases.
- Short MR sequences may improve compliance.
- Intravenous sedation must always be given by an anaesthetist and with extreme caution. Monitoring of $ETco_2$ is advisable.
- Bolus doses of midazolam or low-dose propofol/remifentanil infusion are frequently used.

Children

- Young children cannot lie still without being asleep and conscious sedation may not ensure compliance because of the noise in the scanner.
- Small infants will sleep deeply after a feed.
- Children over 7 years are often compliant without sedation.
- Many anaesthetists recommend general anaesthesia, rather than sedation, for children under the age of 7 years.
- Sedation must always be performed by adequately trained personnel and with extreme care. In some busy paediatric MR units, nurse-led sedation techniques have been developed.
- Sedation techniques include chloral hydrate, benzodiazepines and low-dose propofol infusion.
- Supplemental oxygen should always be given and adequate monitoring established.

Intraoperative MRI

Intraoperative MRI (iMRI) during neurosurgical procedures offers near real-time imaging surgical guidance. Other image-guided neurosurgical techniques are based on scans acquired preoperatively and there is significant brain shift during surgery, making such techniques less accurate. Intraoperative scanning allows the surgeon to scan the patient at an appropriate time during surgery and then conclude the surgical procedure or perform further resection. This approach is associated with improved clinical outcomes and, if repeated operations can be avoided, economic savings.

The successful use of iMRI has been reported in tumour surgery (ventricular tumours, gliomas, particularly low-grade and difficult pituitary tumours), epilepsy surgery (including placement of depth electrodes for monitoring) and deep brain stimulation surgery.

Merging of the MRI suite into an operating theatre creates a great challenge for the anaesthetist. The concerns for safety, physiological monitoring and equipment are the same as in the conventional MRI environment, but there is now the additional focus on complex anaesthesia techniques, prolonged surgical procedures, repeated intraoperative scans, intraoperative thermoregulation and the need for meticulous attention to patient positioning on the operating table and during the transfer into the scanner. With some procedures lasting more than 6 hours, cases of hyperthermia have been reported, possibly due to the RF heating effect of the scanner. Both TIVA and volatile anaesthetic agents have been successfully used in this environment.

The presence of a large multidisciplinary team in the iMRI suite highlights the need for a compulsory safety induction and training, and defined patterns of workflow. During the surgery, an MRI responsible person, usually a senior radiographer, controls the flow of people and equipment through the environment.

Bibliography

Association of Anaesthetists of Great Britain and Ireland. *Provision of Anaesthetic Services in Magnetic Resonance Units.* London: AAGBI, 2002.

Barua E, Johnston J, Fuji J, *et al.* Anaesthesia for brain tumour resection using intraoperative magnetic resonance imaging (iMRI) with the Polestar N-20 system: experience and challenges. *J Clin Anaesth* 2009; **21**: 371–6.

Keengwe IN, Hegde S, Dearlove O, *et al.* Structured sedation programme for magnetic resonance imaging examination in children. *Anaesthesia* 1999; **54**: 1069–72.

Lipson A, Gargolla P, Black P. Intraoperative magnetic resonance imaging: considerations for the operating room of the future. *J Clin Neurosci* 2001; **8**: 305–10.

Medicines and Healthcare Products Regulatory Agency. *Safety Guidelines for Magnetic Resonance Imaging Equipment in Clinical Use.* MHRA Devices Bulletin. London: MHRA, 2007.

Menon D, Peden CJ, Hall A, *et al.* Magnetic resonance for the anaesthetist. Part I. Physical principles, applications, safety aspects. *Anaesthesia* 1992; **47**: 240–55.

Morton G, Gildersleve C. Noise in the MRI scanner. *Anaesthesia* 2000; **55**: 1213.

Peden CJ, Menon D, Hall AS, *et al.* Magnetic resonance for the anaesthetist. Part II. Anaesthesia and monitoring in MRI units. *Anaesthesia* 1992; **47**: 508–17.

Serafini G, Zadra N. Anaesthesia for MRI in the paediatric patient. *Curr Opin Anaesthesiol* 2008; **21**: 499–503.

Sury M, Hatch D, Deeley T, *et al.* Development of a nurse-led sedation service for paediatric magnetic imaging. *Lancet* 1999; **353**: 1667–71.

Cross-references

Complications of position, 743
Day-case surgery, 604
Paediatrics: overview, 552

Anaesthesia for non-craniotomy neurosurgery

Shulpa Reddy and Katharine Hunt

Non-craniotomy neurosurgical operations include stereotactic surgery, insertion of stimulators for neuromodulation, and endoscopic and shunt procedures.

Stereotactic surgery

Stereotactic surgery is an established technique for the diagnosis and treatment of neurological disease. It can be used to facilitate accurate biopsy of an intracranial lesion and to guide the surgeon in 'mini' craniotomy techniques for tumour excision. It is of particular value when treating deep brain lesions or when tissue is closely associated with important functional centres. Stereotaxy is also employed in functional neurosurgery, such as the insertion of deep brain stimulators (DBSs) for disorders including Parkinson disease and dystonia, and during epilepsy surgery (for diagnosis and treatment).

Principles of stereotactic surgery

CT, MRI or digital angiography is used to image the brain and provide a three-dimensional reference to accurately define intracranial lesions. The arrangement of intracranial structures is historically related to an extracranial stereotactic frame which attaches to the head. Frameless stereotaxy is a more recent development whereby the extracranial reference system is made up of small adhesive reference markers (fiducials) attached to the patient's scalp. This is more comfortable for the patient and gives better surgical and anaesthetic access, although it is slightly less accurate than traditional frame stereotaxy.

Preoperative management

Stereotactic procedures can be carried out under local or general anaesthesia. Local anaesthetic techniques require careful preoperative preparation of the patient, but are invaluable in facilitating accurate surgery through intraoperative 'awake' testing. Drugs that inhibit tremor or rigidity may need to be withdrawn in patients undergoing stereotactic procedures for Parkinson disease or other movement disorders as they potentially mask symptoms that are assessed during surgery.

Perioperative management

The procedures may be prolonged and, if so, particular care must be paid to patient positioning and a urinary catheter inserted.

In frameless stereotaxy, the fiducials are attached and brain imaging is performed in advance of surgery with the patient awake, whereas a rigid stereotactic frame is attached to the skull using metal pins and necessitates local or general anaesthesia. This part of the procedure can be very stimulating, so a short-acting opioid may be required. Access to the airway can be challenging when a head frame is being used. If difficulties with the airway arise with the frame in place, an LMA, fibreoptic intubating endoscope or other intubating aids may prove useful.

Awake/sedation techniques for local anaesthesia

Stereotactic procedures which are usually carried out in awake patients include those in which somatotrophic localization is required, e.g. thalamotomy or pallidotomy, DBS insertion, and during some epilepsy and tumour surgery.

Local anaesthetic is applied by the surgeon to sites where frame fixator pins are to be inserted. Several techniques for sedation have been described, including small incremental doses of midazolam and fentanyl or infusions of subanaesthetic doses of propofol and/or remifentanil. Sedation should be used cautiously in all patients because of the potential for loss of airway and ventilatory control, but particularly in patients with raised ICP.

In the sedated patient, $ETco_2$ monitoring may be carried out using oxygen delivery systems with parallel end-tidal sampling ports.

General anaesthesia

There are no specific requirements for stereotactic neurosurgical procedures under general anaesthesia and a standard neuroanaesthetic technique is appropriate. During some procedures it may be necessary to transfer patients between radiology and theatre suites, and TIVA using propofol and/or remifentanil is commonly used during this time.

Postoperative management and complications

Stereotactic surgery has low morbidity and mortality compared with more invasive procedures. The more common risks are associated with DBS insertion and include broken or misplaced leads, infection, seizures, airway obstruction (local anaesthetic technique) perioperative intracranial haemorrhage and air embolism. Patients should be observed for 2–4 hours in a recovery or high-dependency area prior to return to a general neurosurgical ward.

Anaesthesia for neuromodulation

Stimulators that are inserted for neuromodulation include occipital nerve stimulators (ONSs), sacral nerve stimulators and spinal cord stimulators.

Occipital nerve stimulators

Greater occipital nerve stimulators are a means of treating primary headache disorders when medical management has been unsuccessful. The surgical procedure has three phases:

1 subcutaneous implantation of the ONS electrodes
2 confirmation of electrode position
3 implantation of the battery in the pectoral or abdominal region.

Confirmation of the electrode placement is determined by gradually increasing amplitude delivered by an external stimulator while asking the patient to describe the location and quality of the sensation felt. A vibration should be perceived at the base of the skull on the side being tested.

Preoperative management

A thorough airway assessment should be conducted preoperatively owing to the nature of the anaesthetic technique. The patient should be counselled regarding the planned technique, including intraoperative wake-up testing.

Perioperative management

- Full anaesthetic monitoring is applied.
- The patient is positioned in the lateral position with the side where the battery will be inserted uppermost.
- A technique using propofol target-controlled infusion (TCI) and depth of anaesthesia monitoring has recently been described whereby propofol TCI is titrated to achieve the varying levels of anaesthesia required for each stage of the procedure. The aim of phase 1 is to maintain sedation with airway patency without the use of an airway adjunct.
- Oxygenation of the patient during the awake phase (phase 2) can be supported by the use of nasal cannulae, preferably containing end-tidal sampling ports for respiratory monitoring. Large doses of analgesics, including opioids, should be avoided during the awake phase since they have been shown to impair patients' ability to locate the stimulus.
- When the patient is reanaesthetized for phase 3, a LMA is used to facilitate spontaneous ventilation.

Postoperative management

Intraoperative opioids and paracetamol are usually sufficient to achieve postoperative pain relief.

Sacral nerve stimulators

Sacral nerve stimulation was initially developed for patients with urinary retention but is now employed to treat faecal incontinence, constipation and chronic pelvic pain. Sacral nerve stimulators can be inserted under either local or general anaesthesia. An incision is made over the lower back and the electrodes placed in contact with the sacral nerve roots. The wire leads are then tunnelled beneath the skin to the buttock or lower abdomen, where the pulse generator is sited.

Preoperative management

A routine preoperative assessment should be carried out and a determination made whether the procedure will be carried out under local or general anaesthesia.

Perioperative management

Muscle relaxants must be avoided as correct electrode placement is identified using perineal and foot movement to stimulation. Patients are positioned in the prone position and appropriate care must be paid to pressure points.

Postoperative management

This procedure carries a high degree of postoperative discomfort. Opioids, in addition to simple analgesic therapies, will be required.

Endoscopic and shunt procedures

Endoscopic procedures may be carried out for tumour resection (pituitary surgery), and to relieve hydrocephalus. Ventricular shunts are also inserted to relieve hydrocephalus or facilitate cyst drainage, the former being the most common indication.

Hydrocephalus has a variety of causes, which largely fall into two groups:

- obstruction of cerebrospinal fluid (CSF) outflow (non-communicating hydrocephalus)
  - space-occupying lesion
  - SAH
  - spina bifida

- Arnold-Chiari malformation
  - head injury
- failure of absorption of CSF by the arachnoid villi (communicating hydrocephalus)
  - SAH
  - meningitis
  - head injury.

Shunts permit the drainage of CSF to distal sites including peritoneal, atrial and pleural.

Anaesthetic management for endoscopic and shunt procedures

Preoperative

- Patients should be assessed for signs of raised ICP, including headache, vomiting and altered level of consciousness.
- Vomiting can lead to dehydration and electrolyte disturbance.
- Shunt procedures are more common in children who need to be assessed for prematurity and congenital abnormalities.
- Blocked shunts can present as acute cases when patients may have a full stomach or decreased conscious level.

Perioperative management

- Routine anaesthetic monitoring should be instituted in the emergency situation and a rapid sequence induction may be required.
- Patients are typically placed in the supine position, although the lateral position is required for a lumboperitoneal shunt. The head may be held in the three-point pin system to facilitate some shunt and endoscopic procedures.
- Patients may require bolus doses of opioids to cover the period of subcutaneous tunnelling during shunt surgery as it is highly stimulating.

Intraoperative complications

- Hypotension can occur following the release of CSF and reduction in ICP; bradycardias may also occur.
- Subcutaneous tunnelling of the distal portion of the shunt may cause pneumothorax or haemothorax, and there is a significant risk of air embolus during ventriculoatrial shunt creation.

Postoperative management

- Patients should be woken with minimal coughing and straining.
- Analgesia should include regular paracetamol and non-steroidal anti-inflammatory drugs (NSAIDs). Morphine may be required for the initial 24 hours.
- Any new focal neurological signs should prompt an urgent CT scan in order to rule out intracranial haematoma.

Bibliography

Okun MS, Vitek JL. Lesion therapy for Parkinson's disease and other movement disorders: update and controversies. *Mov Disord* 2004; **19**: 375–89.

Pickard JD, Czosnyka M. Management of raised intracranial pressure. *J Neurol Neurosurg Psychiatry* 1993; **56**: 845–58.

Sarang A, Dinsmore J. Anaesthesia for awake craniotomy: evolution of a technique that facilitates awake neurological testing. *Br J Anaesth* 2003; **90**: 161–5.

Suh JH, Vogelbaum MA, Barnett GH. Update of stereotactic surgery for brain tumours. *Curr Opin Neurol* 2004; **17**: 681–6.

Cross-references

Complications of position, 743
Epilepsy, 12
Parkinson disease, 26

Anaesthesia for spine surgery

Michelle Leemans

Anaesthesia for spinal surgery poses many challenges. Complex comorbidities, airway difficulties, significant physiological disturbances and major blood loss are frequent associates. Advances in spinal surgery in association with changing population demographics, including a more elderly case mix, mean that these challenges will become ever more frequent.

Surgical approaches

For most cervical lesions from C3 to C7, an anterior approach to the spine, to the left or right of the trachea, with the patient in the supine position is suitable. Lesions above C3 can be approached through the mouth, at times requiring splitting of the chin, mandible and tongue. Cervical lesions behind the spinal cord or decompression at multiple levels are approached from the posterior aspect with the patient prone.

Accessing the vertebral bodies of the upper thoracic vertebrae is challenging because the major vessels and the heart overlie the vertebral column. Thus, a sternotomy or posterior thoracotomy may be required for anterior approaches. For pathology posterior to the spinal cord, the simpler posterior approach is used. The lumbar and lower thoracic vertebrae are traditionally accessed posteriorly. This is advantageous for decompression and enables a strong and rigid fixation if required. It does, however, entail detachment of major muscle groups and disruption of facet joints. An anterior approach to the lumbar spine is less frequently used and, although it avoids the need for major muscular disruption, it may require the assistance of a vascular surgeon because of the risk of vascular injury.

Patient assessment

Airway

Patients undergoing cervical surgery may have instability owing to trauma, disease or tumour. Alternatively, a disc or osteophyte may compress a nerve root or the spinal cord directly. In these instances, neurological deterioration is possible with forced cervical extension.

Cardiac

The prone position can result in significant changes in cardiac physiology, including obstruction of the inferior vena cava (IVC) and a consequent reduction in venous return and cardiac index. In addition, the associated reduction of systemic vascular resistance from anaesthetic agents can result in profound falls in blood pressure when turning patients into the prone position. Patients with cardiac disease or those with any haemodynamic compromise are particularly at risk.

Respiratory

Providing care is taken to keep the abdomen free, the prone position generally has no adverse effects on respiratory physiology and may, in fact, be beneficial. For patients with pre-existing respiratory disease, difficulties may arise in the postoperative period because of opioid use, pain and periods of immobility. These result in hypoventilation, retention of secretions and subsequent atelectasis and pulmonary infection.

Monitoring

For simple, single-level spinal procedures routine monitoring (including ECG, non-invasive blood pressure monitoring, pulse oximetry, capnography and temperature) is adequate. Arterial blood pressure monitoring is required for complex or prolonged procedures when substantial blood loss is anticipated, and serial blood gas monitoring is required in the presence of significant comorbidities. A central venous catheter (CVC) can assist with fluid balance management or delivery of inotropes/vasopressors. The internal jugular or subclavian routes may be used for thoracic or lumbar procedures, whereas a femoral CVC is more frequently used for cervical approaches. An oesophageal Doppler may be useful for monitoring cardiac output and guiding fluid administration. A urinary catheter is mandatory for long procedures and when significant blood loss is anticipated.

Evoked potential monitoring

Evoked potentials are used during spinal surgery to identify potentially reversible changes in spinal cord function and allow intervention before permanent neurological damage occurs. Somatosensory-evoked potentials (SSEPs) monitor the integrity of the sensory pathway, specifically the dorsal column. SSEPs are recorded from the cerebral cortex using scalp electrodes following electrical stimulation of a peripheral nerve. Motor-evoked potentials (MEPs) allow the integrity of the motor pathways to be assessed. MEP monitoring involves transcranial stimulation (electrical or magnetic) of the motor cortex with the evoked responses being recorded most commonly as compound motor action potentials in peripheral muscles, but occasionally via epidural/intrathecal electrodes or an electrode placed directly on the exposed spinal cord at surgery. SSEP monitoring is relatively routine during complex spinal surgery although MEPs are being increasingly used (in combination with SSEPs), particularly during excision of intramedullary tumours.

SSEPs and MEPs are sensitive to anaesthetic agents. SSEPs are preserved with low/modest dose volatile agents and during intravenous anaesthesia. MEPs are more sensitive and intravenous anaesthesia techniques, with a high-dose opioid component and no muscle relaxant, are required.

Intraoperative considerations

Airway management

Difficult laryngoscopy is common in patients with disease of the upper three cervical vertebrae, and airway access with an alternative to direct laryngoscopy may be required. Patients with limited extension at the craniocervical junction tend also to have poor mouth opening because of a direct effect as well as an association with temporomandibular joint disease.

There is no evidence that any method of airway management has a better outcome than another in patients with an 'unstable' cervical spine. External cervical spine fixation devices make direct laryngoscopy more difficult and an alternative technique (e.g. awake fibreoptic intubation) rather than the application of force should be used.

Positioning

Poor intraoperative positioning can result in cardiorespiratory compromise and pressure injury to face, nerves, viscera and peripheral pressure areas.

In the prone position the torso and pelvis are placed on specially designed mattresses which support the thorax and pelvis while allowing movement of the abdomen during ventilation. Alternatively, pillows can be placed under the thorax and pelvis respectively. Careful positioning is important because pressure on the abdomen can obstruct venous return, increase intra-abdominal pressure and inhibit ventilation. The face, especially the chin, nose and eyes, is particularly vulnerable to pressure injuries and 67% of patients suffering postoperative visual loss have been in the prone position during surgery. The mechanism of injury is probably either direct pressure injury, causing retinal artery occlusion, or ischaemic optic neuropathy, which is less well understood.

Perioperative cerebrovascular events have been documented, as a result of either dissection of the carotid artery or obstructed flow in the carotids. These events occur virtually exclusively in patients whose heads have been turned to the side intraoperatively. Care should therefore be taken to ensure a neutral position with the neck not overextended.

Peripheral nerve injuries are also well documented with ulnar nerve injuries being the most common. Risk factors include the very thin or obese, and male sex. While no particular position seems at greater risk than another, ensuring as natural a position as possible and careful padding of pressure areas seems prudent.

There have been several case reports of liver failure following prone positioning. Although the exact aetiology is unknown, ischaemic hepatitis due to obstructed venous return, hypotension and increased abdominal pressures has been hypothesized. The presentation includes severe metabolic acidosis, increasing lactate levels and elevated liver enzymes. Some patients have developed fulminant hepatic failure.

Blood loss

Massive blood loss can occur during spinal surgery. In the prone position, venous return via the IVC can be obstructed and blood then travels back to the heart via epidural veins leading to the risk of large blood loss from these veins. Although venous bleeding is usually insidious, it can be responsible for major blood loss. Catastrophic bleeding can occur as a result of injury to major vessels, including vertebral or carotid injury during cervical surgery, iliac artery injury during abdominal approaches and penetration of the aorta by misplaced pedicle screws or rongeurs during lumbar microdiscectomy. Adequate large-bore venous access, rapid transfusors, cell salvage and readily available blood and blood products should be available for all major spinal cases.

Temperature

Exposure of patients during prolonged induction of anaesthesia (e.g. during awake fibreoptic intubation), patient positioning and X-raying can lead to pronounced hypothermia prior to the start of surgery. Patients should be kept warm with forced warm air blankets and heated fluids since, hypothermia can contribute to morbidity in terms of coagulopathy and increased infection rates.

Analgesia

Spinal procedures are frequently painful. In addition to pre-existing neuropathic pain, extensive muscle retraction and disruption can lead to muscle injury and ischaemia, resulting in severe postoperative pain.

Anaesthesia for supratentorial surgery

Ian Appleby and Tamsin Gregory

Anaesthesia for supratentorial surgery provides a unique set of challenges in which the anaesthetist's knowledge and skill influence patient outcome. It requires an understanding of the regulation and maintenance of cerebral blood flow, the pathophysiology of intracranial hypertension and the effects of anaesthetic drugs on cerebral perfusion and ICP.

Anatomy and pathology

The supratentorial region of the brain consists predominantly of the cerebral hemispheres and their meninges. Most brain tumours in adults are supratentorial (Box 10.5); patients usually present with seizures, neurological deficits or symptoms of raised ICP. In children, only one-third of tumours are supratentorial; these are predominantly either glioma or craniopharyngioma.

Preoperative assessment and investigations

The indications for supratentorial surgery are shown in Box 10.6.

- All age groups may be involved.
- Cerebral metastases are frequently related to primary tumours in lung, breast, thyroid or bowel. If time permits, CT scans of the chest, abdomen and pelvis should be obtained to identify the primary tumour.
- Meningiomas may be vascular and significant blood loss can occur during surgery.
- Common primary sites for cerebral abscess include the middle ear, paranasal sinuses or lung.
- Routine medication, particularly anticonvulsants and corticosteroids, should be continued in the perioperative period.
- Although patients may be extremely anxious, careful explanation and reassurance are often all that is required and sedative premedication is rarely necessary.
- Existing neurological deficits should be carefully documented so that any postoperative deterioration secondary to oedema or intraoperative damage can be clearly identified.
- Investigations include:
  - plasma glucose: may be raised secondary to steroid use
  - electrolytes: imbalance of plasma sodium is common and may result from complications of the tumour or mannitol
  - clotting studies and blood cross-match
  - CT or MRI: the anaesthetist should always check the imaging to confirm tumour site and size, and any associated oedema and mass effect.

Intraoperative management

Induction of anaesthesia

- Smooth induction with an intravenous anaesthetic agent, usually propofol, and a large dose of a short-acting opioid such as fentanyl or alfentanil avoids coughing, straining and large swings in blood pressure.
- Non-depolarizing muscle relaxants, such as atracurium or vecuronium, are used to facilitate endotracheal intubation.
- If a rapid sequence induction is required, the prompt securing of the airway outweighs the transient rise in ICP caused by succinylcholine.

Box 10.5 Aetiology of supratentorial brain tumours in adults

- Glioma
- Meningioma
- Metastasis
- Craniopharyngioma
- Lymphoma

Box 10.6 Indications for supratentorial surgery

- Burr hole biopsy for histological diagnosis of a lesion
- Craniotomy for excision or debulking or tumour
- Aspiration of cerebral abscess for antibiotic sensitivities

- Orotracheal intubation using a reinforced endotracheal tube fixed with adhesive tape (to prevent obstruction of cerebral venous drainage by ties) is recommended.
- Monitoring for all cases should include ECG, S_po_2, ETco_2, direct arterial blood pressure and core temperature.
- Placement of a central venous catheter should be considered if there is a risk of large blood loss.
- A urinary catheter should be inserted for long cases or if mannitol may be used intraoperatively.

Positioning

The position is dictated by the surgical approach, although the supine position is satisfactory for many cases.

For all patients:

- head-up tilt (10–15°)
- avoid excessive head rotation or flexion since this impairs cerebral venous drainage
- secure the head with a horseshoe headrest or three-point pin fixator (bolus dose of opioid to prevent hypertension during pinning)
- protect the eyes with a waterproof dressing and eye pads
- before draping, check that there are no loose connections/kinks in the breathing circuit and that there is unimpeded access to intravenous cannulae
- the lateral (park bench) position is used for some temporoparietal approaches:
  - the patient is placed on his or her side with abdominal and lumbar supports
  - the lower leg is flexed and the upper leg kept straight with a pillow between the knees
  - the lower arm is flexed and the upper taped along the line of the body.

Maintenance of anaesthesia

There are some theoretical advantages but no proven outcome benefits to the use of TIVA. However, unless the ICP is critically raised, many anaesthetists use a balanced technique with controlled ventilation, opioids and a volatile agent such as sevoflurane.

- Adjust ventilation to maintain P_aco_2 between 4.5 and 5.0 kPa.
- Air–oxygen mix with F_io_2 0.3–0.5. Nitrous oxide should be avoided since it is a cerebral vasodilator and increases ICP.
- Sevoflurane, at doses of up to 1.5 MAC, reduce cerebral oxygen requirements because of decreased metabolic rate and do not affect CO_2 reactivity.
- Remifentanil infusion allows easy control of cardiovascular variables during periods of surgical stimulation and rapid emergence.
- Normothermia should be maintained using a warming mattress, warm air blanket and warmed fluids.
- A balanced salt solution should be used as maintenance fluid, but bear in mind that large volumes of normal saline can produce a hyperchloraemic metabolic acidosis. Blood loss should be replaced with packed red cells and glucose-containing solutions avoided.
- Steroids such as dexamethasone can be given perioperatively to reduce cerebral oedema and prevent postoperative nausea and vomiting.
- All patients should receive prophylactic antibiotics according to local guidelines.
- Deep vein thrombosis (DVT) prophylaxis should include the use of graduated compression stockings and pneumatic calf compression.

Intraoperative management of a tight brain

Bulging dura on removal of the craniotomy flap indicates a 'tight' brain and the following manoeuvres can be used to prevent cerebral ischaemia and improve operating conditions:

- check head position and maintain head-up tilt
- check P_aco_2 4.5–5 kPa
- control blood pressure
- deepen anaesthesia using bolus doses of propofol or thiopental
- consider dexamethasone 8–16 mg if not administered previously
- consider mannitol 20% in 100 mL aliquots.

Emergence

- Emergence should be smooth but rapid to allow early neurological assessment.
- Return blood pressure to normal while the surgeon is securing haemostasis.
- Restore normocapnia and re-establish spontaneous breathing.
- Give analgesia (morphine) and antiemetics (ondansetron, cyclizine).
- Extubate deep to avoid coughing.
- Treat emergence hypertension with labetalol or hydralazine.
- Consider postoperative ventilation only if the patient was severely obtunded preoperatively or there have been intraoperative problems.
- ICP should be monitored if the patient will be sedated and ventilated in the postoperative period.

Postoperative management

- Most postoperative complications occur in the first 6 hours (Box 10.7).

- After supratentorial surgery patients experience moderate to severe pain and analgesia should include:
  - regular paracetamol
  - opioid analgesia either orally or via a PCA
  - non-steroidal drugs are relatively contra-indicated in the immediate postoperative period but can safely be introduced later
  - local anaesthetic infiltration reduces opioid requirements.
- Postoperative nausea and vomiting are common and antiemetics should be prescribed prophylatically.
- Mechanical methods of DVT prophylaxis should be continued until the patient is mobilizing. Low-molecular-weight heparin is used in consultation with the neurosurgeon but is probably safe after 24 hours.

Awake craniotomy

This is the technique of choice for surgical procedures in which lesions are adjacent to or within eloquent areas in the motor and sensory strip, and speech area. It can also be used during epilepsy surgery when intraoperative electrocorticography (ECoG) is being used to define the resection margins precisely and during deep brain surgery to facilitate accurate placement of stimulating electrodes. Awake craniotomy allows the patient's neurological status to be assessed continually during surgery so that maximal resection can be achieved while minimizing the risk of permanent damage.

Preoperative assessment

The key to successful awake surgery is the relationship between patient, surgeon and anaesthetist.

- Identify those patients in whom contraindications to awake surgery exist. These include gross obesity, potential difficult airway, confusion, communication problems, anxiety, extreme response to pain and poor motivation.
- The anaesthetist should explain all the steps of the proposed technique in detail, highlighting that the aim is to provide an awake, lucid and pain-free experience during intraoperative testing.

Box 10.7 Postoperative complications

- Bleeding at the operative site
- Subdural haematoma
- Pneumocephalus
- Remote cerebellar haemorrhage
- Limited mouth opening after frontotemporal craniotomy, which may last up to 3 months

- Determine what neurological function(s) is going to be tested and document baseline responses.
- Explain to patients that they should communicate with the anaesthetist if they feel pain, anxiety or nausea and reassure them that these problems can be dealt with quickly and effectively.

Intraoperative management

Many combinations of sedation, analgesia and anaesthetic techniques have been described, each with their advocates and proposed advantages. They fall into three main categories: local anaesthesia, conscious sedation and asleep–awake–asleep techniques with/without airway instrumentation. The goal is to allow the surgeon to take full advantage of the patient's cooperation during the awake phase while maintaining physiological stability at all times.

The key requirements are optimal analgesia during painful stimuli, prevention of nausea, vomiting and seizures, and patient immobility and comfort during awake testing and resection. Whichever technique is chosen, effective local anaesthesia is essential.

The following is a summary of the authors' own practice:

- All theatre staff should be made aware that an awake craniotomy is taking place and personnel movements through theatre should be kept to a minimum.
- ECG, pulse oximetry and non-invasive blood pressure monitoring are initiated and small-bore intravenous access obtained.
- Anaesthesia is induced with propofol and maintained with either propofol infusion or volatile agents after insertion of an LMA.
- Large-bore intravenous cannula, an arterial cannula and urinary catheter are inserted.
- Before application of a Mayfield head fixator, the neurosurgeon infiltrates the pin sites with local anaesthetic. Anaesthesia can also be briefly deepened if required.
- Following application of the head pins, the anaesthetic agents are discontinued and the LMA removed with the patient still asleep. The patient is allowed to awaken during transfer to the operating table.
- Careful positioning of an awake patient avoids excessive neck rotation and ensures that ankles, knees and back are in the optimal position so that comfort is maximized during the awake phase.
- Once the position is satisfactory, anaesthesia is induced again with propofol and remifentanil infusions titrated to effect. Oxygen (2–4 L min^{-1}) is delivered via nasal prongs and inline CO_2 monitoring commenced.
- Occasionally, it may be necessary to support the airway with gentle chin lift and jaw thrust during the asleep phase, but we try and avoid using airway

adjuncts since these may cause irritation, coughing and even bleeding.

- Give intravenous paracetamol 1 g, dexamethasone 8 mg and ondansetron 8 mg, plus cyclizine 50 mg if there is a high risk of nausea and vomiting.
- Once the patient is asleep, the surgeon performs field blocks of the scalp with a combination of bupivacaine 0.5% and lidocaine 1% with epinephrine, and also infiltrates the incision site.
- Clear surgical drapes should be used to reduce feelings of claustrophobia during the awake phase and positioned to allow continuous and unimpeded access to the patient's airway by the anaesthetist.
- Craniotomy takes place with additional local anaesthetic infiltration of the dura.
- As the dura is being opened the propofol and remifentanil infusions can be discontinued.
- When the patient is fully awake, testing of motor, sensory and speech function can take place.
- Once testing is complete the patient is reanaesthetized for completion of the resection and closure of the craniotomy.
- During closure intravenous morphine (up to 20 mg) is given incrementally with a further 1 g of paracetamol if the procedure has lasted more than 4 hours.
- Anaesthesia is terminated as closure of the wound is completed and the patient is transferred to the recovery room for a period of fully monitored observation.
- After a period of time (4–6 hours in our hospital), the patient can return to the ward and, with appropriate support, may even go home later that day.

Airway management

Whatever anaesthetic technique is chosen, there is always the risk of airway/breathing problems and strategies must be in place to deal with hypoventilation and airway obstruction. It is our practice to have an airway trolley available in theatre with a variety of airway aids, including a fibreoptic laryngoscope. In general, the use of airway instrumentation of any sort increases the risk of coughing, straining and vomiting during 'wake up' and, for this reason, we prefer a simple technique incorporating a single insertion and removal of an LMA.

Complications

These are summarized in Box 10.8.

- Seizures can occur in up to 20% of cases, usually during epilepsy surgery, and can be treated with cortical irrigation with cold saline or bolus doses of propofol. Magnesium up to 10 g given by slow intravenous infusion at the start of surgery may also have some protective effect.
- Intraoperative brain swelling caused by respiratory depression and subsequent hypercapnia may require airway manipulation or the administration of 100 mL 20% mannitol.
- Nausea and vomiting occurs in 10–50% of patients but administration of antiemetics at the start of surgery, adequate analgesia and hydration and limiting surgical traction on the dura and meningeal vessels minimize the risk.
- Loss of patient cooperation terminates any possibility of useful functional testing and thus imposes deepening of anaesthesia to ensure the safe completion of surgery.
- Overall, awake craniotomy is a very safe procedure with minimal mortality and morbidity related to the anaesthetic technique. The conversion rate to general anaesthesia is less than 1% in our institution.

Epilepsy surgery

The aim of epilepsy surgery is to remove an area of cortex which is responsible for the generation of epileptic seizures. Clearly, there is an overlap with 'tumour surgery' since seizures are a frequent presenting symptom of brain tumours. However, formal epilepsy surgery implies resection of brain tissue in patients with medically intractable partial/complex partial seizures who have had surgery identified as the optimal treatment option during a comprehensive and detailed preoperative work-up. This includes:

- clinical history with particular reference to seizure semiology
- non-invasive video EEG recording to record at least two typical seizures and identify their cortical origin
- MRI: the most frequently identified lesion is hippocampal sclerosis
- neuropsychological testing to assess current level of performance and possible effects of planned surgery
- neuropsychiatric assessment to ensure that the patient is emotionally and intellectually capable of withstanding the rigours of the preoperative work-up and the possible psychotic side-effects of surgery.

Box 10.8 Complications of awake craniotomy

- Seizures
- Nausea and vomiting
- Dysphoric reaction
- Respiratory depression
- Airway obstruction
- Air embolism
- Loss of patient cooperation, leading to conversion to general anaesthesia

If all the above data are concordant, i.e. indicating the same origin of the seizures, 'cure' rates of around 80% are achievable with extended temporal lobectomy. If there is any doubt as to the exact localization of the seizure focus, further imaging with SPECT or PET scans, functional MRI, or invasive intracranial EEG recording may be necessary.

Preoperative assessment

As detailed above plus:

- document type and frequency of seizures
- check that anticonvulsant levels are therapeutic; because of an association with coagulation disorders, some centres discontinue sodium valproate 2–3 weeks prior to surgery and replace it with another anticonvulsant
- long-term anticonvulsant therapy may result in mild hyponatraemia, but this should not be corrected acutely
- premedication is generally avoided since benzodiazepines may impair intraoperative ECoG.

Intraoperative management

Epilepsy surgery is usually performed under general anaesthesia, but, if the site of the epileptic focus impinges on eloquent areas, an awake procedure may be required.

- Anaesthesia for epilepsy surgery is similar to that for any other supratentorial procedure.
- If intraoperative ECoG is required, anaesthesia should be maintained with moderate doses of a volatile agent, e.g. sevoflurane ≤1.5 MAC, supplemented with remifentanil. Neuromuscular blockade should be maintained.
- It may occasionally be necessary to administer proconvulsant drugs to stimulate cortical activity; alfentanil and methohexitone have been used successfully.
- Intraoperative seizures may be masked by neuromuscular blockade. Unexpected tachycardia, hypertension or a rise in $ETco_2$ should raise the possibility of seizures. Treatment includes bolus doses of propofol or thiopental and deepening of anaesthesia.

Postoperative care

- Patients should be nursed in a fully monitored recovery/high-dependency unit.
- If there are no complications after 6 hours, patients can be returned to a neurosurgical ward.

Box 10.9 Complications of epilepsy surgery

- Relating to intracranial surgery in general:
  - Haemorrhage
  - Infection
  - Stroke
- Relating to epilepsy surgery in particular:
  - Visual field defect: contralateral superior quadrantopia due to damage of optic radiation as it courses around the temporal lobe
  - Memory problems: verbal if operation on dominant hemisphere, visuospatial if non-dominant
  - Postoperative depressive illness in approximately 30% patients: usually self-limiting and lasts less than 1 year

- Seizures may occur and, if untreated, progress rapidly to status epilepticus. They should be treated aggressively with either propofol boluses (20–40 mg) or lorazepam (0.1 mg kg^{-1}; maximum dose 4 mg) and reloading with phenytoin (15 mg kg^{-1}) if plasma levels are low. Patients should be reintubated if there is any concern about their airway or if general anaesthesia is required to control the seizures. A CT scan is mandatory to exclude a surgical cause of seizures.

Complications of epilepsy surgery

Epilepsy surgery is generally very well tolerated with mortality rates <1% and major morbidity <2%. Complications are shown in Box 10.9.

Bibliography

Batoz H, Verdonck O, Pellerin C. The analgesic properties of scalp infiltrations with ropivacaine after intracranial tumoral resection. *Anesth Analg* 2009; **109**: 240–4.

Bhagat H, Dash H, Bithal P, *et al.* Planning for early emergence in neurosurgical patients: a randomized, prospective trial of low-dose anesthetics. *Anesth Analg* 2008: **107**: 1348–55.

Bilotta F, Rosa G. 'Anesthesia' for awake neurosurgery. *Curr Opin Anaesthesiol* 2009; **22**: 560–5.

Cole C, Gottfried O, Gupta D, Couldwell W. Total intravenous anesthesia: advantages for intracranial surgery. *Neurosurgery* 2007; **61** (Suppl. 5): 369–77.

Dinsmore J. Anaesthesia for elective neurosurgery. *Br J Anaesth* 2007; **99**: 68–74.

Engelhard K, Werner C. Inhalational or intravenous anesthetics for craniotomies? Pro inhalational. *Curr Opin Anaesthesiol* 2006; **19**: 504–8.

Flexman A, Ng J, Gelb A. Acute and chronic pain following craniotomy. *Curr Opin Anaesthesiol* 2010; **23**: 551–7.

Hans P, Bonhomme V. Why we still use intravenous drugs as the basic regimen for neurosurgical anaesthesia. *Curr Opin Anaesthesiol* 2006; **19**: 498–503.

Lauta E, Abbinante C, Del Gaudio A. Emergence times are similar with sevoflurane and total intravenous anesthesia: results of a multicentre RCT of patients scheduled for elective supratentorial surgery. *J Neurosurg Anesthesiol* 2010; **22**: 110–18.

Osborn I, Sebeo J. 'Scalp block' during craniotomy: a classic technique revisited. *J Neurosurg Anesthesiol* 2010; **22**: 187–94.

Randell T, Niskanen M. Management of physiological variables in neuroanesthesia: maintaining homeostasis during intracranial surgery. *Curr Opin Anaesthesiol* 2006; **19**: 492–7.

Sarang A, Dinsmore J. Anaesthesia for awake craniotomy: evolution of a technique that facilitates neurological testing. *Br J Anaesth* 2003; **90**: 161–5.

Skucas A, Artru A. Anesthetic complications of awake craniotomies for epilepsy surgery. *Anesth Analg* 2006; **102**: 882–7.

Talke P, Caldwell JE, Brown R, *et al.* A comparison of three anesthetic techniques in patients undergoing craniotomy for supratentorial intracranial surgery. *Anesth Analg* 2002; **95**: 430–5.

Cross-references

Complications of position, 743
Epilepsy, 12
Raised intracranial pressure/cerabral blood flow control, 791

Anaesthesia for trans-sphenoidal hypophysectomy

Nicholas Hirsch

Anatomy

The pituitary gland lies within the pituitary fossa (sella turcica) of the skull base. The floor of the fossa is formed by the roof of the sphenoid air sinus, the lateral walls by the cavernous sinus (containing the carotid arteries and cranial nerves III, IV and VI) and the roof by the diaphragma sella, through which passes the pituitary stalk. The anterior lobe of the gland secretes growth hormone (GH), adrenocorticotrophic hormone (ACTH), prolactin (PRL), thyroid-stimulating hormone (TSH) and follicle-stimulating and luteinizing hormones (FSH and LH), each of which affects their specific target organ. Production and secretion of these hormones are controlled by peptide hormones secreted by the hypothalamus and that pass to the pituitary via the hypophyseal portal system. The histologically distinct posterior lobe of the pituitary secretes oxytocin and vasopressin (antidiuretic hormone).

Pathology

Adenomas affecting the anterior lobe are common, whereas non-pituitary-derived tumours (e.g. craniopharyngiomas and Rathke's pouch cysts) are rare. Most pituitary surgery is performed via the trans-sphenoidal route, using either a microscope or endoscopic techniques. Pituitary tumours account for 10–15% of intracranial tumours and may present in a variety of ways, as follows.

- Hypersecretion of pituitary hormones (approximately 50% of tumours):
  - GH: results in gigantism in prepubertal individuals and acromegaly in adults
  - ACTH: results in Cushing disease
  - PRL: results in galactorrhoea and secondary amenorrhoea
  - TSH-, FSH- and LH-secreting tumours: very rare.
- Mass effect owing to the presence of large (>1 cm diameter) tumours. These are usually non-hormone secreting and present with:
  - visual field defect (classically bitemporal hemianopia) owing to compression of the optic chiasm
  - hypopituitarism (especially if haemorrhage into the tumour occurs – known as pituitary apoplexy)
  - cranial nerve (III, IV and VI) palsies
  - headache, hydrocephalus (rare).

Preoperative considerations

In addition to the usual preoperative evaluation, attention should be directed to manifestations of hormone hypersecretion syndromes.

- Acromegaly
  - Enlarged jaw and tongue, teeth malocclusion, thickened laryngeal and pharyngeal tissues and thyroid enlargement may pose airway problems. Elective fibreoptic tracheal intubation is indicated if severe airway compromise is present.
  - Obstructive sleep apnoea is common and underdiagnosed.
  - Hypertension occurs in 30% of patients and may be associated with left ventricular hypertrophy.
  - Overt diabetes occurs in 25% of patients and glucose intolerance is common.
- Cushing disease
  - Hypertension occurs in 85% of patients and is often associated with left ventricular hypertrophy and ECG changes (increased QRS voltage and T wave changes).
  - Obstructive sleep apnoea is common.
  - Glucose intolerance or diabetes occurs in 60% of patients.
  - Obesity and gastrointestinal reflux are common and may warrant administration of H_2 receptor antagonists or proton pump inhibitors.
  - High levels of circulating cortisol have an immunosuppressant effect, predisposing to infection.
  - Fragile skin requires careful handling of patients. Bruising occurs easily during cannula insertion.
- Prolactin-secreting tumours
  - Do not usually cause anaesthetically important endocrine disturbance.

Perioperative management

- Full monitoring, including direct arterial blood pressure measurement, should be established.

- Anaesthesia is induced with thiopental or propofol and fentanyl (1–2 μg kg^{-1}).
- Following administration of a suitable non-depolarizing neuromuscular blocking agent the trachea should be intubated with a flexometallic (non-kinkable) tracheal tube. If intubation problems are anticipated a fibreoptic intubation should be considered.
- Following intubation, the patient's lungs should be ventilated to a P_aco_2 of 4.5–5.0 kPa with an oxygen–air–sevoflurane mixture. This maintenance anaesthetic regimen can be supplemented with a remifentanil infusion (0.05–2 μg kg^{-1} min^{-1}).
- After placing a throat pack, a suitable vasoconstrictor (e.g. Moffett's solution or xylometazoline) should be introduced into each nostril to improve surgical conditions.
- If the patient is receiving hydrocortisone replacement for an underactive pituitary gland, 100 mg of hydrocortisone should be given after induction. Dexamethasone should be avoided as it interferes with postoperative hormone investigations.
- A single dose of a prophylactic antibiotic (e.g. cefuroxime 1.5 g intravenously) should be given.
- If the pituitary tumour is large (i.e. with suprasellar extension and a narrow base), a lumbar drain should be inserted into the subarachnoid space (see below).
- The patient should be placed supine on the operating table with a slight head-up tilt.
- Under X-ray control or using an endoscope, the surgeon enters the sphenoid air sinus and reaches the pituitary fossa by removing the bony floor. After incising the pituitary dura, the tumour is removed and nasal packs inserted.
- If there is suprasellar extension to the tumour, the neurosurgeon may request the introduction of 10–40 mL of saline via the lumbar drain. This increases intraventricular pressure and prolapses the suprasellar part of the tumour into the operative field.
- At the end of the procedure neuromuscular block is reversed, the throat pack removed and the trachea extubated following thorough suction of the pharynx and return of spontaneous respiration and airway reflexes.
- The major potential perioperative complications are haemorrhage from the cavernous sinus or carotid arteries and persistent leakage of cerebrospinal fluid (CSF).

Postoperative management

- Many patients spend a few hours in the recovery room where routine neurological observations are performed, although others should be managed in an HDU environment.
- Airway problems may occur, especially in patients with preoperative obstructive sleep apnoea. Nasal continuous positive pressure cannot be used immediately following trans-sphenoidal surgery and continued monitoring in a critical care environment may be required for at-risk patients, particularly during the first postoperative night.
- Morphine sulphate (0.1–0.2 mg kg^{-1} intramuscularly) is the analgesic of choice.
- Diabetes insipidus may occur if there has been damage to the posterior lobe of the pituitary, although this is rare in experienced surgical hands. Diagnosis should be suspected if the patient passes >1 litre of dilute urine (specific gravity <1.005) within 12 hours associated with a plasma sodium of >143 mmol L^{-1}. A plasma osmolality of >295 mOsm kg^{-1} associated with a urine osmolality of <300 mOsm kg^{-1} and a high urine output (>2 mL kg^{-1} h^{-1}) helps confirm the diagnosis. Meticulous fluid replacement (either oral or intravenous) and electrolyte monitoring is required. Diabetes insipidus following pituitary surgery is usually transient and does not require further treatment; however, if it persists, treatment with DDAVP (desmopressin acetate) may be necessary.
- If a CSF leak has been produced during surgery, CSF drainage via the lumbar drain may be required for 24–48 hours.

Bibliography

Nemergut EC, Dumont AS, Barry UT, Laws ER. Perioperative management of patients undergoing transsphenoidal pituitary surgery. *Anesth Anal* 2005; **101**: 1170–81.

Smith M, Hirsch NP. Pituitary disease and anaesthesia. *Br J Anaesth* 2000; **85**: 3–14.

Cross-references

Adrenocortical insufficiency, 46
Complications of position, 743
Diabetes insipidus, 58
Pituitary disorders and hypopituitarism, 78

Anaesthetic and ICU management of the head-injured patient

David Highton and Martin Smith

Intraoperative management

Patients with TBI require anaesthesia for treatment of the primary intracranial pathology or for surgery to associated extracranial injuries.

Preoperative assessment

Most head-injured patients present on an emergency basis and time for assessment may be limited. However, the importance of a rapid yet thorough preoperative check cannot be overemphasized.

Principles of optimal anaesthetic management

- Continue initial resuscitation.
- Maintain cerebral perfusion and oxygenation:
  - mean blood pressure >90 mmHg
  - P_aO_2 >13.0 kPa
  - P_aCO_2 4.5–5.0 kPa
  - ICP <20 cmH_2O.
- Maintenance of low venous pressure - good neck position, head-up tilt.
- Prevent or treat fluid and electrolyte abnormalities.
- Correct coagulation abnormalities.
- Prevent or treat seizures.

Management considerations

Head-injured patients do not have reduced anaesthetic requirements and inadequate anaesthesia allows surgical stimulus to increase CBF, ICP and $CMRO_2$, all of which may be detrimental to the injured brain. The choice of anaesthetic technique depends on the preferences of the individual practitioner, bearing in mind the effects of anaesthetic agents on intracranial physiology as well as the clinical state of the patient (see General principles of neuroanaesthesia, p. 300). Nitrous oxide should be avoided, but a volatile technique using an air–oxygen mix with low-dose sevoflurane is acceptable. Some recommend the use of TIVA with propofol and remifentanil, particularly in the presence of intracranial hypertension. However, there is no firm evidence that one technique is generally better than another so long as these simple principles are followed:

- smooth induction
- haemodynamic stability
- maintenance of cerebral perfusion
- prevention of rises in CBF, ICP and $CMRO_2$
- consideration of requirement for postoperative ventilation
- rapid emergence for neurological assessment if the patient will not be ventilated postoperatively.

Intraoperative problems

Bleeding

Venous bleeding occurs most frequently and can be difficult to control as cerebral venous pressure rises with increasing ICP. Treatment includes reduction in ICP, prevention or correction of venous obstruction and correction of severe hypothermia.

Brain swelling

Acute brain swelling is life-threatening. Treatment includes optimizing the patient's position, discontinuation of the volatile agent, moderate hyperventilation, propofol or barbiturates, CSF drainage and decompressive craniectomy. More aggressive hyperventilation may be life-saving in the acute phase, and the risk of cerebral ischaemia may be minimized by continuous monitoring of cerebral oxygenation or the temporary use of hyperoxia (see below).

Blood pressure

Acute intracranial lesions (particularly extradural and subdural haematoma) are often associated with intense sympathetic stimulation, leading to an increase in systemic vascular resistance and tachycardia. This may mask relative hypovolaemia, which, if untreated, can lead to cardiovascular collapse during surgical decompression. It is important to have a high index of suspicion and initiate early and vigorous fluid therapy. Moderate hypertension (systolic blood pressure ~140 mmHg) should not be treated prior to decompression of an intracranial mass lesion because the high arterial pressure may be required to maintain an adequate CPP in the face of raised ICP.

Coagulopathy

Coagulation abnormalities may be precipitated by ischaemic brain. Hypothermia and massive blood transfusions complicate the picture.

Fluid and electrolyte imbalance

Fluid management can be complicated in head-injured patients by multisystem injury and hypovolaemia. Maintenance of normal or supranormal circulatory volume should be achieved with colloids or crystalloid. Glucose-containing solutions should be avoided unless the patient is hypoglycaemic. Blood loss should be replaced with blood products. Electrolyte abnormalities are common after head injury, and urine output and plasma electrolytes should be monitored closely and treatment initiated as appropriate.

Intensive care management

The aim of the intensive care management of patients with TBI is to prevent and treat secondary ischaemic brain injury using a multifaceted physiological neuroprotective strategy that includes minimizing secondary physiological insults. The ICU management of TBI has undergone extensive revision as evidence accumulates that long-standing and established practices are not as efficacious or innocuous as previously believed. Although it is likely that specialist neurological care, with ICP- and CPP-guided therapy, might benefit patients with severe head injury, there remains a wide variation in clinical practice.

Monitoring

Systemic and cerebral monitoring techniques have been discussed elsewhere.

Treatment

The management of TBI has historically concentrated on a reduction in ICP to prevent secondary ischaemic insults. Although there is limited high-quality evidence that this improves outcome, ICP >20 mmHg is a powerful predictor of poor outcome and consensus guidance recommends that treatment should be initiated if the ICP is >20 mmHg. However, there has been a change in emphasis over recent years, and attention has focused on the maintenance of adequate cerebral perfusion and oxygenation rather than on the reduction of ICP *per se*.

Maintenance of cerebral perfusion pressure

CPP can be maintained using aggressive fluid replacement and cardiovascular support with vasopressors and inotropes to increase mean arterial blood pressure (MAP). However, this approach increases the incidence of cardiovascular complications and acute lung injury. Because of this, the Brain Trauma Foundation now recommends that CPP should be maintained between 50 and 70 mmHg and specifically cautions against CPP >70 mmHg because of excess morbidity and mortality from systemic complications. It is now evident that a CPP threshold exists on an individual basis after TBI, and multimodal monitoring may assist the clinician in selecting the optimal CPP for each patient and in balancing the risks and benefits of particular treatment strategies.

An alternative approach (the Lund concept) adopts a lower CPP target (>50 mmHg) and uses volume-targeted therapy to maintain euvolaemia and oncotic pressure in order to minimize capillary hydrostatic pressure and brain oedema. Lund therapy is not widely practised.

Control of intracranial pressure

Sedation

Intravenous anaesthetic agents are often used to reduce ICP in patients with severe head injury. They produce a dose-dependent reduction in cerebral metabolism, CBF and ICP while maintaining pressure autoregulation and carbon dioxide reactivity. Propofol has become the sedative of choice on the neurointensive care unit, but care must be taken to avoid hypotension. The use of barbiturates is restricted to intracranial hypertension resistant to other interventions since they are associated with significant side-effects. Neuromuscular blocking drugs have no direct effect on ICP, but may prevent rises produced by coughing and straining on the tracheal tube.

Hyperosmolar therapy

Mannitol has been a mainstay of treatment of intracranial hypertension, although it has never been subject to a randomized controlled clinical trial against placebo. Mannitol (0.5 g kg^{-1}) effectively improves elevated ICP, CBF and CPP in certain settings of intracranial hypertension and may improve neurological outcome. ICP-directed treatment is more beneficial than treatment directed by neurological signs or physiological indicators. Prolonged administration may result in passage of mannitol from the blood into the brain, where it might cause increased ICP. Its use should always be discontinued when it no longer produces a significant and sustained reduction in ICP. Plasma osmolarity should also be monitored regularly during mannitol therapy.

Hypertonic saline is an alternative to mannitol and is gaining popularity in the treatment of intracranial hypertension. Its beneficial effects are likely to be related not only to an osmotic effect but also to haemodynamic, vasoregulatory, immunological and neurochemical effects. There are no large, randomized comparisons of hypertonic saline with conventional osmotic agents or long-term functional outcome studies. The optimal osmolar load to lower elevated ICP has also not been defined.

Hyperventilation

Hyperventilation was once the mainstay of treatment of intracranial hypertension. It decreases ICP because of reductions in CBF and CBV secondary to cerebral vasoconstriction. However, empirical and excessive hyperventilation can precipitate regional ischaemia and are associated with adverse neurological outcomes. The routine use of hyperventilation is therefore discouraged, and current guidance recommends $P_{a}CO_2$ targets of 4.5–5.0 kPa. Modest hyperventilation (4.0–4.5 kPa) may be indicated to control intracranial hypertension in selected cases, but should be undertaken in conjunction with cerebral oxygenation monitoring to ensure that hyperventilation does not precipitate cerebral ischaemia.

Therapeutic hypothermia

Moderate hypothermia (33–35°C) is neuroprotective in animal studies, but the results of clinical trials have been disappointing. A prospective, randomized study of moderate hypothermia (33°C) in TBI was terminated early because of increased morbidity in patients over 45 years old treated with hypothermia. There was possible benefit to patients who presented already hypothermic, but older patients had such high rates of medical complications that hypothermia was detrimental regardless of their admission temperature. However, moderate hypothermia is an effective method of reducing raised ICP and is a treatment option in younger patients. Hyperthermia should be avoided and, because brain temperature is higher than core temperature, this potential adverse effect may go unnoticed.

Neurosurgery

Drainage of CSF via an external ventricular drain is an effective means of reducing ICP. Another option for treating refractory intracranial hypertension is decompressive craniectomy – an operation to remove a large area of skull to increase the volume of the cranial cavity and thus decrease its pressure. Although this technique is gaining in popularity, there is divided opinion on the relative benefits and risks.

General aspects of care

Ventilatory support of patients with head injury is vital to ensure maintenance of normal arterial blood gases. Respiratory complications secondary to head injury are common and many patients require advanced ventilatory support within a short period of time. Euvolaemia is the primary resuscitative goal and different fluids may be used to support CPP, with the emphasis on preserving adequate intravascular volume. In the presence of adequate circulating volume, norepinephrine offers predictable and efficient control of blood pressure and CPP.

Head-injured patients have a high calorific requirement and early feeding has been associated with improved neurological outcome. Non-pharmacological methods of thromboembolic prophylaxis should be instituted from admission and LMWH instituted as soon as possible. Disorders of sodium homeostasis are common and should be investigated. Consideration should also be given to seizure control, although routine prophylaxis is controversial and offers no benefit beyond 7 days.

Glycaemic control

Hyperglycaemia exacerbates secondary cerebral ischaemic injury and worsens neurological outcome. The mechanisms underlying this effect include hyperosmolality, lactic acid production, alterations in neuronal pH and increases in excitatory amino acids. The targets for systemic glycaemic control after TBI are not established, and there is accumulating evidence that 'tight' glycaemic control with insulin infusion might result in cerebral hypoglycaemia in a substantial number of patients. Current evidence suggests that systemic glucose levels should not be treated unless >10.0 mmol L^{-1}.

Bibliography

Brain Trauma Foundation. Guidelines for the management of severe traumatic brain injury. *J Neurotrauma* 2007; **24**: S1–S106.

Citerio G, Cormio M. Sedation in neurointensive care: advances in understanding and practice. *Curr Opin Crit Care* 2003; **9**:120–6.

Clifton GL, Miller ER, Choi SC, *et al.* Lack of effect of induction of hypothermia after acute brain injury. *N Engl J Med* 2001; **344**: 556–63.

De Deyne C. Therapeutic hypothermia and traumatic brain injury. *Curr Opin Anaesthesiol* 2010; **23**: 258–62.

Helmy A, Vizcaychipi M. Traumatic brain injury: intensive care management. *Br J Anaesth* 2007; **99**: 32–42.

Himmelseher S. Hypertonic saline solutions for treatment of intracranial hypertension. *Curr Opin Anaesthesiol* 2007; **20**: 414–26.

Lim HB, Smith M. Systemic complications after head injury: a clinical review. *Anaesthesia* 2007; **62**: 474–82.

Prakash A, Matta B. Hyperglycaemia and neurological injury. *Curr Opin Anaesthesiol* 2008; **21**: 265–9.

Smith M. Neurocritical care: has it come of age? *Br J Anaesth* 2004; **93**:753–5.

Wakai A, Roberts I, Schierhout G. Mannitol for acute traumatic brain injury. *Cochrane Database Sys Rev* 2005; (1): CD001049.

White H, Venkatesh B. Cerebral perfusion pressure in neurotrauma: a review. *Anesth Analg* 2008; **107**: 979–88.

Cross-references

General principles of neuroanaesthesia, 300
Head injury, 16
Neuromonitoring, 338
Raised intracranial pressure/cerebral blood flow control, 791

Neuromonitoring

David Highton and Martin Smith

Neuromonitoring allows the early detection of evolving brain injury, provides targets for therapy and may assist in the prediction of outcome. Multiple modalities providing information on pressure, haemodynamics, oxygenation, metabolism and neuronal activity are available, and each has strengths and weaknesses. No ideal monitor exists, but knowledge of the characteristics and limitations unique to each modality aids in their application and interpretation.

Intracranial pressure

ICP cannot be reliably estimated from any specific clinical feature or CT finding and must actually be measured. ICP monitoring is widely used in neurointensive care and provides targets for ICP- and CPP-guided therapy. Changes in intracranial volume and compliance are reflected by an increasing ICP and may herald intracranial changes amenable to treatment, e.g. an expanding mass lesion or cerebral oedema. ICP monitoring also allows determination of CPP (CPP = MAP – ICP) and detection of abnormal ICP waveforms which, with their derivatives, define pathology and physiological processes, including blood flow autoregulation and compensatory reserve.

There are two main methods of monitoring ICP. The gold standard is measurement of global ICP via a catheter placed in a lateral ventricle. This method has the advantage of allowing CSF drainage to reduce ICP but is associated with complications including haemorrhage and ventriculitis. It also requires a surgical procedure for insertion. Fibreoptic and microtransducer devices are miniature probes that can be inserted directly into the brain parenchyma via a cranial access device at the bedside or during neurosurgery. Microtransducers are reliable and associated with low complication rates, but measure localized pressure that may not always reflect global ICP.

Cerebral blood flow

Transcranial Doppler ultrasonography

Transcranial Doppler ultrasonography (TCD) is a non-invasive bedside measure of cerebral arterial flow velocity. Large cerebral vessels are insonated with a 2 MHz ultrasound beam through one of several acoustic windows in the skull, and flow velocity is measured from the Doppler shift caused by red blood cells moving through the field of view. Isolation of specific arterial signals (e.g. the middle cerebral artery) by spatial relationships, direction of flow and response to compression manoeuvres requires experience, is user dependent and is prone to some variability. Long-term recordings are also limited by the need for accurate and immovable Doppler probe fixation, thus realistically restricting TCD to an intermittent monitoring technique.

TCD is non-invasive and, although it does not measure CBF directly, it has diagnostic utility in many circumstances. Provided arterial diameter remains static, flow velocity is related to CBF and can be used to assess flow trends, cerebral vascular reactivity and pressure autoregulation. Flow velocity increases in the presence of cerebral vasoconstriction and TCD is therefore widely used in the evaluation and monitoring of cerebral vasospasm after subarachnoid haemorrhage.

Continuous quantitative cerebral blood flow monitoring

Bedside, quantitative measurement of absolute regional CBF is possible using thermal diffusion flowmetry (TDF). The TDF catheter consists of a thermistor heated to a few degrees above tissue temperature and a second, more proximal, temperature probe. The temperature difference between the thermistor and the temperature probe is a reflection of heat transfer and can be translated into a measurement of CBF.

Cerebral autoregulation

Cerebrovascular autoregulation is frequently impaired after brain injury, rendering the brain more susceptible to ischaemic insults. Established methods of testing static and dynamic cerebrovascular autoregulation are interventional or intermittent and may be difficult to perform in critically ill patients. Monitoring and correlation of spontaneous slow waves in arterial blood pressure and ICP allow calculation of a pressure reactivity index as a novel method of measuring cerebrovascular autoregulation. The pressure reactivity index may be used to define individual CPP targets and offer prognostic information after TBI.

Cerebral oxygenation

Cerebral hypoxia/ischaemia occurs in a wide range of clinical scenarios. Several methods of measuring cerebral oxygenation have been developed to detect hypoxia/ischaemia and guide management.

Jugular venous bulb oximetry

The jugular bulb lies at the superior end of the internal jugular vein and is the final common pathway for venous blood draining from the cerebral hemispheres. Jugular bulb oxygen saturation ($S_{jv}O_2$) is a flow-weighted average of cerebral venous blood and therefore reflects the balance between cerebral oxygen supply and demand. A catheter is directed cephalad within the internal jugular vein so that its tip lies in the jugular bulb. Intermittent samples may be analysed in a co-oximeter and continuous readings are possible if a fibreoptic catheter is used.

The normal range for $S_{jv}O_2$ is 55–75%. Reductions below 50% suggest cerebral hypoperfusion (oxygen demand exceeds supply) and are associated with adverse neurological outcome after head injury. $S_{jv}O_2$ above 85% indicates relative hyperaemia or arteriovenous shunting and is also associated with a poor outcome. Because jugular venous oximetry is a global measure, normal or supranormal values cannot exclude regional ischaemia and limit the sensitivity of the technique.

The jugular venous catheter must be correctly placed to prevent contamination from the extracranial circulation. This is minimal when the catheter tip lies at the level of the first vertebral body on a lateral cervical spine radiograph. Aspiration of blood samples must also be slow to avoid contamination with distal venous blood. $S_{jv}O_2$ also accurately reflects global cerebral oxygenation only if the dominant jugular bulb is cannulated, although, in practice, the right is often chosen.

Brain tissue oxygen tension

Focal brain tissue oxygen tension ($P_{ti}O_2$) can be measured using a small microprobe incorporating a Clark electrode. The probe is inserted into brain parenchyma and measures $P_{ti}O_2$ within a focal area of brain tissue. $P_{ti}O_2$ reflects many variables, but most crucially cerebral oxygen delivery and metabolic rate, as well as arterial PO_2. The normal range of $P_{ti}O_2$ is 3.5–5.0 kPa, but absolute thresholds for abnormality are not well established. $P_{ti}O_2$ may be used to guide treatment after brain injury, and there is growing evidence that $P_{ti}O_2$-directed therapy might improve outcome compared with standard approaches. Reductions in $P_{ti}O_2$ below 1.0 kPa are associated with critical reductions in CBF and adverse neurological outcome after head injury.

Near-infrared spectroscopy

Near-infrared spectroscopy (NIRS) is a non-invasive, real-time, continuous, bedside technique based on the transmission and absorption of near-infrared (NIR) light (700–950 nm) as it passes through tissue. Oxygenated and deoxygenated haemoglobin have characteristic, and different, absorption spectra in the NIR and their relative concentrations in tissue can be determined by their absorption of light at these wavelengths. Modern technology measures absolute cerebral tissue oxygen saturation, a measure of the balance between oxygen supply and demand. However, the utility of this measure is confounded by the optical complexity of the injured brain and changes in systemic physiological variables. Clinical applications are limited by these issues, which are often not appreciated by clinicians. Non-invasive cerebral oximetry using NIRS is gaining popularity for brain monitoring during cardiac surgery and carotid endarterectomy, but there is currently no evidence to support its widespread application as a monitor of cerebral well-being during routine surgical procedures or in critically ill patients on the ICU.

Cerebral microdialysis

Cerebral microdialysis measures local tissue biochemistry and provides unique information regarding the cellular metabolic environment. A miniature catheter is placed intraparenchymally, usually within 'at-risk' or pericontusional brain tissue. Diffusion of molecules across the semipermeable dialysis membrane at the tip of the catheter allows collection of substances from the brain extracellular fluid in the microdialysate. Bedside analysis of the dialysate allows assessment of changes in brain extracellular fluid glucose, glutamate, glycerol and the lactate–pyruvate ratio. Together, these variables monitor tissue hypoxia/ischaemia and cellular energy failure, and biochemical trends can be used to guide individualized therapy after brain injury. Because it measures changes at the cellular level, microdialysis also has the potential to detect cerebral hypoxia/ischaemia before changes can be detected by more conventional monitoring techniques or in clinical status.

Electrophysiological monitoring

Electroencephalography

The EEG is the measurement of spontaneous electrical activity in the cerebral cortex using pairs of between 10 and 20 electrodes applied to the surface of the scalp. Characteristic waveforms are obtained in the normal EEG (Table 10.2) and classic (often diagnostic) changes are described in a variety of clinical situations. The EEG can be used to guide depth of sedation in head-injured patients and to diagnose and guide therapy in those suffering from seizures or status epilepticus.

Table 10.2 Characteristic EEG waveforms

Waveform	Frequency range	Characteristics
Alpha	8–13 Hz	Normal waveform, seen at all ages Disappears with attention, e.g. mental arithmetic
Beta	>13 Hz	Small amplitude, seen in all age groups Augmented by drugs, including barbiturates and benzodiazepines
Theta	3.5–7.5 Hz	Seen in sleep Abnormal in awake adults Known collectively with delta waves as slow waves
Delta	<3 Hz	Seen in deep sleep in adults and infants Abnormal in the awake adult Large-amplitude waves

Measurement and interpretation of EEG requires skilled technicians and physicians and continuous monitoring can be cumbersome. Processed EEG techniques have been developed to allow more user-friendly continuous monitoring during neurocritical care.

Evoked potentials

SSEPs are the electrical response of the cerebral cortex, brainstem and spinal cord to electrical stimulation of a peripheral nerve and are used to assess the integrity of the relevant afferent pathway. Alternatively, in MEP monitoring, the brain and spinal cord is stimulated electrically or magnetically and the evoked response measured in the relevant peripheral muscle. SSEPs and MEPs are often monitored during spinal surgery to confirm the integrity of the spinal cord during manipulation or instrumentation. Brainstem auditory-evoked potentials can be used to assess brainstem function and anaesthetic depth.

Multimodal monitoring

Combining readings from multiple modalities overcomes many of the limitations of individual techniques. Multimodal monitoring allows cross-validation between monitors, artefact rejection and greater confidence to make treatment decisions.

Many challenges exist with the clinical applicability of multimodal monitoring. Communication and synchronization between proprietary devices remains problematic and the difficulties with interpretation, processing and presentation of large datasets should not be underestimated. Optimal monitoring combinations remain a matter of debate but it is likely that the process of miniaturization will eventually result in multiple novel combinations of modalities within a single device.

Bibliography

Dunn IF, Ellegala DB, Kim DH, Litvack ZN. Neuromonitoring in neurological critical care. *Neurocrit Care* 2006; **4**: 83–92.

Friedman D, Claassen J. Continuous electroencephalogram monitoring in the intensive care unit. *Anesth Analg* 2009; **109**: 506–23.

Goodman RC, Robertson CS. Microdialysis: is it ready for prime time? *Curr Opin Crit Care* 2009; **15**: 110–17.

Highton D, Elwell C, Smith M. Noninvasive cerebral oximetry: is there light at the end of the tunnel? *Curr Opin Anaesthesiol* 2010; **23**: 576–81.

Nortje J, Gupta AK. The role of tissue oxygen monitoring in patients with acute brain injury. *Br J Anaesth* 2006; **97**: 95–106.

Smith M. Monitoring intracranial pressure in traumatic brain injury. *Anesth Analg* 2008; **106**: 240–8.

Tisdall M, Smith M. Multimodal monitoring in traumatic brain injury: current status and future directions. *Br J Anaesth* 2007; **99**: 61–7.

White H, Baker A. Continuous jugular venous oximetry in the neurointensive care unit: a brief review. *Can J Anaesth* 2002; **49**: 623–9.

Cross-reference

Raised intracranial pressure/cerebral blood flow control, 791

11 Ophthalmic surgery

Roger M Slater

Bibliography

Eke T, Thomson JR. Serious complications of local anaesthesia for cataract surgery: a 1 year national survey in the United Kingdom. *Br J Ophthalmol* 2007; **91**: 470–5.

Johnson RW. Anatomy for ophthalmic anaesthesia. *Br J Anaesth* 1995; **75**: 80–7.

Moffat A, Cullen PM. Comparison of two standard techniques of general anaesthesia for day-case cataract surgery. *Br J Anaesth* 1995; **74**: 145–8.

Mokashi A, Leatherbarrow B, Slater R, *et al.* Patient communication during cataract surgery. *Eye* 2004; **18**: 147–51.

Royal College of Anaesthetists and Royal College of Ophthalmologists. *Local Anaesthesia for Intraocular Surgery*. London: Joint Working Party of the Royal College of Anaesthetists and Royal College of Ophthalmologists, 2001.

Rubin AP. Complications of local anaesthesia for ophthalmic surgery. *Br J Anaesth* 1995; **75**: 93–6.

Schulenburg H, Sri-Chandana C, Lyons G, *et al.* Hyaluronidase reduces local anaesthetic volumes for sub-Tenon's anaesthesia. *Br J Anaesth* 2007; **99**: 717–20.

Stevens J. A new local anaesthesia technique for cataract extraction by one quadrant sub-Tenon's infiltration. *Br J Ophthalmol* 1992; **76**: 670–4.

Cross-references

Day-case surgery, 604
The elderly patient, 607
Infants and children, 615

Corneal transplant

Roger M Slater

The cornea is the most important focusing element of the eye. Scarring causes impaired focusing. Endothelial cells maintain a clear cornea. Endothelial cell loss occurs with age and with inflammation inside the eye and following eye trauma/surgery. Corneal graft surgery places a new cornea with a full complement of endothelial cells.

Procedure

Penetrating keratoplasty

- A full-thickness disc of cornea is cut out and replaced with donor cornea that is sutured in place.

Lamellar keratoplasty

- The inner layers of the cornea are left intact and the donor cornea is sutured on top.

Patient characteristics

- Atopy associated with the corneal condition of keratoconus.
- Associated connective tissue disorders, such as rheumatoid arthritis, systemic lupus erythematosus (SLE), Wegener's granulomatosis, sarcoidosis.
- Paediatric corneal disease in Down, Alport, Marfan and Goldenhar syndromes, fetal alcohol syndrome, myotonic dystrophy and achondroplasia.

Problems

- Airway is not accessible under the operating microscope.
- Sudden changes in choroidal blood volume and in episcleral venous pressure can compromise the operating field by marked swings in IOP.
- Less suitable for local anaesthesia, in view of risks of coughing and hypertensive responses.

Preoperative assessment

- Identification and optimization of associated or coexisting medical conditions.
- Routine grafts may be managed as day-case procedures.

Anaesthetic management

- Routine monitoring as per AAGBI guidelines.

Local anaesthesia

- For uncomplicated corneal grafts.
- May be appropriate in medically compromised patients.
- Technique used must provide akinesia, IOP control and last for the duration of the surgery (up to 90 minutes).
- Paralysis of the orbicularis orbis is needed to prevent squeezing of the eye.
- *Peribulbar anaesthesia*: 10 mL of a mixture of 2% lidocaine and 0.5% bupivacaine with hyaluronidase 150 units given as an inferolateral and a medial caruncle injection. Ocular compression for 10–15 minutes prior to surgery to reduce IOP.
- *Sub-Tenon's anaesthesia*: 5 mL 0.5% bupivacaine with hyaluronidase 75 units provides lasting anaesthesia and akinesia of the globe. Orbicularis orbis is blocked with a medial caruncle injection of 2–3 mL of the same anaesthetic solution. Ocular compression to reduce IOP.
- *Sedation*: as with all intraocular surgery, patient cooperation is required, but small doses of intravenous benzodiazepine (midazolam 0.5–1.0 mg) or low-dose propofol target-controlled infusion (TCI) (target blood concentration 0.5–1 μg mL^{-1}) can make the procedure more comfortable for the patient. With sedation, oxygen supplementation and careful monitoring are vital as there is limited access to the patient. Careful attention to comfort and warmth ensure a relaxed and still patient.

General anaesthesia

Induction

- TIVA with TCI of propofol and a remifentanil infusion provide excellent operating conditions.
- TIVA also provides rapid and smooth emergence from anaesthesia, with reduced PONV.
- Alternatively, a balanced technique using intravenous induction with propofol, fentanyl or remifentanil infusion, muscle relaxant and volatile agent is suitable.

Airway management

- A reinforced laryngeal mask, unless contraindicated, provides ideal emergence conditions.

- Laryngoscopy and intubation can markedly raise the IOP by raising the systolic pressure. Various methods have been used to obtund this reflex. The use of propofol with an opiate such as alfentanil successfully reduces this rise.
- Insertion of a laryngeal mask causes a lesser rise in the IOP.
- Extubation with coughing or gagging on the tracheal tube causes a rise in the IOP.
- There is minimal coughing and straining in patients recovering with a laryngeal mask *in situ*.

Anaesthetic agents

- All intravenous induction agents apart from ketamine will lower the IOP.
- Propofol produces the most marked reduction in the IOP.
- Ketamine does not lower the IOP and may increase it.
- Inhalation anaesthetics all lower the IOP if there is a normal or low $P\text{CO}_2$.
- Intravenous opioids and benzodiazepines will lower the IOP.
- The non-depolarizing muscle relaxants will reduce the IOP by reducing extraocular muscle tone.
- Succinylcholine will cause a rise in IOP that lasts up to about 10 minutes. However, if it is given following a sleep dose of propofol, the IOP does not rise to above the resting value owing to the reduction in the IOP caused by the propofol.
- The effect of succinylcholine is due to contraction of the extraocular muscles.

Surgical interventions

- Chronic administration of drugs topically or systemically to lower the IOP in chronic glaucoma. These work by affecting aqueous production or drainage, or by constriction of the pupil (Table 11.2).
- To treat acute glaucoma or lower the IOP perioperatively, systemic agents such as 20% mannitol, 30% urea solution or oral glycerol may be used. These are osmotic diuretics and shrink the vitreous volume.
- The lid speculum and traction sutures may press on the eye during surgery and may raise the IOP.
- Intraocular gas bubbles, such as sulphur hexafluoride (SF_6), will expand if the patient is anaesthetized using nitrous oxide. The resultant rise in IOP may compromise perfusion of the optic nerve and retina.

Local anaesthesia

- In a peribulbar block the volume of the local anaesthetic causes an intraorbital pressure increase; this leads to a transient rise in the IOP. Sub-Tenon's block does not cause a significant increase in the IOP.
- Ocular compression following a peribulbar block results in a soft eye, which is preferred during cataract surgery.
- Once the local anaesthetic is effective, the anaesthetic has spread out in the tissues and the extraocular muscles are relaxed, resulting in a lowering of IOP.

Procedure to treat glaucoma (chronically raised IOP)

Surgical trabeculectomy

- A small hole is made through the sclera and into the anterior chamber drainage angle to allow aqueous humour to flow directly to the subconjunctival area, forming a drainage bleb.
- Need to avoid exacerbating any pre-existing ischaemia of the optic nerve head; therefore, take care with peribulbar blockade.

Table 11.2 Drugs for treatment of chronic glaucoma

Drug	Method of action
Miotics Carbachol Pilocarpine	Constrict pupil and open up trabecular meshwork to increase drainage of aqueous. Given topically
β-Blockers Timolol Betaxolol	Reduce rate of aqueous formation. Given topically
Carbonic anhydrase inhibitors Acetazolamide (oral) Dorxolamide (topical)	Reduce rate of aqueous formation
α_2-Adrenoreceptor stimulant Brimonidone (topical)	Reduce rate of aqueous formation
Prostaglandin analogues Latanoprost (topical)	Increases uveoscleral outflow of aqueous

- Sub-Tenon's block may cause an inflammatory response in the conjunctiva and risk blocking the surgical drainage route.
- Options are general anaesthesia (as for cataract surgery; procedure duration 60–90 minutes), peribulbar block with care to avoid raised IOP or subconjunctival-intracameral local anaesthesia.

Bibliography

Eke T. A glaucoma surgeon's view of anaesthesia techniques. *Ophthalmic Anaesth News* 2003; 9: 6–7.

Johnson RW, Forrest FC. *Local and General Anaesthesia for Ophthalmic Surgery*. Oxford: Butterworth Heinemann, 1994.

Murphy DF. Anesthesia and intraocular pressure. *Anesth Analg* 1985; **64**: 520–30.

Saude T. *Ocular Anatomy and Physiology*. Oxford: Blackwell Scientific Publications, 1993.

Vachon CA, Warner D, Bacon D. Succinylcholine and the open globe: tracing the teaching. *Anesthesiology* 2003; **99**: 220–3.

Cross-references

Artificial airways, 642
Total intravenous anaesthesia, 722

Ophthalmic trauma

Roger M Slater

Ophthalmic trauma may result in a spectrum of injury from superficial laceration of the eyelid or cornea to complete disruption of the globe with extrusion of the contents. It may be impossible to assess the extent of the injury until the time of surgery. It may be associated with other injuries. There may be a foreign body present. Ophthalmic trauma is one of the leading causes of monocular blindness.

Procedure

- Exploration and anatomical repair in the first instance.
- Removal of the foreign body, if present.

Patient characteristics

- All age groups.
- May have coexisting medical conditions.
- Patients present as an emergency.
- Trauma is likely to delay gastric emptying.

Problems

- Open eye with full stomach situation.
- Delay before surgery for penetrating eye injury may increase the risk of loss of contents of the globe and increase the risk of infection.
- Associated trauma, particularly of the head and neck.
- Danger of extrusion of the globe contents at induction.

Preoperative assessment

- Assessment of associated injuries as resuscitation and urgent surgery may be required for non-ophthalmic problems.
- If surgery is within 24 hours of injury, treat the patient as having a full stomach.
- Assess the airway for rapid sequence induction.
- Assess and optimize coexisting medical conditions if time allows.

Premedication

- Sedation and antiemetics may be required, especially in tearful children (caution with metoclopramide and risk of extrapyramidal effects in children/young adults).
- Use local anaesthetic cream over the venepuncture site in children.
- Do not attempt to empty the stomach preoperatively in children as crying, struggling or vomiting will increase the IOP.

Anaesthetic management

- Routine monitoring as per AAGBI guidelines.

Local anaesthesia

- Local anaesthesia is appropriate only in simple lid laceration without tear duct involvement.

General anaesthesia

Induction

- There is a conflict between the patient possibly having a full stomach with the need for rapid sequence induction and the need to protect the eye from a rise in IOP.
- Succinylcholine causes a transient rise in IOP.
- Laryngoscopy and intubation also produce a significant rise in IOP.
- *Modified rapid sequence technique*: may be used in experienced hands. Obtain intravenous access. Preoxygenate for 5 minutes without pressing on the eye with the face-mask. Give alfentanil 0.02 mg kg^{-1}, propofol 3 mg kg^{-1} and rocuronium 0.6 mg kg^{-1} and apply cricoid pressure. Intubation can be performed at 60 seconds without coughing.
- *Standard rapid sequence technique*: intubation with succinylcholine, if the anaesthetist is inexperienced or anticipates a difficult intubation. Using propofol as the induction agent (markedly lowers IOP) will protect against any rise in IOP due to succinylcholine. Administration of lidocaine 1.0 mg kg^{-1} prior to induction will attenuate the rise in IOP due to laryngoscopy and intubation.

Maintenance

- With a balanced technique or TIVA.
- Careful monitoring of relaxation to ensure an immobile patient.
- Antiemetic prophylaxis.
- Analgesia with NSAID or opiate.

Emergence and recovery

- Antagonism of the neuromuscular block.
- Extubate when the patient is awake.

Postoperative management

- Antiemetics prescribed for PONV.
- Moderate postoperative pain may require NSAID or opioid analgesia on the first postoperative day.

Bibliography

Lowry DW, Carroll MT, Mirakhur RK, *et al.* Comparison of sevoflurane and propofol with rocuronium for modified rapid-sequence induction of anaesthesia. *Anaesthesia* 2002; **54**: 247–52.

MacEwan CJ. Eye injuries: a prospective survey of 5671 cases. *Br J Ophthalmol* 1989; **73**: 888–94.

Mirakhur RK, Shepherd WFI, Darrah WC. Propofol and thiopentone: effects on intraocular pressure associated with induction of anaesthesia and tracheal intubation (facilitated with suxamethonium). *Br J Anaesth* 1987; **59**: 437–9.

Smith RB, Babinski M, Leano N. The effect of lidocaine on succinylcholine induced rise in intraocular pressure. *Can Anaesth Soc J* 1979; **26**: 482–3.

Cross-references

Emergency surgery, 613
Head injury, 16
Infants and children, 615
Trauma, 801

Strabismus correction

Roger M Slater

Misalignment of the visual axes may result in double vision (diplopia), loss of visual acuity (amblyopia) and loss of binocular vision. This occurs in about 5% of children and treatment usually requires surgical correction. Adults may require strabismus surgery because of thyroid eye disease, trauma, sixth cranial nerve palsy and following strabismus surgery as a child.

Procedure

- Surgery takes 30–90 minutes and is routinely managed as a day case.

Recession

- Weakening an extraocular muscle by moving its insertion on the globe.

Resection

- Strengthening an extraocular muscle by removing a short piece of tendon or muscle.

Adjustable sutures

- Used in some adult patients to allow final adjustments to be made with eye movements postoperatively.

Patient characteristics

- The most common ophthalmic operation carried out in children.
- Infantile strabismus needs early surgery (6–12 months) for the best visual outcome.
- Rare association with primary muscle diseases and malignant hyperthermia.
- Adult patients may have associated medical conditions, such as connective tissue disease, thyroid eye disease and amyloidosis.
- Associated rare conditions: Stickler syndrome, craniosynostosis, Mobius syndrome, incontinentia pigmenti.

Problems

- Airway not accessible under the microscope.
- Avoid succinylcholine:
  - it can trigger malignant hyperthermia in susceptible patients
  - it can cause tonic contracture of extraocular muscles; this interferes with the forced-duction test.
- Oculocardiac reflex.
- Topical epinephrine is often used to reduce bleeding and may be absorbed systemically; however, take care with the dose in small children.
- High incidence of PONV.

Preoperative assessment

- Identification, investigation and optimization of associated syndromes or coexisting medical conditions.
- Assess the patient's suitability for day-case surgery.

Premedication

- Anxiolysis if required (e.g. temazepam 10–20 mg orally in adults, midazolam 0.5 mg kg^{-1} orally in children).
- Apply local anaesthetic cream to the venepuncture site in children.
- Anticholinergic prophylaxis for the oculocardiac reflex is best given intravenously at induction.

Anaesthetic management

- Routine monitoring as per AAGBI guidelines.

Local anaesthetic

- May be used in cooperative adult patients for uncomplicated surgery.
- Topical anaesthesia with 1.0% amethocaine allows optimal adjustment of muscle sutures at the time of surgery. The oculocardiac reflex is not blocked and ECG monitoring and the possible use of anticholinergics is required.
- Sub-Tenon or peribulbar blocks (as for cataract surgery) are suitable and provide protection from the oculocardiac reflex.

General anaesthesia

Induction

- Intravenous or inhalation as appropriate.
- Prophylaxis against the oculocardiac reflex with glycopyrrolate 0.01 mg kg^{-1} intravenously at induction.

- Airway management – use a reinforced laryngeal mask unless this is contraindicated by patient factors.

Maintenance

- TIVA using propofol and remifentanil infusions provides excellent conditions and reduces PONV.
- Non-depolarizing relaxant (e.g. atracurium or rocuronium) if intubation is required. A small dose (half the intubating dose) is required for maintenance with TIVA to ensure a central immobile eye.
- Alternatively, use a balanced technique with fentanyl or remifentanil by infusion, muscle relaxant and volatile agent.

Maintenance

- Ventilation to normal end-tidal CO_2.
- Prophylactic antiemetic (ondansetron 0.01 mg kg^{-1} intravenously).
- Analgesia with diclofenac 2 mg kg^{-1} and/or paracetamol 15 mg kg^{-1} intravenously.
- 1–2 mL 0.5% bupivacaine sub-Tenon block at the end of surgery gives good postoperative analgesia if adjustable sutures are not used.
- Alternatively, give codeine phosphate 1 mg kg^{-1} orally or intramuscularly for more extensive bilateral surgery.

Emergence and recovery

- Reverse neuromuscular block with neostigmine and glycopyrrolate.
- Extubate/remove the laryngeal mask when the patient is awake.

Postoperative management

- Topical amethocaine at the end of surgery for immediate postoperative pain.
- For moderate postoperative pain on the first day, oral paracetamol is usually sufficient.
- Antiemetics are prescribed, but PONV may be delayed until after discharge.

Bibliography

Blanc VF, Hardy JF, Milot J, Jacob JL. The oculocardiac reflex: a graphic and statistical analysis in children. *Can Anaesth Soc J* 1983; **30**: 360–9.

Carrol JB. Increased incidence of masseter spasm in children with strabismus anaesthetised with halothane and suxamethonium. *Anesthesiology* 1987; **67**: 559–61.

Ing MR. Early surgical intervention for congenital esotropia. *Ophthalmology* 1983; **80**: 132–5.

Mirakhur RK, Jones CJ, Dundee JW, Archer DB. IM or IV atropine or glycopyrrolate for the prevention of the oculocardiac reflex in children undergoing squint surgery. *Br J Anaesth* 1982; **54**: 1059–63.

Weir PM, Munro HM, Reynolds P, *et al.* Propofol infusion and the incidence of emesis in paediatric outpatient strabismus surgery. *Anesth Analg* 1993; **76**: 760–4.

Cross-references

Day-case surgery, 604
Infants and children, 615
Malignant hyperthermia: clinical presentation, 770

Vitreoretinal surgery

Roger M Slater

Normal vision requires transparency of the vitreous body and integrity of the retinal layers. These may become disrupted by disease processes and by trauma, resulting in the separation of the photosensitive layer of the retina from the pigment epithelium with visual loss. Diabetes mellitus, myopia and increasing age predispose to retinal detachment. In type 1 diabetes and sickle cell anaemia, abnormal blood vessel growth on the retina can cause vitreous haemorrhages.

Procedure

- There are two types of operation:
  - *External approach* (cryobuckle procedure): location of the retinal holes and treating them externally with cryotherapy while observing with an indirect ophthalmoscope. Traction sutures placed around the recti muscles may stimulate the oculocardiac reflex when pulled up. A silicone sponge or solid explants may be sutured to the globe.
  - *Internal approach* (vitrectomy): three tiny holes are made in the sclera so that instruments can enter the eye; the retina is then treated directly with electrocautery and laser coagulation. Often, agents are used to tamponade the retina such as air, air–gas mixtures (SF_6 or C_3F_8) and silicone oils.
- Vitreoretinal surgery is urgent when the macular is still attached at presentation (macular-on) and in those patients in whom subretinal fluid is likely to rapidly extend. Once the macular has detached, the procedure can be done within 7 days.
- Retinal detachment is frequently associated with areas of weakness in the contralateral eye that could predispose it to the same condition; therefore, laser treatment may be required.

Patient characteristics

- Children with retinopathy of prematurity.
- Adult patients may have associated medical conditions, such as diabetes mellitus and Marfan syndrome.
- Other associated conditions include SLE, sickle cell disease and Stickler syndrome.

Problems

- Remote airway and limited access to the patient because of the vitrectomy equipment.
- Operating theatre is in darkness for much of the surgery.
- Surgery can be lengthy.
- Oculocardiac reflex.
- Midricaine (procaine, atropine and epinephrine mixture for prolonged pupil dilatation) subconjunctival injection may cause cardiovascular effects.
- Laser is frequently used and the anaesthetist has to wear goggles.

Preoperative assessment

- Assessment and optimization of associated medical conditions.

Premedication

- Perioperative management of diabetes if required.
- Anxiolysis with oral temazepam 10–20 mg if required.

Anaesthetic management

- Routine monitoring as per AAGBI guidelines.
- Audio alarms and anaesthetic machine illumination is important in a dark theatre.

Local anaesthesia

- Suitable in cooperative adults for simple detachment and vitreous surgery or in medically compromised patients.
- Sub-Tenon block anaesthesia or two peribulbar block injections (as for corneal graft surgery) provide good operating conditions.
- If the procedure is lengthy, top up of the sub-Tenon block can be given readily by the surgeon.
- Patient comfort is important during lengthy surgery, and sedation with small doses of midazolam (0.5–1.0 mg) or a low-dose propofol TCI (target blood concentration 0.5–1 $\mu g\ mL^{-1}$) can be considered.
- With sedation, oxygen supplementation and careful monitoring are vital as there is limited access to the patient.

General anaesthesia

- General anaesthesia is the preferred technique for prolonged and complicated surgery.

Induction

- TIVA with a TCI of propofol and a remifentanil infusion provides excellent operating conditions and rapid and smooth emergence from lengthy anaesthesia, with greatly reduced PONV.
- Alternatively, a balanced technique using intravenous induction with propofol, fentanyl boluses or a remifentanil infusion, muscle relaxant and a volatile agent is suitable.

Airway management

- A secure airway with either a reinforced laryngeal mask or south-facing endotracheal tube.

Maintenance

- Muscle relaxation (e.g. atracurium or rocuronium). Monitor carefully to avoid sudden movement of the patient during surgery. A remifentanil infusion may also avoid sudden movement and take the place of continuous muscle relaxation.
- Ventilate with oxygen in air and avoid nitrous oxide (nitrous oxide will expand a gas bubble and can result in a dangerous rise in the IOP in the closed eye).
- Careful positioning and padding of the patient.
- Consider active warming and intravenous fluids for prolonged procedures or in at-risk patients.
- Note that cryotherapy may be particularly stimulating.
- Consider prophylaxis against the oculocardiac reflex with glycopyrrolate 0.01 mg kg^{-1} intravenously (note that local anaesthetic eye block usually attenuates this reflex).
- Antiemetic prophylaxis with ondansetron 4 mg intravenously.
- Sub-Tenon block with bupivacaine given by the surgeon provides intraoperative and postoperative analgesia.

Emergence and recovery

- Antagonize the neuromuscular block with neostigmine and glycopyrrolate.
- Extubate when the patient is awake; coughing is usually minimal.

Postoperative management

- Regular paracetamol, NSAIDs, p.r.n. codeine (maximum 240 mg in 24 hours). Intravenous opioids may be required in recovery. Local anaesthesia as part of the general anaesthetic technique can improve patient comfort.
- PONV can be a problem especially after buckling procedures (local anaesthetic block usually reduces this).
- Some patients need to posture postoperatively to ensure that the gas bubble is in the best position to close the retinal break; this may be for 5–10 days.
- Over the following weeks, when a gas bubble is present, the patient should be warned about:
  - avoiding nitrous oxide in general anaesthesia
  - atmospheric pressure changes during aircraft flights.

Bibliography

Charles S, Small KM. Pathogenesis and repair of retinal detachment. In: Easty DL, Sparrow JM (eds) *Oxford Textbook of Ophthalmology*, vol. 2. Oxford: Oxford Medical Publications, 1999, pp. 1261–72.

Mein CE, Woodcock MG. Local anesthesia for vitreoretinal surgery. *Retina* 1990; **10**: 47–9.

Stinson TW, Donlon JV. Interaction of intraocular air and sulphur hexafluoride with nitrous oxide: a computer simulation. *Anesthesiology* 1982; **56**: 385–8.

Watcha MF, White PF. Postoperative nausea and vomiting. *Anesthesiology* 1992; **77**: 162–84.

Cross-references

Diabetes mellitus, 60
Intraocular pressure, 347
Total intravenous anaesthesia, 722

Laryngoscopy and microsurgery of the larynx

Craig R Bailey

The laryngeal inlet is the narrowest part of the upper airway. For safe management, the anaesthetist and surgeon must share responsibility. The anaesthetist needs to understand the nature and types of pathologies commonly encountered and the surgical operating requirements. Surgical work-up can provide valuable information about anatomical abnormalities and assist in planning airway management.

Patient characteristics

- Patients are older with significant comorbidities.
- Squamous cell carcinoma of the larynx is associated with long-standing cigarette and alcohol consumption and disabling cardiorespiratory and hepatic disease.
- Cigarette consumption causes airway hyper-reactivity.

Preoperative assessment

- Routine assessment of associated medical conditions.
- Clinical assessment for respiratory distress and the presence of stridor.
- ENT assessment of the airway, by indirect laryngoscopy and/or fibreoptic nasendoscopy.
- Appropriate investigations dependent upon the history and examination.
- Radiological imaging (CT or MRI) is used to determine the nature and extent of the pathology.

Premedication

- Patients should be warned of possible temporary breathing difficulty postoperatively.
- Premedication is usually unnecessary and may compromise any airway narrowing.
- Antisialagogues may decrease secretions but also make what remains thicker.
- Patients with significant stridor require oxygen during transport. A Heliox mixture can mitigate their symptoms by improving gas flow. Helium is inert, three times less dense than air and eight times less dense than oxygen; therefore, when there is turbulent flow in the upper airway it reduces the work of breathing. It is available from BOC Healthcare (Manchester, UK) as Heliox21, containing 79% helium and 21% oxygen.

Theatre preparation and monitoring

- Monitoring should include ECG, non-invasive blood pressure (BP), S_aO_2, end-tidal CO_2 ($ETCO_2$), airway pressure, disconnect alarm and, where appropriate, neuromuscular function monitoring.
- A difficult intubation trolley with appropriate equipment and tracheal airway access devices (e.g. emergency tracheostomy) may be required and should be available.
- Patient position is with a head-ring, with or without a sandbag beneath the shoulders, with due care as excessive neck extension may cause injury.

General principles of anaesthetic technique

The *main problems* concern sharing the airway with the surgeon to enable access. Prevention of hypoxic brain damage is more difficult when the airway is abnormal. Induction of general anaesthesia in a patient with a compromised airway may result in total obstruction. Generally, supraglottic lesions block the view of the laryngeal inlet, glottic lesions narrow it and subglottic lesions cause narrowing beyond what can be seen during direct laryngoscopy. Neoplastic lesions can be friable and prone to bleeding during instrumentation, obscuring the view further. Airway manipulations may result in laryngeal oedema and a worsened airway at the end of the procedure. The anaesthetist must predict the likely condition of the airway at recovery and anticipate any continued bleeding.

- Tracheal intubation is usually required.
- Muscle relaxants may not be needed to effect tracheal intubation and, in general, should only be administered when assisted ventilation and/or intubation are guaranteed.
- In severely narrowed airways, an urgent tracheostomy performed under local anaesthesia

may be the best option but this can be difficult in a hypoxic, distressed uncooperative patient.

- General anaesthetic techniques include inhalational induction with sevoflurane or a 'quick look' with a small dose of propofol. (In each case the aim is to avoid hypoxaemia and test assisted ventilation and/or intubation conditions.) Alternatively, awake fibreoptic intubation is an option.
- Surgery on the vocal cords (for biopsies or cord stripping) usually requires the patient to be fully relaxed, but assessment of vocal cord movements may need to be considered at some stage.
- Manipulation of the larynx can cause a hypertensive response and cardiac arrhythmias.
- A rapid return of consciousness and protective reflexes should be aimed for whether anaesthesia is of short or prolonged duration.
- Aspiration of blood and surgical debris is possible.

Anaesthetic technique

The choice of anaesthetic technique depends on the condition of the patient at the time of surgery and the individual preferences and expertise of the anaesthetist.

- Cardiovascular stability, avoidance of awareness and a smooth, rapid recovery are essential.
- An intravenous induction is suitable for most patients, followed by maintenance with oxygen, nitrous oxide and a volatile agent with or without an opioid. A total intravenous technique (TIVA) is a useful alternative. This can also be used to avoid the use of muscle relaxants, although hypotension can be a problem in elderly patients.

Airway maintenance

- *Tracheal intubation* is the standard airway management. A microlaryngeal tube is a tube of normal length for adults but small diameter and cuffed. Sizes 4.0–6.0 mm internal diameter are available but have high resistance and can result in difficult ventilation of obese subjects.

The need for optimal access to the vocal cords has led to alternative methods:

- *'Tubeless anaesthesia'* is when there is no tracheal tube between the vocal cords. One method uses intubation lower down the airway, e.g. cricothyroid puncture (usually with jet ventilation). A second uses no tube at all with the patient breathing spontaneously. When no tube is used and the patient breathes spontaneously, local anaesthetic spray to the vocal cords allows a lighter plane of anaesthesia; close cooperation between surgeon and anaesthetist is essential.
- *Tracheal catheter.* Various types of catheter have been used (typical calibre is 14 FG) with insertion through the cords down to the carina to deliver oxygen. Apart from increased aspiration risk, catheters tend to move with the driving gas and cause soft-tissue injury by a flailing effect within the trachea.
- *Venturi jet ventilation* is when an 'injected' driving gas entrains room air. Injectors typically use oxygen as the driving gas. The injector source is firmly attached to a rigid bronchoscope to limit backlash. Ventilation is most effective when the bronchoscope tip is well aligned with the trachea. There is a risk of barotrauma.
- *High-frequency oscillation* uses smaller tidal perturbation at higher rates (60–100 min^{-1}) and requires specialized ventilators to deliver the driving gas, usually via a catheter below the vocal cords. The risk of barotrauma is less than with Venturi ventilation.

With any of the specialized ventilation alternatives, the important considerations are maintenance of a clear conduit for inspiration and expiration and awareness that routine ventilatory monitors, e.g. tidal volume, airway pressures and $ETco_2$, are inaccurate. Hypoventilation and awareness may occur, particularly in patients who are obese or have poor lung compliance. Anaesthetic inexperience and poor technique will also contribute and this is why TIVA is useful because it removes dependence on the breathing circuit to maintain depth of anaesthesia.

Anaesthesia for laser surgery

Lasers (*l*ight *a*mplification by *s*timulated *e*mission of *r*adiation) are used for excision of various laryngeal lesions as they allow precise incisions with an extremely fine zone of coagulation, leading to less postoperative bleeding, minimal tissue reaction and reduced postoperative oedema. Carbon dioxide (the commonest) or neodymium-doped yttrium aluminium garnet (Nd-YAG)-type lasers are available for ENT surgery. Safety training for theatre staff is mandatory to prevent direct and incidental burns and local policies must be adhered to. The eyes are at particular risk, requiring the use of special protective glasses. When more extensive surgery is employed, the usual axial direction of the laser beam down the airway indicates the tissues most at risk from ignition. The tracheal tube itself can catch fire.

Fire precautions and treating a fire

Tracheal tubes will ignite under the right conditions with both oxygen and nitrous oxide supporting combustion. Specially designed, laser-resistant, single use disposable tracheal tubes are recommended. Tube cuffs are at risk of penetration by the laser beam and they have double cuffs filled with saline. The surgeon applies saline-soaked gauze pads to further protect the cuffs and surrounding soft tissue. Wet towel drapes are used around the surgical field. If 'tubeless anaesthesia' is used instead of a laser tube, there may be increased risk of inadvertent laser injury to tissues lower down the airway. Restriction of the laser beam to short bursts rather than continuous cutting is said to reduce the risk of fire.

When fire does occur the first priority is to extinguish it and disconnect anaesthetic gases to avoid further injury. Saline flushing with a syringe can be used to cool tissues and limit secondary damage. The damaged tracheal tube will normally need to be replaced and, for this reason, entirely metallic tubes are available which should be readily to hand. Reactive oedema occurs rapidly. Oxygen administration is resumed as soon as this is considered safe. The patient should be treated as an inhalational burn injury and transferred to an intensive care environment in order to monitor and treat serious complications.

Postoperative complications

- *Immediate*: transient respiratory distress, sore throat, pain, hoarseness, laryngospasm, bleeding, stridor, laryngeal oedema, aspiration of blood and surgical debris.
- *Early*: any or all of the above. Early discharge should only be allowed for carefully selected patients in whom risks are considered minimal.
- *Late*: tissue scarring may occur and the original pathology may progress if appropriate treatment is delayed. When radiation is used in the treatment of malignancy there is an increased risk of reactive laryngeal oedema.

Bibliography

Cinar SO, Costun BU, Cinar U, *et al.* Blood gas changes in patients undergoing laryngeal microsurgery. *Auris Nasus Larynx* 2006; **33**: 299–302.

Werawatganon T, Supiyathon P, Kerekhanjanarong V, *et al.* Intermittent apnoea and total intravenous anesthesia for microscopic laryngeal surgery. *J Med Assoc Thai* 2004; **87**: 547–50.

Cross-references

Awareness, 733
Difficult airway: management, 651
Difficult airway: prediction, 664

Middle ear surgery

Craig R Bailey

Procedures

Middle ear surgery involves careful dissection of small structures, such as the ossicles, using an operating microscope. Surgery may take many hours. Patients are usually admitted on the day of surgery and stay overnight postoperatively.

Preoperative investigations

Assessment and investigations are dictated by the patient's general condition. No specific preoperative considerations arise in these patients, unless controlled hypotension is contemplated. The patient can be of any age.

Principles of the anaesthetic

Surgery will be made impossible by bleeding. The severity of bleeding is related as much to venous as to arterial blood pressure. Attention to the following principles ensures a satisfactory operating field:

- A clear airway is essential. A partially obstructed airway impedes expiration, increases CO_2 levels and raises venous pressure. An armoured endotracheal tube avoids kinking.
- Anaesthesia should be conducted smoothly. The trachea is intubated only after full muscle relaxation. Topical lidocaine spray to the larynx and trachea helps to prevent subsequent responses. Straining and coughing must be avoided as they increase venous pressure and bleeding.
- Venous pressure should be minimized. A head-up tilt of 10–15° helps to minimize bleeding. Avoid extreme lateral head movement by using the lateral tilt facility of the operating table.
- Tachycardia should be avoided. Atropine should not be given. β-Blockers are useful and small doses of labetalol can be titrated intravenously.
- Induced hypotension has been recommended and may be requested by the surgeon. Profound hypotension is unnecessary and may be harmful. A general rule of thumb is not to allow the systolic pressure to drop lower than the preoperative diastolic pressure.

Premedication

Premedication is usually unnecessary.

Anaesthetic technique

The particular choice of anaesthetic agents is not crucial although nitrous oxide is to be avoided. A TIVA technique using propofol and remifentanil and lung ventilation is suitable. The eyes should be protected.

Two important issues arise in middle ear surgery and influence the choice of anaesthetic technique:

- If the surgeon wishes to monitor facial nerve integrity using a nerve stimulator, initial muscle relaxation is allowed to wear off. The patient can then breathe spontaneously and lidocaine spray to the trachea prior to intubation allows the endotracheal tube to be tolerated at light levels of anaesthesia. More commonly, ventilation is controlled using an infusion of remifentanil.
- The middle ear is a closed, air-filled cavity. Nitrous oxide (N_2O) is 30 times more soluble, and hence diffusible, than nitrogen. During the early part of an anaesthetic N_2O will enter a closed cavity faster than nitrogen can leave and pressure will rise. In the recovery period N_2O will diffuse out more rapidly than N_2 can enter and the converse occurs. The position of tympanoplasty grafts can be affected.

The ear is bandaged at the end of the procedure. To prevent displacement of the tracheal tube and trauma to the eyes, the anaesthetist should supervise this.

Monitoring

- Standard minimum monitoring should be applied.
- Neuromuscular function should be monitored continuously.
- Invasive blood pressure monitoring is essential during hypotensive anaesthesia.

Recovery

Nausea, vomiting and dizziness can be a particular problem following these procedures. A suitable antiemetic should be given. Pain is not usually severe.

Bibliography

Degoute CS. Controlled hypotension: a guide to drug choice. *Drugs* 2007; **67**: 1053–76.

Fujii Y. Clinical strategies for preventing postoperative nausea and vomiting after middle ear surgery in adult patients. *Curr Drug Saf* 2008; **3**: 230–9.

Cross-reference

Induced hypotension during anaesthesia, 711

Oesophagoscopy

Craig R Bailey

Procedure

Oesophagoscopy can be performed using a rigid or flexible oesophagoscope. General anaesthesia is required for rigid oesophagoscopy. Sedation is usually adequate for flexible oesophagoscopy in cooperative patients.

Indications for rigid oesophagoscopy

- Removal of a foreign body.
- Assessment and biopsy of lesions of the oesophagus.
- Assessment of lesions of the lower pharynx and the postcricoid region.
- Intubation or dilatation of an oesophageal stricture.
- Endoscopic treatment of pharyngeal pouch.

Patient characteristics

Consideration must be given to the following:

- The oesophagus may be partially or totally obstructed, with food and saliva present above the obstruction. The patient may be suffering from gastro-oesophageal reflux. These factors pose a risk of aspiration.
- Prolonged oesophageal obstruction will cause weight loss, anaemia and dehydration.
- Silent aspiration of oesophageal contents, in the weeks leading up to the oesophagoscopy, can cause pneumonia, basal lung collapse or lung abscess.
- Rarely, a patient with a neurological abnormality such as motor neurone disease presents with dysphagia.

Preoperative investigations and preparation

Investigations are dictated by the patient's general condition, and the indication for surgery. Dehydration should be corrected preoperatively and chest infections treated.

Premedication

Sedation should be avoided. Glycopyrrolate can be given to reduce secretions. Pharmacological means can be used to raise gastric pH. If so, remember that:

- H_2 receptor antagonists and proton pump inhibitors do not neutralize existing acid. They require several hours to be effective.
- Acid is not the only threat. Blood and residual food are still a potential problem.
- The use of such medication does not remove the need to protect the airway during induction.

Principles of the anaesthetic

The following principles apply:

- The airway is shared with the surgeon; close cooperation and communication is required.
- Endotracheal intubation is necessary.
- There is a risk of regurgitation of oesophageal contents and a modified rapid sequence induction is required.
- The endotracheal tube can be compressed, kinked or displaced by the surgeon. A reinforced endotracheal tube prevents kinking and compression. Ventilation by hand allows immediate detection of such events. If a mechanical ventilator is used, careful attention to airway pressure alarms is required.
- Use of an endotracheal tube smaller than usual, and temporary deflation of the cuff, makes it easier to pass the oesophagoscope.
- Coughing, straining and movement during oesophagoscopy makes the procedure difficult and risks oesophageal perforation. The patient should be immobile during surgery.
- Insertion of an oesophagoscope is highly stimulating, and is sustained for several minutes. The result is hypertension, tachycardia and, sometimes, myocardial ischaemia and arrhythmias.
- Biopsy of oesophageal lesions and the presence of varices can cause massive bleeding.
- The operation is of relatively short duration.
- Airway reflexes should be intact at the end of surgery so that the patient can protect his or her airway after extubation.

Anaesthetic technique

- A wide-bore intravenous cannula should be sited.
- Suction apparatus must be checked and switched on.

- Rapid sequence or modified rapid sequence induction with tracheal intubation minimizes the risk of aspiration. The endotracheal tube is moved to the left side of the mouth to facilitate passage of the oesophagoscope. The patient's eyes must be protected.
- Propofol is used for induction and succinylcholine or short-acting non-depolarizing neuromuscular blocking agents to provide muscle relaxation. Anaesthesia is maintained with O_2, air and desflurane. The use of desflurane facilitates prompt recovery of airway reflexes.
- Cardiovascular disturbances are common. Blood pressure may fall profoundly owing to the effect of anaesthetic drugs on a background of undiagnosed hypovolaemia in a cachectic patient. Intravenous fluids and a small dose of vasopressor deal with this problem. Conversely, stimulation can cause hypertension, tachycardia and myocardial ischaemia. Hypertension and tachycardia are treated with small doses of fentanyl. If tachycardia persists and is a problem, a small dose of atenolol or labetalol may be given.

Monitoring

Minimum monitoring standards should be followed. Neuromuscular function should be monitored with a nerve stimulator.

Recovery

The risk of aspiration continues until full recovery. Extubate only when the patient is awake with full recovery of muscle tone. This can be achieved rapidly with modern agents. If there is any doubt as to whether the patient's recovery satisfies these criteria, he or she should be supervised by the anaesthetist in the left lateral, head-down position, with suction available. Instrumentation by either surgeon or anaesthetist may damage lips, mouth or teeth and these structures should be examined after the trachea has been intubated and again postoperatively. Complaints of pain on swallowing should be taken seriously. Perforation of the oesophagus, with pneumomediastinum, surgical emphysema and pneumothorax is a real risk. A chest X-ray should be performed if there is any suspicion of perforation. Intravenous fluids should be prescribed as patients remain starved for several hours postoperatively.

Bibliography

Balci AE, Eren S, Eren NM. Esophageal foreign bodies under cricopharyngeal level in children: an analysis of 1116 cases. *Interact Cardiovasc Thorac Surg* 2004; **3**: 14–18.

Pino Rivero V, Trinidad Ruiz G, Marcos Garcia M, *et al.* Esophagoscopy in adults. Our experience and review of the literature. *Acta Otorrinolaringol Esp* 2003; **54**: 642–5.

Cross-references

Airway and aspiration risk, 640
Disorders of the oesophagus and of swallowing, 177
Fluid and electrolyte balance, 754
Hiatus hernia, 181

Operations on the nose

Craig R Bailey

Nose operations make up a large proportion of the ENT workload. They are often simple and straightforward, e.g. manipulation of nasal bones or polypectomy. Occasionally, the procedures may be more prolonged, e.g. transnasal skull base surgery. As is the case with many ENT procedures, the airway is 'shared'. Cooperation between surgeon and anaesthetist is essential. An unhindered operating field is required and coughing and straining should be avoided.

Common problems

- Patients with polyps often have a history of atopy or the triad of asthma, polyps and aspirin sensitivity.
- Postnasal drip and recurrent chest infections are common.
- Patients with nasal fractures may have sustained other injuries or swallowed a significant amount of blood.
- There is an increasing incidence of patients with obstructive sleep apnoea (OSA).

Preoperative assessment and preparation

- History and examination with particular regard to identifying the problems outlined above.
- Treat chest infections and optimize chronic medical conditions, e.g. asthma.
- Correct hypovolaemia in patients who have bled.
- Investigations are dependent on the patient's current condition.

Premedication

- Most patients do not require premedication but benzodiazepines may be given to the overly anxious.

Nasal vasoconstrictors

Because the nose is highly vascular, some vasoconstriction, in order to decrease bleeding, is advantageous. The following may be used:

- Moffat's solution (a mixture of 10% cocaine, sodium bicarbonate, 1:1000 epinephrine and sterile water).
- Direct injection of local anaesthetic with 1:100 000 or 1:200 000 epinephrine at the start of the procedure.
- Lidocaine 5% and phenylephrine 0.5% spray.
- Less often used vasoconstrictors include ephedrine and xylometazoline.

Perioperative anaesthetic management

- *Minimum monitoring* includes S_po_2, ECG, non-invasive BP, $ETco_2$, disconnection alarm, volatile agent analyser and hypoxia alarm.
- Some operations, such as septoplasty, may be performed under local anaesthesia with sedation in cooperative patients, although most nasal operations require a general anaesthetic.
- A modified rapid sequence induction is required in patients undergoing surgery who have swallowed a significant amount of blood.
- The choice of induction agent will be influenced by factors such as the anaesthetist's preference and patient condition.
- The airway may be secured with an endotracheal tube, commonly a preformed tube or, if no contraindications exist, a single-use flexible laryngeal mask airway. A throat pack is then inserted. All connections must be absolutely secure as, once surgery is under way, access to the airway will be difficult.
- The eyes are protected by simple ointment but not covered in order that the surgeon can check for orbital perforation or damage to the optic nerve.
- Maintenance can be achieved with either inhalation agents and narcotic or a TIVA technique with or without muscle relaxants.
- Nasal surgery is usually performed in the head-up position to reduce bleeding. Hypotension may occur. The thighs are flexed at the hip in order to improve venous return.
- Patients with polyps occasionally receive a preoperative course of steroids. Perioperative steroid cover should be considered.

Safe use of a pharyngeal pack

A throat pack is used to prevent blood and debris contaminating the airway or being swallowed. The most common form of pack is wetted gauze, but some anaesthetists use sponge packs. In a 2 year surveillance period until April 2009, there were

38 incidents involving throat packs which were referred to the National Patient Safety Agency (NPSA) Reporting and Learning System (RLS). On 24 occasions there was unintended throat pack retention and moderate harm occurred in one case, which led to an NPSA safety notice to be issued on 28 April 2009. There should be a two-person check of throat pack insertion and removal and this should be recorded on a whiteboard. The pack should be inserted under direct vision with Magill forceps, and the tail of gauze left to protrude from the mouth to remind the anaesthetist of its presence at the end of surgery and preferably attached to the associated airway. An adhesive label should be applied to the patient or airway as a further reminder. All staff should be fully aware of the insertion of a throat pack and the World Health Organization's surgical safety checklist should be adapted to accommodate insertion and removal of the pack.

When the procedure is complete and the throat pack is removed, direct pharyngoscopy is performed to ensure that the pack has been removed completely and any remaining blood clots or debris are aspirated.

Postoperative management

- Sit the patient up as early as possible to decrease bleeding.
- Encourage the patient to breathe through his/her mouth because nasal packs are often inserted at the end of surgery.
- Plasters and bolsters applied to the nose may make the application of a face-mask difficult.
- Administer oxygen in recovery in a routine fashion, but continuous positive airway pressure is required as soon as possible in patients with OSA.
- Leave the intravenous cannula *in situ* in case of bleeding.
- Repacking may be necessary should bleeding from the nose continue.
- Analgesia will be required. Regular paracetamol with or without a non-steroidal anti-inflammatory drug is often sufficient; opioids are needed following more extensive surgery, but be aware of respiratory depression in patients with OSA.

Bibliography

Bloom JD, Kaplan SE, Bleier BS, Goldstein SA. Septoplasty complications: avoidance and management. *Otolaryngol Clin North Am* 2009; **42**: 463–81.

Harper SJ, Jones NS. Cocaine: what role does it have in current ENT practice? A review of the current literature. *J Laryngol Otol* 2006; **120**: 808–11.

National Patient Safety Agency. Reducing the risk of retained throat packs after surgery. NPSA/2009/SPN001. London: NPSA.

Westreich R, Sampson I, Shaari CM, Lawson W. Negative-pressure pulmonary edema after routine septorhinoplasty: discussion of pathophysiology, treatment and prevention. *Arch Facial Plast Surg* 2006; **8**: 8–15.

Cross-references

Anaesthesia and sleep apnoea syndrome, 98
Induced hypotension during anaesthesia, 711

Tonsillectomy and adenoidectomy

Craig R Bailey

Procedure

Tonsillectomy and/or adenoidectomy procedures are performed through the mouth. A Boyle–Davis gag is used for tonsillectomy. Difficulties may be encountered because of:

- shared airway
- difficult bag–valve–mask ventilation or tracheal intubation in patients with enlarged lymphoid tissue
- poorly placed gag obstructing the tracheal tube or laryngeal mask airway
- postoperative bleeding.

Many centres choose to treat these patients as day cases.

Patient characteristics

- Children and young adults are usually operated on for chronic or recurrent infections.
- Some may have obstructive sleep apnoea or congenital abnormalities, e.g. Down's syndrome.
- Older adults for tonsillectomy may have malignancy and other incidental medical conditions.
- Some have cor pulmonale (right ventricular failure) owing to long-term hypoxia.

Preoperative assessment and investigations

- History of obstructive sleep apnoea (OSA) must be carefully explored. OSA is a clinical condition in which there is intermittent and repeated upper airway collapse during sleep. It occurs more commonly in obese middle-aged male smokers and is suggested by snoring, excessive daytime sleepiness (assessed using the Epworth Sleepiness Scale) restlessness, nocturia and decreased libido. Obesity, large neck circumference and enlarged tonsils on examination are not uncommon, and the gold standard for diagnosis is polysomnography, which shows the number of apnoea/hypopnoea episodes while asleep being quoted as an index. OSA is associated with hypertension and ischaemic heart disease and is being increasingly recognized in children because of the increased incidence of childhood obesity.
- Bleeding disorders are important in the patient or immediate family.
- A thorough airway assessment must be performed.
- Patients presenting on the day of surgery with an acute infection should be deferred. Except in an emergency, patients should be operated upon when well.
- Tests required include full blood count, group and save and clotting studies if indicated by the history.
- Specific consent should be taken if suppositories are planned to be given.

Premedication

- Local anaesthetic gels (EMLA/Ametop) should be applied to those children who request, or whose parents request, an intravenous induction.
- Sedative premedication should not be given to those with airway obstruction or a history of obstructive sleep apnoea.
- An anxiolytic may be useful if there is time or the operation is to be performed at a predictable time.

Perioperative management

- Standard monitoring should be applied to all patients and provision made to assess blood loss.
- Intravenous or inhalational induction can be used.
- Patients are usually intubated with a 'south-facing' pre-formed Ring–Adair–Elwyn (RAE) tube. Some surgeons prefer a nasal tube for tonsillectomy in adult patients.
- Check the length and patency of the endotracheal tube before surgery begins.
- Intubation may be difficult because of large tonsils, but is usually achieved using a non-depolarizing neuromuscular blocking agent.
- Oral tubes must be carefully secured in the midline in order to lie correctly in the Boyle–Davis gag.
- With experienced senior personnel and a regular surgical/anaesthetic team, the reinforced laryngeal mask airway (LMA) may be used for tonsillectomy. Surgeons must avoid soiling of the airway with blood.
- Patients are positioned with the neck extended.
- The eyes must be protected.

- Instrumentation of the postnasal space during adenoidectomy may induce a bradycardia requiring treatment with atropine or glycopyrrolate.
- Peroperative opioid analgesia is usually required, together with intravenous paracetamol and non-steroidal anti-inflammatory drugs (unless contraindicated).
- Extubation can be accomplished either deep or awake, depending on the preference and skills of recovery room staff, but patients should be in the head-down left lateral position.
- Infiltration of local anaesthetic into the tonsillar bed provides good postoperative analgesia.
- Blind or aggressive suctioning of the pharynx may cause bleeding from the tonsillar bed and should be avoided.

Postoperative management

- Non-steroidal analgesics have not been found to significantly increase bleeding in tonsillectomy patients.
- Copious intravenous fluids are not usually required as swallowing is to be encouraged.
- Intravenous cannulae should be left *in situ* in case of early postoperative bleeding.
- Bleeding may not be detected in children until vomiting occurs.

Creutzfeldt–Jakob disease

Transmission of prion-borne diseases, including variant Creutzfeldt-Jakob disease (vCJD), which is acquired from eating beef from cows infected with bovine spongiform encephalopathy (BSE), is theoretically possible with contamination of equipment during surgery on lymphoid tissues. Prions (proteinaceous infectious particles) have been found in tonsillar tissue of patients with no clinical signs of vCJD and are not reliably destroyed by standard surgical sterilization. There have been 168 deaths reported to the Edinburgh Surveillance Unit in the 15 years until 3 May 2010 with a peak of 28 deaths in 2000, which resulted in Department of Health guidelines requiring the use of disposable surgical and anaesthetic equipment for tonsillectomy and adenoidectomy between January and December 2001. These guidelines were rescinded because of an increase in morbidity due to bleeding. The incidence of vCJD has declined significantly since 2000 and only three deaths were recorded in 2009 (www.cjd.ed.ac.uk/figures.htm), although the theoretical risk of developing this degenerative brain disorder must always be borne in mind. Single-use disposable anaesthetic equipment, e.g. endotracheal tube (ETT), laryngoscope blades, bougies and laryngeal mask airways should be used.

Management of the 'bleeding tonsil'

These patients require the skills of senior, experienced anaesthetists.

- Blood loss is difficult to assess because most is swallowed.
- Resuscitation with intravenous fluids and/or blood must be guided by cardiovascular parameters appropriate to the patient's age and size.
- Patients will have a full stomach and a potentially difficult airway with blood in the pharynx and local oedema following recent intubation.
- The anaesthetic record should be studied for any indication of previous airway difficulties.
- Some patients may not have regained consciousness following the first anaesthetic.

Intraoperative management

- Patients should be resuscitated and have full monitoring applied.
- Suction must be immediately available and head-down tilt helps to drain blood away from the larynx.
- A rapid sequence intravenous induction or an inhalational induction with cricoid pressure can be used depending on the skills of the anaesthetist. *Use the technique with which you are most familiar and which will allow the airway to be safely secured.*
- Intubation may require a smaller sized endotracheal tube than originally inserted.
- Volume resuscitation should continue throughout surgery.
- Before awakening, a large-bore nasogastric tube should be carefully inserted to drain stomach contents.
- Patients should be extubated head-down in the left lateral position when fully awake.

Postoperative management

- Patients may require sedation in order to tolerate postnasal space packs if bleeding has occurred after adenoidectomy. This requires observation on a high-dependency unit owing to the risk of airway obstruction.
- Check the haemoglobin and transfuse blood if necessary.
- Patients should be closely monitored for evidence of further bleeding.

Bibliography

Cardwell M, Siviter G, Smith A. Non-steroidal anti-inflammatory drugs and perioperative bleeding in pediatric tonsillectomy. *Cochrane Database Syst Rev* 2005; (2): CD003591.

Johr M. Anaesthesia for tonsillectomy. *Curr Opin Anaesthesiol* 2006; **1a**(3): 260–1.

Cross-references

Anaesthesia and sleep apnoea syndrome, 98
Airway and aspiration risk, 640
Difficult airway: management, 651
Infants and children, 615
Paediatric airway, 675

Tracheostomy

Craig R Bailey

Surgical

This can be an elective or emergency procedure usually performed under general anaesthesia with tracheal intubation (occasionally laryngeal mask airway). Rarely, local anaesthesia is administered in an emergency (e.g. laryngeal trauma).

Indications

- Upper airway obstruction.
- Head and neck surgery, e.g. laryngectomy.
- Laryngeal trauma.
- Failed endotracheal intubation.
- Prolonged tracheal intubation and/or intermittent positive pressure ventilation.
- Facilitate bronchial toilet.
- Prevention of pulmonary aspiration.

Preoperative assessment and investigation

Look for:

- coexisting cardiopulmonary, neurological or muscular disease
- signs of aspiration or airway obstruction (e.g. stridor)
- difficult laryngoscopy and/or difficult face-mask ventilation
- routine investigations plus chest and cervical spine X-rays, CT scans, pulmonary function tests and baseline arterial blood gases.

Preparation and premedication

- Assume a difficult intubation: check equipment and have a plan.
- Various sizes of tracheostomy tubes, sterile catheter mount and suction catheters should be available and checked for correct connectors.
- Minimal dose of anxiolytic if essential.
- Antisialagogue intravenously before induction.
- Continue routine medications.

Induction and maintenance

- Start only when the surgeon is scrubbed and the instruments are ready.
- Use intravenous induction only if confident, otherwise consider inhalational induction or awake fibreoptic intubation.
- Fix the ETT in a way which permits cautious withdrawal.
- Use TIVA for maintenance, careful neck extension, a head-ring and head elevation of 10–15°.
- Clear oropharyngeal secretions.
- The tracheal incision is usually at the third tracheal ring, above the ETT cuff.
- Ventilate manually with 100% oxygen during the tracheostomy tube insertion.
- Retract the ETT until the tip is just above the incision, enabling tracheostomy tube insertion.
- Check position of the tracheostomy and confirm $ETco_2$ trace before reattaching the ventilator.
- Once the correct position of the tracheostomy tube is confirmed, withdraw the ETT completely.
- If local anaesthesia is used, intravenous lidocaine may reduce coughing.

Postoperative management

- Check the chest X-ray (tube position, pneumothorax, surgical emphysema, lobar collapse).
- The patient should be nursed sitting up in an appropriate area (humidified oxygen, suction).
- A selection of endotracheal and tracheostomy tubes and a tracheostomy dilator should be immediately available.
- Tube change is usually only performed after a week in order to allow time for formation of a tract.

Complications

- *Early*: malposition, displacement, bleeding, surgical emphysema, pneumothorax and obstruction (blood, sputum, tracheal wall).
- *Late*: displacement, obstruction, infection, erosion, bleeding, stenosis (cuff or stoma site) and voice changes.

Emergency tracheostomy

- Usually performed under local anaesthesia when the airway is obstructed.
- Needle cricothyroidotomy or a mini-tracheostomy set should be available on every anaesthetic machine.

Percutaneous

- Elective procedure usually performed by a trained intensivist.

- At the bedside: quicker, less traumatic, cost-effective.
- Theatre and transfer not needed.
- Possibly higher incidence of late complications.

Techniques

- Serial dilatation (Ciaglia).
- Single tapered dilatation (Blue Rhino).
- Guidewire dilating (Griggs) forceps or screw (PercuTwist).

Indications

- Prolonged endotracheal intubation.
- To facilitate weaning from the ventilator and aid nursing.

Preoperative assessment

- Coexisting disease, ventilation.
- Consider deferring if the patient is positive end-expiratory pressure dependent or coagulopathic.

Preparation

- Two operators and a bronchoscope are needed.
- Give general anaesthesia with 100% O_2.
- Some advocate change to a smaller ETT or LMA before starting.
- Withdraw the ETT to above the site of the tracheostomy.
- Adjust ventilation or insert a throat pack to compensate for cuff deflation.

Procedure

- Use a head-ring, a sandbag under the shoulders and the head-up position.
- Infiltrate the incision site with lidocaine and epinephrine.
- Site is usually between the first and second tracheal rings.
- Dissect down to the trachea.
- Check the position of the introducer and guidewire bronchoscopically from above.
- Use a high-volume, low-pressure cuffed tracheostomy tube.

Postoperative management

- Adjust ventilator settings.
- Chest X-ray.

Complications

- *Early*: loss of airway, malposition, displacement of the tube, bleeding, infection, surgical emphysema, pneumothorax, occlusion of the tube, oesophageal injury and tracheal injury.
- *Late*: displacement, obstruction, infection, erosion, bleeding, stenosis (cuff or stoma site) and voice changes.

Bibliography

Beltrame F, Zussino M, Martinez B, *et al.* Percutaneous vs surgical bedside tracheostomy in the ICU: a cohort study. *Minerva Anestesiol* 2008; **74**: 529–35.

Durbin Jr CG. Early complications of tracheostomy. *Respir Care* 2005; **50**: 511–15.

Durbin Jr CG. Indications for and timing of tracheostomy. *Respir Care* 2005; **50**: 483–7.

Cross-references

Artificial airways, 642
Difficult airway: management, 651
Difficult airway: prediction, 664

13 Head and neck surgery

Gerhard Schwarz

- Dental abscess — *Gerhard Schwarz*
- Dental surgery — *Isolde Rötzer*
- Face and jaw fractures — *Marianne Hösele*
- Laryngectomy and radical neck dissection — *Gerlinde Mausser*
- Major reconstructive surgery — *Marianne Hösele*
- Operations and the salivary glands — *Gerhard Schwarz*
- Thyroidectomy — *Andreas Schöpfer*

Dental abscess

Gerhard Schwarz

Dental abscesses usually result from infected teeth and cause localized pain and swelling. They may restrict mouth opening and can be associated with pyrexia and malaise. They typically discharge into the buccal sulcus, but may 'point' elsewhere, including extraorally. Their size and possible clinical consequences of fascial or cervical space infection may be underestimated.

The General Dental Council (GDC) and the Royal College of Anaesthetists (RCoA) recommend that, whenever possible, dental procedures are performed under local anaesthesia, in combination with conscious sedation if necessary. General anaesthesia may be clinically justified when local analgesia or patient cooperation are inadequate, or when the stress of surgery while awake would be likely to result in dental phobia.

Deep neck infections and Ludwig's angina

Deep neck infections are found in the submandibular, retropharyngeal or lateral pharyngeal spaces. Ludwig's angina is a bilateral inflammation of the submental, sublingual and submandibular spaces. Causes are infected teeth, oral lesions and injuries. Rarely, a spreading cellulitis with extensive induration and swelling of the anterior neck may occur. Fever, pain, dysphagia, trismus, acute confusional state, swelling of the floor of the mouth and compromise of the airway may be present. This is a potentially life-threatening condition which requires urgent and expert management.

Procedures

- Periradicular surgery (e.g. apicectomy).
- Exodontia (including surgical removal).
- Skin incision and external drainage.

Patient characteristics

The conditions are not limited to those with poor dental hygiene:

- children
- neglected adults
- patients with 'special needs'.

Specific problems

- Patients may be uncooperative.
- May present difficult consent issues.
- Parents or regular care-providers may need to be present at induction.
- Airway problems:
  - shared airway
  - swelling
  - contamination (pus etc.)
  - trismus.

Deep neck infections and Ludwig's angina

- Airway problems are more serious and also include:
  - critical airway patency
  - secretions
  - rigidity
  - distortion.
- Muscle relaxants may not lead to increased mouth opening.
- There is the real potential for a 'can't intubate, can't ventilate' scenario.

Preoperative assessment

- Full general assessment, including appropriate investigations.
- Full airway assessment (including the site of the abscess and restrictions imposed by it).
- Resolve consent issues.
- Risks and options should be understood.

Deep neck infections and Ludwig's angina

- Verbal communication may be difficult (consider using the text display of a mobile phone).
- Comorbidity may be impossible to assess or control fully.
- Special imaging techniques (CT or MRI scans) may be useful.

Premedication

- Routine starvation (nil by mouth) protocols should be observed.
- Consider topical anaesthetic cream (e.g. EMLA or Ametop).

- Oral sedation if needed and if the airway is not compromised.
- Antisialagogue if needed.
- Antiemetic if needed.
- Continue usual cardiorespiratory medication (e.g. salbutamol, glyceryl trinitrate (GTN) etc.).

Theatre preparation

- Skilled assistance is imperative.
- Association of Anaesthetists of Great Britain and Ireland (AAGBI) monitoring standards.
- 'Difficult intubation' equipment, including laryngeal mask airways, anatomically shaped optical (e.g. Airtraq or similar) laryngoscope and a flexible fibreoptic laryngoscope.
- Insufflation of oxygen before induction of anaesthesia.
- For deep neck infections and Ludwig's angina: facilities for immediate emergency tracheotomy are essential (surgeon scrubbed and ready).

Perioperative management

- Topical anaesthesia may allow preliminary drainage of a large 'pointing' abscess.
- Mask anaesthesia for simple exodontia.
- Laryngeal mask for periradicular surgery or external drainage.
- Tracheal intubation if clinically indicated.

Deep neck infections and Ludwig's angina

- Very difficult airway because of airway distortion, trismus and tissue immobility.
- Insufflation of oxygen before induction.
- Strongly consider awake fibreoptic intubation.
- Even careful inhalational induction may result in loss of the airway.

Intraoperative management

- Use propofol and/or sevoflurane for induction and maintenance of anaesthesia.
- Small laryngeal masks are best inserted under direct vision, using a Macintosh laryngoscope.
- Monitor the airway patency continuously and lift the chin or thrust the jaw if needed.
- Advise the surgeon regarding airway care.
- Use an absorbent 'pack' to reduce airway contamination.
- 'Swab count' within the oral cavity.
- Consider antibiotics and watch out for dysrhythmias.
- Avoid opioids unless external drainage is extensive.
- Muscle relaxants are seldom required for uncomplicated abscesses.

Deep neck infections and Ludwig's angina

- Intravenous fluids for volume replacement.
- Extreme caution with induction. It can lead to a 'can't ventilate, can't intubate' situation because of complete airway closure and impossible mask ventilation and intubation.
- Extreme caution with muscle relaxants before airway control (best avoided). If necessary, use agents (rocuronium, vecuronium) which can be rapidly reversed by sugammadex.
- Caution with laryngoscopy and intubation. Abscess rupture, loss of sight, laryngospasm and pus aspiration can occur.
- Tracheotomy can be difficult because of the swelling and can carry over infection to the mediastinum.

Postoperative management

- Position patient to facilitate drainage from the mouth (e.g. lateral).
- Oropharyngeal suction.
- Spontaneous rather than stimulated 'wake up'.
- Remove the airway protection device when awake (consider removing the laryngeal mask with the cuff inflated).
- Ensure the 'swab count' is correct.
- Paracetamol and non-steroidal anti-inflammatory drugs (NSAIDs) (unless contraindicated).

Deep neck infections and Ludwig's angina

- Ventilate electively until the airway is safe.
- Some patients will need ICU/high-dependency unit care for further treatment with antibiotics and fluids.

Outcome

- Simple abscess: full recovery.
- Deep neck infections and Ludwig's angina: may require follow-up surgery.

Bibliography

Atkinson RS, Rushman GB, Davies NJH. Dental anaesthesia. In: Atkinson RS, Rushman GB, Davies NJH (eds) *Lee's Synopsis of Anaesthesia*, 11th edn. Oxford: Butterworth-Heinemann, 1996, pp. 476–87.

Darshane S, Groom P, Charters P. Responsive contingency planning: a novel system for anticipated difficulty in (e.g. by mouth, rectal). Regard additional effects of long-term medication.

- Consider slower gastric emptying because of disease or medical side-effects.
- Avoid known stressors and maintain familiar 'comforts', e.g. allow soft toys.

Theatre preparation

- Skilled assistance.
- AAGBI monitoring standards.
- 'Difficult intubation' equipment, including laryngeal mask airways, optical (e.g. Airtraq or similar) laryngoscope and a flexible fibreoptic laryngoscope.

Patients with 'special needs'

- Consider personal safety issues.
- Consider 'lifting and handling' issues.
- Remove known stressors.
- Consider difficult intubation: macroglossia.
- Nasogastric tube and/or suctioning of feeding tube, e.g. percutaneous endoscopic gastrostomy (PEG) tube.
- Be prepared for the unknown.

Intraoperative management

- Inhalational (sevoflurane) or intravenous induction – caution if difficult airway.
- Flexible laryngeal mask, or tracheal intubation (rarely), needed.
- Sevoflurane, desflurane or propofol (total intravenous anaesthesia (TIVA)) for maintenance of anaesthesia.
- Monitor airway patency continuously and lift the chin or thrust the jaw if needed.
- Advise the surgeon regarding airway care.
- Use an absorbent 'pack' to reduce airway contamination.
- 'Swab count' within the oral cavity.
- Local anaesthesia for postoperative analgesia.
- Consider antibiotics.
- Opioids are seldom required.

Patients with 'special needs'

- Regular care-provider(s) present while awake.
- Flexible approach to induction of anaesthesia.
- Accept goal reduction if intended treatment not possible; try to avoid making next time more difficult.
- Avoid nasal intubation, because patients cannot handle epistaxis. Epistaxis also prevents release from hospital for day-case surgery.
- Beware of using muscle relaxants; if necessary, use a relaxant that is reversible by sugammadex.
- Surgical change of treatment/intervention because of new intraoperative diagnoses makes planning of exact management sometimes impossible.

Postoperative management

- Position the patient to facilitate drainage from mouth (e.g. lateral).
- Oropharyngeal suction.
- Spontaneous rather than stimulated wake-up.
- Remove the airway protection device when awake (consider removing the laryngeal mask airway with the cuff inflated).
- Ensure the 'swab count' is correct.
- Continue paracetamol and NSAIDs (unless contraindicated).

Patients with 'special needs'

- Write detailed notes on what worked and what did not.

Outcome

Patients with 'special needs'

- Are likely to return.
- Often appreciate being treated by staff they recognize.
- May be encouraged to accept minor dental procedures without general anaesthesia only in special cases.
- Day-case surgery:
  - discharge patients when they have recovered to their preoperative status
  - handle each case individually regarding anaesthetic management and discharge
  - work together with the patient's regular care-provider.

Bibliography

Department of Health. *Report of an Expert Working Party on General Anaesthesia, Sedation and Resuscitation in Dentistry.* London: Department of Health, Dental Division, 1991.

Gustavson KH, Umb-Carlsson O, Sonnander K. A follow-up study of mortality, health conditions and associated disabilities of people with intellectual disabilities in a Swedish county. *J Intellect Disabil Res* 2005; **49**(Pt 12): 905–14.

Messieha Z, Ananda RC, Hoffman I, Hoffman W. Five year outcomes study of dental rehabilitation conducted under general anesthesia for special needs patients. *Anesth Prog* 2007; **54**: 170–4.

Royal College of Anaesthetists. *Standards and Guidelines for General Anaesthesia for Dentistry*. London: Royal College of Anaesthetists, 1999.

Royal College of Surgeons of England. *Commission on the Provision of Surgical Services. Guidelines for Day Case Surgery*. London: Royal College of Surgeons of England, 1985.

Cross-references

Day-case surgery, 604
Difficult airway: management, 651
Difficult airway: prediction, 664
Infants and children, 615
Paediatric airway, 675

- Blood loss, fluid balance and urine output.
- Tidal volume, respiratory rate, F_iO_2, $ETco_2$ and disconnect alarm.
- End-tidal agent concentration and depth of anaesthesia monitor.
- Neuromuscular blockade.
- Core and peripheral temperature (groin, big toe).
- An intramucosal pH (pHi) catheter or microdialysis in gastric transposition or flap surgery may be used. (pHi <7.32 or low glucose, high lactate and glycerol indicate ischaemia.)

Bleeding

This is minimized by:

- surgical technique
- infiltration of vasoconstrictors
- smooth induction and recovery
- minimum coughing/straining
- 10–15° head-up tilt (remember risk of air embolism)
- flexion of thighs at the hips improves venous return
- good analgesia/anaesthesia
- controlled hypotension.

To reduce brain volume and facilitate surgery involving the cranium, modest hypocapnia, osmotic diuretics or withdrawing of CSF may be necessary.

Free-flap surgery

Good surgical technique remains a leading factor for graft survival. Optimum anaesthetic management should prevent vasoconstriction and enhance blood flow to the flap. This is achieved and maintained by:

- satisfactory analgesia and P_ao_2
- normotension and cardiac output
- normovolaemia or even slight hypervolaemia
- normothermia and normocapnia
- optimizing blood viscosity
- using Dextran 40 or anticoagulation agents according to the size and function of the anastomosis
- limiting intraoperative fluid replacement by crystalloid infusions and using diuretics to lessen the risk of postoperative pulmonary oedema
- starting β-blocker therapy in high-risk patients preoperatively to minimize the risk of supraventricular tachycardia, if not contraindicated
- minimizing external compression of graft vessels by haematoma or dressings.

Postoperative care

These patients will need care in an HDU/ICU. Intensive care and monitoring give confidence to patients with airway difficulties, a swollen face and inability to see, and allow good analgesia using opioid infusion, PCA or NSAIDs after maxillofacial surgery. Epidural analgesia with or without opioid is useful in surgery involving the thoracoabdominal area. Local anaesthetic infiltration of the donor graft site or its nerves helps in postoperative pain relief.

- The patient is extubated only when awake and when the patient has intact protective reflexes and oozing or bleeding has stopped. Prolonged controlled ventilation is uncommon unless there is coexisting cardiopulmonary disease.
- Perioperative placement of a stomach tube to minimize the risk of vomiting and aspiration pneumonia because of severe dysphagia and to allow early feeding.
- Dexamethasone may be used to reduce postoperative swelling.
- Wire cutters should be readily available if IMF is used. When there has been major surgery to the mouth or upper airway, anticipation of severe postoperative swelling or bleeding dictates the need for tracheostomy.
- Patients may often return to theatre because of early complications, such as airway difficulties, bleeding, compromised blood supply to flaps, and haematoma formation.
- Many patients require repeat procedures, especially those with severe facial deformity and those with malignancy.

Bibliography

Barham CJ. Anaesthesia for maxillofacial surgery. In: Patel H (ed.) *Anaesthesia for Burns, Maxillofacial and Plastic Surgery.* London: Edward Arnold, 1993, pp. 53–77.

Brooks NC, Mostafa SM. Anaesthesia and pain control for head and neck surgery. In: Jones A, Phillips DE, Hilgers JM (eds) *Diseases of the Head and Neck, Nose and Throat.* London: Arnold, 1998, pp. 142–52.

Donlon JV. Eye, ear, nose and throat disease. In: Benumof JL (ed.) *Anaesthesia and Uncommon Diseases*, 4th edn. Philadelphia: WB Saunders, 1998, pp. 38–50.

Goat VA. Anaesthesia for craniofacial surgery. In: Atkinson RS, Adams AP (eds) *Recent Advances in Anaesthesia and Analgesia.* Edinburgh: Churchill Livingstone, 1989, pp. 139–53.

Inglis M, Robbie DS, Edwards JM, Breach NM. The anaesthetic management of patients undergoing free flap reconstructive surgery following resection of head and neck neoplasms – a review of 64 patients. *Ann R Coll Surg Engl* 1988; **70**: 235–8.

Kruse AL, Luebbers HT, Grätz KW, Obwegeser JA. Factors influencing survival of free-flap in reconstruction for cancer of the head and neck: a literature review. *Microsurgery* 2010; **30**: 242–8.

Rojdmark J, Blomquvist L, Malm M, *et al.* Metabolism in myocutaneous flaps studied by in-situ microdialysis. *Scand J Plast Reconstr Surg Hand Surg* 1998; **32**: 27–34.

Smith JE, Suh JD, Erman A, *et al.* Risk factors predicting aspiration after free flap reconstruction of oral cavity and oropharyngeal defects. *Arch Otolaryngol Head Neck Surg* 2008; **134**: 1205–8.

Suh JD, Sercarz JA, Abemayor E, *et al.* Analysis of outcome and complications in 400 cases of microvascular head and neck reconstruction. *Arch Otolaryngol Head Neck Surg* 2004; **130**: 962–6.

Sweeney DB, Sainsbury DA. Anaesthesia for cranio-maxillary-facial surgery. *Curr Anaesth Crit Care* 1992; **3**: 11–16.

Cross-references

Difficult airway: management, 651
Induced hypotension during anaesthesia, 711
Prolonged anaesthesia, 717
Trauma, 801

Thyroidectomy

Andreas Schöpfer

Procedure

Thyroidectomy may be unilateral, subtotal or total. Surgery is performed through a skin crease incision approximately 4 cm above the sternum:

- surgeons should locate and preserve the recurrent laryngeal nerves
- parathyroid glands should be preserved
- in the neck, haemostasis is very important
- suction drains are used to minimize haematoma accumulation
- large retrosternal goitres may require a sternal split to allow complete excision.

Patients' characteristics

Most patients presenting for thyroid surgery are female, and the pathological conditions are listed below. Approximately 10% of nodules will be malignant.

Thyrotoxicosis

- Graves' disease (20–40 years old).
- Multinodular goitre (older patients).
- Toxic solitary nodule.

Carcinoma

- Papillary (30–40 years old).
- Follicular or medullary (older patients).
- Anaplastic.
- Bilateral compressive or cosmetically unacceptable non-toxic goitre.
- Autoimmune thyroiditis.

Preoperative assessment

After general assessment, emphasis should be placed on the following.

Airway assessment

- Tracheal deviation may be marked.
- Some patients may have stridor or respiratory problems when supine.
- Vocal cords movement should be assessed by an otolaryngologist to ensure that pre-existing laryngeal nerve palsy is recognized.

Cardiovascular system

- Hyperthyroidism can cause tachycardia, atrial fibrillation or heart failure.
- Large goitres may obstruct venous drainage.

Eyes

- Lid retraction and exophthalmos mean care is needed to protect the eyes from intraoperative drying or trauma.

Other conditions

Thyroid disease may be part of multiple endocrine neoplasia syndromes, and conditions such as diabetes mellitus, hyperparathyroidism and phaeochromocytoma must be considered.

Preoperative investigation

Thyroid function must be assessed and patients rendered clinically euthyroid prior to surgery. Measure serum thyroxin (tetraiodothyronine (T_4): free, 10–40 pmol L^{-1}; total, 64–160 nmol L^{-1}; and its index 17–47), triiodothyronine (T_3) and thyroid-stimulating hormone (TSH). In another test, thyroid-releasing factor (TRF) is given and the levels of TSH are measured. Failure of TSH to rise indicates hyperthyroidism.

- Other blood tests include full blood count, group and save, serum urea and electrolytes, calcium and phosphate.
- An ECG is important in older or hyperthyroid patients to assess preoperative hormone-suppression regimes.
- Chest X-ray and thoracic inlet views are useful to assess airway compression or deviation.
- With retrosternal disease or severe stridor, a CT or MRI scan will delineate the degree and extent of airway narrowing.
- Surgery must be deferred if patients remain clinically hyperthyroid.
- β-receptor blockade must be continued beyond the day of surgery.

Drug treatment for hyperthyroidism

Carbimazole Inhibits iodination of tyrosyl residues in thyroglobulin.

Propylthiouracil	As carbimazole, but also reduces peripheral de-iodination of T_4 to T_3.
β-blockers	Used to control cardiovascular effects. Propranolol also decreases the peripheral conversion of T_4 to T_3.
Iodine	Potassium iodide is given for 7–10 days preoperatively. It decreases gland vascularity and secretion of thyroxin.

Perioperative care

- Patients often need anxiolytic premedication.
- Use routine monitoring and an intravenous fluid infusion. An arterial line may be required for those with pre-existing cardiovascular disease.
- With massive goitre or airway compromise, a gas induction or awake fibreoptic intubation may be required.
- An intravenous induction and controlled ventilation technique is usually used.
- Use a carefully secured reinforced endotracheal tube.
- Careful neck extension provides surgical access.
- A head-up tilt reduces venous engorgement.
- Endotracheal tube position must be checked after patient positioning as neck extension may change the location of the tube tip.
- The eyes must be protected, as drapes will be placed over the head.
- Surgeons may wish to use a nerve stimulator to locate the laryngeal nerves. In such cases, muscle relaxation cannot be used once intubation is completed.
- An electromyography (EMG) endotracheal tube or invasive techniques using needle electrodes for monitoring the recurrent laryngeal nerve are available.
- In patients with high anaesthetic risks, think about using local anaesthesia.
- Intraoperative monitoring of body temperature: increasing temperature is an indicator for thyrotoxic crises; be aware of hypothermia in hypothyreosis as a result of decreased basal metabolism.
- Supplementation of β-blockade may be needed as manipulation of the thyroid may release more thyroid hormone.
- Prior to wound closure, normotension, head-down tilt and a Valsalva manoeuvre will assist in locating bleeding points.
- Some surgeons request direct laryngoscopy to assess vocal cord movement at the end of surgery. Others prefer a smooth extubation with no hypertensive stimuli. In some centres, the endotracheal tube is replaced by a laryngeal mask airway at the end of surgery. A fibreoptic endoscope is used to assess vocal cord movement.
- Surgical manipulation may kink the trachea. Hence, a reinforced endotracheal tube is needed.

Postoperative care and complications

- Thyrotoxic patients must continue on their preoperative drug regime until T4 levels decrease.
- Serum calcium should be checked to ensure normal parathyroid gland function. Tetany or low serum calcium require calcium supplementation by the intravenous or oral route.
- Postoperatively, recurrent laryngeal nerve palsy (temporary due to oedema, or permanent) will cause the affected vocal cord to lie in adduction. Symptoms range from hoarse voice and dyspnoea to stridor or complete airway obstruction, requiring reintubation and possibly a tracheostomy.
- Early detection of signs of postoperative haemorrhage.
- Neck haematoma and surgical tracheal retraction may cause laryngeal oedema. Removal of wound clips and suture will decompress the neck and trachea prior to urgent evacuation and haemostasis. A gas induction or intravenous induction are suitable techniques. A smaller endotracheal tube may be required. Surgeons should be present in case of the need for an emergency tracheostomy.

Rare complications

- *Tracheomalacia* may be seen following resection of compressive retrosternal thyroid masses. Tracheal collapse may necessitate prolonged intubation.
- *Pneumothorax* is occasionally seen following extensive and difficult resection, requiring insertion of an intercostal chest drain.
- *Thyroid storm* occurs because of uncontrolled release of thyroxin in a thyrotoxic patient and may be triggered by acute illness, surgery or trauma. Signs include hyperpyrexia, tachycardia, hypertension, arrhythmias, vomiting, diarrhoea and altered mental state. Intraoperatively, this may mimic malignant hyperpyrexia. This condition may occur postoperatively if drug treatment is stopped immediately following surgery. The half-life of T_4 is approximately 7 days. This condition can prove fatal and patients must be managed on an ICU. Treatment includes:

  - propranolol intravenously, orally or via a nasogastric tube
  - esmolol may also be used for acute management

- carbimazole or propylthiouracil orally or via a nasogastric tube
- hydrocortisone supplementation intravenously
- oxygen should be given and ventilation may be required
- temperature monitoring and active cooling may be required
- dantrolene use has been reported in these patients.

Bibliography

Hilary Wade JS. Respiratory obstruction in thyroid surgery. *Ann R Coll Surg Engl* 1980; **62**: 15–24.

Mercer EM, Eltringham RJ. Anaesthesia for thyroid surgery. *Ear Nose Throat J* 1985; **64**: 342–75.

Gravenstein N. *Manual of Complications During Anesthesia*. London: JB Lippincott, 1993, pp. 596–601.

Wheeler MH. Malignant goitre/thyroidectomy. *Surgery* 1984; **9**: 200–9.

Chiang FY, Lee KW, Chen HC, *et al.* Standardization of intraoperative neuromonitoring of recurrent laryngeal nerve in thyroid operation. *World J Surg* 2010; **34**: 223–9.

Spanknebel K, Chabot JA, DiGiorgi M, *et al.* Thyroidectomy using local anesthesia: a report of 1,025 cases over 16 years. *J Am Coll Surg* 2005; **201**: 375–85.

Cross-references

Hyperthyroidism, 66
Hypothyroidism, 70
Parathyroid surgery, 546

14

Plastic surgery

Deborah M Nolan

Burns surgery

Deborah M Nolan

Procedures

- 130 000 patients per annum with thermal injury require hospital admission. Half of these are children under 12.
- Major burns surgery should occur in specialized regional units.
- Anaesthesia may be required for tracheostomy, escharotomy, dressing changes or surgery for associated injuries.
- Early surgery improves cosmetic result and removes necrotic tissue.
- Burns are conventionally classified by area (percentage of total body surface area (TBSA) burned) and depth (superficial, shallow and deep dermal, full thickness and full thickness with deep tissue involvement). A major burn in an adult is defined as greater than 20% of TBSA and in children greater than 10% TBSA.
- May be lengthy procedures, e.g. 1–2 hours for burns dressings.

Patient characteristics

- All age groups are affected, but extremes of age are common. Children up to 4 years of age constitute 20% of patients with thermal injury.
- Males predominate in all groups other than the elderly.
- Teenagers are often injured as a result of illicit activity involving, for example, electrocution/petrol.
- May be associated with other injuries.
- May be associated comorbidities, e.g. epilepsy, psychiatric disturbances, history of substance abuse.
- Consider non-accidental injury in every child.
- Adult burns are usually caused by flame, and paediatric burns by scalds.

Preoperative assessment and investigations

- Has there been a history of smoke inhalation?
- Has resuscitation been completed?
- Full blood count, urea and electrolytes, chest X-ray, arterial blood gases, clotting screen and urine output.
- Blood glucose is particularly important in children.
- Check availability of blood and blood products.

Theatre preparation

- A burns theatre may be a relatively isolated site.
- If transferring patients from a burns unit or ITU to theatre, full mobile facilities are required for transfer.
- Large burns require intermittent positive pressure ventilation. An intensive care ventilator may be required to ventilate adequately. Ventilated burns patients may be highly positive end-expiratory pressure dependent.
- Anticipate significant blood loss.
- Warmed rapid infusion systems and forced warmed air blankets.
- Theatre prewarmed to a thermoneutral temperature (approximately 30°C).
- Ideally involve two surgical teams, as well as two anaesthetists.

Premedication

- Preventive analgesia, e.g. for burns dressings.
- Anxiolysis may be required, particularly in children.

Perioperative management

Monitoring

- ECG: placement of electrodes potentially difficult.
- Oximetry:
  - vasoconstriction/burned peripheries may limit use
  - cannot distinguish between carboxyhaemoglobin (COHb) and oxyhaemoglobin; high readings if COHb present.
- Blood pressure: invasive/non-invasive.
- Capnography: increased dead-space in inhalation injury, therefore end-tidal CO_2 ($ETco_2$) may not reflect P_aco_2.
- Central venous pressure (CVP): access may be difficult and pose infection risk.
- Respiratory gas analysis.
- Central temperature.
- Urine output.

Anaesthetic technique

- If there is a possibility of airway oedema consider awake fibreoptic or inhalation induction.

- Repeated fasting required for surgical procedures may interfere with nutritional goals: patients are hypermetabolic. Consider modification of fasting guidelines.
- Anticipate major blood loss, measure Hb intraoperatively and consider dilutional effect on clotting factors.
- Regional techniques are generally not useful in major burns: infection risk, possible coagulopathy and difficult to block sufficient area.
- Hyperkalaemic response to succinylcholine: avoid after 24 hours and arguably up to 1 year postoperatively.
- Induction with propofol has largely superseded ketamine.
- Choice of volatile does not influence outcome.
- Total intravenous anaesthesia.
- Resistance to non-depolarizers develops by 1 week and persists for up to 8 weeks.
- Epinephrine-containing solutions may be applied topically or subcutaneously to decrease bleeding at excision and donor sites.
- EMLA local anaesthetic gel may be applied under dressings.
- Dose requirements of aminoglycosides, cephalosporins, and β-lactams altered owing to increased clearance.
- Meticulous attention to positioning: patients may need to be placed in the prone position.
- Preventive analgesia: usually opiate based.

Dressing changes

- General anaesthesia often appropriate.
- Entonox is useful for short procedures if oxygen requirements are less than 50%: supplement opioids, reduce breakthrough pain and avoid prolonged sedation.
- Ketamine is analgesic and sedative: use limited by hallucinations, but this may be attenuated by use of a benzodiazepine.
- Boluses of shorter acting opioids, e.g. alfentanil and fentanyl, are useful for short procedures.
- Combination with propofol in low-dose infusion: target-controlled infusion at a dose range of 1–2 $\mu g\ mL^{-1}$ is used.
- Further flexibility may be achieved by adding remifentanil: will need supplementation postoperatively.

Postoperative management

- Analgesia: provided by intravenous opioids. Intramuscular or subcutaneous doses are unpredictable in absorption.
- Opioid infusions:
  - caution with accumulation and requires extreme nursing vigilance
  - patient-controlled analgesia with morphine: adults and children, but depends on having use of hands.
- Caution in patients with altered conscious state, e.g. alcohol, drugs,
- Tolerance develops rapidly.
- Caution with non-steroidal drugs: patients prone to renal dysfunction and peptic ulceration.
- Procedural pain associated with dressing changes may be severe.
- Early nutritional supplementation is essential, e.g. 3000–5000 calories per day in adults.

Outcome

- Survival of major burns is age related and decreases over the age of 30. No prospective evaluation in large trials has taken place.
- Worse in the presence of respiratory injury and increasing burn size.
- Results in long-term psychological distress and chronic disability.
- May require frequent subsequent hospital admissions for reconstructive surgery to aid functional recovery.

Bibliography

Black RG, Kinsella J. Anaesthetic management for burns patients. *BJA CEPD Rev* 2001; **1**: 177–80.

Herndon D. *Total Burn Care*, 2nd edn. London: W.B. Saunders.

Hilton PJ, Hepp M. The immediate care of the burned patient. *BJA CEPD Rev* 2001; **1**: 113–16.

Norman AT, Judkins KC. Pain in the patient with burns. *BJA Cont Educ Anaesth Crit Care Pain* 2004; **4**: 57–61.

Ryan CM, Schoenfield DA, Thorpe WP, *et al.* Objective estimates of the probability of death from burn injuries. *N Engl J Med* 1998; **338**: 362–6.

Wilkinson E. The epidemiology of burns in secondary care in a population of 2.6 million people. *Burns* 1998; **24**: 139–43.

Yowler CJ. Recent advances in burn care. *Curr Opin Anaesthesiol* 2001; **14**: 251–5.

Cross-references

Blood transfusion, 735
Fluid and electrolyte balance, 754
Postoperative pain management, 783
Prolonged anaesthesia, 717

Haemangioma

- May be a simple peripheral procedure.
- If involving the face or oral cavity this may be a complicated procedure with associated airway problems, major blood loss and potential for air embolism.
- A cutaneous haemangioma around the face and neck may be associated with a subglottic haemangioma. There is a risk of bleeding into the mouth and airway if this is subject to trauma.

Cystic hygroma

- These are multiloculated cystic swellings. If present in the neck, it may invade the oropharynx and tongue. It can present as an upper airway obstruction in the neonate.
- Intubation can be hazardous: spontaneous ventilation must be maintained until intubation has been achieved. Severe cases will require tracheostomy.
- Postoperative problems include bleeding and respiratory obstruction.

Otoplasty

- This is the procedure for correction of what used to be known as 'bat ears'.
- Correction of prominent ears is often associated with a high incidence of postoperative nausea and vomiting, which can last up to 48 hours; an antiemetic will be required.
- A procedure including local infiltration or nerve block is helpful.

Hypospadias repair

- Anatomical correction of the congenital abnormality of the male urethra.
- Usually undertaken in an infant.
- Spontaneous or controlled ventilation can be used according to length of procedure.
- Caudal block with 0.5–1 mL kg^{-1} of 0.25% bupivacaine provides excellent analgesia that can be extended by adding clonidine, diamorphine or ketamine.

Bibliography

Bosenberg AT, Kimble FW. Infraorbital nerve block in neonates for cleft lip repair: anatomical study and clinical application. *Br J Anaesth* 1995; **74**: 506–8.

Hatch DJ. Airway management in cleft lip and palate surgery. *Br J Anaesth* 1996; **76**: 755–6.

Sommerlad BC. Management of cleft lip and palate. *Curr Paediatr* 1994; **4**: 189–95.

Takemura H, Yasumoto K, Toi T, Hosoyamada A. Correlation of cleft type with incidence of perioperative respiratory complications in infants with cleft lip and palate. *Paediatr Anaesth* 2002; **12:** 585–8.

Cross-references

Infants and children, 615
Paediatric airway, 675
Paediatrics: overview, 552

Peripheral limb surgery

Deborah M Nolan

Procedures

- May be elective or emergency as a result of trauma.
- Examples include surgery for correction of acquired deformities, e.g. Dupuytren's contracture, carpal tunnel syndrome and excision of tumours or skin lesions.
- Replantation of digits or limbs following traumatic amputation may be lengthy procedures.

Patient characteristics

- Entire age range, including early correction of congenital malformations (which may be associated with other anomalies).
- May have associated trauma or alcohol/substance abuse injuries.

Preoperative assessment and investigations

- In trauma situations exclude coexisting injuries.
- Specific assessment for implication of other comorbidities, e.g. in rheumatoid arthritis.
- Full haematology and biochemistry as indicated.
- ECG, chest X-ray and other investigations as indicated.
- Sickle screen important in at-risk populations if a tourniquet is to be used.

Premedication

- Full explanation of procedure and details of any proposed nerve block.
- If the patient is to be discharged while a nerve block is still effective, they should be warned about avoiding hot surfaces.
- Anxiolytic premedication may be useful if timing of admission permits.
- Preoperative analgesia appropriate in recent trauma.

Perioperative management

Monitoring

- ECG.
- S_pO_2.
- Non-invasive BP.
- Capnography: unnecessary for regional blockade.
- If surgery is prolonged, more invasive monitoring may be required.

Technique

- A regional block with or without sedation is usually the most appropriate technique. Reduces physiological disturbance and recovery room time.
- Continuous peripheral nerve blockade is popular for postoperative analgesia and can be placed at the majority of sites where a single shot can be undertaken. Quality of analgesia is superior to opioids.
- Ultrasound-guided regional nerve block facilitates easy and accurate positioning of needles close to the nerves and is being increasingly utilized. Allows neurovascular as well as musculoskeletal structures to be seen, as well as visualization of the injectate with the opportunity to reposition the needle tip if the solution spread is unsatisfactory. Current National Institute for Health and Clinical Excellence guidelines support the use of ultrasound. Clinicians need to be trained in nerve block administration and in ultrasound guidance techniques.
- Establish venous access prior to insertion of a block.
- Suitable for a wide range of procedures.
- In replantation surgery, the associated sympathetic block improves perfusion.

General anaesthesia alone or supplemented by a regional block is also a suitable technique and is useful in the following situations:

- paediatric patients
- prolonged procedures
- uncooperative patients, e.g. learning difficulties, dementia.

Upper limb surgery

Brachial plexus block

- Commonest block for upper limb surgery.
- May be approached using interscalene, subclavian or axillary approaches.
- Ultrasound guidance now being widely utilized.
- Using epinephrine with the local anaesthetic agent increases the intensity and prolongs the duration of the block.

- It is generally accepted practice that a regional block should be inserted prior to induction of anaesthesia. Paediatric practice is an exception.

Peripheral nerve blocks

- Ulnar, median and radial nerve blocks at the elbow and wrist may be used to supplement a brachial plexus block.
- If a digital nerve block is used, epinephrine-containing solutions should be avoided.

Intravenous regional anaesthesia

- Best used for brief (up to 1 hour) minor surgery of hand and forearm, e.g. carpal tunnel release.
- Longer procedures precluded by pain from tourniquet.
- Simple and reliable technique.
- Block resolves rapidly following release of the tourniquet; therefore, confers no postoperative analgesia.

Lower limb surgery

Lumbar and caudal epidural blocks and also spinal blocks are suitable for unilateral or bilateral lower limb surgery.

Peripheral nerve blocks

Used for pain relief following knee surgery and limb fractures.

Examples are:

- three-in-one nerve block (femoral, obturator and lateral cutaneous nerve of the thigh)
- femoral nerve block: easy to master, high success rate
- sciatic nerve block.

Ankle blocks

- Useful for surgery on feet and toes.
- Essentially a block of four sciatic nerve branches, i.e. deep and superficial peroneal, tibial and sural nerves and one cutaneous branch of the femoral nerve (saphenous nerve).

Tourniquet use

- Maximum pressure in the leg should be 300 mmHg.
- Maximum pressure in the arm should be 200 mmHg.
- Maximum tourniquet time 1–2 hours.
- Generally avoided in sickle disease: if use is essential, it should be discussed with a haematologist.

Bibliography

Chapman GA, Johnson D, Bodenham AR. Visualisation of needle position using ultrasonography. *Anaesthesia* 2006; **61**: 148–58.

Liu SS, Salinas FV. Continuous plexus and peripheral nerve blocks for post-operative analgesia. *Anesth Analg* 2003; **96**: 263–72.

Marhofer P, Greher M, Kapral S. Ultrasound guidance in regional anaesthesia. *Br J Anaesthesia* 2005; **94**: 7–17.

New York School of Regional Anaesthesia. See www.nysora.com

Wildsmith JAW, Armitage EN, McClure JH (eds). *Principles and Practice of Regional Anaesthesia*, 3rd edn. Edinburgh: Churchill Livingstone, 2002.

Cross-references

Day-case surgery, 604
Local anaesthetic toxicity, 767
Prolonged anaesthesia, 717
Sickle cell syndrome, 239

15 Thoracic surgery

Mark R Patrick

Bronchopleural fistula

Mark R Patrick

Bronchopleural fistula (BPF) is a direct communication between the tracheobronchial tree and the pleural cavity. Causes of BPF include dehiscence of the bronchial stump, cancer, inflammatory lesions and trauma. In developed countries, dehiscence of the bronchial stump following pneumonectomy is the commonest cause of BPF. The incidence of BPF following pneumonectomy is extremely low in specialized centres.

Minor forms of post-pneumonectomy BPF can be sealed bronchoscopically with fibrin glue. Large fistulas require resuture of the bronchial stump via a repeat thoracotomy.

Preoperative assessment and investigations

- Symptoms relate to fluid from the infected space flowing over to the remaining lung.

Small bronchopleural fistula

- Malaise and low-grade fever.
- Cough with/without haemoptysis, wheeze or dyspnoea.

Large bronchopleural fistula

- Severe dyspnoea and debilitation.
- Coughing up copious amounts of thinnish brown fluid.

Investigations

- Chest X-ray. Loss of pneumonectomy space fluid. Consolidation/collapse of the remaining lung.
- Blood gas analysis to assess hypoxaemia, hypercarbia and acid–base status.

Preoperative preparation

- General resuscitation including oxygen by face-mask.
- Sit the patient up to prevent further spillover.
- Insert a chest drain on the pneumonectomized side.
- Transport the patient to theatre in the sitting position with the drain open.

Premedication

- None required.

Monitoring

- Routine basic monitoring.
- Invasive arterial pressure.
- Central venous pressure.
- Arterial blood gases.
- Core temperature.
- Urine output.

Anaesthetic technique

Classically, it has been advocated that a post-pneumonectomy fistula should be isolated with an endobronchial tube before IPPV is employed. This can be achieved either with awake endobronchial intubation with local analgesia of the airway (with or without fibreoptic bronchoscopy) or with inhalational induction and intubation under deep inhalational anaesthesia. These techniques should be discussed at examinations, but both are fraught with difficulty. Most experienced anaesthetists now use the following technique:

- sit the patient upright with the drain open
- preoxygenate
- use intravenous induction and succinylcholine or rocuronium
- rigid bronchoscopy is usually performed
- insert a double-lumen tube into the remaining bronchus with a fibreoptic bronchoscope
- administer further muscle relaxant
- IPPV via the endobronchial portion of the tube
- place the patient in the lateral position for thoracotomy.

Postoperative management

- Treat as for pneumonectomy.
- Sputum retention, infection, ALI and respiratory failure are common and carry a high mortality. Treat with physiotherapy, antibiotics, ventilation and early tracheostomy.
- Infection in the pneumonectomy space.

Outcome

- Mortality is in the region of 10–20%.

Bibliography

Lauckner ME, Beggs I, Armstrong RF. The radiological characteristics of bronchopleural fistula following pneumonectomy. *Anaesthesia* 1983; **38**: 452–6.

Ryder GH, Short DH, Zeitlin GL. The anaesthetic management of a bronchopleural fistula with the Robertshaw double-lumen tube. *Br J Anaesth* 1965; **37**: 861–5.

Cross-references

Anaesthesia and bronchogenic carcinoma, 86
Bronchiectasis, 109
One-lung anaesthesia, 714
Pneumonectomy, 420
Postoperative analgesia for thoracic surgery patients, 421
Preoperative assessment of pulmonary risk, 625

for postthoracotomy analgesia. *Anesth Analg* 2008; **107**: 1026–40.

Slinger PD, Johnson MR. *Preoperative Assessment for Pulmonary Resection 2005.* See www.thoracicanesthesia.com.

Wright IG. Surgery on the lungs. In: Ghosh S, Latimer RD (eds). *Thoracic Anaesthesia: Principles and Practice.* Oxford: Butterworth-Heinemann, 1999, pp. 73–99.

Cross-references

Anaesthesia and bronchogenic carcinoma, 86
Bronchiectasis, 109
One-lung anaesthesia, 714
Preoperative assessment of respiratory risk, 625

Mediastinal surgery

Mark R Patrick

Mediastinal surgery can be split into two categories:

- diagnostic – mediastinoscopy, mediastinotomy
- therapeutic – excision of tumours and cysts.

Mediastinoscopy and mediastinotomy are used to assess mediastinal lymph node involvement to stage lung cancer. These patients are in the categories outlined for pneumonectomy and lobectomy but the staging procedure is low risk.

Patients with large primary mediastinal tumours are at high risk, mainly from airway obstruction. Such patients may present for minor diagnostic procedures but the airway problems outlined for major mediastinal surgery also apply. Some patients with thymomas have myasthenia gravis. Thymomas are rarely large enough to cause obstruction.

Mediastinoscopy/ mediastinotomy

Mediastinoscopy is the passage of a mediastinoscope into the pretracheal area via a small incision above the suprasternal notch. Biopsies can be taken and nodes palpated digitally. Mediastinotomy is opening of the anterior mediastinum via an incision through the bed of the second costal cartilage. The pleura may be breached.

Preoperative assessment and considerations

- See Preoperative assessment (see Overview), p. 408.
- Assess for tracheal obstruction or deviation with clinical examination (inspiratory stridor), chest X-ray (posteroanterior and lateral) or CT scan.
- Myasthenia is a special case.

Premedication

- None needed.

Monitoring

- Routine basic monitoring.

Anaesthetic technique

- Rigid bronchoscopy is usually performed first.
- Position the patient supine with a sandbag under the shoulders and the neck extended.
- General anaesthesia with an opioid/relaxant technique, supplemented with either a volatile agent or TIVA. Remifentanil, atracurium and desflurane are recommended. Nitrous oxide is not advised.
- There may be airway obstruction.
- If the pleura is breached during mediastinotomy, this is not usually a problem as there is no leak from the lung. IPPV with PEEP keeps the lung expanded.

Postoperative management

- Ensure the relaxant is fully reversed.
- Extubate the patient sitting up.
- Check the chest X-ray for pneumothoraces.

Major mediastinal surgery

Primary anterior and superior mediastinal tumours are most common in young adults. Tumours include thymoma, retrosternal thyroid and teratoma. Ten per cent of patients with myasthenia gravis have thymomas and myasthenia presents its own unique problems. Anterior mediastinal tumours are particularly likely to cause problems during anaesthesia. The greatest of these is compression and obstruction of the airway and vascular structures – most commonly the superior vena cava (SVC). Operative mortality is low in specialized centres with good outcomes following curative resection. Recurrence is a problem with some tumours. These may respond to chemotherapy or radiotherapy. Some tumours (e.g. secondary teratoma) may require reoperation.

Procedure

Surgery is usually performed through a median sternotomy in a supine position, but small tumours may be resectable transcervically. Blood loss can be considerable.

Preoperative assessment and considerations

- Respiratory symptoms, cough, wheeze, stridor or dyspnoea suggest tracheal obstruction.
- Chest X-ray (posteroanterior and lateral) and CT scan to evaluate the trachea.
- Lung function tests with a flow–volume loop.
- Occasionally, echo or pulmonary angiography (involvement of the pericardium or pulmonary artery).
- Myasthenic patients are often receiving steroids and other immunosuppression. Steroid cover may be required.

Pneumonectomy

Mark R Patrick

Pneumonectomy is excision of a whole lung for lung cancer. It is performed via a posterolateral thoracotomy. It is higher risk than lobectomy with an operative mortality of over 6%.

Preoperative assessment

- See Preoperative assessment (see Overview), p. 408.
- Blood must be rapidly available.
- Myasthenic syndrome may be present.

Premedication

- None needed.
- Full explanation about high-dependency care, postoperative monitoring and analgesia, including the benefits and risks of neuraxial blockade.

Monitoring

- Routine basic monitoring.
- Invasive arterial pressure.
- Central venous pressure.
- Core temperature.
- Arterial blood gases.
- Urine output (if epidural analgesia is used or the patient is high risk).

Anaesthetic technique

- General anaesthesia with an opioid/relaxant technique, supplemented with either a volatile agent or TIVA. Remifentanil, atracurium and desflurane are recommended. Nitrous oxide is not advised.
- Regional block (thoracic epidural, paravertebral or epipleural) is routinely used unless contraindicated.
- Rigid bronchoscopy is usually performed first.
- Intubate with a double-lumen endobronchial tube.
- One-lung anaesthesia is used while the chest is open.
- Treat epidural hypotension with a vasoconstrictor, not fluid.
- Catastrophic haemorrhage from the pulmonary artery occurs occasionally.
- The integrity of the bronchial suture line is tested prior to chest closure. The bronchial stump is covered with sterile water and pressure up 30 cmH_2O is exerted by manual compression of the rebreathing bag. Any leak is detected as bubbles.
- Maintenance of normothermia is crucial to postoperative respiratory function. Underbody warming, fluid warming and the use of heat and moisture exchangers are mandatory.

Postoperative management

- Basal drain is placed at surgery.
- Ensure the relaxant is fully reversed (nerve stimulator).
- Extubate in the sitting position, with the patient breathing spontaneously.
- Administer humidified oxygen by face-mask.
- Restrict intravenous fluid.
- Use a vasoconstrictor, not fluid, to treat epidural-related hypotension.
- Never apply suction to a pneumonectomy drain. Most surgeons prefer to leave the drain clamped and to open it for 1 minute every hour to allow blood out. The drain is removed after 24 hours.

Complications

- Haemorrhage into the pleural space: verify by unclamping the drain; replace the volume lost. May need surgical exploration.
- Sputum retention, infection, ALI and respiratory failure: this carries a high mortality after pneumonectomy. Treat with physiotherapy, antibiotics, ventilation and early tracheostomy.
- Infection in pneumonectomy space: this requires draining and may be associated with a bronchopleural fistula.
- Atrial fibrillation: treat with β-blockade with or without amiodarone; digoxin is usually ineffective.

Bibliography

Joshi GP, Bonnet F, Shah R, *et al.* A systematic review of randomized trials evaluating regional techniques for postthoracotomy analgesia. *Anesth Analg* 2008; **107**: 1026–40.

Slinger PD, Johnson MR. *Preoperative Assessment for Pulmonary Resection 2005.* See www.thoracicanesthesia.com.

Wright IG. Surgery on the lungs. In: Ghosh S, Latimer RD (eds). *Thoracic Anaesthesia: Principles and Practice.* Oxford: Butterworth-Heinemann, 1999, pp. 73–99.

Cross-references

One-lung anaesthesia, 714
Postoperative analgesia, 421
Preoperative assessment of respiratory risk, 625

Postoperative analgesia

Mark R Patrick

Pain after thoracotomy is more intense than with any other incision. For this reason, regional block is commonly used, in conjunction with systemic analgesia if needed. All blocks except epidurals usually require additional systemic agents to achieve optimal analgesia. Blocks are usually used for the first 3 postoperative days. The catheter is then removed and systemic analgesia is used. Chronic neuropathic pain is common after thoracotomy. Cryoanalgesia of intercostal nerves is no longer used as its use is associated with a high incidence of neuropathic pain.

Sources of pain

- Chest wall and most of the pleura via the intercostal nerves.
- Diaphragmatic pleura via the phrenic nerves.
- Mediastinal pleura via the vagus nerve.
- Shoulder joint via the spinal nerves C5–C7.

Aims of analgesia

- Reduce distress.
- Improve respiratory function and sputum clearance.
- Reduce complications and length of stay, and improve outcome.

Analgesic techniques

Regional blocks

- Intercostal block.
- Extrapleural block.
- Intrapleural block.
- Paravertebral block.
- Epidural block.

Systemic analgesia

- Parenteral analgesics – opioids (usually patient-controlled analgesia), paracetamol, non-steroidal anti-inflammatory agents (NSAIDs) and tramadol.

Regional anaesthesia

Intercostal nerve block

- Simple to perform but only a 'single shot'; therefore, it has a short duration of action.
- Does not control pain from the diaphragmatic pleura, mediastinal structures and areas supplied by the posterior primary rami.

Extrapleural block

- An indwelling catheter is placed in a pocket of retracted pleura so that the tip lies against a costovertebral joint.
- Local anaesthetic spreads to the paravertebral space providing anaesthesia of both the anterior and posterior primary rami.

Intrapleural block

- Local analgesic agent is deposited between the visceral and parietal pleura via an indwelling catheter.
- Analgesic action is the result of widespread intercostal nerve block.
- Does not spread to the paravertebral space.
- Analgesia is unpredictable because of variable loss of drug into chest drains, binding with blood in the thorax and rapid systemic absorption.
- Cannot be used following pneumonectomy.

Paravertebral block

- A percutaneously inserted catheter at one level allows a considerable spread of the drug between adjacent paravertebral spaces. Alternatively, multiple injections at different levels can be used as a 'one-shot' technique usually coupled with extrapleural block for postoperative analgesia.
- Blocks both anterior and posterior primary rami.
- Provides good analgesia, possibly with fewer side-effects than an epidural.
- Less easy to position accurately and maintain the position compared with an epidural.
- The main disadvantage is inferior reliability compared with an epidural.

Thoracic epidural block

- Considered the gold standard.
- Height of the required block necessitates a thoracic approach (usually about T5–T6).
- Paramedian approach is easier than midline.
- Use weak local anaesthetic solutions in combination with an opioid (usually 0.125% plain bupivacaine with fentanyl 2 $\mu g\ mL^{-1}$ by infusion).
- Provides excellent analgesia.
- Motor block is rarely a problem.
- A urinary catheter is required in most patients.
- Hypotension from a sympathetic block must be treated with a vasoconstrictor (such as a

16 Abdominal surgery

Mark C Bellamy

Overview

Mark C Bellamy

Anaesthesia for abdominal surgery embraces a wide range of disciplines. In many cases, the technique of choice involves general anaesthesia, perhaps in combination with thoracic epidural anaesthesia for postoperative pain relief. Not all intra-abdominal procedures necessitate general anaesthesia. Those confined to the pelvis are frequently carried out under spinal anaesthesia or epidural blockade. Some body surface procedures are adequately carried out using local nerve blocks or infiltration anaesthesia. Inguinal hernia repair falls into this category. Much lower abdominal surgery is performed under a regional block alone – spinal or combined epidural–spinal anaesthesia – or using a regional technique as an adjunct to light general anaesthesia. The more widespread availability of high-quality bedside ultrasound has encouraged increasing use of both single-shot and continuous catheter regional blocks as an alternative to the thoracic epidural. The transversus abdominis plane (TAP) block has emerged as the leading technique in this group, although rectus sheath and other blocks also have a role.

The conduct of anaesthesia for intra-abdominal surgery can have a major bearing on the quality of recovery, including the incidence of complications. Several studies have shown that fluid management and maintenance of adequate perfusion at the level of the tissue bed have a major bearing on surgical outcome in high-risk patients. 'Stroke volume optimization' is supported by an ever-strengthening body of literature, particularly in the field of colorectal surgery. Together with 'enhanced recovery after surgery' (ERAS) protocols, the approach leads to improvements in outcome coupled with a reduction in overall hospital stay. Points of specific interest include:

- splanchnic perfusion
- respiratory function
- cardiovascular function
- temperature regulation
- fluid and electrolyte balance.

Splanchnic perfusion

Patients undergoing major intra-abdominal surgery, especially those who are being operated for bowel obstruction, perforation or other acute conditions, are at high risk of sepsis and multiple organ failure. Similarly, elderly patients and those having major bowel or liver surgery are at risk. Numerous studies have shown that perioperative optimization reduces the risk of subsequent organ failure and postoperative morbidity. Various algorithms and monitoring techniques have been proposed to achieve this. Most are based on the concept of maintaining flow. Techniques which have been shown to be effective in various patient populations include monitoring of cardiac output, stroke volume, central venous oxygen saturation and gastric mucosal intracellular pH. Similarly, several fluid/inotrope regimens have been proposed as 'off-the-shelf' recipes. A number of devices are available as tools to achieve stroke volume optimization, including oesophageal Doppler (potentially difficult to use in upper gastrointestinal (GI) tract surgery, but relatively non-invasive), plethysmographic techniques (non-invasive but less well validated) and a range of proprietary technologies using the arterial waveform by invasive intravascular monitoring (LiDCO, PICCO, Vigileo, pulse pressure variation, etc.). The choice of technology currently seems less important than the use of the technique. Which of these is appropriate in an individual patient depends on the experience of the anaesthetist and clinical judgement, as well as on the available technology.

Respiratory function

Postoperative respiratory function is often impaired following intra-abdominal surgery. First, the use of the supine position, and intraoperative administration of nitrous oxide, may contribute to the development of atelectasis. Second, postoperative pain is associated with chest wall and abdominal splinting. This results in a reduction in functional residual capacity. The consequences of this include impingement of closing volume on tidal volume breathing. This results in ventilation/perfusion mismatch and increased shunting.

The administration of general anaesthesia, together with postoperative analgesic drugs, results in disorganized central control of respiration. Further, opiate analgesics have been shown to suppress rapid eye movement (REM) sleep. After the drugs are discontinued, there is a rebound in REM sleep with consequent hypoxia. There are theoretical reasons why regional blockade may avoid a number of these complications. Although relatively few studies have been able to demonstrate a reduction in the incidence of postoperative respiratory complications when epidural anaesthesia is employed, the pooled data from a number of studies support this view. Moreover, most studies comparing epidural anaesthesia with postoperative opioids report an increase in the quality of pain relief as perceived by the patient. However, the MASTER (Multicentre Australian Study of Epidural Anaesthesia and Analgesia in Major Surgery) study and others have confirmed that these advantages do not confer an overall survival benefit. Epidural analgesia therefore remains a matter of patient and clinician preference. Other approaches involve specific nerve blocks, intravenous paracetamol in an appropriate dose and the use of non-steroidal anti-inflammatory drugs (NSAIDs). Again, there is a growing body of evidence that these approaches may improve the quality of pain relief as well as reducing the rate of respiratory complications. Opioid-sparing techniques offer the additional attraction of improving the quality of postoperative recovery – less nausea and vomiting, earlier restoration of GI tract motility.

Cardiovascular system

A substantial fraction of the cardiac output is delivered to the splanchnic viscera. Venous drainage from the gut and spleen passes into the portal system and on to the liver. Portal venous blood flow represents two-thirds of hepatic perfusion. The remaining one-third is oxygenated blood derived from the hepatic artery. Liver blood flow represents between 25 and 30% of the cardiac output at rest. This increases following food. Any impairment of gut blood flow may therefore result in a reduction in liver blood flow. There are compensatory mechanisms (the hepatic artery buffer response) which normally protect the liver from such effects. Under anaesthesia, the normal buffer response becomes obtunded. Anaesthetic drugs have a differential effect on liver blood flow, with halothane exhibiting the worst profile of the volatile agents, followed by enflurane. Although these two agents have virtually disappeared from UK practice they are still in use in some countries, and it therefore remains an issue in global practice. The two agents sevoflurane and desflurane have a much more benign effect.

Recent work has demonstrated quite clearly that epidural anaesthesia, while protecting against the effects of the stress response, results in a reduction in splanchnic blood flow. This can be offset by restoring normal arterial pressure.

Thermoregulation

Thermoregulation is a major problem in patients undergoing intra-abdominal surgery. Anaesthesia renders the patient poikilothermic. Patients cool rapidly, because of increased heat and water loss across the large surface area of exposed viscera. This can potentially be compounded by the administration of large volumes of inadequately warmed fluids. Patients with a septic illness or a reduced metabolic rate (e.g. those with liver disease) have a reduced production of heat, and therefore tend to cool more quickly and may be difficult to rewarm.

Traditional approaches to maintaining patient warmth in theatre have included maintaining the temperature of the ambient environment close to an isothermic one, i.e. a temperature at which there is no tendency for a transfer of heat between patient and environment. This is a temperature in excess of 24–27°C, and may result in an unacceptable working environment. Warming mattresses, equally, have proved of limited value.

More recently, the advent of forced warm air overblankets has provided a solution to maintaining patient warmth in theatre. Such devices dramatically reduce thermal losses, and may also in some cases actually transfer heat to the patient. Using both upper and lower body devices simultaneously, or a 'whole body' device, is particularly effective.

Devices to humidify gases, including HME (heat and moisture exchanger) filters and circle systems, also help minimize thermal losses. Modern devices include countercurrent fluid warmers which allow delivery of body temperature fluids at very high rates. The universal use of fluid-warming devices is considered mandatory by some. Recent National Institute of Health and Clinical Excellence (NICE) guidance has laid out a practical strategy for approaching the problem of perioperative hypothermia, including universal temperature monitoring, active rewarming and, where appropriate, delaying surgery.

Fluid and electrolyte balance

Patients who present for intra-abdominal surgery may have gross derangement of fluid and electrolytes. Those presenting for elective surgery are particularly at risk in the event of administration of a bowel preparation or laxatives.

Patients presenting for acute surgery may have lost fluids from the central circulating compartment as a result of diarrhoea, vomiting or fluid sequestration into an obstructed intestine. In addition, those patients who suffer an inflammatory process may have lost fluid from the circulating compartment into the so-called 'third space', as a result of altered vascular permeability and colloid oncotic pressure.

These changes can be further exacerbated by handling the gut at surgery. This can result in translocation of bacteria and endotoxin, as well as altered liver blood flow.

Patients who have effusions (including ascites) are particularly at risk of major fluid and electrolyte shifts occurring as a consequence of surgery. Such shifts can precipitate acute haemodynamic decompensation. The anaesthetist must be aware both of the nature and of the severity of any preoperative derangement, together with the contribution likely to be made by surgery. Full assessment should allow correction of fluid and electrolyte abnormalities. Patients with major derangement are likely to require invasive vascular monitoring.

Specific points

Opioids and anastomoses

The debate regarding the contribution of opiates to anastomotic disruption continues. There are differences in basic pharmacology between drugs of this class. While some, including pethidine, are smooth muscle relaxants, others are smooth muscle constrictors, including morphine. The significance of this in clinical practice is unclear. However, most would agree that pethidine is superior to morphine for patients with biliary or ureteric spasm, although it is unclear whether there is any clinical advantage in patients undergoing biliary surgery.

Anticholinesterase drugs

These drugs can increase gut motility and intraluminal pressure. Neostigmine has been used specifically as a prokinetic drug in the treatment of pseudo-obstruction. These effects are only partially blocked by treatment concurrently with vagolytic agents, such as atropine. However, there is no good clinical evidence for an increase in anastomotic failure rate as a consequence of neostigmine use.

Antibiotics

Antibiotics are known to reduce the postoperative infection rate, and in particular the incidence of wound infection. There is no good evidence that the effects of a preinduction antibiotic can be further improved by subsequent doses. The antibiotic used for prophylaxis should be given sufficiently in advance of surgery that adequate tissue levels are obtained at the time of operation. Ideally, it should be given at the time of premedication.

Common antibiotic regimens include the combination of a penicillin or cephalosporin with metronidazole. Choice is likely to be determined by local antibiotic policy so as to manage the emergence of meticillin-resistant *Staphylococcus aureus* (MRSA), *Clostridium difficile* and antimicrobial resistance. Some drugs, particularly the aminoglycosides and streptomycin, may have the additional unwanted effect of perpetuating the effects of neuromuscular blocking agents.

Venous thromboembolism

Intra-abdominal surgery, and in particular pelvic surgery, conveys a significant risk of deep vein thrombosis (DVT). This risk can be minimized by the appropriate use of anticoagulants. Many regimens have been shown to be effective. Most centres currently use a standard dose of a low-molecular-weight heparin.

The risk can be further reduced by the use of support stockings or pneumatic compression boots. Regional anaesthesia and early mobilization can reduce the risk of DVT. Local and national guidelines inform the choice of strategy, and to which patients they should be applied.

Recent work has suggested that low-molecular-weight heparin persists in the circulation over a number of hours. Careful consideration should be given when considering siting a thoracic epidural. This should not be sited in the hours immediately following administration of a dose of low-molecular-weight heparin.

Bibliography

Fearon KC, Ljungqvist O, Von Meyenfeldt M, *et al.* Enhanced recovery after surgery: a consensus review of clinical care for patients undergoing colonic resection. *Clin Nutr* 2005; **24**: 466–77.

National Institute for Health and Clinical Excellence. *Inadvertent Perioperative Hypothermia.* NICE Clinical Guideline CG65, 2008. See http://www.nice.org.uk/nicemedia/pdf/CG65NICEGuidance.pdf.

National Institute for Health and Clinical Excellence. *Venous Thromboembolism: Reducing the Risk.* NICE Clinical Guideline CG92, 2010. See http://www.nice.org.uk/nicemedia/live/12695/47195/47195.pdf.

Rigg JR, Jamrozik K, Myles PS, *et al.* MASTER Anaesthesia Trial Study Group. Epidural anaesthesia and analgesia and outcome of major surgery: a randomised trial. *Lancet* 2002; **359**(9314):1276–82.

Cross-references

Complications of position, 743
Fluid and electrolyte balance, 754
Thrombosis and embolism, 793

Abdominal trauma

Lisa Milligan

General considerations

- Intra-abdominal injuries may carry a high morbidity and mortality. Diagnosis may be difficult or delayed and the severity underestimated.
- A high index of suspicion of abdominal trauma is required in all patients who have sustained serious or high-energy injury.
- The principal cause of death in abdominal trauma is uncontrolled bleeding, particularly from bursting injuries of the liver or spleen.
- Patients often require exploratory laparotomy and repair of the damaged viscera.
- The concept of 'damage control surgery' has been gaining popularity. The least possible is done for the patient with multiple injuries at the first operation. The patient is transferred to the ICU to correct hypothermia, acidosis and coagulopathy, before definitive surgery is undertaken within the next 36 hours.
- Some abdominal injuries (e.g. liver and spleen) do not require surgery and improved outcomes have been shown with conservative management.

Classification

- Blunt: common in road traffic accidents secondary to seat-belt injuries. The spleen is the most vulnerable organ. Liver, pancreas, bowel, kidneys and bladder are injured by greater forces.
- Penetrating: 20% of abdominal injuries in the UK. May be due to low-velocity projectiles, e.g. knives, hand-gun bullets, or high-velocity projectiles, e.g. rifle bullets or shrapnel from bombs or blasts. Impaled objects or weapons must only be removed under controlled circumstances in theatre; 90% of gunshot wounds sustain visceral injuries.

Initial management

- Injuries to the abdomen cannot be managed in isolation and require a multidisciplinary team approach.
- The victim of major trauma will require full assessment and resuscitation before definitive investigations are carried out and the decision to embark on surgery is made.
- By following a system such as ATLS (Advanced Trauma Life Support), the trauma team is able to achieve the stabilization of the injured patient in a consistent and systematic order and life-threatening injuries are treated according to priority.

Primary survey

- An ABCDE approach is followed.
- **A**irway patency is assessed and managed as appropriate, with tracheal intubation if necessary, and the cervical spine is immobilized.
- **B**reathing is assessed and when necessary IPPV commenced. Life-threatening chest injuries are excluded and treated at this stage.
- Intravenous access is obtained and overt external haemorrhage is controlled by compression. Adequacy of the **C**irculation and blood volume is then assessed clinically. It should be remembered that, in young patients, blood pressure is often maintained until the final phase of shock, when catastrophic and sometimes irretrievable falls occur.
- **D**isability and **E**xposure are assessed and managed as appropriate.
- Choice of fluid for resuscitation is controversial; however, ATLS recommends starting with warmed crystalloid solutions. A request for cross-matched blood must be sent immediately. With the exception of imminent exsanguination, there is little indication for the use of O-negative or type-specific blood. Cross-matched blood should be available within 20–30 minutes, particularly in major centres where electronic cross-match/release is practised.
- Excessive fluid resuscitation in penetrating trauma prior to haemostasis may be detrimental. In patients who have sustained major vascular injuries, increasing blood pressure leads to clot disruption and increased bleeding.

Secondary survey

- Once the patient has been stabilized, a full 'top-to-toe' examination is carried out to identify all injuries.
- Constant reassessment and vigilance is required at this stage for on-going life-threatening problems which require immediate treatment.

Investigations

- Routine:
  - haematology: cross-match, full blood count, clotting screen
  - biochemistry: electrolytes, creatinine, amylase

 - radiology: cervical spine, chest X-ray, pelvis
 - ECG.
- Specific to abdominal trauma: erect chest and abdominal X-ray; then, as indicated, proceed to:
  - deep peritoneal lavage
  - CT scan of the abdomen
  - ultrasound scan of the abdomen
    - focused abdominal sonography in trauma (FAST)
  - laparoscopy
  - laparotomy.
- The 'FAST' protocol has gained much in popularity in recent years. Sensitivity ranges between 0.64 and 0.98, but specificity is high, 0.86–1.00. Ultrasound scanning is performed simultaneously with initial assessment and resuscitation. The urinary bladder is filled with saline, then ultrasound is used to look for free fluid in the pericardium, perisplenic and perihepatic areas (including Morrison's pouch), and paracolic gutters. In the absence of fluid, no further immediate radiology is indicated. A positive scan indicates a CT in a stable patient, or laparotomy in an unstable patient. Solid organ trauma is not assessed by ultrasound in this protocol.
- Each of these investigations has its advantages and disadvantages. The choice will depend on the nature of the injury, the stability of the patient and the expertise available in imaging techniques.
- Great care should be exercised when deciding to move a potentially unstable patient from the emergency department to a remote environment, e.g. CT scanner, where staff and resuscitation facilities may be limited.
- There are a few indications for immediate laparotomy:
  - unexplained shock
  - rigid silent abdomen
  - evisceration
  - radiological evidence of free intraperitoneal gas
  - radiological evidence of ruptured diaphragm
  - all gunshot wounds.

Laparotomy for abdominal trauma

When possible the patient should be resuscitated and hypovolaemia corrected prior to induction of anaesthesia. When haemorrhage is ongoing, it may be appropriate to proceed cautiously with anaesthesia in the relatively hypovolaemic patient.

Anaesthetic technique

- Monitoring: standard with/without an arterial line, central venous line, pulmonary artery catheter, temperature, urine output (these may be instituted following induction and surgical control of haemorrhage in life-threatening situations).
- Intravenous access: two large-bore cannulas with/without large-bore central access when feasible. Vasopressors and inotropes should be prepared in advance and intravenous fluids should be running, with a rapid infuser and blood available.
- Induction of anaesthesia: should take place in the operating theatre, with the surgeon scrubbed, so that surgery can commence immediately. Severe cardiovascular decompensation may occur at induction owing to the vasodilatory and myocardial depressant effects of anaesthetic drugs plus the loss of a tamponading effect from the abdominal muscles at the institution of neuromuscular blockade.
- Rapid sequence induction with cricoid pressure is the technique of choice in the unfasted trauma patient. Care must be taken to protect the potentially unstable cervical spine.
- Choice of anaesthetic drugs will depend upon the stability of the patient. Far more important than the actual drug given is the dose of drug used. The intravascular volume is reduced in hypovolaemic patients; therefore, usual doses will result in higher than expected plasma concentrations. Etomidate (0.1–0.3 mg kg^{-1}) is a popular choice for its cardiovascular stability. Ketamine (0.3–0.7 mg kg^{-1}) may also be used; its sympathomimetic effects help to maintain blood pressure, although this may lead to a false sense of security in the patient who already has a maximal endogenous sympathetic drive. It should be avoided in patients with head injuries because of its effects on intracranial pressure.

An alternative technique is high-dose opioid, e.g. fentanyl, combined with a benzodiazepine, e.g. midazolam. This has minimal cardiac depressive action but may result in a decrease in endogenous catecholamine output and the patient will require postoperative ventilation. Succinylcholine or rocuronium are the neuromuscular blocking drugs of choice in rapid sequence induction.

- Intubation may be difficult in patients with facial injuries, cervical spine immobilization and blood in the airway.
- Maintenance of anaesthesia is with cautious amounts of volatile agent in an air/oxygen mixture. Nitrous oxide is avoided in abdominal surgery to prevent bowel distension. Once haemodynamic stability has been achieved, anaesthesia may be deepened.
- Neuromuscular blockade is maintained with an intermediate-acting drug. If rocuronium has been used for intubation, then it is logical to continue

with this. Atracurium may cause histamine release, which will result in vasodilatation compounding hypotension. Cisatracurium is an alternative with greater cardiovascular stability. Pancuronium has some intrinsic sympathomimetic activity and may be preferred in longer cases and those which will require postoperative ventilation.

- A nasogastric tube is inserted and gastric contents aspirated and prophylactic broad-spectrum antibiotics are given to all patients.
- Once control of bleeding has been achieved, the patient's cardiovascular status should improve. Further fluid resuscitation with crystalloid, colloid and blood should be guided by ongoing losses, CVP and urine output. Blood should be taken for arterial gases, haemoglobin concentration, coagulation screen and electrolytes.
- Warming the patient is essential. Hypothermia results in coagulopathy, reduced metabolism of citrate and lactate, hypocalcaemia, increased incidence of cardiac arrhythmias, metabolic acidosis and cardiac arrest. In the longer term, hypothermia impairs immune function, increases the risk of septic consequences and impairs wound healing.

Massive transfusion

- Coagulopathy is common after about one blood volume transfusion owing to dilutional thrombocytopenia, ↓ coagulation factors (~40% of normal), disseminated intravascular coagulation/fibrinolysis.
- Hypothermia causes inhibition of enzyme function and increased fibrinolytic activity.
- Massive transfusion results in metabolic acidosis, hyperkalaemia and impaired oxygen-carrying capacity (↓ 2,3-diphosphoglycerate (DPG)).
- Intraoperative red cell salvage (Cell Saver) provides warm blood with normal levels of 2,3-DPG. It is, however, contraindicated if the blood is contaminated with intestinal contents.
- Coagulopathy is corrected with FFP, cryoprecipitate and platelet transfusions. There is often a delay in obtaining these products, so they should be requested early if their use is anticipated. Recent evidence from the battlefield and in civilian practice suggests that the FFP:blood ratio should be at least 1:1.
- There may be a role for the use of antifibrinolytic and platelet-activating drugs, e.g. tranexamic acid, desmopressin (DDAVP).

Postoperative management

- Patients will require close monitoring in a HDU or ICU.
- Those who have sustained massive blood loss and undergone transfusion are often hypothermic, coagulopathic, acidotic and requiring drugs to support their cardiovascular system. They will benefit from a period of ventilation on the ICU while being warmed and stabilized.
- Oxygen, fluids and analgesia are prescribed. A morphine PCA system is most appropriate for major abdominal trauma where a coagulopathy exists and extradural blockade is contraindicated. However, once the patient's clotting returns to normal, he or she may benefit from the insertion of an epidural.

Liver trauma

- Liver injuries range from trivial to fatal.
- Constitute 45% of abdominal trauma: 30–40% are due to penetrating injuries and 60% are associated with other injuries, especially life-threatening head injuries.
- Liver injuries are graded I–V, from minor lacerations to avulsion from the inferior vena cava.
- Liver injuries may be treated by insertion of packs, which are then removed 1–2 days later, following a period of stabilization, correction of coagulopathy and hypothermia, and transfer to a specialist centre. By this stage haemorrhage will often have stopped.
- Patients may be investigated by angiography, permitting bleeding vessels to be embolized before further surgery to remove packs, or occasionally in a stable patient it is the sole intervention.
- In the most severe liver injuries (grade V) with simultaneous damage to the hepatic veins or vena cava, caval–atrial or caval–caval bypass may be required. Survival from such injuries is less than 10%.
- Stable patients, with a liver injury detected on CT scan, are best managed conservatively in a specialist centre. Transfusion requirements are reduced and there are fewer abdominal complications. In total 34–51% of adult blunt hepatic injuries can be managed conservatively, although in grade V injury only 10% are stable enough.
- Conservative management of solid abdominal visceral injuries is not a passive process, continuous assessment is required. The patient may need emergency laparotomy at any time for potentially exsanguinating haemorrhage. Intensive care monitoring is mandatory.

Splenic injury

- Splenectomy is a relatively simple surgical procedure which has saved many lives. However, it is not necessary for all injuries and splenectomy may occasionally be associated with overwhelming postsplenectomy sepsis.
- Approximately 50% of spleens can be repaired by partial resection, ligation of bleeding vessels and

packing and enveloping the spleen in an absorbable mesh bag.

- If haemostasis is obtained, the incidence of further haemorrhage is <2%.
- In stable patients, conservative treatment is now advocated in a similar manner as in liver trauma. Careful patient selection is required, and laparotomy is undertaken for haemodynamic instability, signs of peritonism or transfusion requirements over 2 units; 50–70% of splenic injuries are now managed conservatively.
- Angiography and embolization techniques have also been employed.
- Observation on an ICU or a HDU is essential, with continual readiness for an emergency operation.
- Patients who have undergone splenectomy are protected by daily administration of oral penicillin V for 2 years and immunized against *Pneumococcus* and *Haemophilus influenzae*.

Bibliography

American College of Surgeons. *ATLS manual*. Chicago: American College of Surgeons, 1997.

Bickell WH, Wall MJ, Pepe PE, *et al.* Immediate versus delayed fluid resuscitation in patients with penetrating torso injury. *N Eng J Med* 1994; **331**: 1105–9.

Bode PJ, Niezen RA, van Vugt AB, Schipper J. Abdominal ultrasound as a reliable indicator for conclusive laparotomy in blunt abdominal trauma. *J Trauma* 1993; **34**: 27–31.

Hishberg A, Mattox KL. Damage control surgery. *Br J Surg* 1993; **80**:1501–2.

Parks RW, Chrysos E, Diamond T. Management of liver trauma. *Br J Surg* 1999; **86**: 1121–35.

Patcher HL, Gram J. The current status of splenic preservation. *Adv Surg* 2000; **34**: 137–74.

Paterson-Brown S. *Emergency Surgery and Critical Care: A Companion to Specialist Surgical Practice*. Edinburgh: WB Saunders, 1997.

Rose AH, Kotzé A, Doolan D, *et al.* Massive transfusion: evaluation of current clinical practice and outcome in two large teaching hospital trusts in Northern England. *Vox Sang* 2009; **97**: 247–53.

Skinner D, Driscoll P, Earlam R. *ABC of Major Trauma*, 3rd edn. London: BMJ Books, 2000.

Smith J. Focused assessment with sonography in trauma (FAST): should its role be reconsidered? *Postgrad Med J* 2010; **86**(1015): 285–91.

Cross-references

Blood transfusion, 735
Emergency surgery, 613
Fluid and electrolyte balance, 754

Anaesthesia for pancreatic surgery

Helen Buglass

The pancreas is an exocrine and endocrine gland situated in the retroperitoneal space in the upper abdomen.

Indications for pancreatic surgery

- Necrotizing acute pancreatitis.
- Chronic pancreatitis.
- Trauma.
- Neoplasia:
  - adenocarcinoma
  - endocrine.

Acute pancreatitis

In recent years, there has been a trend against surgical intervention in acute pancreatitis. Conservative management is the first line, centred around supportive management with critical care support when necessary. Serial radiological imaging of the pancreas, including CT-guided drainage of any abscess or collection, is performed. Antibiotic treatment is reserved for proven infection (not administered solely to patients with an inflammatory reaction, as unguided antibiotic use has been shown to increase mortality).

Surgery is reserved for cases of 'failed' conservative management. The main indication for surgery is necrotizing pancreatitis. The operation of choice is necrosectomy plus lavage. This procedure has reduced the mortality to 24% for this condition.

Minimally invasive radiology-assisted necrosectomy has been described with good results. This has many advantages. Surgery may also be required for complications of acute pancreatitis – persistent pseudocyst, pancreatic abscess and haemorrhage – and increasingly is performed laparoscopically. Epidural analgesia is an excellent method of pain control in the acute episode.

Typical patient characteristics

- Age 40–70 years.
- History of gallstones and associated risk factors.
- Alcohol.
- Trauma.
- Forty per cent idiopathic.
- Drugs: angiotensin-converting enzyme inhibitors, thiazide diuretics, steroids, etc.
- Lipid abnormalities.
- Hypercalcaemia.

Presentation

- Patients can present acutely unwell complaining of epigastric pain.
- Patients are dehydrated and often jaundiced.
- Pleural effusions and acute lung injury can develop.
- Septic shock and multiorgan failure are indicators of necrotizing pancreatitis developing.

Preoperative assessment and investigations

- Full history and examination (patient may be in the ICU).
- Full blood count, electrolytes, liver function tests, coagulation screen, arterial blood gases.
- Chest X-ray and ECG.
- Any further investigations according to coexisting medical conditions.
- If coagulation is deranged, consider giving 10 mg intravenous vitamin K. FFP is reserved for cases of active bleeding.
- Hypovolaemia should be fully corrected

Anaesthetic technique

Preinduction

- Standard monitoring: ECG, pulse oximetry, blood pressure, $ETco_2$, temperature.
- Invasive monitoring: arterial blood pressure, central venous line.
- Rapid sequence induction if not intubated already (gastric stasis is likely).

Induction and maintenance

- Thoracic epidural analgesia is the pain relief of choice when coagulation permits.
- Induction: intravenous induction, muscle relaxation, endotracheal intubation. A nasogastric tube should be inserted if not already present.
- Maintenance: air/oxygen mix with a volatile agent, intermittent bolus of non-depolarizing muscle relaxant, controlled ventilation.

- Analgesia: opioid analgesic or epidural.
- Antagonism of non-depolarizing muscle relaxant at the end of the procedure if the patient is well enough to extubate.

Recovery

- High-dependency unit (HDU) care as minimum.
- Supplemental oxygen via the appropriate method.
- Supportive treatment as surgery causes the release of inflammatory mediators, which can lead to initial clinical deterioration.
- Early commencement of enteral feeding via a nasojejunal feeding tube.
- Postoperative surgical complications include colonic necrosis, fistula formation and bleeding.
- Respiratory and renal complications are common.

Chronic pancreatitis

- Increasing in incidence: 27.4 cases per 1 million of population.
- Indications for surgery are:
  - palliation of pain
  - exclude suspicion of carcinoma
  - bypass or remove the complications of the disease.
- Endoscopic techniques are increasingly being used as an alternative to traditional pancreaticojejunostomy.

Typical patient characteristics

- Alcohol: 60–70% of cases in Western world.
- Tropical pancreatitis.
- Obstructive pancreatitis.
- Hypercalcaemia.
- Hereditary.
- Biliary tract disease.
- Idiopathic.

Presentation

- Chronic abdominal pain radiating to the back.
- Weight loss because of endocrine and exocrine insufficiency.
- Diabetes and associated complications.
- Jaundice is rare.
- Alcohol abuse is common.

Preoperative assessment, investigation and optimization

- History and examination.
- Full blood count, electrolytes, liver function tests, coagulation screen and blood glucose.
- Chest X-ray and ECG.
- Further investigations according to coexisting medical conditions.
- Alcohol intake should be noted and treatment for withdrawal should be commenced.
- Diabetes should be stabilized and converted to an insulin sliding scale perioperatively.
- Multivitamins and vitamin K should be considered perioperatively.

Pancreatic neoplasia

Pancreatic neoplasms comprise a spectrum of exocrine and endocrine tumours, the majority being malignant. Two-thirds of cases arise in the head of the pancreas. The incidence is 10 per 1 million of population, with a 10% 1 year survival. Surgery is by Whipple's pancreaticoduodenectomy or a variant of this, e.g. the pylorus-preserving pancreaticoduodenectomy.

Typical patient characteristics

- Male/female ratio is 1.25:1.
- Smokers.
- Occupational: exposure to β-naphthalene and benzidine.
- Hereditary.
- Diabetes mellitus.
- Chronic pancreatitis.
- Gastrectomy.

Presentation

- Obstructive jaundice, weight loss and abdominal pain.
- Anorexia, nausea and vomiting.
- Impaired glucose tolerance.

Preoperative assessment, investigation and optimization

- History and examination.
- Full blood count, electrolytes, liver function tests and coagulation screen.
- Chest X-ray and ECG.
- Further investigation according to coexisting medical conditions.
- Hypovolaemia should be corrected.
- Diabetes should be stabilized and treatment converted to an insulin sliding scale perioperatively.
- An endocrinologist should be consulted: endocrine tumours are often part of a more complex syndrome.
- Preoperative stenting to relieve jaundice is common, but consider vitamin K 10 mg when the liver function tests remain deranged, even in the presence of normal coagulation.

Anaesthetic technique for Whipple's pancreaticoduodenectomy

This procedure is classically performed as an open procedure. However, in some specialist centres, both simple pancreatectomy and Whipple's procedure (reconstructive pancreatectomy) may be performed laparoscopically in suitable patients. The anaesthetic technique for the laparoscopic variant is essentially similar to that for the open procedure, with the additional consideration of the effects of pneumoperitoneum. The position adopted involves steep lateral tilt and reverse Trendelenburg, with the real possibility of haemodynamic compromise. Procedural duration (and hence appropriate pressure-point padding) is similarly an issue, as the laparoscopic technique is currently one of extended duration in many centres, although this is likely to change as the procedure becomes more familiar.

Preinduction

- Standard monitoring: ECG, pulse oximetry, blood pressure, $ETco_2$, temperature.
- Invasive monitoring: arterial blood pressure, central venous line.

Induction and maintenance

- Thoracic epidural is the pain relief of choice if the coagulation is satisfactory.
- Induction: intravenous induction, non-depolarizing muscle relaxant, tracheal intubation.
- Maintenance: air/oxygen mix with volatile agent, intermittent bolus or infusion of non-depolarizing muscle relaxant.
- Analgesia: epidural preferable, but, when this is not possible, a remifentanil infusion with a loading of morphine at the end of procedure is effective.
- Reversal of non-depolarizing muscle relaxant at the end of the procedure.

Peroperative complications

- Hypothermia: active warming – fluid and blankets.
- Hypovolaemia: large fluid loss perioperatively plus potential large blood losses – maintain central venous pressure (CVP) and monitor haematocrit, transfuse as necessary.
- Hyperkalaemia: surgical manipulation leading to portal vein or hepatic artery obstruction and hepatic ischaemia and intracellular potassium leak – monitor potassium.
- Hypo-/hyperglycaemia: monitor closely; in insulinoma a constant infusion of dextrose infusion has been shown to reduce rebound hyperglycaemia.
- Hypoxia: basal atelectasis or development of acute lung injury – increase F_io_2; add positive end-expiratory pressure – consider facial continuous positive airway pressure or continued ventilation postoperatively.
- Renal dysfunction: hepatorenal syndrome – monitor renal output, maintain circulating volume and mean blood pressure, consider mannitol or a loop diuretic.

Recovery: early

- Oxygen via face-mask.
- HDU care.
- Intravenous fluid then early introduction of enteral (jejunal) feed.
- Analgesia:
  - epidural: low-dose local anaesthetic with opioid
  - intravenous paracetamol
  - intravenous opioid via PCA.
- DVT prophylaxis.
- Monitoring blood glucose: manipulation of insulin and dextrose.

Recovery: late

- The morbidity rate of the operation is high: up to 40%.
- Common complications are basal atelectasis with resultant pneumonia, thromboembolic disease and anastomotic leak.
- Optimizing pain control, physiotherapy, early mobilization and thromboembolic prophylaxis can reduce these.
- Incidence of postoperative diabetes is dependent on the size of pancreatic resection, but is quoted at 50%.
- Operative mortality rate is 5%.

Pancreatic trauma

Deceleration injury is the major mechanism of blunt pancreatic injury. The force required means that, often, other organs are involved (see Abdominal trauma, p. 429).

Bibliography

Manciu N, Beebe DS. Total pancreatectomy with islet cell autotransplantation: anaesthetic implications. *J Clin Anaesth* 1999; **11**: 576–82.

Røsok BI, Marangos IP, Kazaryan AM, *et al.* Single-centre experience of laparoscopic pancreatic surgery. *Br J Surg* 2010; **97**: 902–9.

Cross-references

Complications of position, 743

Fluid and electrolyte balance, 754

Bariatric surgery

Brian J Pollard

The definition of morbid obesity differs slightly between individual authorities. The most commonly accepted definition is that of a person who has a body mass index (BMI) of 40 kg m^{-2} or greater. A further category, the superobese, is sometimes used for those with a BMI of greater than 55 kg m^{-2}. The usual initial treatment options for morbid obesity include dietary and lifestyle changes. Surgery is also available as a later treatment option. The morbidly obese patient may present for gastric banding or bypass surgery. They may also present for surgery unrelated to their weight. In all cases, management strategies are similar.

The incidence of obesity is increasing in the developed world, and morbid obesity has become a significant health problem. Many patients are younger adults, but any age can be encountered.

Patient characteristics

- Any age.
- Males and females equally affected.
- Increased incidence of:
  - diabetes mellitus
  - cardiovascular disease
  - respiratory disease
  - sleep apnoea syndrome.

Preoperative assessment and investigations

- Full history and examination.
- Full blood count and electrolytes.
- Liver function tests (if deranged, coagulation screen).
- Chest X-ray and ECG when warranted.
- Careful assessment of mouth, jaw opening and airway.
- Any further investigations according to coexisting medical conditions.
- Antibiotics as per hospital protocol.

Anaesthetic technique

Preinduction

- Premedication is not usually necessary.
- Consider prophylaxis against gastric acid aspiration.
- Routine standard monitoring: ECG, blood pressure, $ETco_2$, pulse oximetry, temperature as per Association of Anaesthetists of Great Britain and Ireland guidelines.
- Invasive direct blood pressure monitoring is recommended.
- Neuromuscular blockade monitor.
- Adequate intravenous access before starting.
- Discuss fibreoptic intubation with the patient if this technique is indicated.
- Get the patient to position themselves on the operating table before starting and induce anaesthesia in the operating theatre.
- Ensure that the working load of the operating table is correct for a patient of that weight.
- Laparoscopic gastric surgery is often performed with the surgeon standing between the patient's legs and with some head-up tilt. Position a prop (padded roll bar) under the buttocks before starting so that the patient cannot slide down the table when tilted head-up.

Induction and maintenance

- Regional blocks can be challenging. Ultrasound guidance may help. Longer block needles are available.
- Full preoxygenation is important.
- Induction: propofol is recommended.
- Tracheal intubation.
- Relaxants: any short- or intermediate-acting agent is suitable for intubation followed by intermittent boluses guided by neuromuscular monitoring.
- Maintenance: air/oxygen mix with a volatile agent. Desflurane is commonly used owing to its rapid wash-in and wash-out. A propofol infusion (total intravenous anaesthesia (TIVA) or manually controlled) has been recommended. If TIVA is used, the ideal body weight (IBW) or the corrected body weight should be used and not the actual body weight (total body weight (TBW)). The corrected body weight is calculated by:

$$\text{Corrected body weight (Servin's correction)} = \text{IBW} + [0.4 \times (\text{TBW} - \text{IBW})]$$

- Controlled ventilation (higher pressures will be needed and positive end-expiratory pressure is recommended).
- Analgesia: remifentanil has been shown to be useful. Intravenous paracetamol and a NSAID are useful if there is no contraindication.

- Morphine will be required at the end of the procedure as the remifentanil effect wanes.
- Antiemetic prophylaxis: commonly a $5HT_3$ inhibitor and dexamethasone.
- Local anaesthetic infiltration around incisions and laparascopic port sites.
- Reversal of non-depolarizing muscle relaxant as needed at the end of the procedure. If rocuronium has been used then sugammadex may be useful.

Recovery: early

- Oxygen via face-mask.
- Nurse in the semirecumbent position.
- Intravenous fluid until the patient is drinking adequately.
- Analgesia:
  - this depends on the operation and expected analgesic requirements
  - simple oral analgesics may be adequate
  - intravenous opioids via patient-controlled analgesia may be used
  - regional techniques may be used. A continuous epidural infusion of low-dose local anaesthetic and opioid has been used. Patient-controlled epidural analgesia is an option.

Recovery: late

Complications may be secondary to hypoventilation, poor pain control or immobility. Basal atelectasis, deep vein thrombosis and hypoventilation may occur. Optimizing pain control, physiotherapy, early mobilization and thromboembolic prophylaxis can reduce these.

Bibliography

Adams JP, Murphy PG. Obesity in anaesthesia and intensive care. *Br J Anaesth* 2000; **85**: 91–108.

Dowse C, Pyke M. Anaesthesia for obesity surgery. *Anaesth Intensive Care Med* 2008; **9**: 303–5.

La Colla L, La Colla G, Albertin A, *et al.* The use of propofol and remifentanil for the anaesthetic management of a super-obese patient. *Anaesthesia* 2007; **62**: 842–45.

Raeder J. Bariatric procedures as day/short stay surgery: is it possible and reasonable? *Curr Opinion Anaesthesiol* 2007; **20**: 508–12.

Servin F, Farinotti R, Haberer JP, Desmonts JM. Propofol infusion for maintenance of anesthesia in morbidly obese patients receiving nitrous oxide. A clinical and pharmacokinetic study. *Anesthesiology* 1993; **78**: 657–65.

Cross-references

Anaesthesia and sleep apnoea syndrome, 98
Complications of position, 743
Diabetes mellitus, 60
Difficult airway: prediction, 664
Obesity, 189

Colorectal surgery

Lisa Milligan

Procedures

A wide range of surgical procedures are carried out on the lower gastrointestinal tract for a variety of pathologies, including carcinoma, inflammatory bowel disease, diverticular disease, motility disorders, angiodysplasia and bowel obstruction (Box 16.1).

Box 16.1 Common lower gastrointestinal tract surgical procedures

- Appendicectomy
- Anterior resection (left/right hemicolectomy)
- Hartmann's procedure
- Total colectomy
- Panproctocolectomy (abdominoperineal resection)
- Ileorectal pouch formation
- Stoma formation/closure
- Fistula surgery
- Haemorrhoidectomy
- Other perianal surgery, e.g. fissure, haematoma, abscess, carcinoma

Colorectal surgery

Procedures vary in complexity, most involve laparotomy, excision of the affected section of bowel and anastomosis of the remaining segments, with/without stoma formation. Adjacent organs may be involved (e.g. bladder, uterus), requiring a multidisciplinary approach, prolonged anaesthesia and major blood loss. Laparoscopic techniques are now being used for appendicectomy and some bowel resections. The advantages of improved diagnosis, reduced wound size and tissue trauma must be weighed against the problems associated with laparoscopic surgery (see Open and laparoscopic cholecystectomy, p. 451) and increased operating time, and the anaesthetist must be prepared for conversion to laparotomy at any stage. Specific anaesthetic considerations for laparoscopic procedures are covered below, as there are several 'pitfalls for the unwary'.

ERAS protocols allow early mobilization and discharge following colorectal surgery, with rapid restoration of GI tract function. Such programmes consist of a package including:

- admission and discharge planning
- teaching patients stoma care prior to hospital admission
- maintaining GI tract function by continuing feeding until shortly before surgery (high-calorie preoperative drinks)
- low neurohumoral stress response anaesthesia (epidural analgesia, active warming, etc.)
- stroke volume optimization
- avoidance or immediate postoperative removal of the nasogastric tube
- forced early mobilization and diet
- day 1 removal of epidural catheter
- early discharge.

Patients

- All age groups.
- Physiological status depends on:
  - underlying pathology
  - concurrent medical conditions.
- Patients with malignant disease may have significant weight loss, anaemia, bowel obstruction, electrolyte imbalance and metastatic disease.
- Patients are often elderly with one or more of the medical conditions frequently associated with this population, e.g. ischaemic heart disease, hypertension, pulmonary disease, diabetes mellitus, arthritis.
- Patients with inflammatory bowel disease are usually younger but have frequently undergone multiple surgical procedures and may present with severe sepsis due to bowel perforation or 'toxic megacolon'. Steroid therapy may cause immunosuppression and signs of sepsis may be masked.
- Patients of all age groups and levels of fitness present for perianal surgery. Pregnant women can present for urgent haemorrhoidectomy.

Preoperative assessment

- Routine history and examination with special attention to concurrent disease.
- Specific to gastrointestinal pathology:
  - anaemia
  - weight loss
  - diarrhoea and vomiting
  - bowel obstruction
  - sepsis
  - medications (including steroids)
  - metastatic disease.

- Investigations:
  - routine haematology: full blood count with/without clotting screen; group and save or cross-match (depending upon the nature of the surgery and the local transfusion policy)
  - routine biochemistry: creatinine and electrolytes with/without glucose, amylase, liver function tests
  - ECG
  - chest X-ray when indicated by history or examination findings
  - other specialized investigations, e.g. echocardiogram, pulmonary function tests, as indicated by history and examination.

Premedication

- Oral anxiolytic if required, e.g. temazepam.
- Regular medication, especially cardiac drugs, should be continued until the day of surgery, with consideration given to postoperative intravenous regimes.
- Intravenous fluids should be prescribed for patients given 'bowel preparation' or those with diarrhoea or vomiting, to correct hypovolaemia and electrolyte losses prior to surgery.
- Patients with diabetes are commenced on an appropriate intravenous insulin regime.

Perioperative management

- Monitoring: ECG, non-invasive blood pressure, S_pO_2, $ETCO_2$.
- Intravenous access: large-bore access required in major cases in which blood loss is anticipated.
- Arterial line: measure direct arterial blood pressure in cases involving large fluid and blood losses, in patients with significant ischaemic heart disease or arrhythmias, and to obtain arterial blood gases and blood samples.
- Central venous line: to monitor CVP and guide volume replacement, to enable central delivery of drugs, e.g. inotropes, vasopressors and antiarrhythmics, and to allow postoperative intravenous feeding if necessary.
- Following induction of anaesthesia, a nasogastric tube and urinary catheter are inserted.
- Positioning: a variety of positions are used including: Lloyd-Davies, lithotomy, Trendelenburg, prone. Eyes should be taped closed and pressure points protected.
- Temperature: every effort should be made to prevent hypothermia using warming mattresses, forced air warmers and warmed intravenous fluids. Core temperature should be monitored using a nasopharyngeal temperature probe.
- Broad-spectrum prophylactic antibiotics are given at induction of anaesthesia along with steroid cover if indicated (e.g. in patients with ulcerative colitis taking regular steroids).

Anaesthetic technique

In emergency procedures for the 'acute abdomen' in unfasted patients, rapid sequence induction using thiopentone and succinylcholine, with the application of cricoid pressure and tracheal intubation, is the technique of choice (see Section 27, Airway).

For elective major abdominal surgery general anaesthesia with tracheal intubation and controlled ventilation is a well-proven technique.

- Choice of induction agent depends upon the physiological status of the patient and the length of the procedure. In fit patients, propofol or thiopentone may be used. Propofol may be more suitable for shorter cases in which rapid emergence is desirable. In septic, hypovolaemic or haemorrhaging patients and those with significant cardiovascular disease, etomidate may be preferred for its greater cardiovascular stability.
- Maintenance of anaesthesia is usually with a volatile anaesthetic agent; isoflurane or desflurane are suitable choices for longer cases, whereas sevoflurane is often reserved for day cases. Nitrous oxide is avoided to prevent bowel distension. Total intravenous anaesthesia, with propofol and a short-acting opioid, e.g. remifentanil, has also been employed successfully in major abdominal surgery.
- Muscle relaxation is required to facilitate surgical access and IPPV. An agent of intermediate duration of action is chosen, e.g. atracurium or vecuronium. Monitoring of neuromuscular blockade is required to ensure reversal is adequate at the end of the procedure. In the past, there has been concern regarding the use of anticholinesterase drugs, such as neostigmine, for reversal of neuromuscular blockade because of the possibility of increased peristaltic activity and theoretical risk of dehiscence of the bowel anastomosis. Conclusive evidence is lacking and most anaesthetists favour the use of neostigmine to ensure adequate return of respiratory muscle function at the end of surgery. The use of an aminosteroid relaxant reversed with a cyclodextrin is now a viable alternative with theoretical attractions, although, as yet, there is no evidence to demonstrate its superiority.
- Fluid therapy: intravenous infusion of crystalloid solution (e.g. Hartmann's solution) should be commenced via a fluid/blood warmer prior to induction. Fluid balance should be carefully monitored throughout surgery, taking into account

good postoperative analgesia and attenuation of the stress response. Regional techniques may be less suitable for day-case surgery in which urinary retention may prove a concern and early mobilization is required. A low spinal ('saddle block'), aiming to anaesthetize S2–S5, can be performed in the sitting position (difficult in the elderly and in patients with severe perianal pain) using small volumes (0.5–1.5 mL) 0.5% heavy bupivacaine. A caudal extradural block using 15–20 mL 0.5% bupivacaine will provide perianal analgesia. It may be used alone or in combination with general anaesthesia and has been used successfully in day-case surgery. Local blocks, e.g. posterior perineal nerve blockade, and local infiltration have also been used for certain procedures, as sole anaesthetic as well as in combination with general anaesthesia to provide postoperative analgesia.

Postoperative management

- Patients who have undergone major surgery or who have significant concurrent medical problems should be managed in a high-dependency environment with invasive monitoring.
- Oxygen, intravenous fluids and appropriate analgesia should be prescribed and consideration given to antithrombotic prophylaxis.
- Antibiotics are prescribed in conjunction with the surgical team, and provision made for restarting essential medication.
- Day-case patients should be assessed according to unit policy and discharged to the care of a competent adult with suitable analgesia. Clear instructions for follow-up should be given along with contact telephone numbers should problems occur.

Bibliography

Aljafri AM, Kingworth A (eds). *Fundamentals of Surgical Practice*. London: Greenwich Medical Media, 1998.

Amato AC, Pescatori M. Effect of perioperative blood transfusions on recurrence of colorectal cancer: meta-analysis stratified on risk factors. *Dis Colon Rectum* 1998; **41**: 570–85.

Blajchman MA. Immunomodulatory effects of allogenic blood transfusions: clinical manifestations and mechanisms. *Vox Sang* 1998; **74** (Suppl. 2): 315–19.

Buggy DJ, Smith G. Epidural anaesthesia and analgesia: better outcome after major surgery. *BMJ* 1999; **319**: 530–1.

Counihan TC, Favuzza J. Fast track colorectal surgery. *Clin Colon Rectal Surg* 2009; **22**: 60–72.

Jackson IJB. The management of pain following day surgery. *BJA CEPD Rev* 2001; **1**(2) 48–51.

Noblett SE, Snowden CP, Shenton BK, Horgan AF. Randomized clinical trial assessing the effect of Doppler-optimized fluid management on outcome after elective colorectal resection. *Br J Surg* 2006; **93**: 1069–76.

Noblett SE, Watson DS, Huong H, *et al.* Pre-operative oral carbohydrate loading in colorectal surgery: a randomized controlled trial. *Colorectal Dis* 2006; **8**: 563–9.

Schwenk W, Hasse O, NeudeckerJ, Muller JM. Short term benefits for laparoscopic colorectal resection. *Cochrane Database Syst Rev* 2005; (2): CD003145.

Williams B, Wheatley R. *Epidural Analgesia for Postoperative Pain Relief*. Bulletin no. 2. London: Royal College of Anaesthetists, 2000.

Cross-references

Emergency surgery, 613

Complications of position, 743

Open and laparoscopic cholecystectomy, 451

Hernia repair

Lisa Milligan

General considerations

- A hernia is a protrusion of the whole or part of a viscus from its normal position through an opening in the wall of its containing cavity.
- Surgical repair involves excision of the hernia sac and closure of the defect with non-absorbable sutures and/or Prolene mesh. Occasionally, bowel resection and anastomosis is required.

Types of hernia

- Inguinal.
- Femoral.
- Umbilical and paraumbilical.
- Epigastric.
- Incisional.
- Obturator.
- Spigelian.
- Lumbar.
- Gluteal.
- Sciatic.
- Perineal.
- Hiatus.
- Diaphragmatic

Inguinal hernia

- Most common in both sexes, constituting 75–80% of abdominal wall hernias.
- Occur at any age from infancy (especially premature babies) to the elderly.
- Repair early to reduce the risk of strangulation and to minimize stretching of the abdominal wall musculature, hence reducing the recurrence rate.
- Repaired by various techniques of herniorraphy and, in infants, herniotomy.
- Three per cent of hernias recur and patients may present for further repair. Such procedures may be longer and more complex.

Laparoscopic repair

- Extraperitoneal approach; therefore, problems of pneumoperitoneum are avoided. Complexity and the risk of potential complications make it an operation for more experienced laparoscopic surgeons.
- Reduced length of hospital stay and use of analgesia have to be weighed against increased theatre costs.
- A recent meta-analysis confirmed that the patient's experience (pain, rehabilitation time) was superior to the conventional approach, but with a longer operative time and equivalent clinical outcomes. Surgeon experience was a major factor.

Strangulated hernia

- Hernia contents may become constricted by the neck of the sac or by twisting. Symptoms and signs of bowel obstruction indicate the need for urgent surgery. Laparotomy and bowel resection may be required.

Femoral hernia

- Protrusion of the peritoneum into the potential space of the femoral canal.
- Sac may contain abdominal viscera (small bowel) or omentum.
- More common in multiparous women; rare in children.
- Strangulate more readily than inguinal hernias as the femoral canal is small and not distensible.
- Present with symptoms and signs of small bowel obstruction.
- Repair should be undertaken at the earliest opportunity even when asymptomatic.

Umbilical and paraumbilical hernias

- True umbilical hernias only occur in infancy. The most extreme form is exomphalos, in which the midgut fails to return to the abdominal cavity in early fetal life. Surgical repair is required urgently and prognosis is generally poor. A small hernia can occur at the umbilical cicatrix in the first few days of life. Repair is rarely required unless the hernia persists after the age of 18 months.
- Paraumbilical hernias are acquired and associated with middle age, obesity and multiparous women. They occur at a small defect in the linea alba and there is a high risk of strangulation. Repair is recommended even in relatively unfit and obese patients. Mayo's operation is the usual surgical procedure.

Incisional hernias

- Late complication of 10–15% of abdominal wounds; occur between 1 and 5 years postoperatively owing to breakdown of the repair to the abdominal wall muscle and fascia.

- Predisposing factors:
  - obesity
  - distension
  - poor muscle quality
  - inadequate closure technique
  - postoperative wound infection
  - multiple operations through the same incision.
- Usually asymptomatic, but occasionally a narrow-necked hernia may produce pain or strangulation, in which case surgical repair is indicated.

Patients

- All ages: neonates and infants to elderly.
- Can present with any number of concurrent medical problems. The demographics of hernia repair make conditions associated with the elderly particularly common.
- Problems specifically associated with hernias:
  - chronic cough (chronic obstructive pulmonary disease, asthma)
  - chronic constipation
  - obesity (and associated problems, e.g. ischaemic heart disease, diabetes mellitus, sleep apnoea)
  - pregnancy.
- Approximately 50% of patients in the UK undergo day-case hernia repair. Inpatient treatment is required for those with a poor level of fitness, lack of social back-up and complicated hernias. In the USA, 70% of inguinal hernia repairs are performed as a day case, the majority under local anaesthesia, and patients are discharged within 4 hours of surgery.
- Some patients will present as an emergency with the problems associated with bowel obstruction, including:
  - vomiting
  - dehydration
  - hypovolaemia
  - electrolyte and acid-base disturbances

Preoperative assessment

- Routine history and examination, with particular attention to concurrent disease.
- Routine investigations: haematology, biochemistry, ECG, as dictated by local policy.
- Other investigations as indicated by history and examination, e.g. chest X-ray, arterial blood gases, pulmonary function tests.

Premedication

- Sedative premedication is not indicated for day-case patients. An oral anxiolytic, e.g. temazepam, can be prescribed for elective inpatients.
- Oral analgesia may be prescribed as part of a multimodal, pre-emptive analgesic regime.
- Emergency cases can be prescribed an H_2 receptor antagonist, e.g. ranitidine, and prokinetic, e.g. metoclopramide, to reduce the risk of pulmonary aspiration.
- Intravenous fluids should be commenced for patients with a history of vomiting, dehydration, hypovolaemia and electrolyte imbalance.

Anaesthetic management

- Anaesthetic technique depends largely on the type and size of hernia, and whether elective or an emergency case.
- All strangulated hernias with symptoms of bowel obstruction should be treated as an 'acute abdomen'. A general anaesthetic with rapid sequence induction and application of cricoid pressure is the technique of choice.
- For other types of hernia repair, there is a wide choice of anaesthetic technique:
  - general
  - regional
  - local
  - combination of the above
- In all cases standard monitoring is required, along with intravenous access with/without intravenous fluids and broad-spectrum antibiotics.

General anaesthesia

- General anaesthesia is used in preference to regional and local techniques in:
  - anxious patients
  - children
  - obese
  - patients with difficulty lying flat (those with arthritis, congestive cardiac failure).
- For inguinal and femoral hernia repair, where there is no risk of vomiting or regurgitation, a spontaneously breathing technique using a laryngeal mask may be appropriate.
- For abdominal wall hernias, especially large incisional hernias and those involving bowel, muscle relaxation is required and therefore tracheal intubation and positive pressure ventilation is needed.
- Extubation should be achieved where possible with minimal coughing and bucking to protect the hernia repair. The use of drugs, e.g. propofol and sevoflurane, which allow rapid return of consciousness and upper airway reflexes, is recommended. These drugs are also advantageous in day-case surgery.
- Nitrous oxide is not recommended in patients with bowel obstruction.
- Intraoperative analgesia should be multimodal and tailored to the type of hernia repair and amount

of postoperative pain expected. A short-acting opioid, e.g. fentanyl, a NSAID and infiltration of the wound with local anaesthetic may be satisfactory in inguinal and femoral hernia repairs.

- General anaesthesia can be combined with a local block (e.g. inguinal field block) to reduce intraoperative anaesthetic requirements and produce good quality, non-sedative postoperative analgesia.
- In cases where a large laparotomy wound is explored, insertion of an epidural, which can be used for postoperative analgesia, may be beneficial, especially if the patient has concurrent pulmonary disease.

Regional anaesthesia

- Regional techniques (spinal or epidural) are appropriate for the elective repair of hernias provided an intraperitoneal approach is not required.
- Avoids complications of general anaesthesia, reduces stress response and provides good postoperative analgesia.
- Not recommended in emergency cases with bowel obstruction and hypovolaemia.
- May be the technique of choice in high-risk elderly patients.
- Patient must be able to lie flat.
- Sedation may be required, and can be achieved with judicious boluses of midazolam (1–2 mg) or an infusion of propofol (1–2 $\mu g\ kg^{-1}\ hr^{-1}$). Oxygen should be administered by face-mask or nasal cannulas.

Local anaesthesia

- May be used as the sole anaesthetic in day-case surgery or in those patients considered unfit for other anaesthetic techniques. Intraoperative pain has been reported as a problem. May be used in combination with general anaesthesia to reduce anaesthetic requirements and provide postoperative analgesia.
- Gaining popularity as surgical expertise increases.
- Not suitable for the anxious, obese and uncooperative patients, or those with complicated hernias.
- Shown to be the most cost-effective anaesthetic technique in inguinal hernia repair.
- All patients require standard monitoring and intravenous access.

Inguinal field block

- Aims to block:
  - subcostal nerve (T12)
  - iliohypogastric nerve (L1)
  - ilioinguinal nerve (L1).
- Technique: a regional block needle is inserted 2.5 cm inferomedial to the anterior superior iliac spine and advanced through the external oblique aponeurosis. A distinctive 'click' is felt as the needle penetrates the fascia; 10 mL of local anaesthetic (e.g. 0.5% bupivacaine, 0.5–1.0% prilocaine) is infiltrated deep to the aponeurosis, down the inner surface of the ilium through the abdominal muscle layers. A further 10 mL of local anaesthetic is deposited superficial to the external oblique and medial to this point in line with the inguinal ligament. A further injection is made over and around the pubic tubercle in a 'fan' pattern.
- Blockade produces good postoperative analgesia; however, supplementary infiltration, especially around the inguinal ring and hernial sac, is usually necessary during surgery if this is the only anaesthetic employed.

Postoperative management

- Analgesia following hernia repair is best provided by a multimodal approach. A successful regime includes combinations of opioids, simple analgesics (paracetamol) and NSAIDs, along with local block techniques or wound infiltration with local anaesthetic.
- Patients undergoing large or bilateral hernia repairs may prefer a morphine-based PCA system rather than repeated intramuscular injections.
- Those with significant cardiovascular or respiratory disease undergoing major abdominal wall hernia repairs can benefit from insertion of an epidural for postoperative analgesia.
- Oxygen and intravenous fluids should be prescribed and thromboprophylaxis considered.
- Chest physiotherapy is recommended for all patients with respiratory disease.
- Day-case patients must be assessed carefully prior to discharge in accordance with the unit's policy; analgesia should be prescribed and information given regarding follow-up and contacts should problems arise.

Bibliography

Aljafri AM, Kingsnorth A. *Fundamentals of Surgical Practice*. London: Greenwich Medical Media, 1998.

Burkitt HG, Quick CRG, Gatt D. *Essential Surgery: Problems, Diagnosis and Management*. Edinburgh: Churchill Livingstone, 1990.

Callesen T, Bech K, Kehlet H. One-thousand inguinal hernia repairs under unmonitored local anesthesia. *Anesth Analg* 2001; **93**: 1373–6.

Cheek CM, Black NA, Devlin HB, *et al.* Groin hernia surgery: a systematic review. *Ann R Coll Surg Engl* 1998; **80** (Suppl. 1): S1–80.

Jackson IJB. The management of pain following day surgery. *BJA CEPD Rev* 2001; **1**(2): 48–51.

Karthikesalingam A, Markar SR, Holt PJ, Praseedom RK. Meta-analysis of randomized controlled trials comparing laparoscopic with open mesh repair of recurrent inguinal hernia. *Br J Surg* 2010; **97**: 4–11.

Wildsmith JAW, Armitage EN. *The Principles and Practice of Regional Anaesthesia.* Edinburgh: Churchill Livingstone, 1993.

Cross-references

Day-case surgery, 604
Obesity, 189
Obstruction or perforation, 447

Obstruction or perforation

Richard J Harding

These two conditions have multiple aetiologies. They can represent a major anaesthetic and surgical challenge. Gastrointestinal obstruction results in major fluid loss into the bowel lumen. It can be complicated by perforation. Perforation of the gastrointestinal tract results in peritonitis and can produce severe systemic upset.

Patient characteristics

- Neonates to the elderly, but often older age groups with medical comorbidities.
- Often unwell and may have significant pain.
- Invariably hypovolaemic and may have systemic sepsis.
- Associated with underlying pathologies such as malignancy.

Preoperative assessment and investigations

Particular attention should be paid to the following areas:

- presence and severity of comorbid conditions, particularly of the cardiorespiratory system
- state of hydration and serum electrolytes
- evidence of septic/hypovolaemic shock.

Investigations should include:

- full blood count and coagulation screen, particularly if considering epidural analgesia
- urea, electrolytes and creatinine
- cross-match at least 2 units of blood (or follow locally agreed blood ordering schedule)
- arterial blood gases: evidence of metabolic acidosis/high lactate suggests poor tissue perfusion and the need for preoperative resuscitation
- ECG and chest X-ray if clinically indicated.

Preoperative preparation

Patients with bowel obstruction require urgent, but not emergency, surgery. They should be fully resuscitated prior to theatre, and surgery should not be performed precipitously unless the obstruction is complicated by bowel ischaemia or perforation.

Gastrointestinal perforation is a surgical emergency, but patients will still require adequate, and sometimes aggressive, resuscitation prior to surgery.

Any patient who is significantly unwell should be optimized with the aid of invasive monitoring, in a high-dependency area. All patients require a nasogastric tube and a urinary catheter. Adequate analgesia is necessary in all patients. Consider thromboembolic prophylaxis.

Perioperative management

Monitoring

- Routine anaesthetic monitoring.
- Monitoring of core temperature.
- Consider invasive arterial and CVP monitoring in all but the most straightforward of cases. This is particularly important in patients with significant cardiorespiratory disease or poor preoperative condition.
- Monitoring of cardiac output in high-risk cases.

Anaesthetic technique

Such surgery almost always requires general anaesthesia, but this is often supplemented with an epidural, to provide postoperative analgesia. Regional anaesthesia, with a continuous spinal or epidural technique, can be used in selected cases, but adequate anaesthesia can be both difficult to achieve and associated with side-effects such as significant hypotension. An epidural can provide excellent postoperative analgesia, but the following points should be considered:

- there may be a coagulopathy
- intraoperative use may result in profound hypotension since patients are often hypovolaemic and may have severe sepsis
- placement of an epidural catheter in the presence of systemic sepsis; the true risk of an epidural abscess is unknown and this is a risk–benefit decision.

General anaesthesia

Large-bore intravenous access and intravenous fluid administration should be established prior to induction of anaesthesia. Aspirate the nasogastric tube and leave it open to drain freely (consider using a sump-type tube).

Rapid sequence induction is used. There is potential for cardiovascular collapse on induction of anaesthesia if the patient is inadequately resuscitated. Be prepared for this, however adequate resuscitation appears to be.

Choice of agents used is relatively unimportant, but consider drugs with a rapid recovery profile since drug kinetics may be altered in patients who are unwell, particularly in the elderly. Nitrous oxide is best avoided since it can diffuse into an already dilated bowel and may make closure of the abdomen difficult and increase intra-abdominal pressure in the early postoperative period.

Patients with an obstructed or perforated viscus may require very large fluid volumes intraoperatively, including blood transfusion. Fluid warmers and active body warming (e.g. forced warm air overblankets) are mandatory since heat loss will be significant. Patients may require inotropic or vasopressor support.

Postoperative management

All but the most straightforward cases should be managed in a HDU or ICU in the early postoperative period. This is particularly true if an epidural catheter has been sited. Significant fluid loss and fluid shifts are likely to continue in the postoperative period, owing to redistribution and sequestration. There is potential for deterioration, most commonly because of sepsis or respiratory complications.

Patients require good quality analgesia. Both epidurals and opioid-based regimes are suitable.

Care should be taken using NSAIDs if upper gastrointestinal tract perforation or renal compromise are present: this includes a substantial proportion of patients suffering a perforated or obstructed viscus.

Bibliography

Callum KG, Gray AJG, Hoile RW, *et al. Extremes of Age: the 1999 Report of the National Confidential Enquiry into Perioperative Deaths.* London: NCEPOD, 1999.

Harper SJ. NCEPOD: caring to the end? *J Intensive Care Soc* 2010; **11**: 88–9.

National Confidential Enquiry into Patient Outcome and Death. *Caring to the End? A Review of Patients Who Died in Hospital Within Four Days of Admission.* London: NCEPOD, 2009. See www.ncepod.org.uk/2009dah.htm.

Paterson-Brown S. *Emergency Surgery and Critical Care: A Companion to Specialist Surgical Practice.* London: WB Saunders, 1997.

Pearse RM, Harrison DA, James P, *et al.* Identification and characterisation of the high-risk surgical population in the United Kingdom. *Crit Care* 2006; **10**: R81.

Cross-references

Emergency surgery, 613
Fluid and electrolyte balance, 754

Oesophagogastrectomy

Richard J Harding

Surgery for malignant lesions of the oesophagus and stomach

There are several surgical approaches for oesophageal surgery, which are determined by the anatomical position of the tumour and by surgical preference:

- 'Ivor Lewis' oesophagectomy: upper midline laparotomy followed by right thoracotomy for tumours in the middle and lower thirds of the oesophagus
- left thoracoabdominal oesophagectomy: for tumours of the lower third and cardia
- three-stage oesophagectomy: upper midline laparotomy, right thoracotomy and left- or right-sided cervical incision; for tumours of the upper and middle thirds
- pharyngolaryngo-oesophagectomy: for tumours of the hypopharynx and cervical oesophagus; usually an ENT procedure
- transhiatal oesophagectomy: oesophagectomy without thoracotomy; rarely used
- thorascopic surgery is becoming more popular
- gastric surgery is performed via an upper midline laparotomy.

This chapter will concentrate on the anaesthesia for oesophagectomy. The majority of cases are performed either open or by a combination of laparoscopy and thoracotomy. Some centres now practise a fully 'minimally invasive' technique – laparoscopy (reverse Trendelenburg), thoracoscopy/video-assisted thoracic surgery (VATS) (prone) and a neck incision for removal of the specimen and anastomosis.

Patient characteristics

- Elderly.
- High prevalence of tobacco and alcohol consumption.
- Patients frequently suffer from smoking-related conditions, particularly ischaemic heart disease and chronic obstructive pulmonary disease.
- Patients are often malnourished secondary to dysphagia and the presence of a malignancy. Surgery on malnourished patients carries a high morbidity and mortality.

Preoperative assessment and investigations

Adequate staging of the tumour is essential to ensure that proposed surgery is appropriate. Assessment of the severity of comorbid disease, particularly of the cardiorespiratory system, and assessment of nutritional status are important as these influence the choice of anaesthetic technique.

Investigations

- Full blood count.
- Urea, electrolytes and creatinine.
- ECG.
- Chest X-ray.
- Lung function tests and arterial blood gases if the patient has respiratory disease and one-lung ventilation is required.
- Further cardiovascular testing, such as echocardiography, should be considered.
- Many centres employ additional tests of global cardiorespiratory function, including the shuttle walk test, or formal cardiopulmonary exercise testing (CPX). Results of CPX testing have so far proved disappointing; in one recent study, there was no significant increase in cardiopulmonary or other complications, unplanned ICU admission rates or length of hospital stay in patients with an anaerobic threshold (AT) less than 11 mL min^{-1} kg^{-1}. Overall area under the receiver operating characteristic curve was less than 0.63 for the ability of either AT or $\dot{V}o_2$max to predict poor outcome.

Preoperative preparation

Attention should be given to the nutritional state of the patient. Both enteral and parenteral nutrition have a role and currently there is interest in the addition of immunomodulatory substances to these. Maximum medical treatment of comorbid conditions should be implemented. Patients with poor respiratory function may benefit from admission to allow preoperative physiotherapy and treatment of infection.

Thromboembolic prophylaxis and premedication are administered.

Perioperative management

Monitoring

- Routine anaesthetic monitoring.
- Urinary catheter.
- Core temperature.
- Invasive arterial pressure and CVP monitoring.
- Monitoring of cardiac output in high-risk cases.

Patients can be haemodynamically unstable during thoracotomy and arterial lines are also useful for assessing the adequacy of one-lung ventilation. Central lines should be sited ipsilateral to the side of the thoracotomy, owing to the risk of pneumothorax or vessel damage.

Anaesthetic technique

The technique chosen most commonly involves a general anaesthetic supplemented by epidural analgesia. A balanced anaesthetic technique is used. Agents with rapid recovery profiles are useful to avoid prolonged postoperative respiratory depression. Unlike the volatile agents, propofol does not inhibit hypoxic pulmonary vasoconstriction, and may therefore confer a small benefit. A double-lumen endobronchial tube is inserted to allow one-lung ventilation, which may be prolonged. A left-sided tube is usually employed for oesophageal surgery. Correct positioning is vital and should be checked fibreoptically. Active patient warming is required. Some anaesthetists prefer to use a single-lumen tube with an endobronchial blocker.

Special points

With multilevel approaches to the oesophagus, such as the Ivor Lewis operation, several intraoperative changes of patient position are required. This risks displacement of the double-lumen tube, loss of invasive lines and patient injury.

- Tube position needs to be checked after each change of position.
- Surgery can be prolonged and involve significant fluid and blood loss.
- Manipulation of mediastinal structures can impede cardiac filling and produce arrhythmias.

Postoperative management

In most cases, the aim is early extubation and admission to a HDU. However, some patients will need ventilation on the ICU. Adequate analgesia is vital to avoid respiratory complications. Analgesia can be provided by an epidural, paravertebral catheter, intercostal nerve blocks or an opioid-based technique. Epidural analgesia is the most popular technique in the UK. Complete analgesia can sometimes be difficult to achieve because the surgery involves many dermatome levels. A multimodal approach is advisable.

Other key therapies

- Aggressive physiotherapy.
- Thromboembolic prophylaxis.
- Early institution of enteral nutrition, often via a surgically sited jejunostomy, reduces the incidence of postoperative complications.
- A high index of suspicion is required for surgical complications, the most important of these being anastomotic breakdown.

Outcome

- Oesophagectomy has an operative mortality of approximately 10%.
- Outcome is improved by performing oesophagectomies in specialist centres with experienced teams.

Complications

- Respiratory complications occur in 25% of patients after oesophagectomy.
- Cardiovascular complications (including arrhythmias, especially atrial fibrillation) occur in approximately 10%, and thromboembolic complications in <10%. Anastomotic leaks occur in approximately 10%, and chylothorax in 3%. These have a high mortality if not aggressively managed. Early systemic inflammatory response syndrome or sepsis, unexplained infiltrates on chest X-ray, etc. should always raise the possibility of an anastomotic leak.
- After surgery 1 year survival is approximately 50%, with a 5 year survival of 20%.

Bibliography

Braga M, Gianotti L, Nespoli L, *et al.* Nutritional approach in malnourished surgical patients: a prospective randomised study. *Arch Surg* 2002; **137**: 174–8.

Forshaw MJ, Strauss DC, Davies AR, *et al.* Is cardiopulmonary exercise testing a useful test before esophagectomy? *Ann Thorac Surg* 2008; **85**: 294–9.

Gray AJG, Hoile RW, Ingram GS, Sherry KM. *The Report of the National Confidential Enquiry into Perioperative Deaths 1996/1997.* London: NCEPOD, 1998.

Griffin SM, Raimes SA. *Upper Gastrointestinal Surgery: A Companion to Specialist Surgical Practice.* London: W.B. Saunders, 1997.

Sherry KM. How can we improve the outcome of oesophagectomy? *Br J Anaesth* 2001; **86**: 611–13.

Vaughan RS. Pain relief after thoracotomy. *Br J Anaesth* 2001; **87**: 681.

Cross-references

Complications of position, 743
Mediastinal surgery, 417
One-lung anaesthesia, 714

Open and laparoscopic cholecystectomy

Helen Buglass

The incidence of gallstones is approximately 12% in men and 24% in women in the UK. The standard treatment for symptomatic gallstones is now laparoscopic cholecystectomy. There are relatively few absolute contraindications, and most surgeons proceed with laparoscopic surgery even after acute cholecystitis, previous surgery and in patients with common bile duct stones. Additionally, a minority of patients with impacted duct stones may benefit from endoscopic retrograde cholangiopancreatography and sphincterotomy.

The main indications for open cholecystectomy are:

- patients unfit to tolerate pneumoperitoneum (although surgical techniques using laparoscopic retractors require a lower intra-abdominal pressure)
- intraoperative conversion to an open technique
- previous upper abdominal surgery (relative)
- cholecystectomy performed at the same time as another open procedure.

Typical patient characteristics

- Age 40–50 years.
- Female/male ratio is 5:1.
- History of hypercholesterolaemia or haemolytic disease.
- Obesity and its complications.
- Majority are performed electively.

Preoperative assessment and investigations

Elective cholecystectomy

- History and examination.
- Full blood count and electrolytes.
- Liver function tests (if deranged, coagulation screen).
- Chest X-ray and ECG when warranted.
- Any further investigations according to coexisting medical conditions.

Acute cholecystectomy

- Patients can present acutely unwell, jaundiced and/or dehydrated.
- Special attention should be paid to renal function.
- Hypovolaemia should be fully corrected with crystalloid and colloids according to clinical need.
- If coagulation is deranged, 10 mg intravenous vitamin K with/without fresh-frozen plasma (FFP) should be considered
- Antibiotics as per hospital protocol.

Anaesthetic technique

Preinduction

- Routine standard monitoring. ECG, blood pressure, end-tidal CO_2 ($ETco_2$), pulse oximetry, temperature as per Association of Anaesthetists of Great Britain and Ireland guidelines.
- Occasionally, invasive monitoring dependent on any comorbidity or intercurrent condition.
- Rapid sequence induction may be indicated in the acute state.

Induction and maintenance: open cholecystectomy

- Thoracic epidural is the pain relief of choice when coagulation is satisfactory.
- Alternatives include intercostals or field blocks.
- If a midline incision is employed, rectus sheath block may be a suitable alternative.
- In the acute state, with normal coagulation but deranged liver function tests, vitamin K preoperatively is advisable.
- Induction: standard intravenous induction, non-depolarizing muscle relaxation, endotracheal intubation.
- Maintenance: air/oxygen mix with a volatile agent, intermittent bolus of non-depolarizing muscle relaxant, controlled ventilation.
- Analgesia: opioid analgesics, plus intravenous paracetamol and a NSAID, particularly when epidural analgesia is not used.
- Historically, morphine was avoided as it was thought to cause painful contraction of the sphincter of Oddi. This is not now thought to be the case, although some continue to use pethidine for its supposed smooth muscle relaxant properties. Hyoscine may occasionally be requested by the surgeon when duct exploration or intraoperative cholangiography proves difficult.
- Reversal of non-depolarizing muscle relaxant at the end of the procedure.

Box 16.3 Perioperative complications of laparoscopic cholecystectomy

- Cardiovascular collapse: raised intra-abdominal pressure leads to decreased venous return, increased systemic vascular resistance and reduced cardiac output. Further compromised by reverse Trendelenburg (head-up) position
- Gas embolism: sudden fall in $ETco_2$, cardiovascular collapse, hypoxaemia. Differential diagnosis of above. In principle, CO_2 is rapidly absorbed leading to resolution
- Direct surgical trauma: vascular or visceral injury (increased risk after gas insufflation of stomach by intermittent positive pressure ventilation (IPPV), reduced by insertion of nasogastric tube)
- Severe dysrrhythmias: severe bradycardia on inflation related to vagal stimulation due to peritoneal stretch. Many anaesthetists use prophylactic anticholinergics
- Hypercarbia: ventilation can become difficult particularly in obese patients
- Haemorrhage: difficult to access
- Pneumothorax, mediastinal emphysema: present with cardiovascular collapse
- Hypothermia: owing to the large volumes of gas used. Monitor temperature and actively warm.
- Postoperative nausea and vomiting

Recovery: early

- Oxygen via face-mask.
- Intravenous fluid until the patient is drinking adequately.
- Analgesia:
  - intravenous opioid via patient-controlled analgesia (PCA)
  - regional technique; continuous epidural infusion of low-dose local anaesthetic and opioid; patient-controlled epidural analgesia is a popular option
  - paravertebral blocks and intercostal blocks are occasionally used.

Recovery: late

- Complications may be secondary to poor pain control, obesity or immobility. These include basal atelectasis with resultant pneumonia, and DVT. Optimizing pain control, physiotherapy, early mobilization and thromboembolic prophylaxis can reduce these.
- Operative mortality is substantially below 1%. Factors increasing the risk of postoperative mortality are advancing age and acute surgery.

Induction and maintenance: laparoscopic cholecystectomy (Box 16.3)

- Induction: standard intravenous induction, non-depolarizing muscle relaxation, endotracheal intubation. In some centres, controlled ventilation via the laryngeal mask airway is used. While this may be appropriate in some cases, its general applicability may be limited by body habitus.
- Maintenance: air/oxygen mix with a volatile agent, or a propofol infusion in those at greatest risk of postoperative nausea and vomiting (PONV). Intermittent bolus of non-depolarizing muscle relaxant, controlled ventilation.
- Analgesia: opioid analgesic, usually fentanyl, plus paracetamol and a NSAID unless specifically contraindicated. TAP block and/or local infiltration to port sites may prove beneficial.
- Antiemetic prophylaxis: commonly, a $5HT_3$ inhibitor and dexamethasone, particularly in day-case surgery.
- Reversal of non-depolarizing muscle relaxant at the end of the procedure
- This can be a deceptive operation which can finish very suddenly and quickly: watch the screens and be aware of surgical progress.

Recovery: early

- Oxygen via face-mask.
- Intravenous fluid until the patient is drinking adequately.
- Analgesia: regular paracetemol supplemented with codeine or a NSAID.

Recovery: late

- Possible as day-case procedure.
- Delayed owing to conversion to open technique, 4%. Incidence of bile duct injury, 0.3%.
- Mortality rate, <0.4%.

Bibliography

Adams JP, Murphy PG. Obesity in anaesthesia and intensive care. *Br J Anaesth* 2000; **85**: 91–108.

Andersson L, Lindberg G, Bringman S, *et al.* Pneumoperitoneum versus abdominal wall lift: effects on central haemodynamics and intrathoracic pressure during laparoscopic cholecystectomy. *Acta Anaesthesiol Scand* 2003; **47**: 838–46.

Hirvonen EA, Poikolainen EO. The adverse effects of anaesthesia, head up tilt, and carbon dioxide pneumoperitoneum during laparoscopic cholecystectomy. *Surg Endosc* 2000; **14**: 272–7.

Cross-references

Complications of position, 743
Day-case surgery, 604

17

Gynaecological surgery

Giorgio Capogna and Silvia Stirparo

Fertility surgery

Giorgio Capogna and Silvia Stirparo

Procedure

The most common procedure for fertility surgery is probably for egg retrieval. Very occasionally, a general anaesthetic may be required for embryo replacement, but this is rare.

More extensive procedures may be necessary in the early diagnosis of infertility and these might include hysteroscopy, laparoscopy or laparotomy. These may be of a minor diagnostic nature to check for tubal patency or more extensive with tubal reconstruction or for adhesiolysis.

The procedures may form part of an *in vitro* fertilization programme, e.g. egg retrieval (transvaginally or laparascopically) and gamete intrafallopian transfer (GIFT).

An operating microscope may be used during tubal surgery and the procedure may be lengthy.

Patients are generally young, highly motivated and knowledgeable about their treatment, and as such often request further information and an explanation of the anaesthetic procedure.

Except for procedures which require a laparotomy, the patient is likely to be managed on a day-case basis.

For egg retrieval and embryo replacement, ovarian or endometrial stimulation may have been undertaken by carefully controlled hormonal therapy. The procedure may have to be performed within a specific time window.

Some centres use general anaesthesia for egg retrieval and some use sedation techniques (but administered by an anaesthetist).

Patient characteristics

- The patients are generally young, physically fit, women of American Society of Anesthesiologists grade 1 or 2.
- Infertility may sometimes be associated with specific psychological problems ranging from anxiety/stress disorders to compulsive/obsessive neuroses. Such women need a sympathetic and understanding approach.
- Occasionally, there may be an associated endocrine disorder.
- Very occasionally, a patient may appear as an urgent case following a failed attempt under local analgesia and sedation. It is essential to determine exactly what drugs have already been administered so as to avoid potentially harmful interactions

Preoperative assessment

- There may be a history of a recent large (1 litre) oral fluid intake to fill the bladder to facilitate a preoperative pelvic ultrasound scan.
- The patient may have had many previous anaesthetics.
- The risk of postoperative nausea and vomiting (PONV) is high in this patient population.

Premedication

- Usually unnecessary.
- If the patient is very anxious, a short-acting benzodiazepine is suitable.

Theatre preparation

- Routine equipment and machine check.
- Lithotomy position is likely to be required and so check leg supports, personnel for lifting the two legs simultaneously, etc.
- Bulky video and ultrasound equipment may be used by the gynaecologist.
- If the laser is to be used, arrange appropriate eye protection.

Anaesthetic technique

- For diagnostic hysteroscopy, laparoscopy, etc., any appropriate technique is suitable.
- For egg retrieval, the evidence that any sedative drug, anaesthetic drug or technique is associated with higher conception rates is inconclusive. Halothane should be avoided but all other inhalational agents appear to be equally acceptable. It has been suggested that some NSAIDs may impair embryo development and the gynaecologist may request that these be avoided. A good general rule is to keep it as simple as possible and use as few drugs as possible.
- As the patient is likely to be a day case, avoid succinylcholine and use short-acting agents.
- Total intravenous anaesthesia (TIVA) is favoured by many.

- Nitrous oxide may increase nausea and vomiting but there is no evidence that it is detrimental to embryo development as a component of the anaesthetic (although some gynaecologists request that it not be used). Tracheal intubation is usually only necessary for laparotomies, laparoscopies or patients who are at risk from regurgitation. A laryngeal mask is usually suitable for airway management.
- A spinal or epidural may be used. Motivated patients may like to take an active interest in the proceedings. Careful explanation and counselling is necessary if using a central block in a day-case patient.
- Many centres now use a sedation technique and low-dose propofol TIVA together with small doses of midazolam and a short-acting opioid are suitable.

Intraoperative monitoring

- Standard minimal monitoring should be used even if sedation and not anaesthesia is the technique.

Complications

Unexpected collapse may be due to:

- sudden extreme bradycardia secondary to peritoneal distension or traction on pelvic structures
- blood loss from an unrecognized laceration to a major pelvic blood vessel; such blood loss may be retroperitoneal and thus unseen
- venous gas embolism
- tension pneumothorax.

Postoperative management

Pain relief usually requires only oral paracetamol with or without codeine. A NSAID may be administered if the gynaecologist has no objection. Opioids may be required in a small number of patients. Any available antiemetic drug is suitable and is recommended if the patient is a day case.

Bibliography

Bokhari A, Pollard BJ. Anaesthesia for assisted conception. *Eur J Anaesthesiol* 1998; **15**: 391–6.

Bokhari A, Pollard BJ. Anaesthesia for assisted conception: a survey of UK practice. *Eur J Anaesthesiol* 1999; **16**: 225–30.

Critchlow BM, Ibrahim Z, Pollard BJ. General anaesthesia for gamete intrafallopian transfer. *Eur J Anaesthesiol* 1991; **8**: 381–4.

Cross-references

Complications of position, 743
Day-case surgery, 604
Hysteroscopy and laser surgery, 456
Laparoscopy, 458
Premedication, 619

Hysteroscopy and laser surgery

Giorgio Capogna and Silvia Stirparo

These procedures include direct examination of the uterine cavity using a fibreoptic endoscope, often followed by other intrauterine surgical interventions. Uterine distension is necessary for visualization. The use of an irrigation fluid also permits removal of blood and detritus and the dissipation of heat. Distension is usually achieved with a fluid (saline, glycine, dextran). CO_2 may very occasionally be used.

Office-based techniques using miniature hysteroscopes are currently being developed in some countries. These new techniques have developed following technological advances in medical instrumentation. They require only minimal (or no) cervical dilatation and thus the patients do not require anaesthesia and in many cases do not require sedation either.

- Complications – fluid:
  - absorption and circulatory overload
  - dilutional hyponatraemia and hypoproteinaemia,
  - transurethral resection (TUR) syndrome
  - disseminated intravascular coagulation
  - anaphylaxis
- Complications – CO_2:
  - abdominal distension during long procedures (leak via the fallopian tubes)
  - CO_2 absorption - acidosis, arrhythmias
  - CO_2 embolism.

The laser

The commonest lasers in gynaecological use are the neodymium-yttrium-aluminium-garnet (Nd-YAG) and CO_2 lasers.

All staff concerned should be familiar with the national guidelines on the safe operation of medical lasers and also local policies. Although the laser should only be operated in the surgical field, precautions must be taken to protect against injury from inadvertent operation:

- patient eye protection
- staff eye protection
- designated operating theatre with locked doors and covered windows (if any)
- removal/covering of reflective surfaces
- no casual access
- extra eye protection outside in case of need.

Intrauterine hysteroscopic laser surgery is carried out under fluid uterine distension. Procedures include endometrial destruction and removal of benign intrauterine pathology.

Complications include uterine perforation, haemorrhage (usually controlled with the laser but may necessitate laparotomy if the uterus is perforated) and heat transmission (not clinically important at typical power settings for intrauterine surgery).

Patient characteristics

- May be any age from mid-teens onwards.
- No particular medical disorder is associated with the need for hysteroscopic laser surgery except for anaemia.
- The procedure may be performed as a day case; therefore, check suitability (medical status, home circumstances, etc.).

Preoperative assessment and investigations

- Check for anaemia.
- Other investigations as indicated by the patient's medical status.

Premedication

- Not usually required. Anxiolysis with a benzodiazepine may be valuable.
- Consider an antiemetic.
- Antibiotic prophylaxis may be given with the premedication or on induction of anaesthesia in at-risk patients.

Theatre preparation

- Familiarity with policies on the use of the laser is essential.
- Availability of patient protection: eye pads, foil, etc.
- Availability of staff eye protection: goggles.

Perioperative management

- Minimal monitoring standards apply (ECG, NIBP, S_po_2, F_io_2, $ETco_2$).

- Fluid balance (including uterine distension fluid) may need to be measured.
- Temperature if the procedure is prolonged.

Anaesthetic technique

- Resuscitation equipment should be available.
- General anaesthesia with either spontaneous or controlled respiration is commonly used.
- Choice of maintenance technique depends on the patient's medical condition and the anaesthetist's preference.
- Regional: epidural or spinal are suitable. Light sedation may be needed (e.g. midazolam) with oxygen via face-mask.
- Local: paracervical, intracervical and intrauterine local block may be given by the surgeon. These are not favoured by all gynaecologists. Sedation may be needed (e.g. midazolam).
- Analgesia, e.g. ketorolac or alfentanil.
- Position patient in the lithotomy position.

Fluid balance

- Measurement of fluid instilled and retrieved can be difficult, but in longer procedures should be attempted because of the possible effects of fluid absorption.
- Sample protocol:
  - 1000 mL absorbed: continue surgery
  - 1500 mL absorbed: end surgery as soon as possible
  - 2000 mL absorbed: stop surgery.
- Excessive blood loss is rarely a problem.
- Watch for signs of TUR syndrome, especially with extensive surgery and high intrauterine pressures.

Postoperative management

- Any postoperative discomfort may usually be managed by NSAIDs.
- Gynaecological procedures are associated with an increased incidence of PONV and an antiemetic should be prescribed.

Bibliography

Department of Health and Social Security. *Guidelines on the Safe Use of Lasers in Medical Practice.* London: DHSS, 1984.

Di Spiezio Sardo A, Bettocchi S, Spinelli M, *et al.* Review of new office-based hysteroscopic procedures 2003–2009. *J Minim Invasive Gynecol* 2010; **17**: 436–48.

Morrison LMM, Davis J, Sumner D. Absorption of irrigating fluid during laser photocoagulation of the endometrium in the treatment of menorrhagia. *Br J Obstet Gynaecol* 1989; **96**: 346–52.

Osborne GA, Rudkin GE, Moran P. Fluid uptake in laser endometrial ablation. *Anaesth Intensive Care* 1991; **19**: 217–19.

Van Boven MJ, Singelyn F, Donnez J, Gribomont BF. Dilutional hyponatraemia associated with intrauterine endoscopic laser surgery. *Anesthesiology* 1989; **71** :449–50.

Cross-references

Complications of position, 743
Day-case surgery, 604
Transurethral resection of the prostate syndrome, 805

Minor gynaecological procedures

Giorgio Capogna and Silvia Stirparo

Minor gynaecological procedures are common and include dilatation and curettage (D&C), evacuation of retained products of conception (ERPC) and suction termination of pregnancy (TOP). Other minor procedures are often added, e.g. hysteroscopy or cystoscopy, and these can lengthen the procedure, possibly quite considerably.

Procedures

- Short in duration.
- Often undertaken as day cases.
- Normally performed in the lithotomy position.
- Involve an initial period of intense surgical stimulation for dilatation of the cervix.
- May be diagnostic (e.g. D&C for postmenopausal bleeding) or therapeutic (e.g. ERPC).

Patient characteristics

- May be of any age from puberty onwards.
- Are generally young and fit for TOP and ERPC.
- They may have significant comorbidities (e.g. cardiac abnormalities) which are possibly related to the reason for the TOP.
- Those for ERPC who are beyond the first trimester of pregnancy or who have symptomatic gastro-oesophageal reflux require precautions against aspiration of gastric contents.
- Many patients for D&C are elderly with various comorbidities and perhaps malignant disease.

Preoperative assessment and investigations

- Assess the adequacy of resuscitation if a patient for ERPC has vaginal bleeding as this may have been considerable and be continuing.
- If urgent then determine when and what was the last oral intake and what analgesia has been given as this may warn of the possibility of a full stomach.
- What is the length of gestation if relevant and are there any symptoms of reflux?
- Investigations (e.g. chest X-ray, ECG, electrolytes, coagulation profile), as clinically indicated.
- Measure haemoglobin if actively bleeding, but remember that following acute blood loss there may be no change in the haemoglobin for several hours.
- Enquire about any coexisting diseases.
- Enquire about any limitation of knee and hip movement (needed for the lithotomy position).
- If planned as a day case, ensure that appropriate procedures are in place for subsequent care.

Premedication

- Anxiolysis is rarely required but a short-acting benzodiazepine may be useful if necessary.
- H_2 antagonists and sodium citrate if at risk of regurgitation.
- Has a prostaglandin pessary been given? This may increase requirements for postoperative analgesia.

Theatre preparation

- Routine equipment and machine check.
- Adequate personnel to ensure simultaneous lifting and lowering of legs to avoid injuries to hips and knees.
- Remember when positioning to avoid nerve injury due to pressure on the medial or lateral lower leg from lithotomy poles.

Perioperative management

- Minimal monitoring standards apply ($F_{I}O_2$, $S_{p}O_2$, ECG, non-invasive blood pressure (NIBP) monitoring, end-tidal CO_2 ($ETco_2$)).
- General anaesthesia is usually the technique of choice because these operations are short and quite stimulating.
- Regional techniques are acceptable in selected patients.
- For TOP or ERPC, uterine relaxation should be avoided if possible by selecting a total intravenous technique or using a low concentration of volatile agent.
- Intravenous induction with spontaneous ventilation using a volatile agent (with or without N_2O) and a short-acting opioid, e.g. alfentanil or fentanyl, to obtund the response to cervical dilation is a suitable technique.
- Rapid sequence induction and tracheal intubation are necessary if there is risk of regurgitation.

- Oxytocics may be requested by the gynaecologist. Synthetic oxytocin (e.g. Syntocinon) is preferred. Products containing ergometrine (e.g. Syntometrine) should be avoided as these may cause hypertension, bronchospasm, nausea and vomiting, especially if given intravenously. Oxytocin may cause a fall in arterial pressure, which can be minimized by giving it slowly and limiting the dose to 5 units.
- Non-steroidal anti-inflammatory drugs (NSAIDs) are useful for postoperative analgesia, especially if prostaglandin pessaries have been used as these cause painful uterine contractions. A suitable dose of a NSAID may be given with the premedication or a suppository (remember the consent) during the procedure.
- Antiemetics may be needed in view of the high incidence of PONV in patients undergoing gynaecological surgery.
- There is little evidence that concentrations of volatile agents of 0.5 MAC or less lead to a clinically significant increase in blood loss during TOP or ERPC. Any uterine relaxation will be rapidly reversed by the administration of an oxytocic.

Postoperative management

- Nurse in the lateral position with supplemental oxygen until awake.
- If the trachea was intubated, then extubate awake in the lateral position.
- Male recovery staff should have chaperones in view of the possibility of inappropriate patient behaviour during recovery.
- Simple analgesics are usually adequate. Postoperative pain is usually minimal but may be greater in those patients who normally experience painful menstruation or who have received a prostaglandin pessary.
- If the patient's condition allows and domestic circumstances are suitable, most patients may be allowed home on the day of surgery with appropriate day-case procedure advice.

Cross-references

Complications of position, 743
Day-case surgery, 604
Premedication, 619

18 Obstetric anaesthesia

Giorgio Capogna and Silvia Stirparo

communication with a haematologist and arrangement of an intensive care bed should be expedited.

Puerperal cardiomyopathy

- Onset can be between 6 months of gestation and 6 months postpartum.
- More common in multiple pregnancies and in multiparous and older women.
- Presents as dyspnoea, palpitations and pulmonary and/or peripheral oedema, all of which are features of normal pregnancy.
- Diagnosed by cardiomegaly and reduced left ventricular function on echocardiography.
- Treatment includes delivery, anticoagulation, conventional heart failure drugs and occasionally heart transplantation.
- Fifty per cent spontaneous and full recovery, but sudden death can occur.

Acute fatty liver of pregnancy

- Rare, but potentially fatal.
- Associated with male fetuses, obesity and multiple pregnancies.
- Usually presents after 30 weeks' gestation with nausea, anorexia, abdominal pain and malaise.
- Often coexists with features of mild pre-eclampsia.
- Can be hard to distinguish from the HELLP syndrome, but differentiated by hypoglycaemia and marked hyperuricaemia.
- Early delivery usually reverses the disease process.
- Early consultation with intensivists and hepatologists is essential.
- Fulminant hepatic failure with encephalopathy may necessitate transfer to a liver unit for multisystem support and even hepatic transplant.

Bibliography

Nelson-Piercy C. *Handbook of Obstetric Medicine*. Oxford: Isis Medical Media, 1997.

The Eclampsia Trial Collaborative Group. Which anticonvulsant for women with eclampsia? Evidence from the collaborative eclampsia trial. *Lancet* 1995; **345**: 1455–63.

The MAGPIE Trial Collaborative Group. Do women with preeclampsia, and their babies, benefit from magnesium sulphate? The MAGPIE Trial: a randomised placebo controlled trial. *Lancet* 2002; **359**: 1877–89.

Walker JJ. Pre-eclampsia. *Lancet* 2000; **356**: 1260–5.

Cross-references

Amniotic fluid embolism, 730
Blood transfusion, 735
Cardiomyopathy, 136
Fluid and electrolyte balance, 754
Thrombosis and embolism, 793

19 Urology

Iurie Acalovschi

Laser resection of prostate

Iurie Acalovschi

The relatively new technique of laser resection of the prostate is being undertaken in a few centres. In this procedure, the prostatic tissue is resected with the histological prostate architecture being preserved by using a high-powered (60–80 W), pulsed, solid-state holmium:YAG laser, or vaporized by the 'photoselective' high-powered potassium-titanyl-phosphate (KTP) lasers.

Procedure

- The patient is placed in the lithotomy position.
- Resection of the prostate is performed endoscopically.
- There is no need for a non-conductive irrigant during the procedure, so saline can be used.
- Fewer blood transfusions are needed as laser therapy results in significantly less bleeding.

Patient characteristics

- Over 50 years of age; male.
- High incidence of chronic disease.
- ASA status 1–4.
- Because of advanced age, the patients have a relatively high prevalence (30–60%) of both cardiovascular and pulmonary disorders. Anticoagulant therapy is not uncommon in this patient population. Long-standing obstruction can lead to impaired renal function. Urinary tract infection can complicate large residual volumes of urine.

Preoperative assessment and investigation

- Exclude associated conditions.
- Systematic review for intercurrent illness.
- Discuss anaesthetic technique.

Premedication

If a premedicant is required, then a short-acting benzodiazepine is suitable.

Perioperative management

Theatre preparation

- The patient is placed in the lithotomy position.
- Protective goggles should be available for all staff and also the patient.
- A means to evacuate the smoke plume is required.

Monitoring

- Routine; minimal monitoring.
- $ETco_2$.
- Blood loss.
- Core temperature.

Anaesthetic technique

Either general or regional anaesthesia provides good operating conditions for transurethral resection of the prostate (TURP). Because the systemic complications of the classical TURP syndrome are diminished, general anaesthesia may be used, even on an ambulatory basis. In patients with severe chronic obstructive pulmonary disease, regional anaesthesia is preferred. In high-risk patients, caudal and saddle block spinal anaesthesia has been successfully used. The anaesthetic should be one of rapid recovery and minimal interference with postoperative urinary voiding.

The TURP syndrome

The introduction of laser technology for endoscopic resection of prostate tissue has nearly eliminated the risk of the TURP syndrome. The minimal fluid absorption reduces the incidence of excessive intravascular volume and minimizes the risk of electrolyte abnormalities. As it is unimportant whether the irrigant can conduct electricity or not then normal saline may be used. As a consequence, the risk of solute toxicity by absorbing large quantities of glycine, mannitol or sorbitol is avoided. The required irrigation pressures are much less than for a classical TURP.

Outcome

Holmium laser techniques require an average of 18–27 hours of postoperative catheterization and hospital stays of 1–2 days. For KTP laser therapy, the majority of patients are treated in an ambulatory setting and do not require an indwelling catheter postoperatively. Compared with the TURP technique, reoperations are more often required.

Bibliography

Barber NJ, Muir GH. High-power KTP laser prostatectomy: the new challenge to transurethral resection of the prostate. *Curr Opin Urol* 2004; **14**: 21–5.

Hanson RA, Zornow MH, Conlin MJ, Brambrink AM. Laser resection of the prostate: implications for anesthesia. *Anesth Analg* 2007; **105**: 475–9.

Kuntz R. Current role of lasers in the treatment of benign prostatic hyperplasia (BPH). *Eur Urol* 2006; **49**: 961–9.

Tan AH, Gilling PJ. Lasers in the treatment of benign prostatic hyperplasia: an update. *Curr Opin Urol* 2005; **15**: 55–8.

Cross-references

Blood transfusion, 735

Fluid and electrolyte balance, 754

The elderly patient, 607

Transurethral resection of the prostate syndrome, 805

Nephrectomy

Iurie Acalovschi

This operation involves the removal of a kidney with or without part of the ureter. In cases of radical nephrectomy for renal cell carcinoma besides removal of kidney, the excision of the ipsilateral adrenal gland and a regional lymphadenectomy are performed. Considering the size and location of the tumour, an open or a laparoscopic technique may be used. Thermal ablative therapies, including renal cryosurgery and radiofrequency ablation have emerged recently as treatments of localized renal cell carcinoma or for high-risk patients. In selected patients, cryoablation has been successfully performed using the laparoscopic approach. There is potential for considerable blood loss.

Nephrectomy may be performed for tumour, hydronephrosis, chronic infection and, rarely, for staghorn calculi which cannot be treated by other means. Patients with renal tumours may have pulmonary metastases. In 5–10% of patients, the tumour is associated with thrombus extending into the renal vein, vena cava and/or right atrium. Paraneoplastic syndromes (hypertension, polycythaemia, hypercalcaemia, non-metastatic hepatic dysfunction) are found in 20% of patients with renal cell carcinoma.

The laparoscopic approach is gaining popularity. It is becoming preferred to the open approach in many centres and may be advantageous with respect to recovery and duration of hospital stay.

The open operation may be carried out via a dorsal incision or an anterior subcostal, flank, midline or thoracoabdominal incision. In cases of chronic infection, the patient may be debilitated with low plasma albumin. The majority of patients with renal cell carcinoma are anaemic. These patients may range from ASA 1 to 4.

Nephrectomy may also be carried out as the first stage in a renal transplant. The donor patient has one kidney removed and this is then prepared and preserved for transplantation shortly afterwards. The recipient is often in another nearby operating theatre or follows on in this theatre. In this operation, the patient is likely to be fit and well with no comorbidities. It must be remembered that this patient is otherwise devoid of any kidney disease and does not need the operation except for the act of donating a kidney.

Preoperative assessment

- Exclude associated conditions.
- A systematic review of other medical conditions is essential.
- Evaluate the degree of renal impairment.
- Establish the extent of the lesions and the type of ablative therapy.
- Patients with suspected or proven urinary tract infection should receive 48 hours of antibiotic therapy.
- Ensure the availability of blood.

Premedication

A short-acting benzodiazepine is useful. An analgesic premedication may be useful.

Perioperative management

Theatre preparation

Careful positioning of the patient for this operation is important. Usually, the patient is placed laterally on the operating table with the side of operation uppermost. The surgeon may request that the table be moved to the flexed position such that the head and feet are both lowered to facilitate surgical access. In cases of radical nephrectomy for excision of tumour thrombus, a thoracoabdominal approach may be necessary. Cardiopulmonary bypass to prevent embolization may be required in these cases. For laparoscopic nephrectomy three approaches may be used: transperitoneal, retroperitoneal and hand-assisted. Fluids should be warmed. When a large tumour is to be resected preoperative blood transfusion may be required in anaemic patients.

Monitoring

The potential for blood loss during this operation may be an indication for invasive monitoring in certain patients. A CVP line and an intra-arterial line are recommended in such circumstances. In addition to routine monitoring, blood loss, temperature and urine output are useful.

Anaesthetic technique

General endotracheal anaesthesia with controlled ventilation is normally used. The positioning of the patient on the side results in a ventilation/perfusion mismatch between the lungs. Intermittent positive pressure ventilation is mandatory. In addition, there is a risk of surgical disruption of the pleura during the dissection. General anaesthesia is indicated in laparoscopic renal surgery, which also requires controlled ventilation. In cases of abdominal laparoscopic nephrectomy, the use of N_2O should be avoided if possible.

The combination of general anaesthesia with epidural analgesia via a low thoracic or high lumbar catheter is useful to provide postoperative analgesia. If an epidural is not possible, intercostal nerve blocks from T9 to T12 are a useful supplement to general anaesthesia and will give some postoperative pain relief.

In renal cell carcinoma with thrombus, anaesthetic management is complex and may require massive blood transfusion (up to 50 units of packed red blood cells, plasma and platelets). Large-bore intravenous cannulae and a catheter should be placed.

Complications

- Pneumothorax may occur during thoracoabdominal or flank incisions. At the end of the procedure, several large-volume breaths may be given to attempt to detect any pleural leak. If there is a pneumothorax, the pleural injuries should be repaired and a chest tube or drain inserted.
- In patients with partial nephrectomy, complications include haemorrhage, urinary fistula, urethral obstruction and renal insufficiency.

Postoperative management

Open nephrectomy is a painful operation and requires optimal postoperative pain relief. This is best provided by continuous epidural infusion of a mixture of opioids and low-dose local anaesthetics. Nephrectomy by the laparoscopic approach results in much less postoperative pain and routine analgesics are often sufficient. There is a risk of atelectasis in the dependent lung and postoperative physiotherapy is essential.

Long-term outcome depends largely on the aetiology of the renal damage and the type of procedure. After radical nephrectomy, postoperative complications occur in approximately 20% of patients and the operative mortality rate is approximately 2%.

In cases of laparoscopic nephrectomy, the postoperative pain requirements are four times less than with open incisions and hospital stay is decreased by 50%. For patients with comorbidities, laparoscopic nephrectomy may be preferable and minimally invasive.

Bibliography

Conacher ID, Soomro NA, Rix D. Anaesthesia for laparoscopic urological surgery. *Br J Anaesth* 2004; **93**: 859–64.

El Galley R, Hammontree L, Urban D, *et al.* Anesthesia for laparoscopic donor nephrectomy: is nitrous oxide contraindicated? *J Urol* 2007; **178**: 225–7.

Sener M, Torgay A, Akpek E, *et al.* Regional versus general anesthesia for donor nephrectomy: effects on graft function. *Transplant Proc* 2004; **36**: 2954–8.

Cross-references

Blood transfusion, 735
Complications of position, 743
Kidney transplantation, 522

Percutaneous nephrolithotomy

Iurie Acalovschi

Percutaneous nephrolithotomy is a procedure whereby stones in the renal tract are removed with a rigid or flexible endoscope via ultrasound-guided puncture and fluoroscopy-controlled placement of the endoscope. A guidewire is inserted through a hollow needle and advanced into the collecting system. Then tract dilation is performed over the guidewire. At the completion of access tract dilation, a working sheath is left in place to accommodate the endoscope and drain the irrigation fluid. The procedure is particularly indicated in patients with staghorn calculi, and lower pole calculi larger than 10 mm. Patients with stones resistant to extracorporeal shockwave lithotripsy should also be treated with this process. Small calculi are removed through the endoscope under direct vision using a forceps or a stone basket. Stones larger than 1 cm require fragmentation by use of an intracorporeal lithotripsy device. The most efficient are the ultrasonic and the pneumatic rigid lithotripters.

Patient characteristics

Patients are generally of any age, ASA 1–4, with the potential for compromised renal function. Morbidly obese patients in whom shockwave lithotripsy is impractical or technically impossible may also need to be treated in this way.

Preoperative investigations

- Exclusion of commonly associated medical conditions.
- Review of renal function.
- Bacteriological evaluation of the urine. Urinary calculi may harbour bacteria.
- Antibiotic prophylaxis.
- Correction of an existing coagulopathy.
- Antiplatelet medication should be discontinued 7 days before procedure.

Premedication

This is often not needed, but a short-acting benzodiazepine may be useful in some patients.

Perioperative management

Positioning

Traditionally, the patient is placed in the prone position with the stone-containing side elevated:

- ensure that there is enough man-power to turn the patient
- protect the eyes, shoulders, knees, elbows
- place the arm with intravenous access above the head (beware of brachial plexus strain)
- the other arm with the BP cuff may be placed by the side
- place a pillow(s) under the chest and pelvis to free the abdomen for ventilation
- place a pad under the flank to prevent a mobile kidney from rotating anteriorly in the prone position
- turn the head to the side to be punctured in order to prevent neck strain.

In high-risk patients, in order to minimize the haemodynamic and respiratory changes, a full lateral or a supine anterolateral position may be used. It prevents the discomfort and ventilation difficulties of the prone position, particularly in obese patients.

Monitoring

In addition to routine monitoring, estimation of blood loss and core temperature are useful.

Anaesthetic technique

General anaesthesia is a suitable technique when a lengthy procedure is planned. Muscular paralysis is usually required because the patient will be placed prone or lateral and coughing must be avoided during renal puncture. An armoured (reinforced) tracheal tube should be used if placed prone.

Spinal anaesthesia is safe and effective in selected patients. Intrathecal low-dose bupivacaine and fentanyl offer reliable neuraxial block. Combined spinal–epidural anaesthesia with a sensory block above T6 is an attractive alternative to general anaesthesia. It has the advantage of shorter hospital stay, better patient satisfaction and superior postoperative pain relief.

Local anaesthesia by delivering the local anaesthetic through the access track combined with sedation is safe and effective in selected patients.

Complications

Bleeding is the most significant complication. The kidney is a very vascular organ and tears in the parenchyma may occur if the rigid scope is not handled with care. Bleeding requiring transfusion is rare. Most reports quote 3%. About 0.5% of cases may require balloon tamponade of the tract or arterial embolization.

Extravasation of irrigation fluid may result from a tear in the pelvicalyceal system. It is important, therefore, that normal saline is used as the endoscopic irrigation fluid. Water and glycine can cause fluid intoxication because they are absorbed from the peritoneum.

Pleural complications can result from an intercostal puncture to reach an upper calyceal calculus. The pleura may be entered and either a minor pleural reaction is seen or, following endoscopy, there could be a massive collection of irrigation fluid and air within the thoracic cavity.

Infection is the most serious complication and may be seen in 0.3–2.5% of cases. Stones containing infection may be disintegrated at percutaneous nephrolithotomy, releasing bacteria into the urine and, therefore, potentially into the bloodstream. Bacteraemia is unavoidable, but the time of the endoscopy should be limited to 1 hour if a large infected stone is being disintegrated and to 1.5 hours for a non-infected stone. If Gram-negative septicaemia is suspected, the patient should be treated aggressively immediately.

Postoperative management

Intravenous fluids should be given to increase urine output and flush out any gravel via the nephrostomy left *in situ*. Analgesia, as required, with opioids and/or non-steroidal anti-inflammatory drugs if renal function is normal. Peritubal infiltration of 0.25% bupivacaine solution is efficient in alleviating postoperative pain.

Bibliography

Atallah MM, Shorrab AA, Abdel Magled YM, Demian AD. Low-dose bupivacaine spinal anaesthesia for percutaneous nephrolithotripsy: the suitability and impact of adding intrathecal fentanyl. *Acta Anaesthesiol Scand* 2006; **50**: 798–803.

Jonnavithula N, Pisopati MV, Druga P, *et al.* Efficacy of peritubal local anesthetic infiltration in alleviating postoperative pain in percutaneous nephrolithotomy. *J Endourol* 2009; **23**: 857–60.

Karacalar S, Bolen CY, Sarihasan B, Sarikaya S. Spinal epidural anesthesia versus general anesthesia in the management of percutaneous nephrolithotripsy. *J Endourol* 2009; **23**: 1591–7.

Mehrabi S, Karimzadeh Shirazi K. Results and complications of spinal anaesthesia in percutaneous nephrolithotomy. *Urol J* 2010; **7**: 22–5.

Munohar T, Jain P, Desai M. Supine percutaneous nephrolithotomy: effective approach to high-risk and morbidly obese patients. *J Endourol* 2007; **21**: 44–9.

Cross-references

Blood transfusion, 735
Complications of position, 743
Transurethral resection of the prostate syndrome, 805

Radical prostatectomy

Iurie Acalovschi

Radical retropubic prostatectomy is the normal surgical therapy for prostate cancer. The retropubic approach is mostly used nowadays. The procedure can be performed by open laparotomy and the prostate is removed together with pelvic lymph nodes, seminal vesicles, ejaculatory ducts and part of the bladder neck. The laparoscopic approach can also be used and robotic surgery has been introduced lately. The retropubic approach can also be used for resection of a benign hypertrophic prostate, too large for transurethral resection.

Patient characteristics

- Over 50 years of age.
- High incidence of chronic disease.
- ASA grades 2–4.

Preoperative assessment and investigations

- Identification and assessment of chronic disease.
- Deep vein thrombosis prophylaxis (elasticated stockings are recommended; patients are not routinely heparinized because it is felt that, on balance, the decreased haemostasis may do more harm than good).
- Blood transfusion availability, as radical prostatectomy is often associated with significant operative blood loss.
- Antibiotic prophylaxis.
- Assessment of the suitability for spinal or epidural analgesia. This is a particularly valuable technique to use in conjunction with general anaesthesia for radical prostatectomy because it provides excellent postoperative analgesia, reduces the perioperative blood loss and decreases the quantity of inhalational agent required.

Premedication

- An opioid premedicant is suitable. It has the advantage of pre-empting the nociceptive stimulus, although if an epidural technique is contemplated this is not necessary.
- A benzodiazepine is a suitable alternative and will provide anxiolysis and amnesia.

Perioperative management

The patient is usually placed supine in a hyperextended position which places the pubis above the head. A steep Trendelenburg position is required for the laparoscopic approach.

Theatre preparation

- Patient positioning requires care since surgery is often lengthy.
- Body temperature should be maintained with a warming mattress, warm air overblanket, warmed intravenous fluids and a ventilator circuit humidifier. Because of the potential for massive blood loss, a large-bore intravenous access and invasive monitoring are advisable.

Monitoring

In addition to routine monitoring, invasive BP via an arterial line (for a radical prostatectomy), core temperature, fluid balance, blood loss, CVP (for radical prostatectomy).

Anaesthetic technique

The combination of epidural and general anaesthesia with a muscle relaxant and volatile agent is a suitable technique. Retropubic prostatectomy can be performed under neuraxial analgesia alone if a T6 sensory level is achieved. In cases where a laparoscopic approach is used, general endotracheal anaesthesia is required because of the necessity for controlled mechanical ventilation imposed by the abdominal distension and the steep Trendelenburg position. The insufflated carbon dioxide spreads into the retroperitoneal space and increases the intra-abdominal and intrathoracic pressures.

The intraoperative blood loss varies with the length of surgery and grade and stage of malignancy. In some cases transfusion of up to 6 units could be necessary. It has been suggested that fibrinolysins, which exacerbate bleeding, are released by prostatic handling. When using the laparoscopic approach the amount of bleeding and need for transfusion are much reduced. Less blood loss and a lower frequency of pulmonary emboli are associated with regional anaesthesia. Transversus abdominus plane (TAP) block is now being used in some centres as an alternative to an epidural block.

Postoperative management

- When compared with the open surgical approach, laparoscopic radical prostatectomy is associated with shorter operating times, lower urinary leakage rates, lower stricture rates and lower blood loss.

- If an epidural infusion is already in situ, then a combination of local anaesthetic and an opioid will provide excellent analgesia.
- Postoperative blood loss and urine output should be monitored.
- Thrombophlebitis with pulmonary embolism is a major cause of postoperative mortality.
- With good case selection, the 5 year survival is 95%. Operative mortality is low.

Bibliography

Biki B, Mascha E, Moriarty DC, *et al.* Anesthetic technique for radical prostatectomy effects cancer recurrence: a retrospective analysis. *Anesthesiology* 2008; **109**: 180–7.

Dunet F, Pfister C, Deghmani M, *et al.* Clinical results of combined epidural and general anesthesia procedure in radical prostatectomy management. *Can J Urol* 2004; **11**: 2204

Lepage JY, Rivault O, Karam G, *et al.* Anaesthesia and prostate surgery. *Ann Fr Anesth Reanim* 2005; **24**: 397–411.

Remzi M, Klingler HC, Tinzl MV, *et al.* Morbidity of laparoscopic extraperitoneal versus transperitoneal radical prostatectomy versus open retropubic radical prostatectomy. *Eur Urol* 2005; **48**: 83–9.

Cross-references

Blood transfusion, 735
Epidural and spinal anaesthesia, 707
Preoperative assessment of pulmonary risk, 625
Regional anaesthesia techniques, 719
The elderly patient, 604
Thrombosis and embolism, 793

Transurethral resection of prostate

Iurie Acalovschi

Ninety-five per cent of prostatectomies are performed endoscopically. The patient is placed in the lithotomy position. Electrocautery resection is performed by passing an electrically powered cutting-coagulating loop through a special cystoscope (resectoscope). Continuous irrigation of the bladder with a solution of 1.5% glycine or a mixture of 0.54% mannitol and 2.7% sorbitol is used during the resection. The operation may be performed as a repeat procedure. Patients may present with haematuria or may have long-standing obstruction, increasing the risk of renal failure. Urinary tract infection can complicate large residual volumes of urine. These patients have a higher incidence of cardiopulmonary problems, hypertension, obesity and diabetes mellitus.

Patient characteristics

- Over 50 years of age, male.
- High incidence of chronic disease.
- ASA status 1–4.

Preoperative assessment and investigation

- Systematic review of intercurrent illness.
- In patients with cardiovascular comorbidities, anticoagulant therapy is common and the risk for bleeding is increased.
- Discuss anaesthetic technique and decide on suitability for regional anaesthesia.
- The anticoagulation medications may prevent regional anaesthesia.
- Prostatic bleeding can be difficult to control through the cystoscope. Cross-matched blood should be available for anaemic patients or patients with a large gland (>45 g).

Premedication

If a premedicant is required, then anxiolysis with a benzodiazepine is suitable for patients having a regional technique. For general anaesthesia, analgesic premedication may be preferred.

Perioperative management

- Warm irrigating fluid should be used in order to maintain core temperature.
- The patient should be given antibiotics according to the hospital policy. This is usually gentamicin or a cephalosporin.

Monitoring

- Mental status if awake.
- Routine minimal monitoring.
- $ETco_2$.
- Estimation of blood loss.
- Core temperature.

Anaesthetic technique

This operation can be conducted using a regional technique: either spinal or epidural anaesthesia with a T10 sensory level. Spinal anaesthesia is commonly used, although a number of patients prefer to be asleep during the operation. There are advantages to a regional technique:

- These patients often have intercurrent chest disease and may benefit postoperatively from not having a general anaesthetic.
- In the awake patient, the evaluation of mental status is the best monitor of the onset of the transurethral resection of the prostate syndrome and of bladder perforation.
- Low-dose diluted bupivacaine with fentanyl 25 μg or sufentanil 5 μg can provide adequate anaesthesia without haemodynamic instability in elderly patients. Spinal anaesthesia, however, reduces CVP, potentially resulting in greater absorption of irrigating fluid than with general anaesthesia.
- Degenerative changes in the spine of elderly patients may make neuraxial anaesthesia technically difficult. The possibility of vertebral metastasis in patients with carcinoma represents a contraindication to regional anaesthesia.
- If a general anaesthetic is to be used, paralysis and ventilation is not specifically required for this operation, which can be performed with the patient breathing spontaneously through a laryngeal mask. Some authors have reported carrying out TURP under local anaesthesia alone.

The TURP syndrome

This is caused by the absorption of the irrigating fluid during resection of the prostate. Symptoms include hypertension, headache, visual disturbances, dyspnoea, mental changes, seizures and circulatory collapse. The manifestations are those of circulatory fluid overload, hyponatraemia, reduced blood osmolality and toxicity from the solute in the irrigating fluid.

Postoperative management

The TURP syndrome can develop intraoperatively or at any stage in the postoperative period and the nursing staff should be aware of this. The initial postoperative period is not characterized as particularly painful, the most painful period being the time when the urinary catheter is removed.

Outcome

The reported hospital mortality is 0.2–6% and may be as low as 0.5–1% in specialist centres. There is evidence of increased intermediate and long-term mortality and morbidity with TURP compared with open prostatectomy, and with other minimally invasive surgery in this age group. Increased morbidity may be found after resections exceeding 90 minutes, gland size greater than 45 g and age older than 80 years.

Bibliography

Gehring H, Nahm W, Baerwald J, *et al.* Irrigation fluid absorption during transurethral resection of the prostate. Spinal vs general anaesthesia. *Acta Anaesthesiol Scand* 1999; **43**: 458–63.

Graverstein D. Transurethral resection of the prostate (TURP) syndrome: a review of pathophysiology and management. *Anesth Analg* 1997; **84**: 438–46.

Hawary A, Mukhtar K, Sinclair A, Pearce I. Transurethral resection of the prostate syndrome: almost gone but not forgotten. *J Endourol* 2009; **23**: 2013–20.

Kim SY, Cho JE, Hong JY, *et al.* Comparison of intrathecal fentanyl and sufentanil in low-dose dilute bupivacaine spinal anesthesia for transurethral prostatectomy. *Br J Anaesth* 2009; **103**: 750–4.

Cross-references

Blood transfusion, 735
Epidural and spinal anaesthesia, 707
Fluid and electrolyte balance, 754
The elderly patient, 604
Transurethral resection of the prostate syndrome, 805

20
Vascular surgery

Andrew J Mortimer and Rachel A Stoeter

- Overview — *Andrew J Mortimer and Rachel A Stoeter*
- Abdominal aortic reconstruction: elective open repair — *Rachel A Stoeter and Andrew J Mortimer*
- Abdominal aortic reconstruction: emergency repair — *Rachel A Stoeter and Andrew J Mortimer*
- Abdominal aortic reconstruction: endovascular aneurysm repair — *Rachel A Stoeter and Andrew J Mortimer*
- Carotid endarterectomy — *Rachel A Stoeter and Andrew J Mortimer*
- Leg revascularization and amputations — *Rachel A Stoeter and Andrew J Mortimer*

Overview

Andrew J Mortimer and Rachel A Stoeter

Vascular surgery comprises the major operations of aortic reconstruction, carotid endarterectomy and leg salvage procedures either by arterial grafting or by amputation of the distal limb when gangrene or infection is present. The commonest underlying pathological condition is atherosclerotic disease of the main conducting arteries, often with associated aneurysm formation.

Ruptured aneurysms usually present with abdominal or flank pain and cardiovascular collapse. Unruptured aneurysms are frequently asymptomatic, although they can cause vague symptoms of abdominal and back pain due to both stretching and direct pressure. Carotid artery disease may present with transient ischaemic attacks (TIAs) or stroke. Peripheral arterial occlusive disease causes ischaemic symptoms, when the oxygen delivery is insufficient to satisfy tissue oxygen consumption.

Abdominal aortic aneurysm (AAA) conventionally refers to an aorta diameter of ≥30 mm. They occur in 1.5% of all people over 50 years old and most commonly in males, in smokers and in those with hypertension, hyperlipidaemia and a family history. A national screening programme using ultrasonography is currently being introduced for all men from their 65th birthday. Once the aneurysm diameter reaches 55 mm, surgery is usually offered. The risk of rupture increases exponentially as the size of the aneurysm increases. Emergency surgery for rupture carries a mortality risk of around 40%, compared with a mortality of around 5% for elective open repair.

Carotid endarterectomy (CEA) aims to reduce the risk of cerebral ischaemic events and is usually offered to those who are symptomatic with carotid artery stenosis >70%, within 2 weeks of presentation.

The commonest symptom of peripheral vascular disease (PVD) is intermittent claudication, occurring when blood flow is reduced by ≥75% (this corresponds to a ≥50% reduction in arterial diameter as seen on an angiogram). The presence of persistent leg pain at rest indicates that blood flow is reduced by ≥90% (which corresponds to a ≥70% reduction in arterial diameter as seen on an angiogram). A patient in this condition requires urgent treatment, usually by amputation.

Assessing perioperative risk

Risk factors and predictors

The American College of Cardiology (ACC) and American Heart Association (AHA) have produced guidelines for evaluating cardiac risk in non-cardiac surgery. They use clinical factors in addition to functional capacity and surgical risk stratification to predict cardiac risk. High-risk surgery includes aortic and other major vascular surgery plus peripheral vascular surgery; intermediate risk surgery includes carotid endarterectomy and endovascular aneurysm repair. The majority of patients are elderly with a greater male preponderance (5:1). Younger patients often have a family history, are smokers or have a history of diabetes mellitus. Most vascular patients are American Society of Anesthesiologists (ASA) grade 3 or above and usually have one or more comorbidities.

A preoperative history of cardiac ischaemia is important, but greater emphasis is placed on cardiac failure as a predictor for postoperative morbidity and mortality. Several prediction tools have been developed to quantify risk, including those of Goldman, Detsky and Lee. The Lee Revised Cardiac Index uses six predictive factors to determine perioperative cardiac risk: high-risk surgery, ischaemic heart disease (IHD), congestive cardiac failure (CCF), renal insufficiency, insulin-dependent diabetes mellitus (IDDM) and cerebrovascular disease (CVD). Advanced age (>70 years) and hypertension are also recognized factors. Although chronic obstructive pulmonary disease (COPD) is not classed as a risk factor, it increases hospital stay and the need for postoperative ventilation.

Comorbidities

- IHD: manifests as angina or myocardial infarction (MI). Perioperative myocardial infarction occurs mostly in the first postoperative week, with the greatest risk on the third postoperative day.
- CCF: considered more important than IHD in predicting perioperative morbidity and mortality.
- KI (kidney injury): causes of renal impairment are multifactorial. Serum creatinine >176.8 μmol L^{-1} (2 mg dL^{-1}) indicates a high-risk patient.
- IDDM: patients with diabetes constitute a large number of those undergoing peripheral arterial reconstruction. Both macro- and microvascular complications result. Amputation of toes and limbs is commonly undertaken to control infection, which may be adversely affecting diabetic management. Good glycaemic control is essential in the perioperative period. Metformin may worsen lactic acidosis.

- CVD: cerebrovascular disease is a marker of the presence of atherosclerosis, which may be complicated by a perioperative stroke.
- HTN (hypertension): hypertensive disease results in left ventricular hypertrophy requiring higher filling pressures to achieve adequate cardiac output and can progress to heart failure. In the brain and kidneys, autoregulation of blood flow is shifted to the right. The widespread increase in arteriolar resistance means that patients manifest exaggerated intraoperative haemodynamic changes.
- COPD: preoperative lung function tests are rarely of help. Perioperative nebulizers and physiotherapy should be considered.

Functional capacity

The following can be used to assess functional capacity:

- Medical history, including metabolic equivalents (METs) and scoring systems (e.g. the Duke Activity Status Index), has been used to assess a patient's maximum physical activity. Exercise can be limited by claudication and mobility, although, if a patient can climb two flights of stairs, equivalent to >4 METs, they may not require further testing.
- Cardiopulmonary exercise testing (CPET): current opinion considers a patient to be high risk if his or her anaerobic threshold (AT) is <11 mL kg^{-1} min^{-1}.

Concurrent medication

Patients are usually taking medication from one or more of the following groups: antianginal, antihypertensive, antiarrhythmic, antiplatelet, anticoagulant and bronchodilator agents.

Most drugs should be continued perioperatively. However, there are some that require further consideration.

- Clopidogrel: should be stopped 5–7 days before planned surgery
- Warfarin: this needs to be stopped at least 3 days prior to planned surgery with an INR (international normalized ratio) check
- Heparin: patients may be on a heparin infusion or low-molecular-weight heparin (LMWH); consider timing of neuraxial blockade in relation to this
- Angiotensin-converting enzyme inhibitors: consider omitting on the day of surgery to minimize intraoperative hypotension
- Statins: must be continued as cardiac risk increases if stopped
- Beta-blockers should be continued.

Other considerations

- CPET: currently used as the gold standard for combined assessment of functional capacity of both cardiac and respiratory systems. CPET helps determine an individual's physiological reserve in order to predict his or her ability to cope with the stress of surgery and postoperative recovery. It also aids decision-making with regards to whether surgery should proceed and procedure choice.
- Coronary revascularization: percutaneous cardiac intervention (PCI) and coronary artery grafting should only be done prior to non-cardiac surgery if these interventions are deemed necessary irrespective of the proposed vascular operation.
- PCI (angioplasty, bare metal stents and drug-eluting stents): perioperative patient management should be a multidisciplinary decision because of the balance of risk between haemorrhage and thrombosis. Risks relate to the type of stent, their medical management and the timing of the percutaneous intervention to proposed surgery.
- Perioperative optimization: the best methods of reducing cardiac complications are still unknown. Possible interventions include:
  - smoking cessation, weight loss and improving exercise tolerance
  - optimal medical treatment of concurrent conditions
  - potential medical interventions
    - β-blockers: the role of perioperative β-blockade has been under scrutiny for over 20 years. β-blockers can improve cardiovascular stability but have the disadvantage of causing hypotension and bradycardia. It is suggested that, where indicated, β-blockers should be started at least a week before elective surgery and the dose titrated to achieve a resting heart rate between 60 and 80 beats per minute, while avoiding hypotension
    - statins: should be continued perioperatively as they increase plaque stability, reduce the inflammatory response and low-density lipoprotein cholesterol
    - perioperative preconditioning: there is current interest in the potential role of ischaemic preconditioning to reduce perioperative ischaemia of the myocardium and other organs, by increasing their tolerance to ischaemia. This may possibly be achieved by volatile agents and by intermittent arterial cross-clamping during aortic surgery.
- Hypothermia: inadvertent hypothermia, when the core temperature falls below 36.0°C, should be

avoided in order to reduce the complications of infection, delayed healing, bleeding, arrhythmias and protracted hospital stay. Preoperative warming of the patient should be considered. Intraoperatively, active patient warming should be carried out with the use of fluid warmers and forced air blankets.

- Central venous catheter (CVC): cannulation of an internal jugular vein should be performed for operations in which significant blood loss may occur, using a portable ultrasound device.
- Endovascular aneurysm repair (EVAR): choice of EVAR versus open AAA repair (see Abdominal aortic reconstruction: endovascular aneurysm repair, p. 511).
- CEA: choice of local anaesthesia (LA) versus general anaesthesia (GA) (see Carotid endarterectomy, p. 513).

Bibliography

American Heart Association. ACC/AHA Guidelines on Perioperative Cardiovascular Evaluation and Care for Noncardiac Surgery. Executive Summary: A Report of the American College of Cardiology/ American Heart Association Task Force on Practice Guidelines. *Circulation* 2007; **116**: 1971–96.

American Heart Association. ACCF/AHA Focused Update on Perioperative Beta Blockade: A Report of the American College of Cardiology Foundation/ American Heart Association Task Force on Practice Guidelines. *Circulation* 2009; **120**: 2123–51.

Atkinson D, Carter A. Pre-operative assessment for aortic surgery. *Curr Anaesth Crit Care* 2008; **19**: 115–27.

Crider BA, Mortimer AJ. Anesthesia for vascular surgery. In: Healy TEJ, Knight PR (eds) *A Practice of Anesthesia*, 7th edn. London: Arnold, 2003, pp. 765–87.

Garrioch MA, Pichel AC. Reducing the risk of vascular surgery. *Curr Anaesth Crit Care* 2008; **19**: 128–37.

Loveridge R, Schroeder F. Anaesthetic preconditioning. *Cont Educ Anaesth Crit Care Pain* 2010; **10**: 38–42.

National Institute for Health and Clinical Excellence. *Inadvertent Perioperative Hypothermia. The Management of Inadvertent Perioperative Hypothermia in Adults.* Clinical Guidance no. 65. London: NICE, 2008. See www.nice.org.uk/CG065

Pichel AC, Serracino-Inglott F. Anaesthetic consideration for endovascular abdominal aortic aneurysm repair (EVAR). *Curr Anaesth Crit Care* 2008; **19**: 150–62.

Sakalihasan N, Limet R, Defawe OD. Abdominal aortic aneurysm. *Lancet* 2005; **365**: 1577–89.

Scott, T. Perioperative myocardial protection. *Cont Educ Anaesth Crit Care Pain* 2009; **9**: 97–101.

Smith TB, Stonell C, Purkayastha S, Paraskevas P. Cardiopulmonary exercise testing as a risk assessment method in non cardio-pulmonary surgery: a systematic review. *Anaesthesia* 2009; **64**: 883–93.

Abdominal aortic reconstruction: elective open repair

Rachel A Stoeter and Andrew J Mortimer

This is a major surgical procedure aimed at reducing the mortality from rupture of an aneurysm, or the symptoms of claudication in occlusive disease. The operation is classed as high risk by the ACC and the AHA with a perioperative cardiac risk of >5%. Outcome depends on age and coexisting disease. Mortality is around 5%, with perioperative myocardial infarction being the principal cause.

Aneurysm formation is linked to an imbalance of protease inhibitors, leading to a reduction in elastin and collagen in the arterial wall.

Most patients are elderly with significant comorbidities, carrying the major risk of perioperative cardiopulmonary morbidity and mortality. The procedure involves aortic cross-clamping with resultant haemodynamic and ischaemic complications. In 90% of patients, a tube graft or a bifurcation graft is inserted below the origin of the renal arteries.

Preoperative assessment and investigations

Goals

- To identify and evaluate patient comorbidities.
- To optimize the patient's condition when possible.
- To help make informed decisions for best management.

A full and thorough anaesthetic history should be taken, examination performed and investigations completed. Risk factors/predictors, functional capacity assessment and scoring systems can be used to help determine perioperative risk (e.g. the Lee Revised Cardiac Index and guidelines by the AHA/ACC assessing cardiac risk in patients for non-cardiac surgery).

Risk factors and predictors

See Overview, p. 502.

Functional capacity

See Overview, p. 502.

Emphasis is placed on assessment of cardiorespiratory functional capacity since major abdominal surgery leads to a large inflammatory response, which may require up to a 50% increase in resting $\dot{V}O_2$ to survive.

Investigations

- General:
  - full blood count (FBC), urea and creatinine, electrolytes, glucose
  - group and save sample (if cell salvage is not available, up to 6 units of blood should be cross-matched).
- Cardiac:
  - resting cardiac evaluation (does not give functional status or indication of response to stress):
    - 12 lead ECG
    - echocardiography
  - stress cardiac evaluation:
    - exercise ECG (effort dependent and requires mobility)
    - dobutamine stress echocardiography.
- Respiratory:
  - chest X-ray
  - consider possible respiratory function tests, although not a test of reserve function (peak expiratory flow rate, forced expiratory volume in 1 second (FEV_1)/forced vital capacity (FVC) ratio).
- Combined assessment of functional cardio-respiratory reserve:
  - CPET: useful as it measures both the cardiac and respiratory elements of exercise.

Preoptimization

See Overview, p. 502.

Ideally, the patient should be seen 1 month preoperatively and risk factors assessed. Explanation to the patient about the procedure, anaesthetic management and postoperative care is important. Surgery should take precedence over time taken for lifestyle changes since delays could increase the risk of aortic rupture.

Perioperative management

The aim is to maintain the balance of myocardial and end-organ oxygen supply and demand by the avoidance of tachycardia, hypotension, hypoxia and hypothermia.

Abdominal aortic reconstruction: emergency repair

Rachel A Stoeter and Andrew J Mortimer

A ruptured or leaking aortic aneurysm is fatal if untreated and emergency repair is the patient's only chance of survival. Emergency surgery in a specialist unit is required because perioperative morbidity and mortality is very high. Overall mortality is over 60%. For those surviving to surgery, it is around 40%, compared with 5% for elective procedures. In certain patients, surgical intervention may be inappropriate. Scoring systems can be used to predict mortality but does not replace overall clinical judgement. Effective analgesia and nursing care should be provided if surgery is not appropriate to ensure death is peaceful and dignified. Poorer outcomes are more likely with advanced age (>76 years), raised creatinine (>190 μmol L^{-1}), haemoglobin <9 g dL^{-1}, loss of consciousness, and an ischaemic ECG (Hardman index).

The clinical presentation of a ruptured AAA ranges from severe abdominal/lumbar pain with a palpable pulsatile abdominal mass to complete cardiovascular collapse and sudden death. Ideally, patients are transferred to a specialist vascular unit. If cardiovascularly stable, a CT scan of the abdomen is performed, whereas the severely compromised patient is taken directly to theatre. Emergency EVAR is an alternative to open repair, but requires CT assessment. When the rupture is retroperitoneal, the haemorrhage may be slowed by a tamponade effect.

Preoperative assessment, investigations and preoptimization

Goals

- Rapid assessment and preoptimization with appropriate fluid resuscitation, alongside timely surgical intervention.

Assessment, investigation and preoptimization are likely to be carried out simultaneously to ensure timely transfer to theatre. Ultimately, the need is for control of blood loss by aortic cross-clamp application. A second experienced anaesthetist is required to assist, although the procedure may need to commence while awaiting their arrival.

Resuscitation requires large-bore peripheral access. Judicious fluid and blood product infusions are required – a normal blood pressure is not the target, rather a blood pressure to ensure adequate myocardial and cerebral perfusion. Excessive fluid resuscitation risks greater haemorrhage with clot dislodgement and dilutional coagulopathy. Consider arterial line insertion, although this should not delay commencement of surgery. Ensure adequate pain relief.

Formal detailed assessment and investigations are rarely possible, but attempts should be made to establish the severity of any coexisting disease. Recent hospital admissions and their documented findings in hospital records may prove useful.

Investigations

- General:
  - FBC, urea and creatinine, electrolytes, glucose
  - coagulation
  - request urgent cross-match of red cells, fresh-frozen plasma and platelets; if available, emergency cell salvage may be used to minimize allogeneic blood transfusion requirements.
- Cardiac:
  - a 12 lead ECG may be helpful when a differential diagnosis of aneurysm leak/rupture and massive myocardial infarction is being considered.

Perioperative management

The aim is to ensure anaesthesia while attempting cardiovascular stability and normothermia.

Preinduction

- Reassure the patient, maintain a calm environment.
- Transfer the patient into the operating theatre, with high-flow face-mask oxygen.
- Monitoring as per AAGBI guidelines.
- ECG: leads II and V5, ST analysis.
- No time should be wasted in attempting to set up invasive arterial monitoring or a central venous line at the beginning; it is important for the surgeon to cross-clamp the aorta as soon as possible.
- Colloid, blood products and rapid infusers with fluid warmers should be prepared; if cross-matched

blood is not yet available, group O negative blood should be.

- Draw up induction drugs and have available a vasopressor (metaraminol, norepinephrine) and an inotrope (epinephrine).
- The patient should be positioned on the operating table with both arms out for access.
- During skin preparation and draping, the patient is preoxygenated.

Induction and maintenance

During rapid sequence induction, care must be taken to minimize hypotension. As soon as the airway is secured with an endotracheal tube, instruct the surgeon to proceed. Cardiovascular collapse should be anticipated, as the abdominal tamponade effect is lost at laparotomy. A balanced anaesthetic technique with IPPV delivering volatile anaesthesia in 100% oxygen, with either sevoflurane or isoflurane, is appropriate. TIVA with propofol and remifentanil is an acceptable alternative. Nitrous oxide should be avoided because of its myocardial depressant effect and expansion of air emboli.

Once the aorta has been cross-clamped a degree of haemodynamic stability may occur, facilitating the insertion of invasive monitoring lines.

Intraoperative monitoring

- As per AAGBI guidelines with:
  - ECG: leads II and V5, ST analysis
  - invasive arterial blood pressure monitoring
  - central venous catheter insertion post induction
  - cardiac output monitor, depends on availability and preference.
- Serial arterial blood gases.
- Near patient coagulation testing, e.g. TEG.
- Core temperature monitoring.
- Urinary catheter.

Specific points

- Continued haemorrhage is common and large volumes of blood may need to be administered, resulting in a dilutional coagulopathy. Choice of blood products can be guided by point-of-care testing, such as TEG, and may require a haematologist's input.
- Aortic cross-clamp application leads to an increase in blood pressure proximal to the cross-clamp. Should hypertension occur, it may be reduced by an increase in the volatile agent or the use of a vasodilator (GTN).
- Aortic cross-clamp release may cause severe hypotension. This may be due to the reduction in afterload along with severe ischaemia-reperfusion injury and metabolic acidosis. Controlled cross-clamp release by the surgeon is the best option. Previous fluid loading will help reduce the impact. Further fluid use and vasopressor/inotropic support can be administered guided by trends in invasive pressure and/or oesophageal Doppler monitoring.
- Heat loss must be minimized by humidifying inspired gases, warming intravenous fluids, using a warming mattress and a forced air warming blanket.
- Give broad-spectrum antibiotic prophylaxis (e.g. cefuroxime or co-amoxiclav).
- Positioning: supine, ensure potential pressure areas are padded, a table break may be required to improve surgical access.
- A nasogastric tube is required because postoperative ileus is common.

Postoperative management

- HDU/ITU care is required to optimize the cardiovascular, renal and respiratory systems and ensure maintenance of normothermia and blood coagulation.
- Analgesia is usually intravenous morphine. (Regional anaesthesia may occasionally be considered after correction of coagulopathies.)
- Close monitoring of renal function is required as renal failure is common, often due to acute tubular necrosis.

Perioperative complications

Surgical

- Uncontrolled haemorrhage.
- Ischaemic limb because of embolization.
- Ischaemia of the gastrointestinal tract or spinal cord.
- Intra-abdominal hypertension (intra-abdominal pressure (IAP) ≥12 mmHg) and abdominal compartment syndrome (IAP ≥20 mmHg).

Medical

- Myocardial infarction.
- Kidney injury.
- Respiratory failure.
- Coagulopathy, DIC.

Bibliography

Crider BA, Mortimer AJ. Anesthesia for vascular surgery. In: Healy TEJ, Knight PR (eds) *A Practice of Anesthesia*, 7th edn. London: Arnold, 2003, pp. 765–87.

Preinduction

- Reassure the patient, maintain a calm environment.
- Peripheral intravenous access with large-bore cannulae.
- Monitoring as per AAGBI guidelines.
- ECG: leads II and V5, ST analysis.
- Insertion of an intra-arterial line under local anaesthetic: use right radial artery as may need left axillary artery.
- RA is carried out where applicable.

Induction and maintenance/regional with/without sedation

Care must be taken to avoid haemodynamic instability, especially at induction, laryngoscopy, tracheal intubation and with the potential effects of RA. The goal is to ensure that normoxia, normocapnia, normotension, normothermia and normoglycaemia are maintained throughout the operation.

Maintenance may be achieved with inhalational anaesthesia (sevoflurane/isoflurane) or TIVA with propofol and remifentanil with IPPV. Sedation may be carried out with propofol, remifentanil or midazolam.

Intraoperative monitoring

- As per AAGBI guidelines with:
  - ECG: leads II and V5, ST analysis
  - invasive arterial blood pressure monitoring.
- Core temperature monitoring.
- Urinary catheter.

Specific points

- Heat loss must be minimized by humidifying inspired gases, warming intravenous fluids, using a warming mattress and a forced air warming blanket.
- Give broad-spectrum antibiotic prophylaxis (e.g. cefuroxime or co-amoxiclav).
- Intravenous heparin, 5000 IU, is administered after the femoral artery is exposed.
- Positioning: supine, ensure potential pressure areas are protected/padded.
- Potential remote site surgery concerns.
- Be prepared for possible conversion to open repair.

Postoperative management

- Nurse on HDU for first 24 hours or equivalent care on a specialist vascular ward.
- Analgesia: paracetamol with/without morphine. Requirements may be minimal owing to intraoperative local anaesthetic infiltration made by the surgeon/regional technique where applicable.
- Avoid NSAIDs (renal impairment).
- Early mobilization is encouraged.

Perioperative complications

Surgical

- Endoluminal leaks from either the proximal or distal anastomosis.
- Maldeployment of stent.
- Graft thrombosis.
- Graft migration.
- Arterial rupture.
- Aortic injury from instruments, occlusion or embolization.
- Distal organ embolization and ischaemia: lower limb and renal.
- Conversion to open repair.
- Graft infection.

Medical

- Kidney injury: particular risk from radiographic contrast or ischaemia.
- Myocardial ischaemia.
- Respiratory failure.
- Postimplantation syndrome (often self-limiting): fever, leukocytosis, raised C reactive protein, rarely disseminated intravascular coagulopathy (DIC) and shock.
- Sepsis.

Bibliography

Nataraj V, Mortimer AJ. Endovascular abdominal aortic aneurysm repair. *Cont Educ Anaesth Crit Care Pain* 2004. **4**: 91–4.

Pichel AC, Serracino-Inglott F. Focus on: Vascular anaesthesia. Anaesthetic considerations for endovascular abdominal aortic aneurysm repair (EVAR). *Curr Anaesth Crit Care* 2008; **19**: 150–62.

Sakalihasan N, Limet R, Defawe OD. Abdominal aortic aneurysm. *Lancet* 2005; **365**: 1577–89.

Cross-references

Abdominal aortic reconstruction: elective open repair, 505

Monitoring, 690

Preoperative assessment of cardiovascular risk in non-cardiac surgery, 621

Vascular surgery: overview, 502

Carotid endarterectomy

Rachel A Stoeter and Andrew J Mortimer

Carotid artery disease causes symptoms of cerebral ischaemia, which may reverse within 24 hours (TIAs) or last >24 hours (cerebrovascular accident (CVA) or stroke). It is caused by atheromatous plaques, leading to narrowing at the carotid bifurcation, reducing cerebral blood flow and initiating platelet or clot embolism into the distant cerebral vessels.

The aim of CEA is to reduce the risk of cerebral ischaemic events, with greater benefit seen in patients with symptomatic disease. It is a prophylactic operation but carries a high morbidity (6%) and mortality (3%) owing to the patient population and perioperative complications. The majority of deaths are due to stroke or MI. Significant haemodynamic changes may occur, compromising cerebral and myocardial perfusion.

The incision is made along the anterior border of the sternocleidomastoid muscle, the carotid and internal jugular vessels are dissected and cross-clamps applied sequentially to the internal, common and external carotid arteries. Following the endarterectomy, the artery may be closed directly or, more commonly, increased in diameter by a patch angioplasty.

Controversy exists in the fields of patient selection, anaesthetic technique and cerebral monitoring during the operation.

In symptomatic patients, the general consensus is that surgery should be performed in those with carotid stenosis >70%. In asymptomatic patients, the operation may not be as beneficial.

The surgery may be carried out under LA or GA. Each technique has advantages and disadvantages. A decade ago, it had been presumed that LA would lead to better outcomes; however, the General Anaesthesia versus Local Anaesthesia for Carotid Surgery (GALA) trial failed to demonstrate this.

At the time of cross-clamping there is a risk of cerebral hypoperfusion and ischaemia, with blood flow to the ipsilateral hemisphere being dependent on the collateral supply from the circle of Willis. In order to try to prevent this ischaemia, a shunt may be inserted between the common carotid artery and the internal carotid artery. However, the shunt may become kinked and can cause embolic complications or damage to the arterial wall. The need for shunt insertion is determined either by surgical preference or from the estimated cerebral perfusion, guided by cerebral monitoring. There is no ideal cerebral monitor. Some surgeons shunt routinely whereas others never use shunts.

Preoperative assessment and investigations

Goals

- To identify and evaluate patient comorbidities.
- To optimize the patient's condition when possible.

A thorough anaesthetic history should be taken, examination performed and investigations carried out. It is important to document preoperative neurological status.

Risk factors, predictors and scoring systems can be used to help determine perioperative risk. Functional capacity should be considered.

Risk factors and predictors

See Overview, p. 502.

Hypertension is commonplace and carries the risk of perioperative haemodynamic instability with reduced cerebral perfusion and potential haemorrhage.

Functional capacity

See Overview, p. 502.

Investigations

- General:
  - FBC, urea and creatinine, electrolytes, glucose
  - group and save sample.
- Cardiac:
  - ECG; other cardiac investigations as indicated.
- Respiratory:
  - chest X-ray.

Preoptimization

See Overview, p. 502.

Although preoptimization may be possible in some patients, others must undergo surgery without such delay. If patients present with uncontrolled hypertension, (systolic blood pressure >180 mmHg and/or diastolic pressure >110 mmHg) delaying surgery may be considered until adequately treated. In symptomatic patients, the general consensus is that urgent surgery should be performed within 2 weeks of onset of presentation of symptoms.

Perioperative management

The aim is to ensure adequate cerebral and myocardial perfusion via maintenance of blood pressure, P_aO_2, P_aCO_2

and normothermia throughout the procedure. Some authorities advocate keeping mean arterial pressure 20% above baseline at the time of cross-clamping for optimal cerebral blood flow. Adequate venous drainage should be ensured.

The procedure may be carried out under GA or LA, or a combination.

Preinduction

- Reassure patient, maintain a calm environment.
- Peripheral intravenous access.
- Monitoring as per AAGBI guidelines.
- ECG: leads II and V5, ST analysis.
- Insertion of an intra-arterial line under local anaesthetic.

Anaesthetic technique

- GA.
- GA with LA.
- LA:
  - deep plus superficial cervical plexus block
  - superficial cervical plexus block alone.
- LA with sedation.

Carotid endarterectomy under general anaesthesia with/without local anaesthesia

Induction and maintenance

Care is needed to prevent or minimize haemodynamic instability, in particular at high-risk times such as induction, laryngoscopy, intubation, cross-clamp application, surgical stimulation of carotid sinus and extubation. Haemodynamic stability may be achieved using a volatile agent (sevoflurane/isoflurane) or TIVA. Attenuation of pressure responses may be achieved with opiate boluses or a remifentanil infusion. The aim is to reduce cerebral metabolic rate for oxygen ($CMRo_2$) and therefore O_2 demand. Nitrous oxide should be avoided because of its propensity to increase cerebral metabolic rate, cerebral blood flow (CBF) and impairment of CO_2 response of the cerebral vasculature. It also worsens air emboli. An endotracheal tube is used, either regular or reinforced. Lack of access to the airway intraoperatively must be remembered. Supplementation with LA may be used. Hypotension must be avoided as it risks cerebral hypoperfusion – vasopressors may be required. Analgesia with LA and paracetamol is usually adequate.

GA advantages

- Provides more controlled operating conditions.
- Avoids need for patient compliance.
- Reduces $CMRo_2$.
- Volatiles or propofol may potentially confer neurological and cardiac ischaemic protection.
- Reduces catecholamine release and stress response of surgery.
- Allows greater cardiovascular control/pharmacological manipulation.

GA disadvantages

- Reduces CBF.
- May lead to more frequent, unnecessary shunt use with associated complications.
- Risks failure to detect cerebral ischaemia after cross-clamp application.
- Haemodynamic fluctuations associated with induction/laryngoscopy/extubation.

An alternative technique is to use superficial cervical plexus block in combination with GA.

Carotid endarterectomy under local anaesthesia

LA requires blockade of the C2–4 dermatomes. Some cover of cranial nerve V (mandibular branch) may be needed for surgical retraction. Supplemental local infiltration into the carotid sheath may be required.

C2–4 cover can be achieved by:

- superficial cervical plexus block alone (provides adequate analgesia in most patients)
- deep cervical plexus block (increases risk of complications; see below)
- combination of the above.

Intraoperative supplementation by the surgeon with LA may be required, as may sedation. If sedation is needed, it can be difficult to determine between oversedation and ischaemia, and the benefit of awake direct cerebral monitoring is lost. Otherwise, titratable sedation is required, which is ideally rapidly reversible so that sedation can be stopped at the time of cross-clamping.

LA advantages

- Allows direct cerebral function monitoring: considered the gold standard.
- Reduces unnecessary shunt insertion.
- Avoids the haemodynamic instability associated with induction, laryngoscopy, intubation and extubation.
- Preserves cardiovascular and cerebrovascular autoregulation.

LA disadvantages

- Lack of direct haemodynamic control.
- Poor access to airway.
- No cerebral or cardiac ischaemic protection.
- Requires patient compliance.
- May be claustrophobic, uncomfortable and stressful for the patient.
- May provide inadequate analgesia requiring supplementation, sedation or GA.

- Conversion to GA is likely to be hurried and uncontrolled.
- Possible inadvertent injection into the vertebral artery or subarachnoid space, phrenic nerve block with respiratory compromise and haematoma formation (greater risk with deep cervical block).
- Potential greater stress response, increasing cardiac and $CMRo_2$ consumption with possible ischaemia.

Intraoperative monitoring

- As per AAGBI guidelines with:
  - ECG: leads II and V5, ST analysis
  - invasive arterial blood pressure monitoring
  - with/without cerebral function monitoring.
- Core temperature monitoring.
- Cardiac output monitoring if clinically indicated.

Cerebral function monitors

An awake patient is the gold standard for monitoring cerebral function intraoperatively, via assessment of motor, verbal and cognitive function. However, use of sedation will impede this. There is no ideal assessment of adequacy of cerebral perfusion during cross-clamping but options may include the following:

- transcranial Doppler of the middle cerebral artery
- near infrared spectroscopy measuring oxygen saturation of the cerebral hemisphere at risk
- processed EEG: includes bispectral index (frontal lobe monitor) and compressed spectral array.

Specific points

- Heat loss must be minimized by humidifying inspired gases, warming intravenous fluids, using a warming mattress and a forced air warming blanket
- Give broad-spectrum antibiotic prophylaxis (e.g. cefuroxime or co-amoxiclav).
- Intravenous heparin, 5000 IU, is administered prior to cross-clamping.
- Position: reverse Trendelenburg; head turned away from operating side; shoulders raised with support between shoulder blades; head ring. Ensure potential pressure areas are protected/padded.
- Surgical stimulation of the carotid sinus may cause bradycardia plus hypotension and rarely asystole. Treatment includes removal of the surgical stimulus, administration of vagolytic drugs and injection of lidocaine around the carotid sinus nerve.

Postoperative management

- Patients are at risk of cerebral and cardiovascular instability postoperatively. They therefore require initial close observation via a HDU bed, or a similarly closely monitored bed on a specialist vascular ward, for 24 hours. Most complications tend to occur in the first 12 hours postoperatively, with embolism being the most common cause. If neurological deterioration occurs, this needs immediate investigation and possible re-exploration.
- Analgesia with LA and paracetamol will usually suffice.

Perioperative complications

Surgical

- Haematoma and oedema: potential airway compromise.
- CVA.
- Nerve damage: hypoglossal nerve > recurrent laryngeal nerve > superior laryngeal nerve, marginal mandibular nerve and great auricular nerve injuries (most likely because of traction; usually transient).

Medical

- Myocardial ischaemia.
- Labile BP: postoperative hypertension may occur, possibly because of baroreceptor dysfunction. Marked hypertension may injure the myocardium and lead to hyperperfusion syndrome. Hypotension is also a risk.
- Hyperperfusion syndrome: leads to a significant increase in blood flow and the following may result: headache, hypertension, seizures, neurological deficit, cerebral oedema, subarachnoid haemorrhage, intracranial haemorrhage and death.

Bibliography

Benington S, Pichel AC. Focus on: Vascular anaesthesia. Anaesthesia for carotid endarterectomy. *Curr Anaesth Crit Care* 2008; **19**: 138–49.

GALA Trial Collaborative Group. General anaesthesia versus local anaesthesia for carotid surgery (GALA): a multicentre, randomised controlled trial. *Lancet* 2008; **372**: 2132–42.

Howell SJ. Carotid endarterectomy. *Br J Anaesth* 2007; **99**: 119–31.

Spargo JR, Thomas D. Local anaesthesia for carotid endarterectomy. *Cont Educ Anaesth Crit Care Pain* 2004; **4**: 62–5.

Cross-references

Monitoring, 690
Regional anaesthetic techniques, 719
Vascular surgery: overview, 502

Leg revascularization and amputations

Rachel A Stoeter and Andrew J Mortimer

Peripheral revascularization is classed as high-risk surgery (ACC/AHA) with perioperative cardiac complications being the most frequent. The greatest risk is in patients requiring emergency surgery for proximal arterial occlusion with limb-threatening ischaemia, where time is limited for preoperative management. Even when the limb ischaemia is chronic, the 12 month mortality is around 35%. Surgery, although relatively non-invasive, is usually prolonged and is carried out on patients with significant comorbidities. Almost all patients with significant peripheral vascular disease are current or previous cigarette smokers. In severe cases, acute limb ischaemia is a preterminal event and surgery may be inappropriate.

Acute limb ischaemia, presenting with a pale, pulseless, paraesthetic leg, is usually caused by an embolism and is often managed with surgical embolectomy under local anaesthetic. Further surgery to improve the arterial blood supply may include angioplasty, thrombolysis, stenting and bypass grafting – this is usually carried out under general anaesthesia. Ideally, revascularization should be performed within 6 hours of the onset of critical ischaemia.

Chronic limb ischaemia, presenting with symptoms of claudication, is due to atheromatous disease. These patients are more likely to have an established collateral circulation. The surgical procedures commonly encountered are femoropopliteal or femorofemoral bypass grafting.

Patients may present for repeated procedures in an attempt to salvage ischaemic limbs, sometimes culminating in progressive proximal amputation in the following sequence: (1) toes; (2) forefoot; (3) below knee; and (4) above knee. Risk increases with the number of procedures carried out. Many patients are diabetic, with infected and necrotic tissue disturbing blood sugar control.

Preoperative assessment, investigation and preoptimization

Goals

- Preoperative goals and preoptimization will depend on the urgency of surgery. For emergency procedures, investigations are likely to be limited to blood tests and an ECG.

A full history should be taken and appropriate examination performed. When time is available, and if appropriate, risk factors and predictors can be more formally assessed, as can functional capacity.

Risk factors and predictors

See Overview, p. 502.

Functional capacity

See Overview, p. 502.

Investigations

- General:
  - FBC, urea and creatinine, electrolytes, glucose
  - group and save sample
  - coagulation studies as needed.
- Cardiac:
  - 12 lead resting ECG; consider other tests as appropriate.
- Respiratory:
  - chest X-ray.

Perioperative management

The aim is to ensure anaesthesia with cardiovascular stability, avoiding hypoxia, hypercarbia, hypothermia and hyper/hypoglycaemia.

The choice of anaesthetic technique includes:

- GA: volatile agent or TIVA
- RA: single-shot spinal epidural, CSE or femoral and sciatic nerve blocks
- combined GA and RA.

GA is often preferred because of uncertainty over the duration of surgery. Central and peripheral RA have the advantage of reducing opiate requirements postoperatively.

Preinduction

- Reassure patient, maintain a calm environment.
- Intravenous access.
- Monitoring as per AAGBI guidelines.
- ECG: leads II and V5, ST analysis.

- Consider insertion of an intra-arterial line under local anaesthetic.
- RA is carried out where appropriate.

Induction and maintenance

Aim to maintain cardiovascular stability, especially at induction, laryngoscopy, intubation and extubation. The airway may be maintained with an endotracheal tube or a laryngeal mask airway.

Maintenance is with either volatile anaesthetic (sevoflurane/isoflurane) or TIVA with propofol and remifentanil.

Intraoperative monitoring

- As per AAGBI guidelines with:
  - ECG: leads II and V5, ST analysis
  - possible invasive arterial blood pressure monitoring.
- Core temperature monitoring.
- Urinary catheter.
- Cardiac output monitoring and CVC if clinically indicated.

Specific points

- Blood loss is usually minimal, apart from in patients on clopidogrel.
- Heat loss must be minimized during a prolonged procedure by humidifying inspiratory gases, warming intravenous fluids, using a warming mattress and forced air warming blanket.
- Give broad-spectrum antibiotic prophylaxis (e.g. cefuroxime or co-amoxiclav).
- Intravenous heparin, 5000 IU, is administered for reconstructive procedures.
- Positioning: supine, ensure potential pressure areas are padded/protected.

Postoperative management

- Although high-risk patients, the majority will return to the vascular ward. Some will require HDU care.
- Analgesia includes regular paracetamol and opiates or RA where applicable.
- Avoid NSAIDs (renal impairment).

Perioperative complications

Surgical

- Persistent ischaemia.
- Progression to gangrene with localized or systemic infection.
- Repeat surgery.
- Poor wound healing.
- Reperfusion injury following revascularization of a critically ischaemic limb may cause hyperkalaemia, cardiac arrhythmias or arrest, myoglobinuria and acute kidney injury.
- Compartment syndrome.

Medical

- Myocardial ischaemia.
- Rhabdomyolysis.
- Kidney injury.
- Respiratory failure.
- Unstable diabetic control.

Bibliography

Barbosa FT, Cavalcante JC, Jucá MJ, Castro AA. Neuraxial anaesthesia for lower-limb revascularization. *Cochrane Database Syst Rev* 2010; (1): CD007083.

Tovey G, Thompson JP. Anaesthesia for lower limb revascularisation. *Cont Educ Anaesth Crit Care Pain* 2005; **5**: 89–92.

Cross-references

Emergency surgery, 613
Monitoring, 690
Vascular surgery: Overview, 502

21 Transplantation

Richard Wadsworth

Heart transplantation

Andrew Roscoe

Procedure

- Median sternotomy with cardiopulmonary bypass (CPB), using bicaval venous cannulation.
- Orthotopic transplant: anastomoses of left atrium with native pulmonary veins, right atrium with inferior vena cava (IVC) and superior vena cava (SVC), main pulmonary artery and ascending aorta.

Patient characteristics

- End-stage heart failure (New York Heart Association grade 4) with life expectancy less than 1 year.
- Peak $\dot{V}o_2$ <14 mL kg^{-1} min^{-1}.
- Majority have ischaemic or dilated cardiomyopathy.
- Often have biventricular pacemaker/implantable cardioverter defibrillator (ICD).
- Decompensated, urgent inpatients usually receiving intravenous inotropes, with intra-aortic balloon pump (IABP) support. Increasing use of preoperative ventricular assist device (VAD) insertion as 'bridge to transplant'.
- May have undergone sternotomy for prior cardiac surgery.
- Absolute contraindications:
  - malignancy
  - active infection (suspended from transplant list until treated)
  - severe comorbidity (not amenable to multiorgan transplant procedure)
  - fixed elevated pulmonary vascular resistance (PVR)
  - substance abuse (including tobacco) within previous 6 months
  - mental illness/inability to comply with postoperative medication.
- Relative contraindications:
  - age >70 years old
  - BMI >30 kg m^{-2}
  - renal dysfunction with estimated glomerular filtration rate (GFR) of <40 mL min^{-1}
  - significant cerebral or peripheral vascular disease.

Preoperative assessment and investigations

Patients are often receiving high doses of anti-heart failure medications: angiotensin-converting enzyme inhibitors, angiotensin receptor antagonists, β-blockers, diuretics and warfarin anticoagulation.

- Check electrolytes and international normalized ratio (INR).
- Calculate transpulmonary gradient (TPG):

  TPG = mean pulmonary artery pressure − pulmonary capillary wedge pressure

- TPG >10: benefit from inhaled nitric oxide (iNO) therapy after CPB.
- Renal dysfunction common secondary to low cardiac output (CO).
- Preoperative creatinine >220 μmol L^{-1} associated with doubled postoperative mortality.
- Preoperative haemofiltration may be used to optimize renal function and fluid balance.
- Patients with intrinsic renal failure may be suitable for heart–kidney transplant.
- Hepatic congestion and dysfunction possible due to right ventricular (RV) failure.

Premedication

- Oxygen by facemask.
- Sedative medication usually unnecessary. Sedation may cause hypoventilation, hypercapnia and pulmonary hypertension, precipitating RV failure.

Perioperative management

Theatre preparation

- Intravenous fluid warmer. Forced air-warming device.
- Heparin drawn up in advance in case of cardiovascular collapse and emergency institution of CPB.
- Cross-matched blood readily available if re-sternotomy.
- Pacemaker technician to deactivate ICD: external defibrillator pads essential.

Monitoring

- Wide-bore venous access and invasive arterial monitoring prior to induction.
- Five-lead ECG, S_po_2, end-tidal CO_2 (ETco$_2$), nasopharyngeal temperature, urinary catheter.
- Central venous pressure (CVP) and pulmonary artery (PA) catheter sheath: PA catheter may be floated after CPB.

- Transoesophageal echocardiography (TOE): category IIa indication.
- Consider depth of anaesthesia monitor (e.g. bispectral index): high risk of awareness.

Physiological goals

- Avoid bradycardia: CO becomes rate dependent in end-stage cardiac failure.
- Avoid increasing systemic vascular resistance (SVR): small increases in SVR cause large reductions in stroke volume.
- Avoid excess fluid administration: heart towards end of Starling curve.
- Avoid negative inotropy: high-dose fentanyl cardiovascularly stable.
- Avoid hypoxaemia/hypercapnia: precipitate RV failure owing to increased PVR.

Induction

- Preoxygenation.
- Midazolam, etomidate or propofol.
- High-dose fentanyl. Use of remifentanil has been described.
- Pancuronium, rocuronium or vecuronium. Atracurium if significant hepatic or renal dysfunction.
- Other medications:
  - prophylactic antibiotics
  - methylprednisolone
  - antifibrinolytic (aprotinin or tranexamic acid)
  - vitamin K (patients on warfarin).

Maintenance

- Intermittent positive pressure ventilation (IPPV) with O_2/air mixture.
- Inhalational agents have more consistent pharmacokinetics than intravenous drugs in patients with end-stage heart failure.

Weaning from cardiopulmonary bypass

- Target heart rate 90–100 beats per minute: achieved with isoprenaline, dopamine or pacing.
- Epicardial pacing wires routinely inserted: risk of atrioventricular block.
- TOE required to assess ventricular function and filling.
- Risk of RV failure increases as ischaemic time extends beyond 4 hours.
- Avoid excess fluid administration: stiff ventricles easily fluid overloaded.
- Left ventricular (LV) dysfunction: dopamine, dobutamine or epinephrine.
- RV dysfunction: milrinone, enoximone and/or levosimendan (with norepinephrine).
- Low threshold for IABP insertion.
- Consider iNO/nebulized prostacyclin to reduce RV afterload.
- Severe graft dysfunction may necessitate VAD insertion.

Postoperative management

- Bleeding is a common complication: low threshold for use of blood products.
- Insert nasogastric tube for early administration of enteral immunosuppression.
- Cardiac function/haemodynamics monitored by PA catheter or TOE.
- Majority of cases extubated within 24 hours and managed similar to routine cardiac surgery patients.

Outcomes

Actuarial survival figures are:

- 85% at 1 year
- 70% at 5 years
- 50% at 10 years.

Long-term mortality caused by infection, organ rejection, cardiac allograft vasculopathy (accelerated coronary artery disease), renal failure and malignancy (secondary to immunosuppression).

Bibliography

Cheitlin MD, Armstrong WF, Aurigemma GP, *et al.* ACC/AHA/ASE 2003 guideline update for the clinical application of echocardiography: summary article. *J Am Soc Echocardiogr* 2003; **16**: 1091–110.

Mehra MR, Kobashigawa J, Starling R, *et al.* Listing criteria for heart transplantation: International Society for Heart and Lung Transplantation guidelines for the care of cardiac transplant candidates 2006. *J Heart Lung Transplant* 2006; **25**: 1024–42.

Mets B. Anesthesia for left ventricular assist device placement. *J Cardiothorac Vasc Anesth* 2000; **14**: 316–26.

Quinlan JJ, Firestone S, Firestone LL. Anesthesia for heart, lung and heart-lung transplantation. In: Kaplan JA (ed.) *Cardiac Anesthesia*, 4th edn. Philadelphia: WB Saunders, 1999, pp. 991–1013.

Taylor DO, Stehlik J, Edwards LB, *et al.* Registry of the International Society of Heart and Lung Transplantation: twenty-sixth official adult heart transplant report – 2009. *J Heart Lung Transplant* 2009; **28**: 1007–22.

Cross-references

Kidney transplantation, 522
Lung and heart–lung transplantation, 530

Kidney transplantation

Swati Karmarkar

Kidney transplantation is at present the renal replacement therapy of choice for patients with established renal failure (ERF) who are considered fit for major surgery. ERF is defined as chronic kidney disease with a GFR <15 mL min^{-1} 1.73 m^{-2} or which has progressed so far that renal replacement therapy is needed to maintain life. Transplanted kidneys come from deceased heart-beating donors, non-heart-beating donors or living donors.

The commonest cause of ERF is diabetes mellitus, which accounts for approximately one-fifth of cases. Other causes include glomerulonephritis, pyelonephritis, renovascular disease, polycystic kidney disease and hypertension. The pathophysiological consequences of ERF affect many systems throughout the body. Cardiovascular disease is up to 20 times more common in these patients. Long-term dialysis is itself associated with increased morbidity and mortality.

Patient selection and evaluation

Most patients with ERF are considered for transplantation unless they have significant contraindications. Patients with a suggestive family history or those over 50 are screened for the presence of pre-existing cancer. All patients are tested for the presence of viral diseases such as hepatitis B and C and HIV. Emphasis is placed on evaluation and optimization of the cardiovascular system as cardiovascular disease is the main cause of mortality following transplantation. Echocardiography is undertaken routinely; dobutamine stress echocardiography or thallium dipyridamole stress tests are considered especially in patients with diabetes. If reversible ischaemia is demonstrated, then coronary angioplasty, stenting and revascularization are considered before activation on the transplant list. In patients with significant cardiovascular comorbidity, a physiological stress test such as cardiopulmonary exercise testing (CPET) is performed. An anaerobic threshold <11 mL min^{-1} kg^{-1} combined with inducible ischaemia would place the patient at highest risk for postoperative adverse cardiovascular events. A few studies have shown that optimizing nutrition, especially serum phosphorus, may improve CPET results for patients with ERF.

The matching process

Donor and recipient matching, whether living or cadaveric kidney donation, is divided into three distinct areas: blood group and type matching, tissue type matching and the final cross-match. Six antigens (major histocompatibility complexes), at three loci (A, B and DR), are considered during tissue matching. Although the best outcomes may still be achieved with a six-antigen match, major developments in immunosuppression have ensured that even fully mismatched organs could have a favourable outcome, especially in living donor transplantation. A lymphocytotoxicity cross-match between donor lymphocytes and recipient serum is the final test performed. If the cross-match is positive then the risk of hyperacute rejection necessitates consideration of the next potential recipient.

Preoperative assessment

To keep cold ischaemia time to the minimum (less than 24 hours), there is often limited time available for preoperative assessment on the day of surgery. The anaesthetic assessment should concentrate on:

- reassessing comorbidities
- fluid and electrolyte imbalance, including signs of systemic volume overload, hyperkalaemia (>5.5 mmol L^{-1}) and acidosis
- haematological status.

Any abnormalities in these could necessitate dialysis, pharmacological correction or blood transfusion before the procedure.

Surgical procedure

The anastomoses are an extraperitoneal procedure. A curvilinear incision is made from above the symphysis pubis to the anterior superior iliac spine. The donor kidney is placed in the iliac fossa, below the native kidney, which is typically left *in situ*. The iliac vessels are exposed extraperitoneally and anastomoses are made between the renal vein and the external iliac vein and between the renal artery and the common, external or internal iliac artery. This will mean a period of vascular cross-clamping of the iliac artery and vein on the side of the implant. The ureter of the transplanted kidney is anastomosed to the bladder. A critical point in the operation is when the vascular clamps are removed and the transplanted kidney is reperfused.

Anaesthesia and perioperative management

Technique

- General anaesthesia is considered the technique of choice.
- A combined spinal–epidural technique without sedation has been used successfully in patients considered to be at high risk for general anaesthesia, usually because of poor respiratory function. Concerns with the routine use of regional anaesthesia are an increased risk of epidural haematoma (uraemic thrombasthenia and thrombocytopathy, residual dialysis anticoagulation) and infection (long-term immunosuppression).

Monitoring

- A five-lead ECG.
- Non-invasive blood pressure (NIBP) monitoring is adequate in most cases. Care is taken not to place the NIBP cuff on the same side as an arteriovenous (AV) fistula.
- A central venous catheter is inserted for intraoperative CVP monitoring and postoperative venous access. This is usually kept in place for 3 days for postoperative fluid management. Routine use of ultrasound guidance is advocated owing to distorted anatomy from previous central lines and hypovolaemia following dialysis The right internal jugular vein is preferred as the risk of stenosis is least at this insertion site. The femoral veins are avoided as the transplanted kidney is anastomosed to the external iliac veins.
- Cardiac output monitoring, such as oesophageal Doppler monitoring, is used to optimize fluid management and graft perfusion.
- Temperature monitoring is mandatory in order to maintain normothermia to optimize graft function.
- Neuromuscular junction monitoring is essential owing to decreased clearance and potential for drug accumulation and residual neuromuscular blockade.

Positioning

- Supine.
- Warming mattress, fluid warmer and forced air-warming blanket.
- AV fistula sites are protected.
- Graduated compression stockings and pneumatic compression devices for thromboembolism prophylaxis.

Induction and maintenance of anaesthesia

- Peripheral intravenous access can be difficult. Intravenous cannulae are not inserted in the same arm as a working AV fistula. Use of existing dialysis lines is avoided.
- Both intravenous induction with volatile-based maintenance and total intravenous anaesthetic (TIVA) techniques have been used.
- Isoflurane and desflurane are not nephrotoxic and are considered the volatile agents of choice. Exposure to <4 minimum alveolar concentration (MAC) hours of sevoflurane is not associated with renal toxicity. Studies of fluoride pharmacokinetics in patients with chronic kidney disease have proved sevoflurane to be a safe alternative.
- TIVA is a suitable option as the pharmacokinetics of propofol and remifentanil are not significantly altered in chronic kidney disease.

Muscle relaxants

- Use of cisatracurium or atracurium is advocated as they have an organ-independent elimination pathway.
- Vecuronium and rocuronium can cause prolonged neuromuscular blockade, especially with repeated doses, and should be used cautiously. Interpatient variability is increased in patients with ERF. Sugammadex has been shown to provide effective and complete reversal of rocuronium blockade in patients with renal impairment. However, further studies are awaited on the safety and efficacy of this drug in patients with ERF.

Rapid sequence induction and hyperkalaemia

- Succinylcholine can be safely used if the serum potassium (K^+) is less than 5.5 mmol L^{-1}. If above this level, surgery may have to be delayed while the potassium level is treated by dialysis.
- Medical management using an insulin–dextrose infusion is instituted only if K^+ is more than 6.5 mmol L^{-1} or if there are hyperkalaemia-related ECG changes.
- A modified rapid sequence induction with rocuronium may be used in case of emergency surgery along with institution of medical management of hyperkalaemia.

Fluid management and graft optimization

- Intraoperative volume expansion increases renal blood flow and improves graft function. Most patients are hypovolaemic on induction owing to recent dialysis and fluid removal. It is important to maintain a mean arterial pressure at 70–80 mmHg to optimize graft perfusion. The CVP is maintained between 10 and 12 mmHg.
- Normal saline was the crystalloid of choice, but recent concerns over the impaired ability to excrete large amounts of sodium immediately postoperatively leading to volume overload and the development of hyperchloraemic acidosis following administration of large volumes of normal saline have led to balanced salt solutions (e.g. compound sodium lactate) being favoured.
- Colloid solutions containing gelatin are used to maintain graft perfusion and avoid hypotension.
- Fluids containing hydroxyethyl starch have adverse effects on renal function in transplant recipients.
- Prior to revascularization 1 g of methylprednisolone is given to prevent hyperacute rejection and mannitol (0.5–1.0 g kg^{-1}) as a free radical scavenger and osmotic diuretic.

Analgesia

- Intraoperative analgesia by intermittent boluses of fentanyl or by a remifentanil infusion. The pharmacokinetics of short-acting opioids (e.g. fentanyl, alfentanil and remifentanil) is unaltered in ERF.
- Fentanyl patient-controlled analgesia (PCA) pumps are commonly used to manage postoperative pain.
- Transverse abdominal plane blocks at induction with continuous local anaesthetic infusion catheters placed postoperatively are also used to decrease total amount of fentanyl used.
- Non-steroidal anti-inflammatory drugs (NSAIDs) are avoided to prevent renal impairment and hyperkalaemia.
- Paracetamol is safe to use without dose adjustment.

Postoperative care

Postoperative care is usually on a ward staffed by nurses and clinicians with specialist expertise. Patient parameters and graft function are optimized using protocol-driven regimens encompassing fluids, pain relief and immunosuppression.

Immunosuppression

- Immunosuppression strategies aim to prevent graft rejection.
- This usually consists of triple therapy with a calcineurin inhibitor (e.g. ciclosporin, tacrolimus), an antiproliferative agent (e.g. azathioprine, mycophenolate mofetil) and a steroid.
- Current regimens adopt a steroid-sparing and calcineurin inhibitor minimization approach.
- Primary immunosuppression strategy includes induction therapy with two 20 mg doses of basiliximab, the first dose of which is given at induction of anaesthesia, followed by tacrolimus monotherapy.
- There is a significant shift towards dual-agent maintenance immunosuppression in a large number of patients. Different strategies are adopted for patients who are perceived to have a higher risk of rejection (recipients from non-heart-beating donors, previous failed transplant) or those with delayed graft function (need for dialysis in the first week) postoperatively.

Living donor kidney transplants

Living donor kidney transplants now represent over 30% of the total kidney transplant programme. The main benefits over deceased donor transplantation include over 95% primary graft function, shorter waiting times, planned elective surgery and better patient and graft survival.

Living donors can be:

- blood relatives of the recipient
- living genetically unrelated donors (partners/spouses); outcomes are equal to genetically related donations
- ABO incompatible if antibodies are removed by plasmapheresis before and after surgery.

In addition:

- altruistic non-directed donation allows an individual to donate a kidney to a stranger via the national matching and allocation system
- paired/pooled donation pairs an incompatible donor/recipient couple anonymously with another couple in the same situation in another centre in order to exchange suitably matched organs between couples. Simultaneous donor operations are performed with direct telephonic contact between the two centres with the donor kidney being sent to the centre where the compatible recipient is transplanted.

Donor selection

- All living donors must make a voluntary and informed decision and the donor is given the option to withdraw at any time. An independent assessor also assesses the donor to ensure a totally altruistic donation.
- Medical assessment of the potential donor is extensive and is performed by a clinician who is not part of the transplant team. In order to determine that the donor in his/her lifetime will not develop clinically significant renal impairment as a result of unilateral nephrectomy, the donor must have sufficient kidney function prior to donation to have an effective GFR (37.5 mL min^{-1} 1.73 m^{-2}) at the age of 80 years, independent of the age at which he/she donated.
- Absolute contraindications for donation include diabetes mellitus, malignancy and hypertension with evidence of end-stage organ damage.
- Obesity and old age are relative contraindications.
- Recipients often receive their transplant earlier in the course of their disease, sometimes before dialysis. So, they have fewer associated comorbidities, but are more likely to develop hyperkalaemia perioperatively.

Procedure

- The donor kidney nephrectomy and kidney transplant either are performed simultaneously in neighbouring operating theatres or both operations are performed sequentially by the same anaesthetic and surgical team. The small difference in ischaemic time has no demonstrable effect on outcome.
- The donor kidney nephrectomy is performed either laparoscopically or as an open procedure in the partial or full lateral position with a lumbar break.
- A laparoscopic nephrectomy takes longer to perform but causes less tissue trauma and is associated with less postoperative pain and shorter recovery and hospital stay.
- Both approaches have similar complication rates (1–2%).

Anaesthetic considerations

- Donors are hydrated with 1–2 litres of crystalloid the night before surgery.
- General anaesthesia is the method of choice, often combined with an epidural in open procedures.
- Invasive arterial blood pressure monitoring is recommended as haemorrhage and cardiovascular instability following major vascular haemorrhage is a potential complication.
- The donor kidney must be kept well perfused during its retrieval. A positive fluid balance is maintained up to 10 mL kg^{-1} h^{-1} over surgical losses, especially in laparoscopic nephrectomy, to counteract the compressive effects of the pneumoperitoneum.
- Urine output should be at least 1.5–2 mL kg^{-1} h^{-1}.
- Mannitol (0.5–1.0 g kg^{-1}) is given prior to kidney retrieval.
- Postoperative analgesia is provided with an epidural or PCA combined with abdominal field blocks.
- There may be a short period of decreased renal function in donors, which prompts some centres to use a fentanyl PCA and avoid NSAIDs. The mortality from donor nephrectomy is 1:3000. The incidence of chronic wound pain is 3.2%.

Outcome and complications

Kidney transplantation is a life-changing procedure in a group of patients who often have multisystem comorbidities. A year after surgery 94% of living donor kidneys and 88% of kidneys from deceased donors are functioning effectively. Graft survival after living donor transplants is over 90%. Possible complications are:

- transplant rejection (hyperacute, acute or chronic)
- infections and sepsis due to the immunosuppressant drugs
- post-transplant lymphoproliferative disorder
- imbalances in electrolytes, including calcium and phosphate, which can lead to bone problems.

Bibliography

British Transplantation Society; The Renal Association. *United Kingdom Guidelines for Living Donor Kidney Transplantation*. See www.bts.org.uk

Craig RG, Hunter JM. Recent developments in the perioperative management of adult patients with chronic kidney disease. *Br J Anaesth* 2008; **101**: 296–310.

Jankovic Z. Anaesthesia for living-donor renal transplant. *Curr Anaesth Crit Care* 2008; **19**: 175–80.

Jankovic Z, Sri-Chandana C. Anaesthesia for renal transplant: recent developments and recommendations. *Curr Anaesth Crit Care* 2008; **19**: 247–53.

Mazze RI, Callan CM, Galvez ST, *et al*. The effects of sevoflurane on serum creatinine and blood urea nitrogen concentrations: a retrospective, twenty two center, and comparative evaluation of renal function in adult surgical patients. *Anesth Analg* 2000; **90**: 683–8.

Older P, Hall A. Symposium on anaesthesia: preoperative evaluation of cardiac risk. *Br J Hosp Med* 2005; **66**: 452–7.

Rela M, Jassem W. Transplantation from non-heart-beating donors. *Transplant Proc* 2007; **39**: 726–72.

Staals LM, Snoeck MMJ, Driessen JJ, *et al.* Multicentre parallel group, comparative trial evaluating the efficacy and safety of sugammadex in patients with end stage renal failure or normal renal function. *Br J Anaesth* 2008; **101**: 492–7.

UK Transplant. See http://uktransplant.org.uk/ukt/default.jsp

Cross-references

Chronic kidney disease, 203
Fluid and electrolyte balance, 754
Nephrectomy, 492

Liver transplantation

Zoka Milan

Procedure

- Laparotomy by subcostal (right or bilateral) incision with or without an upper middle incision (Mercedes incision).
- Surgery is divided into three phases:
  - dissection phase, with skeletonization of native liver
  - anhepatic phase with removal of native and implantation of donor liver
  - reperfusion phase with graft revascularization with portal blood, haemostasis, completion of hepatic arterial anastomosis and biliary drainage.
- Orthotopic liver transplantation (OLT) is the replacement of a whole diseased liver with a deceased (heart beating or non-heart beating) donor liver.
- Alternatives include living donor, auxiliary, split or reduced graft liver transplantation and ABO-incompatible grafts.

Box 21.1 United Network for Organ Sharing (UNOS) exclusion and listing criteria for transplantation for acute liver failure

- Exclusion
  - Age >70 years old (relative)
  - Certain malignancies outside the liver
  - Severe cardiac, lung or multiple organ failure
  - Severe infection
  - Uncontrolled septic shock
  - Brain death
- UNOS listing criteria
  - Life expectancy without a liver transplant <7 days
  - Onset of encephalopathy within 8 weeks of the first symptom of liver disease
  - Absence of pre-existing liver disease (except for the diagnosis of fulminant Wilson disease)
  - Residence in the ITU
  - At least one of the following: ventilator dependence, renal replacement treatment, or INR >2.0

INR, international normalized ratio.

Patient characteristics

Patients are aged from 1 week to 70 years and fall into two distinct patient groups.

Acute liver failure (ALF)

- Jaundice and encephalopathy developing in a patient with no history of chronic liver disease.
- Hyperacute liver failure: encephalopathy within 7 days of onset of jaundice.
- Acute liver failure: encephalopathy in 8–28 days from onset of jaundice.
- Subacute liver failure: encephalopathy in 5–12 weeks from onset of jaundice.

Exclusion and listing criteria for transplantation for acute liver failure are presented in Box 21.1.

Chronic liver disease (CLD)

A wide variety of congenital and acquired disease in both adults and children may lead to end-stage liver disease. Transplantation is frequently required in order to prolong and/or improve quality of life.

Commonly associated pathology

- Central nervous system:
  - encephalopathy (CLD)
  - cerebral oedema (80% of ALF).
- Respiratory:
  - restrictive defect due to massive ascites (CLD)
  - hepatopulmonary syndrome (hypoxaemia and intrapulmonary shunting) (CLD)
  - pulmonary hypertension (1% of CLD) (pulmonary artery pressure >50 mmHg contraindication to transplantation)
  - adult respiratory distress syndrome, non-cardiogenic pulmonary oedema (ALF).
- Cardiovascular:
  - hyperdynamic circulation (high cardiac output and low SVR)
  - hyporeactive circulation
  - cirrhotic cardiomyopathy (cardiac dysfunction manifest during stress)
  - reduced effective circulating volume.
- Renal:
  - prerenal or renal failure (ALF)
  - hepatorenal syndrome (CLD).
- Electrolytes/metabolic:
  - hyponatraemia, hypomagnesaemia, hyperkalaemia (CLD), metabolic acidosis
  - hypoglycaemia (ALF).

- Haematology:
  - anaemia, thrombocytopenia (hypersplenism), platelet dysfunction (CLD)
  - reduced/defective synthesis of vitamin K-dependent clotting factors (ALF, CLD)
  - hyperfibrinolysis with/without low grade disseminated intravascular coagulopathy (ALF, CLD).

The Model for End-Stage Liver Disease (MELD), Paediatric End-Stage Liver disease (PELD) and UK End-Stage Liver Disease (UKELD) scores are numerical scales that are currently used for liver allocation. Scores are based on objective and verifiable medical data and represent the risk of a patient dying while waiting for a liver transplant.

Preoperative assessment

A multidisciplinary approach is essential to assess risk, aimed at precisely defining the multisystem involvement. Occult cardiovascular disease is a major cause of perioperative death and complications; rigorous cardiac work-up includes routine echocardiography, cardiopulmonary exercise testing and dobutamine stress echo and angiography when indicated.

Preoperative preparation

- Detailed patient and relative counselling.
- When an organ becomes available, liaison with the donor team is essential.
- Success is dependent on support services such as blood bank and laboratory services, anaesthetic technical back-up and clinical perfusionists for rapid infusion devices, cell saver and bypass equipment (<5% of liver transplants; Fig. 21.1). Patient-warming devices and monitoring must be available and ready.

Perioperative management

Monitoring

- ECG, S_pO_2, $ETCO_2$.
- Invasive arterial pressure, CVP.
- Core temperature, urine output and blood loss.
- Pulmonary artery catheter or lithium dilution cardiac output (LiDCO), pulse contour continuous cardiac output (PiCCO) or TOE for haemodynamic monitoring.
- Intracranial pressure (ALF).

Blood samples

- Arterial gases with electrolytes, glucose and lactate hourly.
- Mixed venous gases.
- Full blood count and clotting screen.
- Thromboelastography.

Intravenous access

- Wide-bore venous access is mandatory for rapid infusion.
- Internal jugular access is safer than subclavian in the presence of severe coagulopathy.
- Large-bore bypass lines if venovenous bypass is used (Fig. 21.1).

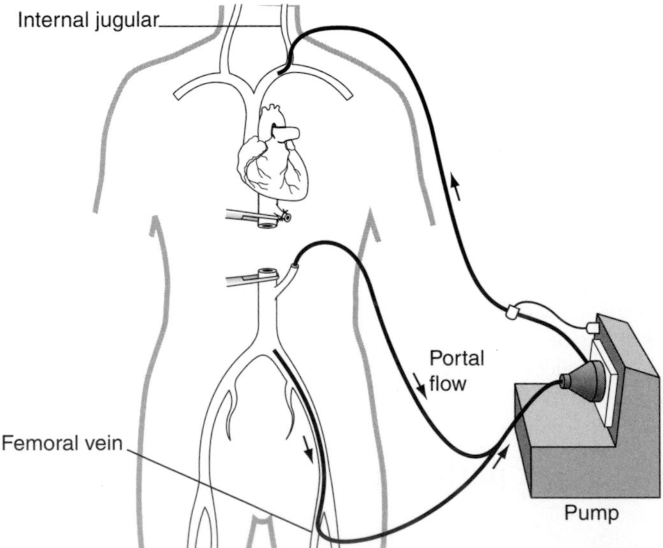

Figure 21.1 Venovenous bypass.

Anaesthetic technique

- Rapid sequence induction is advisable if the patient is not fully fasted, or in the presence of massive varices and ascites.
- Induction with narcotic (fentanyl or remifentanil) and sleep dose of propofol.
- Insert a wide-bore nasogastric tube and a fine-bore enteral feeding tube for early postoperative enteral nutrition.
- Maintenance with oxygen/air/desflurane, narcotic and relaxant infusion.
- TIVA for ALF to decrease raised intracranial pressure.
- IPPV, pressure controlled, with positive end-expiratory pressure (PEEP).
- Aim to maintain renal perfusion.
- Maintenance of cardiac output and oxygen transport, especially in the anhepatic phase. Intraoperatively, cardiac output increases, especially on reperfusion with profound systemic vasodilation. Adequate volume loading is essential. Pressor inotropes are occasionally required, as guided by cardiac output and SVR. Beware of the deleterious effects of vasoconstrictors on already limited oxygen extraction.
- Intraoperative monitoring of coagulation and appropriate blood product replacement. Ionized calcium concentration will fall owing to administered citrate and will require supplementation.
- Prophylactic antibiotic administration and intraoperative doses of immunosuppression.

Postoperative management

- 95% of patients with CLD are extubated at the end of the procedure.
- In ALF, ITU stay may be prolonged and continuous invasive monitoring is recommended.
- Early liver function is monitored by resolution of metabolic and lactic acidosis and resolution of coagulopathy (falling INR).
- Early complications include bleeding (now <5%) and hepatic artery or portal vein thrombosis (<1%), which will require early re-exploration.
- Poor initial graft function is treated with all-organ support.
- Primary non function of the liver is rare in UK centres (1–2%), but will entail emergency retransplantation. Initial poor function is relatively common with the increasing use of 'marginal' donors.
- Acute rejection, suggested by changes in aspartate transaminase and INR and confirmed by biopsy if coagulation permits. Treat with additional steroids and/or modification of the immunosuppressive regime.
- Ciclosporin or tacrolimus may be introduced early if renal function is satisfactory.

Outcome

- Patients with acute liver failure are selected for OLT if their chances of survival with medical treatment are <10%. One year survival following emergency OLT is currently 60–80%.
- Patients with chronic liver disease currently have a 1 year survival of 90% and 5 year survival of 76% following OLT.
- Quality of life is improved; the majority of patients are severely incapacitated prior to transplantation.
- The majority of deaths in the early postoperative period are due to sepsis. Later deaths are due to complications of immunosuppression, chronic rejection or recurrence of the primary liver disease.
- Retransplantation will be required in 5–10% of patients.

Bibliography

Jankovic Z, Taylor C, Duncan B. *et al.* Haemodynamic changes during liver transplantation: predictive value for outcome and effect of marginal donors. In: Knudsen KH (ed.) *Liver Transplantation*. New York: Nova Biomedical Books, 2009, pp. 191–207.

NHS Blood and Transplant. *Statistics: Transplants Save Lives*. See www.uktransplant.org.uk/ukt/statistics/statistics.jsp

Ozier Y, Klinck JR. Anesthetic management of hepatic transplantation. *Curr Opin Anaesthesiol* 2008; **21**: 391–400.

United Network for Organ Sharing. See www.unos.org.

Cross-references

Chronic liver disease, 174
Previous liver transplant, 192

Lung and heart–lung transplantation

Andrew Roscoe

Procedure

- Heart–lung transplant (HLT) performed through median sternotomy or clam-shell (transverse sternobithoracic) incision, with CPB.
- HLT anastomoses: right atrium (RA) to SVC and IVC, ascending aorta and trachea.
- HLT is becoming a very uncommon procedure (fewer than 10 in the UK in 2008).
- Lung transplant (LT):
  - single-lung transplant (SLT) via thoracotomy
  - bilateral sequential lung transplant (BSLT) via a clam-shell incision.
  - anastomoses: main bronchus, pulmonary artery and pulmonary vein cuff to left atrium.
- SLT usually performed off CPB.
- BSLT may be performed on or off CPB.
- Some evidence that elective use of CPB is detrimental to outcomes.
- Living donor lobe transplant involves two donors (usually one lower lobe from each) providing organs for BSLT for recipient (usually child or small adult): common in Japan.

Donor organs

- Significant shortage of donor lungs (less than 20% of donors of other organs have lungs suitable for donation). Approximately 30% on the waiting list die before receiving a transplant.
- Use of marginal donors, non-heart-beating donors and *ex vivo* reconditioning designed to increase the donor pool.

Patient characteristics

- HLT: majority for congenital heart disease.
- End-stage pulmonary disease when transplant provides survival benefit.
- Indications:
  - emphysema (chronic obstructive pulmonary disease or α_1-antitrypsin deficiency): 43%
  - idiopathic pulmonary fibrosis (IPF): 21%
  - cystic fibrosis (CF): 16%
  - primary pulmonary hypertension (PPH): 3%
  - sarcoidosis: 3%
  - bronchiectasis: 3%
  - others: 11%.
- SLT: 55% for emphysema; 30% for IPF.
- BSLT: 27% for CF; 25% for emphysema; 15% for IPF; 5% for PPH.
- Emphysema: forced expiratory volume in 1 second (FEV_1) <20% predicted.
- IPF: diffusing capacity (DLco) <39% predicted.
- CF: O_2 dependent with hypercapnia and pulmonary hypertension.
- PPH: cardiac index (CI) <2 L min^{-1} m^{-2} and RA pressure >15 mmHg.
- Patient may have had previous thoracic surgery, e.g. lung volume reduction surgery.
- Absolute contraindications:
  - malignancy (except locally resectable cutaneous basal cell carcinoma or squamous cell carcinoma)
  - chronic non-pulmonary infection (e.g. HIV)
  - severe comorbidity (not amenable to multiorgan transplant procedure)
  - severe chest wall deformity
  - substance abuse (including tobacco) within previous 6 months
  - mental illness/inability to comply with postoperative medication.
- Relative contraindications:
  - age >65 years old
  - BMI >30 kg m^{-2}
  - severe osteoporosis
  - colonized with resistant organisms (*Burkholderia cepacia* in CF patients)
  - dependent upon invasive ventilation or extracorporeal membrane oxygenation (ECMO).

Preoperative assessment and investigations

- Airway: determine ease of intubation and size of double-lumen tube (DLT) required.
- Respiratory:
  - chest X-ray/CT scan may provide anatomical information
  - arterial blood gases on air provide baseline measurement

– pulmonary function tests differentiate between restrictive and obstructive defect
– ventilation–perfusion (V/Q) scan displays differential blood flow to each lung.

- Cardiac:
  – right heart catheter measures PA pressures
  – echocardiogram displays LV and RV function.
- Renal: patients should have normal kidney function.
- Liver:
  – mild dysfunction may be present owing to congestion from RV failure
  – hepatic failure (in some CF patients) amenable to lung and liver transplant.
- Consent patients for postoperative insertion of thoracic epidural/paravertebral catheter for analgesia.

Premedication

- Oxygen by facemask.
- Bronchodilator therapy.
- Sedative medication is avoided as it can exacerbate hypoxaemia and hypercapnia, precipitating acute pulmonary hypertension and RV failure.

Perioperative management

Theatre preparation

- Intravenous fluid warmer. Forced air-warming device.
- Left-sided double-lumen tube: patients with IPF usually have contracted thoracic cavity and require a smaller DLT than expected.
- Fibreoptic bronchoscope (FOB) to confirm the position of the DLT.
- Heparin drawn up in advance in case of cardiovascular collapse and emergency institution of CPB.

Monitoring

- Wide-bore venous access and invasive arterial monitoring prior to induction.
- ECG, $S_{p}O_2$, $ETCO_2$, CVP, PA catheter, nasopharyngeal temperature and urinary catheter.
- TOE: category IIb indication.
- Consider depth of anaesthesia monitor (e.g. bispectral index): high risk of awareness.

Physiological goals

- Avoid severe hypoxaemia and hypercapnia: tolerated limits are extended based on baseline arterial blood gas measurement.
- Cardiovascular stability.
- Obstructive defects:
  – low inspiratory pressure, no PEEP, long expiratory phase
  – risk of dynamic hyperinflation and gas-trapping.
- Restrictive defects:
  – high inspiratory pressure, high PEEP, low tidal volume
  – ventilation strategy similar to patients with acute respiratory distress syndrome.
- Infective disease: may require repeated suctioning to remove sputum plugs.
- Pulmonary hypertension:
  – maintain positive chronotropy/inotropy (epinephrine)
  – avoid hypercapnia/high intrathoracic pressures
  – may require iNO or urgent institution of CPB.

Induction

- Preoxygenation.
- Midazolam, etomidate or propofol.
- Fentanyl. Use of remifentanil has been described.
- Pancuronium, rocuronium or vecuronium. Atracurium if significant hepatic dysfunction.
- Other medications:
  – prophylactic antibiotics
  – methylprednisolone
  – antifibrinolytic (aprotinin or tranexamic acid) if use of CPB.
- Single-lumen endotracheal tube for HLT.
- Left-sided DLT for SLT or BSLT.
- Advantage of DLT in BSLT with CPB: allows ventilation and oxygenation of first transplanted lung, while second lung being implanted.

Maintenance

- IPPV with O_2/air mixture. Avoid N_2O because of increases in PVR.
- Intravenous drugs (e.g. propofol TIVA) may provide more consistent pharmacokinetics than inhalational agents in patients with profound V/Q mismatch and air leaks.
- Indications for CPB:
  – severe pulmonary hypertension
  – unmanageable haemodynamic instability
  – unable to tolerate one-lung ventilation (OLV).
- If CPB used: heart remains warm and beating throughout.
- Without CPB: the lung with the least perfusion (from V/Q scan) is explanted first, with OLV of the contralateral native lung. After completion of the first side, the transplanted lung undergoes OLV and the second native lung is explanted. Once implanted, both lungs are ventilated with protective lung strategy.
- Advantages of CPB:
  – avoidance of OLV (and hypoxaemia/hypercapnia)
  – limited duration of haemodynamic instability.
- Disadvantages of CPB:
  – heparinization and increased bleeding

- crystalloid fluid loading causing pulmonary oedema
- systemic inflammatory response to CPB
- reduced allograft function.

Fluid management

- Keep crystalloid administration to minimum: the lung allograft is prone to low-pressure pulmonary oedema as a result of ischaemia-reperfusion microvascular leak, re-expansion injury and absence of lymphatic drainage.
- Blood and blood products transfused as indicated.

Weaning from CPB

- HLT:
  - similar to heart transplant
  - TOE essential to monitor ventricular function and filling.
- BSLT:
  - protective lung ventilation strategy to avoid barotrauma
  - use minimal tolerated F_iO_2 to reduce free radical injury
  - TOE to assess RV function and pulmonary vein anastomotic sites
  - right ventricle may require inotropic support (milrinone or enoximone).
- Severe primary graft dysfunction: consider iNO/ temporary ECMO.

Postoperative management

- Change DLT for single-lumen tube: surgeon will pass large bronchoscope to assess bronchial anastomoses.
- Insert nasogastric tube for early administration of enteral immunosuppression.
- Insertion of epidural catheter once coagulopathy excluded.
- Early extubation is beneficial.
- Maintain restrictive fluid administration regimen.
- HLT: note loss of carinal reflex and lack of cough on suctioning.
- *Beware SLT for emphysema!*
- IPPV through single-lumen tube will preferentially ventilate compliant native emphysematous lung, leading to dynamic hyperinflation, gas-trapping and eventually cardiac compression and arrest.
- Often require differential lung ventilation via DLT or double-lumen tracheostomy.

Outcomes

- HLT:
  - 63% 1 year survival
  - 42% 5 year survival
  - 28% 10 year survival.
- LT: BSLT patients have better survival than SLT.
- Actuarial survival figures are:
  - 1 year: 80% overall; 78% (SLT); 81% (BSLT)
  - 3 years: 63% overall; 61% (SLT); 66% (BSLT)
  - 5 years: 52% overall; 47% (SLT); 56% (BSLT)
  - 10 years: 29% overall; 21% (SLT); 37% (BSLT).
- CF patients have better outcomes: 40% 10 year survival.
- Emphysema: BSLT has better outcome than SLT – 32% vs 19% 10 year survival.
- Long-term mortality caused by infection, chronic rejection (bronchiolitis obliterans), renal failure and malignancy (secondary to immunosuppression).

Bibliography

Cheitlin MD, Armstrong WF, Aurigemma GP, *et al.* ACC/AHA/ASE 2003 guideline update for the clinical application of echocardiography: summary article. *J Am Soc Echocardiogr* 2003; **16**: 1091–110.

Christie JD, Edwards LB, Aurora P, *et al.* The Registry of the International Society of Heart and Lung Transplantation: Twenty-sixth Official Adult Lung and Heart-Lung Transplantation Report – 2009. *J Heart Lung Transplant* 2009; **28**: 1031–49.

Myles PS. Pulmonary transplantation. In: Kaplan JA, Slinger PD (eds) *Thoracic Anesthesia*, 3rd edn. Philadelphia: Churchill Livingstone, 2003, pp. 295–314.

Orens JB, Estenne M, Arcasoy S, *et al.* International guidelines for the selection of lung transplant candidates: 2006 update. A consensus report from the Pulmonary Scientific Council of the International Society of Heart and Lung Transplantation. *J Heart Lung Transplant* 2006; **25**: 745–55.

Cross-references

Heart transplantation, 520
Liver transplantation, 527
One-lung anaesthesia, 714

Pancreas transplantation

William R Macnab

Procedure

Pancreas transplantation improves quality of life, stabilizes or improves secondary complications of diabetes mellitus and has long-term survival advantage in patients with type 1 diabetes. There are three main categories of pancreas transplantation: simultaneous pancreas and kidney transplant (SPK), pancreas transplant alone (PTA) and pancreas after kidney (PAK). SPK is by far the most common procedure. There are other procedures such as segmental transplant of the tail from live donors and islet cell transplant. The surgery takes approx 5–7 hours via a laparotomy and midline incision. The surgical technique involves placing the graft in the peritoneum. The systemic venous drainage is obtained by anastomosing donor portal vein to recipient iliac vein or vena cava. Pancreas graft arterial revascularization typically is accomplished using the recipient's right common or external iliac artery. Drainage of pancreatic exocrine secretions is achieved by the donor duodenum being anastomosed to the jejunum or bladder. The former technique is performed in the majority of cases as it is associated with significantly fewer urological and metabolic complications. In a SPK, the pancreas is implanted first. The native pancreas is not removed. The benchwork to prepare the pancreas takes about 2 hours. The goal should be to implant the graft as soon as possible, keeping the cold ischaemic times to ideally less than 12 hours.

Patient characteristics

There is a national protocol for assessment of pancreas transplant patients. All have type 1 insulin-dependent diabetes mellitus. Patients for SPK have diabetes and end-stage chronic renal failure or a predictive date for dialysis within 6 months. For PTA, patients will have diabetes with significant diabetic complications, e.g. life-threatening complications of hypoglycaemic unawareness or of frequent and severe hypoglycaemia. For PAK, patients will have diabetes and stable function of a previous renal allograft and fulfil the criteria for PTA. Patients with poor cardiac reserve and untreatable coronary artery disease are excluded. The average waiting time for a pancreas transplant is 2–3 years once listed.

Preoperatively

Extensive preoperative work-up, clinical assessment and investigations will have been done, including:

- echocardiography
- assessment of cardiovascular reserve, e.g. CPET, 6 minute walk, myocardial perfusion scan or stress echocardiography.

On admission, patients require a full history and examination with particular reference to cardiac, renal and diabetic pathology. They require the following up-to-date investigations on the day of surgery:

- full blood count
- urea, electrolytes and calcium
- clotting
- ECG
- four units of blood cross-matched.

Premedication

Cardiac medications should be given (but usually omitting angiotensin-converting enzyme inhibitors and angiotensin II receptor blockers) and gastric acid prophylaxis should be considered. A standard insulin and glucose sliding scale should start preoperatively. Anxiolysis can be prescribed if required and appropriate.

Perioperative management

- Establish intravenous access, 16 G or above. Do not use any arm with a fistula.
- Thoracic epidural.
- Tranversus abdominis plane blocks/catheters or wound catheters could be used if an epidural is not used.
- Immunosuppression and broad-spectrum antibiotics.
- Warming equipment.
- Monitoring:
  - routine monitoring, ideally with five-lead ECG and ST analysis
  - arterial line; inserted awake if significant autonomic dysfunction
  - central venous line is essential

- oesophageal Doppler or other monitor of cardiac output to optimize patient
- neuromuscular monitoring
- core temperature
- urinary catheter
- nasogastric tube.
- Induction:
  - induction agent titrated to patient response; rapid sequence if warranted
  - relaxant: atracurium or cisatracurium is the usual choice
  - volatile agent: isoflurane or desflurane as they are metabolized least
  - opiates: fentanyl or remifentanil
  - take care to obtund the hypertensive response with appropriate agents.

Take baseline bloods for arterial gases, blood sugar and central venous saturation. Near-patient tests of coagulation can be helpful during the operation. Monitor gases and near-patient parameters regularly throughout the procedure.

Maintenance

The aim is to keep the patient's fluid optimized and to maintain an appropriate perfusion pressure, normothermia and normal biochemical parameters. The goal is to optimize graft perfusion and function. Maintenance with oxygen and air and a volatile agent is usual, but TIVA can be used.

Fluid management

- Aim to keep well filled: CVP 12–16 mmHg and optimize stroke volume.
- Crystalloid: balanced salt solution should be used to avoid hyperchloraemic acidosis caused by large volumes of 0.9% saline.
- Colloids: hetastarch has been shown to improve graft vessel flow in patients with functioning kidneys. Some prefer to avoid Gelofusine because of concerns of graft oedema.
- Blood: aim for a haemoglobin >8 g dL^{-1}.
- 10% mannitol (0.5 g kg^{-1}) prior to reperfusion of the graft.

Reperfusion

Aim for a well-filled circulation prior to unclamping of vessels. Stop the insulin sliding scale on reperfusion of the pancreas. Monitor blood glucose every 15 minutes for the first hour and then every 30 minutes until the patient stabilizes. Surgeons should be made aware of any significant rise in glucose >12.

Postoperatively

- Patients will be nursed in a critical care unit postoperatively.
- Postoperative analgesia: epidural or PCA with or without local anaesthetic infusions.
- Fluid management is aggressive to aid graft perfusion. Aim to keep well filled.
- Maintenance with balanced salt solutions (e.g. rate = last hour's urine output + 50 mL), with fluid challenges of crystalloid or colloid to maintain CVP or maximize stoke volume. Transfuse when necessary (e.g. if Hb < 8 g dL^{-1}).

Complications

Complications include early and late rejection, graft thrombosis, pancreatitis, haemorrhage, anastomotic leak, local and systemic infection, systemic inflammatory response syndrome and side-effects of the immunosuppression.

Outcome

The survival rates at 1 year after transplantation are 84% (SPK) and 71% (pancreas only). Overall, 1 year survival is 95–100%.

Bibliography

Koehntop DE, Beebe DS, Belani KG. Perioperative anaesthetic management of the kidney pancreas transplant recipient. *Curr Opin Anaesthesiol* 2000; **13**: 341–7.

Larson-Wadd K, Belani KG. Pancreas and islet cell transplantation. *Anesthesiol Clin North Am* 2004; **22**: 663–74.

Pichel AC, Macnab WR. Anaesthesia for pancreas transplantation. *Cont Educ Anaesth Crit Care Pain* 2005; **5**: 149–52.

Rabbatt CG, Treleaven DJ, Russell JD, *et al.* Prognostic value of myocardial perfusion studies in patients with end-stage renal disease assessed for kidney or kidney-pancreas transplantation: a meta-analysis. *J Am Soc Nephrol* 2003; **14**: 431–9.

UK Transplant Kidney and Pancreas Advisory Group. *National Protocol for Assessment of Kidney and Pancreas Transplant Patients.* Bristol: NHS Blood and Transplant, 2003. See www.uktransplant.org.uk

Cross-references

Anaesthesia for pancreatic surgery, 433
Chronic kidney disease, 203
Diabetes mellitus, 60

22 Orthopaedics

Stuart White

Overview

Stuart White

Approximately 850 000 orthopaedic operations were performed in England and Wales in 2008–9, 25% of which were performed as emergency surgery. Elective orthopaedic surgery is associated with ever-improving functional outcome and low mortality, with advances in prosthesis technology allowing surgeons to perform an expanding number of procedures for a greater proportion of the population. Conversely, trauma surgery is associated with higher morbidity and mortality, and may extend beyond purely orthopaedic injury.

Joint replacement

Arthroplasty restores joint function, improves quality of life and reduces the pain associated with osteoarthritis. As the demography of Western populations ages, arthroplasty is an increasingly common operation. For example, the number of hip and knee replacements (the commonest types of arthroplasty) recorded by the National Joint Registry has increased by 50% in 5 years, from 106 904 in 2004–5 to 160 027 in 2008–9. In addition, the prevalence of both primary arthroplasty after trauma and revision arthroplasty is increasing. Revision arthroplasty can be a complex, lengthy procedure involving considerable blood loss and physiological insult.

Arthroscopy

Arthroscopy is a very commonly performed procedure, performed as both a diagnostic and a definitive intervention. Compared with open procedures, arthroscopy markedly improves perioperative outcome (reduced pain, blood loss, infection rates, etc.) and reduces inpatient length of stay. For example, of approximately 67 000 knee arthroscopies performed in England and Wales in 2008–9, 93% were day-case procedures.

Spinal and pelvic surgery

Decompressive laminectomy and discectomy aim to correct the pain and loss of function that result from spinal nerve impingement. Prone positioning and haemorrhage, particularly with multilevel procedures, can be problematic. More extensive surgery, such as scoliosis correction, tumour resection and posterior pelvic surgery, can be associated with massive haemorrhage (necessitating transfusion and/or cell salvage) and spinal cord damage (necessitating cord function monitoring using evoked responses).

Internal and external fixation

Internal fixation is used to restore correct anatomy in unstable fractures, promoting bone healing and allowing earlier rehabilitation and return to function. Distal long-bone fracture plate fixation is a very common procedure, usually performed on a younger, fitter patient group. The frequency of internal fixation for smaller hand and feet bones has increased with improved prosthetic technology. Intramedullary 'nailing' procedures reduce the soft-tissue damage and non-union related to tibial, femoral and humeral fractures, but are associated with an increased incidence of fat embolization syndrome compared with plating procedures. External fixation involves the use of external rods and frames to maintain bone anatomy and minimize soft tissue injury, either as a definitive procedure or until such time as internal fixation can be attempted.

Problems in orthopaedic anaesthesia

Bleeding

Interruption of bone vasculature, either through trauma or surgery, results in steady haemorrhage, which may be further increased by associated soft-tissue damage, anticoagulant medication and hypothermia. Blood loss is commonly underestimated, particularly in longer procedures not amenable to tourniquet use. Careful assessment of swab weights and suction loss gives an indication of blood loss, but consideration should be given to near patient monitoring of haemoglobin levels (e.g. use of a HemoCue) during longer procedures, spinal/pelvic/tumour surgery and revision arthroplasty, together with the use of cell salvage and reinfusion drains.

Infection

Osteomyelitis leads to chronic morbidity, mortality and reoperation. Although certain patients are more susceptible to perioperative infection, e.g. patients with cancer and diabetes, rigid adherence to infection control procedures and the maintenance of sterility is essential. Prophylactic antibiotics reduce prosthesis-related infection by skin pathogens, and should be administered immediately prior to surgery. Deep infection may require repeated surgical irrigation under anaesthesia.

Venous thromboembolism

Tissue trauma, dehydration, immobility and hypercoagulability render the orthopaedic patient particularly susceptible to venous thromboembolism (VTE) in the perioperative period, especially those with comorbidities such as diabetes, cancer and obesity or those who smoke. Fatal pulmonary embolism may occur in up to 1.7% of patients after knee arthroplasty and 2% of patients after hip arthroplasty. Mortality is reduced through the prophylactic use of fitted graduated compression stockings, perioperative anticoagulation, adequate hydration and early mobilization. Central neuraxial blockade reduces the incidence of VTE.

Age

Two-thirds of arthroplasties involve patients over 65 years old. Increasing age is associated with increasing comorbidity and polypharmacy, the effects (and side-effects) of which may be compounded by age-related reductions in physiological reserve. Reduced mobility and muscle power make rehabilitation after surgery more problematic.

Positioning

For some orthopaedic procedures (e.g. shoulder and spinal surgery), surgical access is improved by positioning the patient other than supine. The anaesthetist must be aware of the specific problems associated with each position, in order to avoid pressure- and traction-related nerve compression or ischaemia and other patient injury.

Tourniquets

Although blood loss is reduced and surgical view improved, the use of tourniquets can cause nerve and soft-tissue damage, VTE, pain and reperfusion injury, particularly in longer procedures with high inflation pressures involving patients with peripheral vascular disease.

Thermoregulation

Heat loss of approximately 1°C can result from a combination of laminar airflow ventilation, patient exposure, wound exposure and administration of cold intravenous fluids. Children and the elderly are more susceptible to intraoperative hypothermia, increasing the risk of haemorrhage, wound infection and postoperative shivering. Active warming is essential for all at-risk patients and those undergoing surgery for more than 30 minutes, and may include the use of fluid warmers, warming mattresses and forced air warming devices.

Bibliography

Boezaart AE. *Anaesthesia and Orthopaedic Surgery.* New York: McGraw-Hill Professional, 2006.

National Institute of Health and Clinical Excellence. Reducing the Risk of Venous Thromboembolism (Deep Vein Thrombosis and Pulmonary Embolism) in Patients Admitted to Hospital. London: NICE, 2010. See http://guidance.nice.org.uk/CG92/Guidance/pdf/English

Cross-references

Blood transfusion, 735
Complications of position, 743
Fat embolism, 751
Metabolic and degenerative bone disease, 253
Rheumatoid disease, 255
Scoliosis, 258
Spinalcord surgery, 36
The elderly patient, 607
Thrombosis and embolism, 793

Arthroscopy

Stuart White

Procedure

Arthroscopy involves the insertion of a rigid, fine-bore arthroscope through a small, periarticular incision into a joint cavity, in order to examine the anatomy of the joint. A magnified image is relayed via a camera attached to the arthroscope onto a video screen. Up to three further incisions may be made to allow the introduction of other instruments into the joint cavity to assist the removal of tissue or debris. Avoiding open surgical exposure of the joint dramatically reduces recovery time and postoperative pain and immobility, which makes arthroscopy suitable as a day-case procedure.

Knee (with/without meniscectomy) and shoulder (with/without subacromial decompression) arthroscopy are common procedures, although wrist, ankle and hip arthroscopy are increasingly performed.

Patient characteristics

Patients usually fall into one of two categories: (1) young, fit sportsmen and women presenting for damage assessment and/or cartilage repair after injury and (2) older patients presenting for diagnosis and assessment of osteoarthritic joint damage prior to definitive arthroplasty.

Preoperative assessment and investigations

Younger sportspeople present few problems. The assessment of older patients should include consideration of whether overnight inpatient stay would be of benefit, particularly for patients with comorbidities.

Premedication

Seldom required and may delay recovery of day cases.

Theatre preparation

Arthroscopy of hip, knee and ankle and wrist is performed with the patient supine. Elbow arthroscopy is usually performed with the patient in the lateral position and the arm draped over a support. Shoulder arthroscopy may be performed in the 'deckchair' position or in the lateral position with traction applied to the forearm (in which case, the risk of ipsilateral brachial plexus damage must be minimized by supporting the head in a neutral position).

Perioperative management

Monitoring

- ECG, S_pO_2, non-invasive BP, inspired/expired gas analysis for general anaesthesia, temperature.
- Irrigation fluid administered: pressurized extravasation can occur in significant volumes.
- Tourniquet time (particularly arthroscopic cruciate ligament reconstruction).

Regional anaesthesia

Regional anaesthesia is suitable for knee, elbow, shoulder and wrist arthroscopy, and provides good postoperative analgesia, although day-case patients should be provided with additional analgesia to take after discharge as nerve blockade recedes. Low-dose spinal anaesthesia has been used successfully for knee arthroscopy, without delaying hospital discharge as a result of associated urinary retention.

Knee

Intra-articular 20 mL plain bupivacaine (0.375%) and to skin incisions. Opioids provide no additional analgesia. Epinephrine may be added to reduce bleeding. Intra-articular magnesium may improve analgesia.

Shoulder

Ultrasound-guided interscalene brachial plexus block (either as a single-shot or catheter technique inserted into the awake patient) provides better analgesia than intra-articular/subacromial injection of local anaesthetic, but is associated with a small risk of significant complications.

General anaesthesia

Standard techniques suitable for day surgery are adequate.

Postoperative management

Patients should be provided with advice and additional simple analgesics prior to discharge, in the event of experiencing postoperative pain after local anaesthetics have worn off.

Outcome

Recovery and return to function normally occurs within 7 days.

Bibliography

Fredrickson MJ, Krishnan S, Chen CY. Postoperative analgesia for shoulder surgery: a critical appraisal and review of current techniques. *Anaesthesia* 2010; **65**: 608–24.

Cross-references

Day-case surgery, 604
Local anaesthetic toxicity, 767
Metabolic and degenerative bone disease, 253
Orthopaedics: overview, 536
Regional anaesthetic techniques, 719
Rheumatoid disease, 255
Thrombosis and embolism, 793

Manipulation under anaesthesia

Stuart White

Procedure

Manipulation under anaesthesia (MUA) is performed to:

- relocate dislocated joints
- correct fracture deformity
- improve the mobility of 'fixed' joints
- effect adhesiolysis and improve mobility after arthroplasty.

Patient characteristics

Although anyone may present for MUA, the procedure may be urgent – and therefore the patient unprepared – if there is considerable pain, or if there is a risk of distal ischaemia because of vascular impairment (e.g. of the foot after ankle fracture).

Preoperative assessment and investigations

Emergency patients may not be fasted, and require antacid prophylaxis. Patients with fractures may have other injuries. Occult blood loss from long-bone fractures can be considerable, and not apparent prior to the induction of anaesthesia.

Premedication

For emergency patients and as indicated by history and examination.

Theatre preparation

MUA may be performed in the anaesthetic room, and occasionally in the accident and emergency department.

Perioperative management

Monitoring

- S_ao_2, ECG, non-invasive BP.

Anaesthetic technique

Regional or general anaesthesia may be used. General anaesthesia avoids any contention that post-MUA neuropraxia may have resulted from regional anaesthesia, rather than the original injury or manipulation.

Adhesiolysis is usually achievable under propofol sedation, although local anaesthetic catheter placement and infusion may be necessary if continuous passive movement is intended postoperatively.

Distal fracture reduction requires general or regional anaesthesia, particularly if Kirschner ('K') wires are required for fracture stabilization. Proximal fracture reduction or joint relocation under general anaesthesia may require the administration of a small dose of non-depolarizing neuromuscular blocker (e.g. 15 mg rocuronium) to facilitate manipulation with propofol or general anaesthesia.

Postoperative management

MUA for adhesiolysis is very painful. Regional anaesthesia and patient-controlled analgesia should be considered.

MUA for fracture/relocation usually relieves pain, with simple analgesics only required postoperatively.

Cross-references

Blood transfusion, 735
Fat embolism, 751
Regional anaesthetic techniques, 719
Local anaesthetic toxicity, 767
Metabolic and degenerative bone disease, 253
Thrombosis and embolism, 793
Total hip arthroplasty, 543

Repair of fractured neck of femur

Stuart White

Approximately 77 000 hip fractures occur in the UK each year. Although the prevalence is decreasing, the incidence is increasing as the population ages.

Procedure

Subcapital, transcervical or basicervical fractures of the neck of femur may interrupt the retinacular blood supply of the femoral head, leading to avascular necrosis, pain and loss of mobility, necessitating hemiarthroplasty (or, in younger patients, primary total arthroplasty).

Capital blood supply is preserved in intertrochanteric and subtrochanteric fractures, favouring internal fixation using a dynamic hip screw (DHS), cannulated screws or a proximal femoral nail.

Surgical repair is pain-relieving, and reduces the complications associated with the prolonged immobility of conservative management.

Patient characteristics

- Patients have a mean age of 81 years.
- Ninety-five per cent of hip fractures occur after simple falls in patients over 60 years of age with osteoporotic bones.
- Seventy-five per cent are female, median American Society of Anesthesiologists (ASA) grade 3.
- Twenty-five per cent of patients have two or more significant comorbidities – valvular heart disease, dysrhythmia, chronic obstructive pulmonary disease, cerebrovascular disease, renal dysfunction – all of which may alter anaesthetic management.
- Forty per cent have cognitive impairment, complicating the process of consent.
- Polypharmacy is common.

Preoperative assessment

Careful history and examination is necessary. Preoperative blood loss from the fracture may cause preoperative anaemia (40%) and dehydration; intravenous fluids should be routinely administered prior to surgery. Routine blood tests should always be performed – full blood count (FBC), urea and electrolytes, group and save/cross-match.

Additional investigations (e.g. echocardiography) should rarely delay surgery: the risks of prolonged delay (>48 hours) between hospital admission and operation (increased mortality and overall length of stay) must be balanced against the benefits derived from additional preoperative investigations.

Premedication

Simple analgesia and antacids, as required. Sedative and anticholinergic drugs should be avoided, as they increase the risk of perioperative confusion.

Perioperative management

Monitoring

- Standard: ECG, non-invasive BP, $S_{p}O_{2}$, $ETCO_{2}$, temperature, fluid balance.
- Additional:
  - invasive BP is underutilized for hip fracture patients, and should be used for patients with valvular heart disease and heart failure
  - postoperative bedside haemoglobin measurement avoids delay in treating common (90%) postoperative anaemia
  - oesophageal Doppler is useful for guiding fluid therapy in patients under general anaesthesia. Lithium dilution techniques (e.g. LiDCO) may prove beneficial for patients receiving regional anaesthesia.

Anaesthetic technique

Meta-analysis has not found major differences in outcomes between regional and general anaesthesia, although regional anaesthesia appears to be associated with reduced blood loss, postoperative confusion and VTE, and is cheaper (although no quicker) to administer.

Regional anaesthesia, most commonly subarachnoid/spinal anaesthesia, may be technically difficult in the elderly. Spinal anaesthesia may be administered with the patient seated or, more commonly, in the lateral position with the affected side downmost. Sedation (e.g. midazolam 1–2 mg) and femoral nerve blockade may be administered prior to turning the patient. Spinal anaesthesia-related hypotension is less prevalent if the patient is preadministered intravenous fluids, and a lower dose of subarachnoid local anaesthetic (e.g. 1–2 mL 0.5% 'heavy' bupivacaine) is administered. Avoiding relative

(>20% fall in mean arterial pressure) and absolute (<90 mmHg systolic blood pressure) hypotension may require vasopressor administration (titrated boluses of 3 mg ephedrine or 0.5 mg metaraminol); care should be taken to avoid excessive administration of intravenous fluids in this instance. Additional opioids (e.g. fentanyl 20 μg) may be added to the injectate to prolong postoperative analgesia.

The induction of general anaesthesia should be sympathetic to the patient's age and comorbidities, with reduced doses avoiding sudden hypotension. General anaesthesia may be augmented by a number of lower limb regional blocks – psoas compartment (lumbar plexus) block, fascia iliaca block, femoral nerve/'three-in-one' block, block of the lateral cutaneous nerve of the thigh. Ideally, paralysis should be avoided.

Operative blood loss is moderate (200–300 mL). Patients should receive warmed fluids and additional warming (mattress/forced air warming). Pressure care is essential. Antibiotic prophylaxis should be administered.

Problems associated with prosthesis insertion

Prosthesis insertion (particularly during hemiarthroplasty) may be associated with bone cement implantation syndrome (see below).

Postoperative management

Postoperative hypoxia is common, and additional nasal oxygen should routinely be administered.

Intravenous fluid therapy should be continued until the patient is eating and drinking. Severe hypoxaemia can occur after general anaesthesia if patients do not receive added oxygen.

Simple analgesia (paracetamol 1 g four times a day) is often sufficient; opioids should be used with caution particularly in patients with renal disease (halve the dose and frequency of administration). Codeine is very constipating in this patient group. Non-steroidal anti-inflammatory drugs (NSAIDs) should be used cautiously, as they worsen renal impairment and increase the risk of gastrointestinal bleeding.

Outcome

Thirty day mortality rates vary, being approximately 8–12%. Length of inpatient stay varies, but is approximately 15–25 days. Both outcomes are unaffected by type of anaesthesia, which is likely only to affect early postoperative complications, such as hypoxia, hypotension, anaemia, electrolyte disturbance, pain relief and mobility.

Bibliography

Association of Anaesthetists of Great Britain and Ireland. *Anaesthesia for Hip Fracture Surgery*. London: AAGBI, 2010.

Parker MJ, Handol HHG, Griffiths R. Anaesthesia for hip fracture surgery in adults. *Cochrane Database Syst Rev* 2004; (4): CD000251.

Maxwell MJ, Moran CG, Moppett IK. Development and validation of a preoperative scoring system to predict 30 day mortality in patients undergoing hip fracture surgery. *Br J Anaesth* 2008; **101**: 511–17.

Murray JM, Derbyshire S, Shields MO. Lower limb blocks. *Anaesthesia* 2010; **65**: S57–66.

Cross-references

Blood transfusion, 735
Fat embolism, 751
Local anaesthetic toxicity, 767
Metabolic and degenerative bone disease, 253
Rheumatoid disease, 255
The elderly patient, 604
Thrombosis and embolism, 793
Total hip arthroplasty, 543

Total hip arthroplasty

Stuart White

Procedure

Total hip arthroplasty (THA) involves replacement of both the acetabulum (using a cemented prosthesis) and the head/neck of the femur (using a stemmed, modular prosthesis, cemented into place in 70% of procedures) to treat the pain and loss of function usually due to chronic osteoarthritis, but increasingly in selected patients after hip fracture (with or without avascular necrosis) and patients with rheumatoid arthritis or ankylosing spondylitis. A posterior or anterolateral incision (L4–S3) is made.

Minimal access arthroplasty through a medial incision may become more common in future. Hip resurfacing is a less invasive procedure. Revision procedures are becoming more prevalent as patients approach the natural lifespan of various prostheses and more prostheses are inserted.

Patient characteristics

Usually aged over 50 years (including very active elderly), ASA 1–4, with or without comorbidity.

Preoperative assessment and investigations

Full history and examination is required. Relative immobility may mask myocardial ischaemia, necessitating ECG assessment. Anaemia is not uncommon: FBC, urea and electrolytes and group and save required.

Premedication

Seldom necessary in the elderly, and likely to cause confusion. If essential, give a minimal dose of a benzodiazepine.

Theatre preparation

The procedure takes about 1.5 hours and involves elderly patients; therefore, sympathetic positioning (usually lateral) and thermal care (warmed fluids, theatre and mattress/forced air warmer) are required.

Blood loss measured during THA varies between 300 mL (primary simple arthroplasty) and 1500 mL (complex revision), and is doubled in the first 24 hours postoperatively. HemoCue assessment of haemoglobin level postoperatively is useful.

Perioperative management

Monitoring

- Standard: ECG, non-invasive BP, S_pO_2, $ETco_2$, temperature, fluid balance/blood loss.
- Additional:
  - invasive BP should be considered for ASA grade 3 and 4 patients.
  - oesophageal Doppler is useful for guiding fluid therapy in patients under general anaesthesia who are undergoing revision surgery. Lithium dilution techniques (e.g. LiDCO) may prove beneficial for patients receiving regional anaesthesia.

Anaesthetic technique

The technique selected should cause the minimum impact on the comorbid state of the patient.

Regional anaesthesia is the method of choice, as it is associated with reductions in the duration of surgery, intraoperative blood loss, the need for transfusion, postoperative nausea and vomiting, and the incidence of VTE compared with general anaesthesia.

Spinal and epidural techniques may be difficult in the elderly (look at hip X-rays for the lower spine); positioning may be impeded by pain. Single-shot spinal anaesthesia, with or without supplemental nerve block for postoperative analgesia, is preferred to epidural anaesthesia, unless the patient has a high risk of cardiopulmonary complications. Epidural anaesthesia usually requires urinary catheterization of the patient.

Sedation should be offered to the patient if appropriate: boluses of midazolam or a propofol infusion (1–2 mg kg^{-1} h^{-1}) are effective. Supplemental oxygen should be administered.

General anaesthesia may be a patient choice, or may be necessary if regional anaesthesia or block is contraindicated (e.g. previous spinal fusion, severe scoliosis). Ideally, paralysis should be avoided.

Spinal anaesthesia and general anaesthesia may be augmented by a number of lower limb regional blocks – psoas compartment (lumbar plexus) block, fascia iliaca block, femoral nerve/'three-in-one' block, block of the lateral cutaneous nerve of the thigh; postoperative analgesia may be extended by the insertion of local anaesthesia infusion catheters.

24 Paediatrics

George H Meakin

Overview

George H Meakin

The fundamental differences between paediatric patients and adults concerning anaesthesia are discussed elsewhere (p. 615).This section deals with the practical aspects of anaesthetic management.

Preoperative preparation

Before admission

The child and the parents should be given a clear explanation of the proposed surgery and admission procedures at the initial outpatient clinic visit. They should be supplied with suitable written information regarding the proposed surgery and anaesthesia, as well as instructions on preoperative fasting requirements (Table 24.1).

Preadmission care may include attendance at a clinician or nurse-led preoperative assessment clinic. Preadmission assessment has been shown to decrease cancellations on the day of surgery. Preadmission services that include age-appropriate psychological preparation using books, videos, play therapy and/or a tour of the hospital may be useful in reducing children's anxiety.

The preoperative assessment should include a full birth history, including the duration of pregnancy, any perinatal problems and the presence of congenital and/or acquired diseases and allergies. Details of previous anaesthetics and a family history of anaesthetic problems should be obtained. Blood tests and other investigations should be performed when indicated and sickle cell screening should be performed in susceptible ethnic groups. A physical examination should be performed, the airway assessed and the presence of any loose, usually deciduous, teeth noted.

Telephone contact on the day before surgery provides an opportunity to confirm attendance, reinforce preoperative instructions and detect reasons for late cancellation, such as family problems or an acute infection.

After admission

The child should be admitted to a dedicated children's day-case unit or hospital ward staffed by medical and nursing staff trained in dealing with children and their families. The facility should be suitably decorated, and toys, books, videos and a play therapist should be available. All children should be weighed and have their pulse rate, blood pressure and temperature recorded on admission.

The anaesthetist should see the child and the parents before the operation to confirm the adequacy of, or perform, the preoperative assessment, confirm compliance with fasting guidelines, discuss anaesthetic techniques and postoperative pain treatments, and obtain verbal consent for invasive procedures such as suppositories and nerve blocks. A major aim of the interview should be to allay anxiety and provide reassurance to the parents and the child.

- All communication should be comprehensible to the child and the parents and all questions should be answered truthfully, but tactfully.
- The possible modes of induction (intravenous/inhalation) should be discussed and the wishes of the child and parents complied with where possible.
- If intravenous induction is planned, a topical local analgesic preparation such as EMLA cream or Ametop gel should be applied over possible venepuncture sites.
- Selected children may benefit from oral sedative premedication (e.g. oral midazolam, 0.5 mg kg^{-1}, maximum 20 mg, 30–45 minutes preoperatively).
- The child should be allowed to wear suitable clothing of their own to theatre.
- A parent should be invited to accompany the child at induction of anaesthesia and their role in the anaesthetic room discussed.

Children with a history of upper respiratory tract infection within 4 weeks of operation are at

Table 24.1 Preoperative fasting times for different types of liquids and solids

	Minimum fasting period (h)			
	Clear fluids*	Breast milk	Formula or cow's milk	Solids
<3 months	2	4	4	6
>3 months	2	4	6	6

*A clear fluid is one you can read newsprint through.

increased risk of respiratory complications during or after anaesthesia. Ideally, elective surgery should be postponed for 4–6 weeks, but this is not always practical as symptoms tend to recur. Moreover, many children with recurrent symptoms will be suffering from allergy. If a decision is made to proceed, it may be prudent to intubate and ventilate the patient during anaesthesia to minimize the risk of coughing or laryngospasm. Careful monitoring and supplemental oxygen will be required during recovery. When signs of lower respiratory tract infection are present, elective surgery must be postponed for 4–6 weeks to allow hyperactive airways to return to normal.

Management of anaesthesia

Induction

Inhalation induction of anaesthesia is often more convenient for infants and toddlers, who frequently have poor venous access and difficulty cooperating with an intravenous induction. Inhalation induction is also rapid in these very young patients owing to a relatively large minute volume ventilation in relation to the functional residual capacity and a relatively high cardiac output. Sevoflurane is used most commonly because of its relative lack of pungency, rapid uptake and elimination and reduced incidence of cardiovascular effects. For older children with visible veins, intravenous induction of anaesthesia with thiopental or propofol is quicker and creates less operating room pollution.

Airway management

The laryngeal mask (LM) is the most common method of managing the airway in children aged over 1 year undergoing relatively short procedures under anaesthesia with spontaneous ventilation. It may also be used for short procedures in some infants aged 6–12 months depending on the experience and preference of the anaesthetist. The appropriate sizes of LM for paediatric patients together with their maximum inflation volumes are given in Table 24.2. Overinflation of the cuff must be avoided as it may cause trauma to the pharynx and larynx or herniation of the cuff. The LM is usually inserted during moderately deep anaesthesia without the aid of a muscle relaxant. It can be left *in situ* at the end of the case and removed by the recovery nurse when the child is fully awake.

Despite the popularity of the LM, tracheal intubation remains the 'gold standard' for paediatric airway management, especially when controlled ventilation is required.

In contrast to adults, infants and children are intubated with the head in a neutral position as raising the head on a pillow does not improve the view of the larynx. The most effective manoeuvre is the application of external pressure at the level of the cricoid cartilage to push the larynx into view.

In infants, a flat-blade laryngoscope such as the infant Magill, which passes posterior to the epiglottis, may be more suitable than a curved one, since it flattens out the U-shaped curvature of the epiglottis and can be used to lift it forwards to expose the larynx. In children aged over 1 year, laryngoscopy can usually be accomplished using a medium sized Macintosh blade with the tip placed in the vallecula.

Since the narrowest part of the larynx before puberty is the cricoid ring, cuffed tracheal tubes are not usually required in infants and children. The correct sized tube is one that passes easily through the cricoid ring and leaks minimally or not at all in the working range 0–20 cm H_2O. The following formula may be used as a guide in children aged 2 years and over:

Tube size (internal diameter in mm) = [Age (years)]/4 + 4.5

Tube sizes in infants and children aged less than 2 years have to be memorized. A normal neonate weighing 3 kg usually requires a 3 mm tracheal tube; premature and low-weight babies may require a 2.5 mm tube. Other tube sizes can be interpolated.

Many anaesthetists cut tracheal tubes to a length which allows the tip of the tube to be placed in the mid-trachea, while 2–3 cm protrudes from the mouth for fixation. The following formula may be used to estimate orotracheal tube length in children aged over 2 years:

Orotracheal tube length (cm) = [Age (years)]/2 + 13

Orotracheal tube lengths for patients aged less than 2 years have to be memorized. The length for a

Table 24.2 Laryngeal mask sizes for paediatric patients

Size	Weight (kg)	Maximum inflation volume (mL)
1.5	5–10	7
2.0	10–20	10
2.5	20–30	15
3.0	30–50	20
4.0	>50	30

neonate is 10 cm, and for a 1 year old is 12 cm; other tube lengths can be interpolated. The position of the tracheal tube should be checked by auscultation of both lung fields.

Maintenance of anaesthesia

In general, infants are poor candidates for anaesthesia with spontaneous ventilation because of poor pulmonary mechanics. In most of these patients, the combination of tracheal intubation and balanced anaesthesia with full doses of muscle relaxants, controlled ventilation, minimum concentrations of volatile anaesthetics and reduced doses of opioids will be required. This regimen provides ideal surgical conditions with minimal cardiovascular depression and rapid return of laryngeal reflexes at the conclusion of anaesthesia.

Children aged over 1 year undergoing long or complex surgery will also benefit from balanced anaesthesia. However, for many children undergoing operations lasting less than 30–40 minutes, simple inhalation anaesthesia with 66% nitrous oxide in oxygen and sevoflurane (2–3%) may be adequate. This may be combined with an opioid analgesic, local infiltration or a regional block to provide analgesia in the postoperative period.

Anaesthetic breathing systems

Anaesthetic breathing systems may be classified into those which do not contain a chemical means of absorbing carbon dioxide and those which are equipped with such units. In the past, concerns about resistance to breathing and apparatus deadspace with the use of absorber systems led paediatric anaesthetists to use mainly non-absorber breathing systems. However, concerns for economy and environmental pollution since the mid-1990s has greatly increased the use of circle absorber systems in paediatric anaesthesia.

The Jackson Rees T-piece is a popular non-absorber breathing system for paediatric anaesthesia owing to its compact size, low resistance to breathing and low apparatus deadspace. The low compression volume of the T-piece gives a good 'feel' for the lung compliance in infants and young children and facilitates hand ventilation even in the face of a decrease in lung compliance or partial respiratory obstruction. Notable disadvantages of the system include its high fresh gas requirements (3–8 L min^{-1}) and the inability to scavenge waste gases. However, the practical advantages of the T-piece can outweigh its disadvantages when the system is used for induction of anaesthesia and anaesthesia of short duration.

The main advantages of circle absorber systems are economy in the use of anaesthetic agents and gases, conservation of heat and moisture in the respiratory tract and reduced operating room pollution. These advantages are most evident when the circle system is used for maintenance of anaesthesia of intermediate to long duration. Fears that these systems invariably impose unacceptable resistance to breathing and apparatus deadspace for paediatric use appear to have been unfounded. Moreover, the ready availability of anaesthetic gas monitors and oxygen saturation monitors has greatly improved the safety of low-flow anaesthesia techniques. The main disadvantage of circle systems in paediatric anaesthesia is their high compression volume, which gives a poor 'feel' for the lung compliance in infants and young children and may make it difficult to hand ventilate these patients in the event of an unexpected decrease in lung compliance. Accordingly, a system with a low compression volume, such as the T-piece, should always be readily available when using a circle system in children.

Monitoring

Routine monitoring should include:

- ECG
- non-invasive blood pressure
- pulse oximetry
- respiratory gases.

A range of paediatric cuffs must be available for measurement of blood pressure; the correct sized cuff is one which covers two-thirds of the upper arm. Temperature measurement is mandatory in infants and young children, who are at especially high risk of developing hypothermia. Heating devices such as electric underblankets and warm air blowers should be available to counter heat loss in these patients.

Intravenous therapy

Intravenous fluids are given during surgery to correct the preoperative fasting deficit, satisfy maintenance requirements and replace intraoperative losses (e.g. third-space losses and blood). In most children aged over 1 month all these requirements should be managed initially by giving an isotonic fluid (e.g. normal saline or Hartmann's solution). Neonates, and some other high-risk patients, should receive a glucose-containing maintenance fluid and/or have their blood glucose monitored during surgery.

The fasting deficit can usually be treated by giving a bolus of 10 mL kg^{-1} of Hartmann's solution after induction. Maintenance fluid requirements can be calculated from the patient's weight using Holliday and Segar's equation (p. 617). Third-space loss may be as little as 1–2 mL kg^{-1} for neurosurgery and 6–10 mL kg^{-1} h^{-1} in major laparotomy. Clinical signs such as heart rate, blood pressure and capillary refill time can be used to guide replacement, but when large fluid shifts are anticipated central venous pressure measurement is essential.

Blood loss should be estimated and replaced initially with isotonic fluid or colloid. Blood transfusion is indicated if the Hb decreases to 7.0 g dL^{-1}, which corresponds to a haematocrit of 25%.

Postoperative management

At the conclusion of anaesthesia, the child should be turned into the lateral position and transported, breathing oxygen, to a fully equipped recovery room. Details of the operative procedure and any special instructions should be given to the recovery nurse assuming care of the child. Recovery room protocol should include airway maintenance, provision of oxygen therapy, monitoring of oxygen saturation, pulse, respiration and blood pressure, and the completion of a postanaesthetic recovery chart. Once the child is awake, a parent should be called to the recovery room. The anaesthetist should check that the patient is pain free and that postoperative fluids and analgesics have been ordered before the child is returned to the surgical ward.

Bibliography

Association of Anaesthetists of Great Britain and Ireland Safety Guideline. *Pre-operative Assessment and Patient Preparation: The Role of the Anaesthetist.* London: AAGBI, 2010. See www.aagbi.org/publications/guidelines/docs/preop2010.pdf.

Association of Paediatric Anaesthetists of Great Britain and Ireland. *Consensus Guideline on Perioperative Fluid Management in Children.* London: APA, 2007. See www.apagbi.org.uk/sites/apagbi.org.uk/files/Perioperative_Fluid_Management_2007.pdf.

Bingham R, Lloyd-Thomas A, Sury M (eds) *Hatch and Sumner's Textbook of Paediatric Anaesthesia.* London: Hodder Arnold, 2008.

Motoyama EK, Davis PJ (eds) *Smith's Anesthesia for Infants and Children.* Philadelphia: Mosby, 2006.

Cross-reference

Infants and children, 615

Circumcision

Davandra Patel

Procedure

Circumcision is excision of the foreskin from around the penis. It is usually performed on an elective day-case basis.

Patient characteristics

Approximately 12 200 boys each year in England are circumcised in the hospital setting (3.8% of boys <15 years old). Pathological phimosis is the only absolute indication for circumcision. This affects 0.6% of boys, with a peak incidence at 11 years of age, and is rarely encountered before the age of 5. In addition, many procedures are performed by non-medical practitioners for religious and cultural reasons.

Preoperative assessment

- Exclude active respiratory tract infection with productive cough or pyrexia.
- Exclude those with a recent exposure to childhood infections.
- Ensure no history of bleeding diathesis or anaesthetic problems.

Preoperative investigations

None necessary unless clinically indicated.

Preoperative preparation

- Fasting of solids (including milk) for 6 hours and clear fluids for 2 hours.
- Obtain informed consent and explain to parents if a local anaesthetic procedure and/or rectal analgesics are to be used during surgery.
- A parent should be invited to accompany the child at induction of anaesthesia.

Premedication

- Topical local anaesthetic preparation (e.g. EMLA cream or Ametop gel) over possible venepuncture sites.
- Oral paracetamol 20 mg kg^{-1} and/or ibuprofen 5 mg kg^{-1}, 30–45 minutes before operation to enhance intraoperative and postoperative analgesia.
- If anxiolytic required, oral midazolam (0.5 mg kg^{-1}) may be given 30–45 minutes before surgery.

Perioperative management

Routine non-invasive monitoring.

General anaesthesia

- Intravenous or inhalation induction.
- Spontaneous ventilation via LM for children aged over 1 year.
- Intermittent positive pressure ventilation (IPPV) via tracheal tube for children aged under 1 year.
- Intravenous paracetamol 15 mg kg^{-1} if not given as premedication.

Local anaesthesia

- The local anaesthetic block should be performed after induction to provide intra- and postoperative analgesia.
- Penile nerve block using plain 0.25% levobupivacaine (1–3 mL) for babies aged less than 1 year and plain 0.5% levobupivacaine (3–5 mL) for those aged over 1 year (Box 24.1)

Box 24.1 Penile nerve block

- The nerves lie deep and superficial to Buck's fascia and may be separated by a midline septum
- Supine position
- Aseptic technique
- A 21 G regional block needle is used
- Palpate the lower border of the symphysis pubis with the index finger and retract the penis
- Insert the needle between finger and the arch of the pubis until there is a slight 'give' or bone is struck; if bone is struck, 'walk' the needle inferiorly until it is free
- Local anaesthetic solution should be injected either side of the midline by directing the needle from a single puncture
- Aspirate before injecting deep and superficial to Buck's fascia
- Minimal swelling should be seen
- Analgesia should last about 4–6 hours

Box 24.2 Caudal extradural block of the sacral nerves

- The sacral hiatus is located by placing the child on his side with legs flexed at the hips. The posterior superior iliac spines are located with the thumb and middle finger, and an equilateral triangle formed with the index finger will reliably locate the sacral hiatus at the lower end of the vertebral column
- A 22 G cannula or a regional block needle is used
- The cannula or needle is advanced through the sacrococcygeal membrane at the apex of the hiatus until a 'give' is felt. The cannula or needle should be advanced only a few millimetres to avoid dural puncture
- A single-shot caudal block does not cause hypotension in children
- Analgesia should last about 4–6 hours and up to 12 hours with caudal additives

- Alternatively, a single-shot caudal extradural block, using 0.25% levobupivacaine (0.5 mL kg^{-1}), is suitable (Box 24.2).
- Clonidine (1–2 μg kg^{-1}) or preservative-free ketamine (0.5 mg kg^{-1}) additives may be used to prolong the caudal block.

Postoperative management

- Good postoperative analgesia is essential for smooth recovery; be prepared to supplement with oral or intravenous opioids.
- Provide an information leaflet, contact details and oral analgesia on discharge.

Outcome

Discharge may be delayed by:

- failure to micturate (more likely with inadequate analgesia; penile block has a higher failure rate than caudal)
- bleeding
- unsteady when walking (occasionally with caudal epidural, but should delay discharge in young children)
- nausea and vomiting.

Bibliography

Peutrell J, Mather SJ. *Regional Anaesthesia in Babies and Children*. Oxford: Oxford University Press, 1996.

Rickwood AMK, Walker J. Is phimosis over diagnosed in boys and are too many circumcisions performed in consequence? *Ann R Coll Surg Engl* 1989; **71**: 275–7.

Shankar KR, Rickwood AMK. The incidence of phimosis in boys. *Br J Urol* 1999; **84**: 101–2.

Cross-references

Infants and children, 615

Local anaesthetic toxicity, 767

Congenital diaphragmatic hernia

Andrew J Charlton

Presentation

The incidence of congenital diaphragmatic hernia is 1 in 2–4000 live births. It is probably a primary defect of lung growth, and right-sided hernia (10%) is associated with higher mortality.

Congenital diaphragmatic hernia presents with respiratory failure at birth or, now more often, at antenatal ultrasonography. Patients have bilateral pulmonary hypoplasia (normal side affected by mediastinal shift during growth) and tend to revert to fetal circulation with severe right–left shunting.

Death occurs because of:

- inadequate gas exchange surface
- fixed high pulmonary vascular resistance (decreased vascular cross-sectional area, normal cardiac output)
- reversible pulmonary hypertension (abnormal muscularity of vessels)
- pneumothorax
- additional anomalies (5%) and complications of intensive therapy.

Resuscitation

Mask inflation distends herniated viscera, worsening mediastinal shift and risking pneumothorax. Use immediate tracheal intubation, with muscle relaxants to facilitate IPPV. Nasal intubation aids secure fixation and ventilator compliance. Pass a nasogastric tube to deflate the gut and keep on free drainage.

Preoperative preparation

Surgery often worsens lung mechanics and is not an emergency. Time (days) should be taken to stabilize and improve gas exchange by meticulous medical management aiming to avoid trigger factors for pulmonary vasoconstriction (hypoxia, hypercarbia, acidosis) and allow the normal physiological fall in pulmonary vascular resistance to occur. Precise indicators of the optimal time for surgery have not been established.

Monitoring

Peripheral arterial cannulation allows arterial pressure and blood gas monitoring with minimal disturbance. Published predictive indices require postductal oxygen values. Pulse oximeters placed pre- and postductally may demonstrate the variability of shunting.

Ventilation

- Risk of pneumothorax from high inflation pressures and asynchrony.
- Muscle relaxants (such as atracurium or cisatracurium) by infusion give optimal control and decrease oxygen consumption. Continue until weaning after surgery.
- 'Gentle ventilation strategies' (peak airway pressure <25 mmHg) reduce barotrauma.
- No firm evidence for benefit from individual treatment modalities (e.g. surfactant, high-frequency oscillatory ventilation, nitric oxide (iNO), extracorporeal membrane oxygenation (ECMO)).
- Protocolized care may improve institutional survival.

Acid–base status

Metabolic acidosis should be corrected with buffers. Moderate alkalosis by systemic alkalinization (to pH 7.5–7.6) or hyperventilation (to $P_{a}co_{2}$ 30–35 mmHg) may enhance pulmonary circulation.

Pulmonary circulation

Refractory hypoxaemia may respond to pulmonary vasodilators. iNO 10–20 p.p.m. has superseded other agents. Oral sildenafil is undergoing clinical trials.

Fluid balance

Preoperative restriction (6 mL kg^{-1} per 24 hours) avoids fluid retention. Initial maintenance fluid should contain 5–10% glucose (e.g. 0.18% NaCl with 10% glucose), switching to parenteral nutrition by 48 hours. Circulating volume should be maintained with plasma or blood (maintain Hb above 14 g dL^{-1}).

Sedation

Lability in response to handling (unusual) may be helped by a narcotic (e.g. morphine) infusion.

Surgery

Usually undertaken via an upper abdominal incision, which permits correction of gut malrotation. In about 5% of cases, closure can only be achieved with a prosthetic patch or latissimus dorsi muscle flap. Such patients are often slower to wean. Thoracoscopic surgery may be possible.

Anaesthesia

- Surgery causes little disturbance if delayed to permit inspired oxygen requirement to stabilize below 50%.
- The exact pattern of preoperative ventilation should be continued.
- Volatile agents should be avoided: risk of cardiovascular depression.
- Fentanyl in large doses (up to 25 μg kg^{-1}) obtunds the response to surgery (even with 100% oxygen) and has a negligible cardiovascular effect. An alternative is a remifentanil infusion.
- Monitoring must include ECG, direct or indirect arterial pressure, pulse oximetry, capnography and body temperature.
- A glucose-containing maintenance fluid should be used in place of parenteral nutrition intraoperatively and for 24 hours postoperatively. Blood glucose should be monitored. Intraoperative losses can be replaced with an isotonic fluid (e.g. Hartmann's solution or 0.9% NaCl) or 4% human albumin. Red cell transfusion is rarely required.

Postoperative care

General intensive care with attention to fluid and nutritional requirements (enteral or parenteral) must continue. Weaning from IPPV in severe cases may take months. After tracheal extubation a period on continuous positive airway pressure is usual. The most severely affected survivors have little respiratory reserve, require long-term oxygen therapy and may die in infancy from respiratory infection.

Extracorporeal membrane oxygenation

ECMO has little impact on survival statistics. Consider in severely ill patients (oxygenation index (OI) >0.4; OI = $F_{I}co_2$ × mean airway pressure/$P_{a}o_2$) who have a reversible (additional) pathology. Transport to an ECMO centre is hazardous.

Outcome

Current management has evolved without controlled trials. Reported mortality in large series ranges from 29 to 55% (but note case selection bias). Most survivors become functionally normal. The most severely affected may exhibit chronic lung disease and developmental impairment.

Bibliography

Moyer V, Moya F, Tibboel R, *et al.* Late versus early surgical correction for congenital diaphragmatic hernia in newborn infants. *Cochrane Database Syst Rev* 2002; (3): CD001695.

Robinson PD, Fitzgerald DA. Congenital diaphragmatic hernia. *Paediatr Resp Rev* 2007; **8**: 323–5.

Sakai H, Tamura M, Hosokawa Y, *et al.* Effect of surgical repair on respiratory mechanics in congenital diaphragmatic hernia. *J Pediatr* 1987; **111**: 432–8.

Tracy ET, Mears SE, Smith PB, *et al.* Protocolized approach to the management of congenital diaphragmatic hernia: benefits of reducing variability in care. *J Pediatr Surg* 2010; **45**:1343–8.

Cross-reference

Infants and children, 615

Tracheo-oesophageal fistula and oesophageal atresia

Stephen Greenhough

Procedure

Tracheo-oesophageal fistula (TOF) and oesophageal atresia repair is performed as follows:

- left lateral position (right side up)
- axillary skin crease or axillary longitudinal incision
- extrapleural approach, if possible
- requires compression collapse of right lung
- in the presence of oesophageal atresia, closure of TOF and either primary oesophageal anastomosis or gastrostomy with or without oesophagostomy is required.

Patient characteristics

- Generally less than 1 week old.
- Incidence of 1 in 3500 live births.
- 30% of babies are premature.

There are several different combinations of fistula and atresia. The three most common are oesophageal atresia and lower pouch fistula (80%), oesophageal atresia with no fistula (10%), and TOF with no oesophageal atresia (2%) (Fig. 24.1).

Common associations with TOF

- Polyhydramnios during pregnancy.
- Increasing antenatal diagnosis.
- Up to 30% of babies are premature or low birth weight.
- 30–50% have additional anomalies as part of the VACTERL association: vertebral, anal, cardiac, tracheo-esophageal (US spelling), renal and limb anomalies.

Preoperative assessment and investigations

Routine

- Haemoglobin.
- Urea and electrolytes.
- Cranial ultrasonography.
- Single X-ray of chest and abdomen.
- Cross-match blood.

Specific

- Rectal examination.
- Renal ultrasonography.
- Echocardiography.
- Blood gases if indicated, especially if premature.

Preoperative management

- Replogle tube to prevent aspiration of saliva.
- A small number of premature babies may require positive pressure ventilation. If lung compliance is

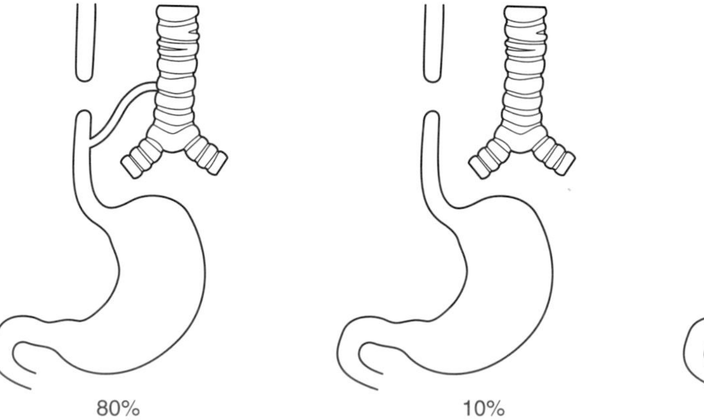

Figure 24.1 Common presentations of oesophageal atresia.

low and the fistula large, immediate surgery may be the only method of achieving adequate ventilation.

Theatre preparation

- High theatre temperature.
- Warming blanket.
- Humidification of inspired gases.

Perioperative management

Induction

- In the operating theatre.
- Thiopental and atracurium.

Tracheoscopy

- Requires a ventilating bronchoscope to identify the fistula position.
- A small percentage of patients will have upper and lower pouch fistulae.
- In some units, flexible fibreoptic bronchoscopy is an alternative.

Monitoring

- ECG.
- S_aO_2.
- Non-invasive blood pressure.
- $ETCO_2$.
- Core temperature.

Care should be taken with placing the monitors. The axillary artery in the uppermost arm may be compressed by surgical traction.

Maintenance

- Oxygen and nitrous oxide with 0.5–2% sevoflurane and fentanyl 1–2 µg kg^{-1}.
- Inspired oxygen may occasionally need to be increased during lung collapse.

Special considerations

Many authors stress the importance of tracheal tube placement relative to the fistula in order to prevent excessive quantities of gas being forced into the stomach. In the author's unit, this risk is believed to be overstated and normal length tracheal tubes are sited irrespective of fistula position. Gastric distension is much more commonly the result of overvigorous ventilation with high airway pressures; gentle hand ventilation is the best way of avoiding this. Lung collapse is produced by surgical retraction, which has the advantage of compressing both alveoli and blood supply together, making ventilation–perfusion mismatch uncommon. This method of collapsing the lung does, however, commonly result in intermittent tracheal obstruction owing to overenthusiastic retraction by the assistant. Hand ventilation using a Jackson Rees T-piece allows obstruction to be detected instantly and also allows reinflation of the compressed lung periodically during periods of surgical inactivity.

Immediate postoperative period

Although TOF repairs can be managed without elective postoperative ventilation, it may be difficult to predict which patients will require ventilation and which will not. In order to decrease the risk of collapse requiring emergency ventilation, often during the hours of darkness, patients with TOF repair in the author's unit are electively ventilated overnight. A small number of patients, particularly preterm babies, may require longer periods of ventilation. It is common surgical practice to request ventilation for difficult TOF repairs for periods of between 5 and 10 days postoperatively. In ventilated babies, care should be taken with both tracheal suction and physiotherapy to avoid the risk of disruption of the repair.

Outcome

- Good in TOF with no other abnormalities.
- Overall survival is about 90%.
- If there are associated anomalies, the mortality rate is much higher.
- A small number have tracheal weakening at the site of the fistula and may require aortopexy, tracheopexy or, in severe cases, tracheoplasty before extubation is possible.

Bibliography

Goh DW, Brereton RJ. Success and failure with neonatal tracheo-oesophageal anomalies. *Br J Surg* 1991; **78**: 834–7.

Keckler SJ, St Peter SD, Valusek PA, *et al.* VACTERL anomalies in patients with esophageal atresia: an updated delineation of the spectrum and review of the literature. *Pediatr Surg Int* 2007; **23**: 309–13.

Waterston DJ, Bonham-Carter RE, Aberdeen E. Oesophageal atresia: tracheo-oesophageal fistula. A study of survival in 218 infants. *Lancet* 1962; **1**: 819–22.

Cross-references

Infants and children, 615

25 Cardiac surgery

Akbar Vohra

Aortic valve surgery

Akbar Vohra

Aortic stenosis

Physiological considerations

Aortic stenosis can be either congenital (in which case the valve is abnormal and bicuspid in over 50% of cases) or acquired (usually from rheumatic involvement of a previously normal valve). In the absence of other valvular disease, aortic stenosis is almost always congenital in origin. If it is of rheumatic aetiology, there is usually involvement of the mitral valve as well. The normal aortic valve area (AVA) is >2.0 cm^2. 'Severe' aortic stenosis has an AVA of <1 cm^2 and 'moderate' aortic stenosis has an AVA of 1.0–1.4 cm^2.

As aortic stenosis develops, there is a progressive increase in outflow obstruction to the left ventricle. Systolic pressures within the left ventricle rise and a pressure gradient develops between the left ventricle and the aorta. Increased systolic chamber pressure stimulates parallel replication of sarcomeres with consequent wall thickening and concentric ventricular hypertrophy. The consequences of this are twofold. First, the ventricle relaxes poorly during diastole, so LVEDP rises and higher filling pressures are needed to maintain cardiac output. The ventricle becomes increasingly dependent on atrial contraction to ensure diastolic filling and the atrium (in sinus rhythm) contributes up to 40% of left ventricular end diastolic volume (LVEDV) in aortic stenosis compared with 10–15% in normal patients. The sudden onset of atrial fibrillation (which suggests a rheumatic aetiology) can precipitate a major fall in cardiac output. Second, the balance between myocardial oxygen supply and demand becomes precarious. This is because increased myocardial bulk and high cavity pressures increase myocardial oxygen demand, while increased wall thickness and raised LVEDP predispose to subendocardial ischaemia. The relationship between diastolic time (determined by heart rate), LVEDP and the systemic diastolic pressure available for coronary perfusion (determined by cardiac output and SVR) is therefore critical. Coincident coronary artery disease is a serious added risk factor for these patients.

With aortic stenosis there is usually a long (can be up to 50 years or more) asymptomatic period and sudden death may be the first presenting feature. The most common symptoms are syncope, angina, dyspnoea and dysrhythmias. When symptoms finally occur the stenosis is severe. Their significance, particularly signs of left ventricular failure, are ominous and if the stenosis is not surgically corrected death occurs within a few years.

The ECG will show left ventricular hypertrophy (LVH) if aortic stenosis is significant, often with ST segment changes of left ventricular strain. Unless there is left ventricular failure (LVF) the chest X-ray will show a normal transverse diameter of the heart. If LVF has supervened there will be cardiomegaly and lung field changes. Specialist investigation is by coronary angiography and ultrasound.

General anaesthetic principles

Anaesthetic technique is similar to that described under Coronary artery bypass grafting, p. 580. The physiological objective is to maintain the basic haemodynamic state by carefully managing heart rate, filling pressure and systemic blood pressure. Give antibiotic prophylaxis.

Hypotension

Very dangerous. Caused by low cardiac output, hypovolaemia or vasodilatation. It implies that a ventricle generating high intracavity pressures is being perfused by a low-pressure arterial system. Needs immediate correction with an α-agonist, while the underlying cause is remedied.

Tachycardia

Dangerous. Produces myocardial ischaemia (sometimes acute LVF), and reduces cardiac output by increasing dynamic impedance of stenosis. Treat cause (light anaesthesia, hypovolaemia, etc.). Do not give β-blockers. Persistent dysrhythmias affecting cardiac output may need d.c. synchronized cardioversion.

Bradycardia

Moderate degrees tolerated. Reduces dynamic impedance of stenosis. If severe with very low diastolic pressures, use tiny doses of glycopyrrolate and avoid overcorrection at all costs.

Preload on left ventricle

Must be maintained to ensure filling of hypertrophied ventricle.

Afterload on left ventricle

Changes have little effect on valve pressure gradient and hence left ventricular load, but the effect on systemic blood pressure in the aortic root significantly changes coronary perfusion.

Monitoring

Invasive arterial monitoring is mandatory prior to induction. ECG monitoring must be able to detect left ventricular ischaemia and diagnose dysrhythmias; use V_5 and standard lead 2 leads. In practice, it may be difficult to interpret 'ischaemic' changes owing to pre-existing ST abnormalities caused by LVH (strain pattern).

The CVP is a poor indicator of left ventricular filling when left ventricular compliance is reduced. A flotation catheter, however, may cause severe and persistent dysrhythmias as it passes through the right ventricle.

Persistent ischaemia in the face of appropriate corrective measures necessitates early institution of CPB. In the event of cardiac arrest, defibrillate immediately. Only internal massage is effective because of valve stenosis, and emergency bypass may be required. Do not commence anaesthesia unless a theatre and bypass facilities are immediately available.

Intraoperative care, management of bypass and postoperative care are as described elsewhere under Coronary artery bypass grafting, p. 580 and Postoperative care of adult patients after cardiopulmonary bypass, p. 589.

Aortic regurgitation

Physiological considerations

Aortic regurgitation may be acute or chronic. Chronic causes are rheumatic valve disease, connective tissue disorders or a congenital bicuspid valve. Acute aortic regurgitation is most commonly caused by infective endocarditis or trauma. The basic problem is volume overload of the left ventricle caused by blood leaking through the incompetent aortic valve during diastole. The degree of regurgitation is determined by the size of the regurgitant orifice and the diastolic time interval. Systemic vasodilatation, increased inotropy and tachycardia all contribute to increased forward flow in patients with aortic regurgitation and may explain the phenomenon of mild exercise tolerance with symptoms at rest. Over a period of time, eccentric left ventricular hypertrophy, gross cardiomegaly and impaired oxygen supply result.

Mild to moderate degrees of chronic regurgitation are well tolerated and there is a long asymptomatic period. Symptoms, when they arise, are usually those of LVF or angina. The life expectancy of patients with significant aortic regurgitation is about 9 years. Sudden death is rare. In acute aortic regurgitation there is a sudden volume overload of the left ventricle with a dramatic rise in the LVEDP. Ventricular dilatation enlarges the mitral valve annulus resulting in functional mitral regurgitation. Pulmonary oedema is marked and refractory. Very severe aortic regurgitation with gross distortion of the valve ring can result in dissection, which may involve the coronary arteries.

General anaesthetic principles

Anaesthetic technique is as for coronary artery bypass grafting (CABG). Only severe aortic regurgitation is a major anaesthetic risk. If there is an associated dissection, refer to the appropriate section. Remember antibiotic prophylaxis.

Bradycardia

Allows time for back flow into the ventricle and increases regurgitant fraction. Treat carefully with glycopyrrolate or a very small dose of epinephrine, dobutamine or isoprenaline.

Tachycardia

If mild, it is well tolerated, because it increases dynamic impedance of reverse flow through valve.

Preload

This needs to be maintained to keep the dilated ventricle full.

Afterload

This needs to be kept low to enhance forward flow. A balance has to be found between good cardiac output and an aortic perfusion pressure adequate to perfuse the coronary arteries of the dilated ventricle.

Monitoring

As for aortic stenosis. In severe cases, use of a pulmonary artery flotation catheter allows one to maximize cardiac output by afterload reduction, while maintaining preload by titrating fluid replacement to pulmonary artery capillary wedge pressure.

Principles of intra- and postoperative management are as for CABG and ICU care.

Bibliography

Kaplan JA, Reich DL, Lake CL, Konstadt SN (eds) *Kaplan's Cardiac Anesthesia*, 5th edn. Philadelphia, PA: WB Saunders.

Cross-references

Aortic valve disease, 126
Elective surgery, 610
Premedication, 619

Cardiopulmonary bypass: principles, physiology and biochemistry

Akbar Vohra

The objective of cardiopulmonary bypass (CPB) is to allow surgery on the heart and great vessels while the rest of the body is perfused with oxygenated blood and the products of metabolism are removed. Bypass necessitates anticoagulation with heparin (usually 3–4 mg kg^{-1}) and haemodilution. Abnormal surface interactions between blood, air and plastics damage cells and denatures proteins. Air and particulate microemboli may enter the bypass circuit via suction, so blood filters are essential.

The CPB circuit

This is shown diagrammatically in Fig. 25.1. Venous cannulae are inserted into the right atrium, the venae cavae or, more rarely, the femoral vein or pulmonary artery. The large-bore venous return line drains blood, under gravity, from the patient on the table to the reservoir of the bypass machine on the floor. The reservoir is either a rigid casing or a bag (soft-cell). Blood is then pumped through the oxygenator, where it is oxygenated and carbon dioxide is removed. In addition, a heat exchanger allows heating and cooling of the blood. The pumps driving the flow may be compression roller devices or use centrifugal force (centrifugal pumps). The blood is returned to the body via an aortic or, more rarely, a femoral cannula after passing through a filter. The arterial cannula is always inserted first.

There are additional auxiliary roller pumps, which feed blood into the circuit. One (sometimes called the 'coronary sucker' or 'cardiotomy sucker') acts as a sucker to return blood in the operative field to the bypass circuit. The other (sometimes called the 'vent') aspirates gently from the left ventricle, or pulmonary artery to prevent ventricular distension, and from the aortic root when retrograde cardioplegia is used. During bypass when the heart is arrested and there is no effective ejection, blood draining from the bronchial and thesebian veins and retrogradely across the aortic valve collects in the left ventricle. Ventricular distension causes mechanical damage, impairs subendocardial perfusion and can result in subendocardial infarction.

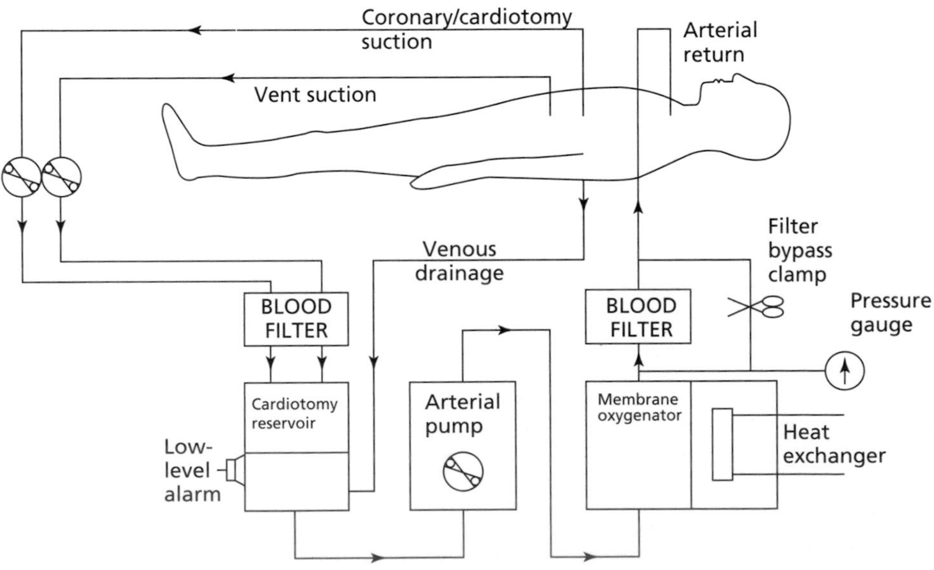

● **Figure 25.1** The cardiopulmonary bypass circuit.

Poor venous return is occasionally a problem and can result from kinks, air locks, drainage tube malposition, decreased circulating blood volume, sequestration of blood into body cavities or into the tissues or from vasodilator therapy. When the heart is rotated by the surgeons operating on the circumflex arteries, not only can venous return be impaired but also venous drainage from the brain may be sufficiently obstructed to cause jugular venous hypertension with an acute rise in central venous pressure (CVP). This obviously needs immediate correction. Complications of aortic cannulation are embolization (from air and wall debris), haemorrhage, dissection and malposition (abutting the aortic wall), and this can be detected by high arterial supply line pressures in the presence of normal flow rates. It is usually amenable to repositioning. Complications of venous cannulae are haemorrhage, reduction of venous return, arrhythmias and atrial or caval damage.

Management of anticoagulation

The activated clotting time should be kept three times greater than the baseline, or over 450 seconds, by the use of heparin. The patient must be anticoagulated adequately before the arterial return cannula is inserted, or a clot will form on its tip and within its lumen. At the end of bypass, the action of the heparin is reversed with protamine. Protamine is a potent vasodilator, and decreases in blood pressure should be anticipated and treated. No blood must be returned to the pump via suction after this. If it is, clot formation can occur in the pump, making an emergency return to bypass impossible and preventing the blood being used later for autotransfusion.

Aprotinin was frequently used for patients with a high risk of bleeding. Regimes ranged from 500 000 to 2 000 000 KIU to the patient and 2 000 000 KIU in the pump and occasionally a 500 000 KIU h^{-1} infusion. This was withdrawn from routine use owing to data suggesting increased morbidity and mortality, although its reintroduction has recently been suggested. Some units now use tranexamic acid (2 g bolus followed by infusion) as an alternative. Problems of graft occlusion associated with these two drugs are as yet inconclusive.

Thromboelastography

Thromboelastography (TEG) is a method of evaluating the formation and breakdown of a clot. A small amount of blood is placed into the machine to obtain values for the following parameters:

- *R time* is the period of time to initial fibrin formation.
- *K time* is a measure of the speed to reach a certain level of clot strength.
- α measures the rapidity of fibrin build-up and cross-linking (clot strengthening).
- *Maximum amplitude (MA)* represents the ultimate strength of the fibrin clot.
- *LY30* measures the rate of amplitude reduction 30 minutes after MA.

It may be used to evaluate platelet function, plasma factors and activators/inhibitors of coagulation. Thus, it may be of use as a guide to appropriate therapy for postoperative bleeding. However, standard cups will not indicate the level of platelet inhibition due to aspirin or clopidogrel. The specialized cups for aspirin and clopidogrel effect are available.

Temperature, flow and pressure on CPB

There are many controversies surrounding the management of CPB. For instance, some centres routinely use normothermic bypass whenever possible, whereas others invariably use hypothermic bypass. The advantages claimed for normothermic bypass are reduced bypass time (no cooling or warming needed), reduction in postoperative clotting dysfunction and reduced postoperative cooling (afterdrop) and shivering with its increased metabolic demand and tissue hypoxia. For normothermic bypass, flow rates of greater than 2.2 L min^{-1} m^{-2} are usually used. Hypothermic bypass reduces metabolism and oxygen consumption falls by a factor of 2.5 (known as the Q10), for every 10°C fall in temperature. Moderate hypothermia (25–30°C) is commonly used for adult coronary and valve work, with an associated reduction in flow rate. For some operations (e.g. on the aortic arch), circulatory arrest is needed. The brain will tolerate approximately 1 hour of arrest during deep hypothermia at 15–18°C. Even moderate hypothermia permits a brief (approximately 12 minutes) period of circulatory arrest, which may be life-saving if there is a catastrophic mechanical failure or circuit disruption.

Management protocols vary considerably in relation to the perfusion pressure to be maintained on bypass. As far as the heart is concerned, when the aorta is clamped and the heart protected by cardioplegia, myocardial perfusion pressure is irrelevant. If the aorta is not cross-clamped the heart is least likely to suffer ischaemic damage if it is kept empty, beating and well perfused. During intermittent cross-clamping techniques, the fibrillating ventricle consumes more oxygen than the beating but unloaded heart. At normothermia, with autoregulation, cerebral blood flow is maintained at 50 mmHg mean perfusion pressure. Under hypothermia, with reduced metabolic demand, lower perfusion pressures can be tolerated and many regard 40 mmHg as satisfactory. A number of retrospective studies indicate no relationship between hypotension during bypass and postoperative neurological dysfunction. There is a greater correlation with ascending aorta calcification. Typical UK practice is to fix the flow rate and then keep the mean perfusion pressure above 50 mmHg and below 80 mmHg. Pharmacological management of blood pressure centres around the use of α-agonists (metaraminol, phenylephrine, norepinephrine) and smooth-muscle relaxants (sodium nitroprusside, glyceryl trinitrate and phentolamine).

The use of pulsatile flow is controversial and outcome data on its benefits are lacking. Physiological models would suggest that such flow improves perfusion and oxygen uptake; achieving it requires intermittent roller pump action or external reservoir compression, both of which add complexity to the circuit. It is not commonly used.

Biochemical and haematological control of CPB

For adult patients, the CPB is primed with 1.5–2 litres of balanced asanguinous salt solution (e.g. 1000 mL Gelofusine plus 800 mL Hartmann's solution and 200 mL mannitol 10%), to which heparin is added. This causes significant haemodilution with a reduction in the total oxygen-carrying capacity per millilitre. On the other hand, by reducing viscosity, haemodilution improves blood rheology and prevents microcirculatory sludging during hypothermia. Most anaesthetists consider a haematocrit of >15% to be satisfactory for bypass.

Oxygen flow into the oxygenator should be sufficient to maintain an arterial P_ao_2 of over 14 kPa. If this produces unacceptable hypocapnia then carbon dioxide will need to be added to the oxygenator gas flow to reduce carbon dioxide washout. Some centres now use in-line electrodes to monitor both arterial and venous blood gas status, the oxygen saturation in the venous line being used to confirm acceptable blood flow rates, with the arterial–venous difference across the pump confirming satisfactory oxygenator function. Guidelines for minimal monitoring during bypass must be followed.

There is controversy over the optimum method of blood gas management during hypothermic CPB. The α-stat method aims to achieve a pH of 7.4 and a P_aco_2 of 40 mmHg when blood drawn from the hypothermic patient is measured at 37°C: the pH stat method aims to achieve a pH of 7.4 and a P_aco_2 of 40 mmHg when blood drawn from the hypothermic patient is measured at the *in vivo* temperature. A comparison between the two methods is shown in Table 25.1. Alpha-stat management is thought to preserve autoregulation and coupling of flow and metabolism in the brain better than pH stat, and therefore is currently gaining favour.

The most important electrolyte to monitor on CPB is potassium, because correct levels optimize contractility and suppress dysrhythmias. High levels can be reduced by haemofiltration, diuresis, and insulin and dextrose and countered by calcium. Low levels can be corrected by giving incremental doses of 10–20 mmol of potassium chloride. These need correcting near the end of the bypass phase, just prior to coming off bypass.

Temperature measurements on bypass

It is vital to measure the body temperature on bypass. The temperature of the nasopharynx is generally used to approximate to that of the brain. Thorough rewarming is essential. Normal central blood temperatures at the end of bypass after the patient has been rewarmed do not, however, represent the temperature in peripheral, poorly perfused tissues. After the discontinuation of CPB an 'afterdrop' is usually seen, which is caused by the opening up of cold, vasoconstricted tissue beds, particularly muscle. This can lead to post-bypass shivering with its high metabolic load.

Table 25.1 α stat versus pH stat blood gas management

In *vivo* temperature (°C)	Measured and reported at 37°C				Corrected to in *vivo* temperature			
	pH_a	v_aco_2 (mmHg)		pH_a	P_aco_2 (mmHg)			
	α stat	pH stat	α stat	pH stat	α stat	pH stat	α stat	pH stat
37	7.40	7.40	40	40	7.40	7.40	40	40
33	7.40	7.34	40	47	7.44	7.40	35	40
30	7.40	7.30	40	54	7.50	7.40	29	40
27	7.40	7.26	40	62	7.55	7.40	26	40
23	7.40	7.21	40	74	7.60	7.40	22	40
20	7.40	7.18	40	84	7.65	7.40	19	40

Reproduced with permission from Hindman BJ, Lillehaug SL, Tinker JH. Cardiopulmonary bypass and the anesthesiologist. In: Kaplan JA (ed.) *Cardiac Analgesia*, 3rd edn. Philadelphia: Saunders, 1993, pp. 919–50.

Bibliography

Fergusson DA, Hébert PC, Mazer CD, *et al*; BART Investigators. A comparison of aprotinin and lysine analogues in high-risk cardiac surgery. *N Engl J Med* 2008; **358**: 2319–31.

Mangano DT, Tudor JC, Dietzel C, for the Multicenter Study of Perioperative Ischemia Research Group and the Ischemia Research and Education Foundation. The risk associated with aprotinin in cardiac surgery. *N Engl J Med* 2006; **354**: 353–65.

Cardiopulmonary bypass: sequelae

Akbar Vohra

During CPB, normal physiology and biochemistry are significantly altered by changes in blood pressure and flow, temperature and haemodilution. The blood is in contact with abnormal surfaces in the oxygenator, heat exchanger, reservoir, tubing, cannulae and filters. These factors can lead to systemic and cerebral complications. Fortunately, the incidence of serious morbidity from them is sufficiently low (0.5–1%) for CPB to be regarded as a safe procedure in the majority of patients. There is, however, a much higher incidence of more minor and subtle effects which are usually temporary and which the patient may not notice.

Blood flow, pressure and temperature are abnormal during CPB. At the onset of CPB using a crystalloid prime there can be a sharp drop in the blood pressure. This is caused by the lower systemic flow and the sudden fall in blood viscosity as the crystalloid is pumped into the circulation. Subsequently during bypass the systemic vascular resistance (SVR) usually gradually increases towards the normal range. A further reduction may be seen when the cross-clamp is removed, particularly in patients receiving blood cardioplegia.

Although the endocrine response cannot be separated from that due to anaesthesia and surgery, during CPB there is a generalized increase in serum catecholamine levels in excess of those seen in operations not utilizing CPB. There is no pulmonary metabolism of norepinephrine; renin secretion is increased, and with this follows angiotensin activation and aldosterone secretion. Vasopressin levels increase considerably during CPB and remain elevated for up to 48 hours following surgery. These increased levels of catecholamines, angiotensin and vasopressin, together with local tissue vasoconstrictor agents, lead to arteriolar constriction. A mild hyperglycaemia may be seen following CPB, owing to increased gluconeogenesis, peripheral insulin resistance, a decrease in serum insulin and raised adrenocorticotropic hormone and cortisol levels.

Total body water is increased at the end of CPB, the extra water being contained in the extracellular and extravascular spaces. Haemodilution and the increased capillary permeability resulting from activation of inflammatory mediators are the major factors causing this fluid shift.

Damaging effects of the CPB circuit

The exposure of blood to abnormal surfaces during CPB causes platelet activation and aggregation, the net effect being a reduction in platelet numbers and impairment in function of those which remain. Platelet damage is probably the most important factor in the bleeding diathesis associated with CPB. Proteins are denatured by contact with foreign surfaces, and this can lead to activation of various clotting and fibrinolytic cascades with consumption of clotting factors, microcoagulation, fibrin generation and complement activation. The complement cascade results in the production of powerful anaphylotoxins which increase capillary leakage, mediate leukocyte chemotaxis and facilitate leukocyte aggregation and enzyme release. There is mechanical damage to leukocytes and erythrocytes from the shear stresses caused by turbulence from the pumps, suckers, abrupt changes in velocity of blood flow and cavitation around the cannula tip. Damage to blood produces fibrin microemboli, aggregates of denatured protein and lipoproteins and platelet and leukocyte aggregates. Particulate emboli in spilt blood are aspirated by suckers and returned to the bypass circuit. There can be significant air emboli during aortic cannulation, during filling of the beating heart after removal of the aortic cross-clamp and during discontinuation of CPB despite meticulous de-airing techniques. In about 1 in 1000 procedures a critical incident will occur from malfunction of the extracorporeal circuit.

Specific organ damage associated with CPB

Heart

CPB, *per se*, has only a minor effect on cardiac dysfunction unless there has been inadequate myocardial protection or perfusion. Post-bypass cardiac function is more closely related to the preoperative condition of the heart and the success of surgery.

Lungs

Abnormalities of lung function following CPB are frequent, with clinical manifestations of atelectasis and pulmonary oedema. Acute lung injury leading to adult respiratory distress syndrome (ARDS) occurs in less than 1% of patients. A reduction in functional residual capacity with an increased A–a difference may persist for up to 10 days. Sputum retention and ineffective coughing, which contribute to pulmonary morbidity, are consequences of the surgery and postoperative care rather than the CPB.

Kidneys

Renal dysfunction occurs to some degree in 1–4% of patients following CPB. It is usually due to acute tubular necrosis and, although potentially reversible, is associated with a high mortality. Factors associated with an increased risk of renal failure are pre-existing renal impairment, long bypass times and low cardiac output. Drugs such as aminoglycoside antibiotics and non-steroidal anti-inflammatory drugs (NSAIDs) may be contributory.

Gastrointestinal tract

Gastrointestinal tract complications develop in less than 2% of patients following CPB, but the associated mortality is high. The commonest problem is upper gastrointestinal bleeding and is maximal on the 10th postoperative day. Hyperbilirubinaemia has been reported in up to 20% of patients. Rare complications are ischaemic bowel and ischaemic pancreatitis.

Neurological

These can be divided into global, focal or neuropsychological complications. Global damage often presents as a prolonged depression of conscious level unrelated to sedation and is seen in up to 3% of patients. In serious cases there are frequently signs of widespread neurological dysfunction present. Patients in coma for over 24 hours have a high mortality, and poor prognostic signs include extensor posturing, the absence of motor responses and seizures. Choreoathetosis is a rare but serious complication occurring almost exclusively in paediatric patients who have had total circulatory arrest. Sensorineural hearing loss is often missed clinically, but up to 13% of patients have been reported to have a hearing loss of greater than 10 dB following CPB.

Focal events or strokes (defined as a focal central nervous system deficit of relatively sudden origin that lasts for more than 24 hours) are the major cause of persisting neurological disability following cardiac surgery. They are usually seen as an acute hemiparesis or visual field defect and have been reported as occurring in 1–6% of patients after coronary artery bypass grafting. Approximately 70% of cardiac-related strokes occur intraoperatively and 30% in the early postoperative period. Acute focal deficits due to air emboli usually resolve steadily over the first 24 hours. Membrane oxygenators have been shown to produce fewer microemboli than bubble oxygenators, and there are fewer microvascular occlusions seen in the retinal microcirculation when using a membrane oxygenator than when using a bubble oxygenator.

The most important risk factors for cerebral damage during CPB are increasing age, a previous cerebrovascular event, pre-existing carotid or cerebrovascular disease, aortic atherosclerosis, valve surgery, left ventricular thrombus, poor preoperative cardiac function, the occurrence of microemboli and long bypass times. Current evidence suggests that the best way to reduce the sequelae of CPB is to perform the surgery meticulously and expeditiously, with minimum suction of shed blood, using a membrane oxygenator and a 40 mm main arterial filter.

Bibliography

Kaplan JA, Reich DL, Lake CL, Konstadt SN (eds). *Kaplan's Cardiac Anesthesia*, 5th edn. Philadelphia, PA: WB Saunders.

Cross-reference

Cardiopulmonary bypass: principles, physiology and biochemistry, 568

Congenital heart disease: general principles

Sally Wilmshurst

Many patients are now surviving beyond childhood and presenting for revision surgery to the regional adult congenital heart disease centres. Common surgical interventions include revision surgery for pulmonary valve incompetence or stenosis; right ventricular outflow obstruction at the subvalvular or pulmonary artery level requiring new conduits and valve replacement are necessary. Residual atrial and ventricular septal defects are also relatively common. The usual problems of surgery for revision cardiac surgery apply. These patients are usually young adults and occasionally have other medical syndromes.

Congenital heart disease first needs to be classified and the basic principles of anaesthesia for cardiac surgery explained. An understanding of the lesions and surgery are also helpful when anaesthetizing children with heart disease for non-cardiac surgery.

Epidemiology

The incidence is eight per 1000 live births:

Ventricular septal defect (VSD)	20%
Atrial septal defect (ASD)	10%
Tetralogy of Fallot (TOF)	6%
Transposition of the great arteries (TGA)	5%
Coarctation	5%

There is an association with other 'midline' abnormalities, e.g. tracheo-oesophageal fistula and imperforate anus. It can also occur as part of a number of syndromes, including those with airway involvement, e.g. Down syndrome (in 40%) or Pierre Robin syndrome. Congenital heart disease may result from teratogenic exposure, e.g. maternal alcohol (25%) or rubella (35%).

Classification

Shunts

In shunts, blood moves between the oxygenated and deoxygenated sides of the circulation.

Left-to-right

- ASD.
- VSD.
- Atrioventricular septal defect.
- Patent ductus arteriosus (PDA).
- Partial anomalous pulmonary venous drainage.

Right-to-left

- TOF.
- Double-outlet right ventricle.
- TGA.
- Total anomalous pulmonary venous drainage.
- Pulmonary atresia.
- Tricuspid atresia.
- Truncus arteriosus.

Obstructive lesions

- Aortic coarctation.
- Aortic stenosis (valvar, subvalvar and supravalvar).
- Pulmonary stenosis.
- Interrupted aortic arch.

Single ventricle

- Congenital, e.g. hypoplastic left heart syndrome, double inlet left ventricle.
- Acquired as result of a surgical strategy, e.g. Glenn, Fontan.

Other congenital heart diseases

- Congenital complete heart block.
- Inherited cardiomyopathies.

General principles

Minor lesions can present as an incidental finding, such as a heart murmur on routine cardiac examination. Neonates constitute 25% of the practice, many of whom have duct-dependent disease and are maintained on intravenous prostaglandin E_1 (Prostin). These are often antenatally diagnosed with improvements in screening and imaging.

Palliation versus repair

Repair implies a return to normal physiology and normal life expectancy. Palliative surgery aims to improve quality and quantity of life, or allow growth so that a more definitive repair can be attained later.

Differences between children and adults

Children are smaller and have immature physiology and pharmacokinetics, especially neonates. The cardiac pathology is more varied and there is less comorbidity. Palliative procedures and 'open' surgery are more common and cyanosis and pulmonary hypertension is more often present.

CPB in children

Haemodilution is greater (the smallest pump prime volume possible is around 300 mL) and multiple venous cannulae are often required. Aortopulmonary collaterals may be present, affecting emptying of the heart. Deep hypothermic arrest is more commonly used. Modified ultrafiltration (MUF) is used in small children to remove excess fluid and inflammatory mediators, thereby reducing transfusion requirements and lung injury.

Preoperative assessment

History

Cardiac symptoms

Failure to thrive, tachypnoea, poor feeding and sweating are all features of cardiac failure. Squatting and blue lips may signify cyanotic spells. Blackouts and chest pain may occur, although a history of pain is difficult to obtain in the younger child.

Other history

It is important to obtain a drug history, especially for cardiac medication and anticoagulant therapy, ascertain any allergies and take the usual general and anaesthetic history.

Examination

Cardiac signs

Shortness of breath, sweating, tachycardia, raised jugular venous pressure and hepatomegaly are seen in cardiac failure. In addition to routine observations, blood pressure needs to be measured in all four limbs in the presence of a coarctation and saturation measured pre- and postductally. Capillary refill time is useful, especially if the patient is acutely unwell.

Other systems

Features of coexisting diseases or syndromes should be noted. An assessment of the respiratory system and any end-organ damage should be made. If airway difficulties are anticipated, a detailed assessment should be undertaken prior to anaesthesia.

Investigation

The following investigations may be available.

Cardiac

- ECG.
- Echocardiogram.
- Reports from catheter studies/cardiac CT/cardiac MRI.
- Chest X-ray.

Blood test

- Full blood count.
- Renal, especially if taking diuretics or antihypertensive therapy.
- Clotting.
- Ensure the patient is appropriately cross-matched.

Anaesthetic considerations

Preoperative visit

During the preoperative visit, the child and parents are given a detailed explanation of the anaesthetic and postoperative care including:

- requirement for premedication
- type of induction
- monitoring, including TOE if required
- blood transfusion
- postoperative ICU
- analgesia and sedation.

Conduct of anaesthesia

Intravenous or inhalational induction is used, although inhalational is preferred in small children and neonates. Maintenance is usually with moderate- to high-dose fentanyl (10–50 $\mu g\ kg^{-1}$) and volatile anaesthesia. Both isoflurane and sevoflurane have ischaemic preconditioning properties. Long-acting muscle relaxants can be used for long cases in which postoperative ventilation is expected. Inotropes may be required pre- or post-CPB, depending on the type of surgery.

Monitoring

Standard monitoring

- Three or five lead ECG.
- Pulse oximetry (pre- and postductal may be required).
- End-tidal capnography (beware large arterial to end-tidal gradient with low pulmonary blood flow states).
- Ventilation and volatile agent monitoring.
- Urine output.
- Core and peripheral temperature.
- Invasive pressure monitoring.
- Arterial line (site may be important if duct-dependent, Blalock–Taussig (BT) shunt or in the presence of vascular abnormalities).
- Central venous line (usually right internal jugular or femoral).
- Surgically sited lines, e.g. left atrium or pulmonary artery.

Other monitors

- Near infrared spectroscopy (NIRS).
- TOE.

Transoesophageal echocardiography

This is becoming increasingly the standard of care for paediatric bypass cases. Paediatric 8 Hz multiplane probes are suitable for infants >3 kg. TOE is used to assess anatomy before and after bypass, to look for air after cardiotomy and to estimate cardiac function. Complications are rare.

Special circumstances

Neonates

Neonates often have duct-dependent lesions. They have immature physiology, pharmacology and haemostasis. The myocardium is sensitive to the extracellular calcium concentration and they have a fixed, rate-dependent cardiac output. On bypass, there is massive dilution of haemoglobin and clotting factors.

Redo sternotomy

Congenital lesions are often repaired or palliated in stages. Scar tissue forms during healing and components of the heart may become attached to the back of the sternum and be damaged during reopening. Bleeding is expected and ventricular fibrillation can occur owing to excessive diathermy near to the heart. The patient must be prepared for emergency initiation of bypass via the femoral vessels if the heart becomes damaged on opening. Externally placed defibrillation pads are used.

Fast-track cardiac surgery

Simple surgery may be suitable for a shorter intensive care stay, including lesions such as ASD and VSD and conduit replacements. Early extubation is performed, either in theatre or early on the ICU and anaesthesia needs to be tailored to allow this.

Cyanotic patients

Right-to-left shunting lesions result in cyanosis; if this is chronic, patients can become polycythaemic and coagulopathic through a variety of mechanisms. There is a risk of thrombosis and cerebral infarction if the haematocrit is >60%. Avoiding long preoperative fasting and dehydration is important.

Bibliography

Bingham R, Lloyd Thomas A, Sury M (eds). *Hatch & Sumner's Textbook of Paediatric Anaesthesia*, 3rd edn. London: Hodder Arnold, 2007.

Eliot May L. *Pediatric Heart Surgery: A Ready Reference for Professionals*. Milwaukee: Maxishare, 2008.

Lake CL, Booker PD. *Pediatric Cardiac Anesthesia*, 4th edn. Philadelphia: Lippincott, Williams & Wilkins, 2004.

Cross-references

Cardiopulmonary bypass: principles, physiology and biochemistry, 568

Infants and children, 615

Congenital heart disease: management of specific lesions

Sally Wilmshurst

Anaesthesia for left-to-right and right-to-left shunts

Shunts, whether left-to-right or right-to-left, are managed under anaesthesia by manipulating the relative systemic (SVR) and pulmonary (PVR) vascular resistances.

Raising SVR increases left-to-right shunt, whereas lowering SVR or raising PVR increases right-to-left shunt. General anaesthetic agents usually lower SVR. The SVR can be raised using vasopressor agents such as phenylephrine or metaraminol. PVR is raised by hypoxia, acidosis, cold, hypercarbia, excessive ventilation pressures and drugs such as norepinephrine and dopamine. PVR is kept to a minimum by normoxia, hypocarbia and alkalosis, and drugs such as milrinone and nitric oxide, which is used as a treatment for pulmonary hypertension.

In addition, great care must be taken to avoid air or particulate emboli which may enter the arterial circulation. Severe shunts require endocarditis prophylaxis as per local guidelines.

Atrial septal defects

Several different types of ASD exist; the commonest requiring closure is the ostium secundum defect. They commonly coexist with other cardiac lesions. Isolated ASDs usually present incidentally, usually in older children, and are generally well tolerated. Pulmonary hypertension may develop in later life owing to long-standing high pulmonary blood flow and vascular damage.

Anaesthetic considerations

The main anaesthetic issues are discussed above. Some are suitable for device closure in the catheter laboratory. Surgery is usually straightforward and the patient may be suitable for 'fast-tracking'. Occasionally, rhythm problems may occur because of atrioventricular node damage.

Ventricular septal defects

Several different types of VSD occur according to the location within the ventricular septum (membranous or muscular) and the area of the ventricular cavity (inlet, outlet, apical, subvalvar) in which they lie. VSDs commonly occur in complex cardiac lesions. Small muscular VSDs may close spontaneously, and small perimembranous VSDs may be occluded by tricuspid valve tissue and be insignificant, or cause mild progressive aortic regurgitation. Larger lesions cause significant left-to-right shunting, pulmonary overload and heart failure and present early.

Over time, the shunt can reverse owing to chronic injury to the pulmonary vascular bed, leading to pulmonary hypertension and eventually Eisenmenger syndrome.

Anaesthetic considerations

The main anaesthetic implications are discussed above. In addition, the pulmonary vasculature may be reactive. Very small babies may be unsuitable for early VSD repair and a band is used on the pulmonary artery to minimize shunting. Surgical repair of a VSD can result in damage to the ventricular conducting tissue from suturing in the patch, especially with perimembranous lesions. Temporary or even permanent pacing may be required.

Postoperative cardiac dysfunction may occur, especially if the ventricle has been opened.

Device closure in the catheter laboratory is becoming more common.

Patent ductus arteriosus

Failure of the arterial duct to close is common, especially in preterm babies. In older children, it can be incidental and asymptomatic. Larger ducts can cause severe heart failure and pulmonary hypertension. Diastolic blood pressure is usually low in the presence of a significant duct. In preterm babies, left-to-right flow can cause low cardiac output, failure to wean from ventilation and necrotizing enterocolitis. Medical management involves treatment of heart failure and the use of indometacin to close the duct.

In older children, the duct can be occluded using a device in the catheter laboratory.

In younger children, or in those with a large lesion, surgical closure is performed via a thoracotomy.

Anaesthetic considerations

The general anaesthetic issues are discussed above. Catastrophic bleeding can occur if the duct or nearby vessels are damaged; therefore, cross-matched blood should be available. In neonates, the duct can be difficult to distinguish from the aorta or pulmonary artery and these can be mistakenly ligated. Monitoring of postductal blood pressure, saturation and end-tidal capnography should confirm that the duct has been ligated. Diastolic blood pressure will rise after ligation of a large duct.

After repair

After correction of an ASD, VSD or PDA, children are generally well. Endocarditis prophylaxis is not required in the absence of a residual lesion.

Tetralogy of Fallot

This relatively common condition has the features of a VSD, a malaligned aorta over-riding the VSD, right ventricular outflow tract obstruction and right ventricular hypertrophy. A spectrum of outflow tract obstruction severity occurs, from absent pulmonary valve to pulmonary atresia. The presence of β-adrenergic receptors in the outflow tract causes intermittent worsening of right-to-left shunting during pain and stress, which manifests as cyanotic spells. Typically, children squat during a cyanotic spell to increase the SVR and reduce right-to-left shunting. Preoperative β-blockers may be prescribed. Some children are asymptomatic and never become noticeably cyanosed.

Surgical repair involves closure of the VSD, and relief of the outflow tract obstruction. Sometimes pulmonary valve replacement or a patch to enlarge the valve is required. Surgical repair usually takes place around 6 months of age but severe cases may be managed with a BT shunt as a neonate. Some centres perform full neonatal repair.

Anaesthesia considerations

The degree of shunting can be controlled as above. Some patients are cyanotic and prolonged fasting and dehydration should be avoided. Cyanotic spells occurring under anaesthesia can be managed with:

- vasopressor therapy, e.g. phenylephrine 4 μg kg^{-1}
- fluid bolus
- opiate analgesia
- β-blockade, e.g. propranolol 0.1 mg kg^{-1}.

Cyanotic spells can occur even if there is no history, especially during line insertion and surgical manipulation. An audible pulse oximeter is useful as a warning.

Surgical complications include damage to the conducting system and junctional ectopic tachycardia (JET). Postoperative complications include myocardial dysfunction, JET and restrictive right ventricular physiology, leading to pleural and pericardial effusions, low cardiac output and renal failure.

After repair

Long-term complications include pulmonary regurgitation and ventricular dilatation and further surgery is usually required in early adulthood. Children who present for non-cardiac surgery after repair should be well from a cardiac point of view, but may require endocarditis prophylaxis if prosthetic material is present within the repair, or a residual valve gradient or VSD exists.

Transposition of the great arteries

In this condition, the great arteries arise from the wrong ventricle. It usually presents as desaturation when the arterial duct closes early in life. Reopening of the duct with Prostin is necessary for mixing of oxygenated and deoxygenated blood and balloon atrial septostomy is often performed to improve mixing and to allow withdrawal of Prostin. Variants include TGA with intact ventricular septum and TGA with VSD. Coronary anatomy can be variable.

In 'congenitally corrected TGA', the atria also drain to the wrong ventricular chamber, but the venous return reaches the correct great artery.

Surgical repair is undertaken early in life, while the PVR remains high in the neonatal period. Delayed repair results in a left ventricle that cannot cope with a systemic afterload. Surgery can be delayed in the presence of a VSD but accelerated pulmonary hypertension is a risk.

Surgical repair involves transection and switching of the great arteries, and transplanting the coronary arteries to the new aorta which is formed from the pulmonary artery stump. It is long surgery and bleeding from extensive aortic suture lines is expected. Post-bypass ischaemia can occur as a result of coronary problems, and the left ventricle can have difficulty coping with the systemic afterload, so left atrial pressure is usually continually monitored after bypass and on ICU. Fluid and blood products must be carefully administered as they can result in elevated left atrial pressure.

Often, the chest is left open for a few days postoperatively.

After repair

Cardiac anatomy is usually restored to normal after repair, although sometimes pulmonary artery stenosis can occur.

Coarctation of the aorta

A coarctation of the aorta may present in the neonate as a duct-dependent obstruction to the circulation, or in later childhood as a result of systemic hypertension or a murmur. Collaterals develop in older children. The narrowing often occurs at the site of the arterial duct tissue.

Repair may be urgent or scheduled and usually involves a thoracotomy. Occasionally, a long section of the aorta is involved and repair takes place on CPB with circulatory arrest.

Anaesthetic considerations

Maintenance of arterial duct patency with Prostin may be required in the neonate. The site of blood pressure monitoring depends on the level of the coarctation, head and neck blood pressure is measured proximal to the obstruction and femoral pulses may be impalpable.

During surgical repair the aorta is cross-clamped and fluid loading is necessary prior to unclamping. Long cross-clamp times can result in spinal cord ischaemia. Hypertension can develop rapidly after repair and may need nitrate or nitroprusside therapy.

After repair

Recoarctation is common and can often be managed in the catheter laboratory.

Single-ventricle (Fontan) circulations

In some situations, a single-ventricle circulation is created surgically in which the ventricle supports the systemic circulation and pulmonary blood flow comes directly from the systemic veins. The single ventricle can be a right or a left ventricle. Lesions requiring a Fontan strategy include hypoplastic left heart syndrome and tricuspid atresia.

A single ventricle is created in stages by creating a superior vena cava to pulmonary artery communication (Glenn) at around 6 months of age, followed by a total cavopulmonary connection during early childhood when the inferior vena cava is also connected (Fontan). For hypoplastic left heart syndrome, early neonatal surgery is also performed.

Early complications include high systemic venous pressure leading to head and neck swelling and pleural and pericardial effusions. Late complications include ventricular failure, arrhythmias, thrombosis and protein-losing enteropathy.

Anaesthetic considerations

Preoperatively patients are often cyanotic, so long fasting times and dehydration must be avoided or thrombosis can occur in existing shunts. Because surgery is staged, precautions must be taken for redo surgery (see above). Pulmonary blood flow is passive and reversed during intermittent positive pressure ventilation and PEEP; therefore, minimal ventilator settings and an early return of spontaneous ventilation is optimal.

After repair

An increasing population of single-ventricle patients are presenting for non-cardiac surgery. Some patients will be taking long-term anticoagulant therapy. Occasionally, a communication is left between the inferior vena cava and right atrium (fenestration), in which case paradoxical air embolus, desaturation and endocarditis remain a risk.

Careful positioning is essential to maintain systemic venous return as flow into the pulmonary arteries is passive. Overventilation and atelectasis must be avoided or spontaneously ventilating strategies used.

Bibliography

Bingham R, Lloyd Thomas A, Sury M (eds). *Hatch & Sumner's Textbook of Paediatric Anaesthesia*, 3rd edn. London: Hodder Arnold, 2007.

Eliot May L. *Pediatric Heart Surgery: A Ready Reference for Professionals*. Milwaukee: Maxishare, 2008.

Lake CL, Booker PD. *Pediatric Cardiac Anesthesia*, 4th edn. Philadelphia: Lippincott, Williams & Wilkins, 2004.

Cross-references

Atrial septal defect, 129

Cardiopulmonary bypass: principles, physiology and biochemistry, 568

Infants and children, 615

Tetralogy of Fallot, 169

Coronary artery bypass grafting

Akbar Vohra

Physiological considerations

Coronary artery disease (CAD) is the leading cause of death in Western societies and coronary artery bypass graft (CABG) surgery constitutes 50–60% of most cardiac surgical programmes. The heart extracts oxygen to a greater extent than any other organ with only minimal increases in oxygen extraction possible; therefore, any increase in oxygen demand must be met by increasing flow. In health, this is done by autoregulation and in the absence of CAD maximal flow is four to five times as great as at rest. The coronary arteries arborize on the surface of the heart to form a mass of smaller epicardial arteries from which 'B' branches perforate directly through the myocardium to reach the endocardium (Fig. 25.2). These vessels are subject to torsion and pressure during muscular contraction which in the left ventricle results in the majority of useful myocardial perfusion occurring during diastole. The only collateral circulation exists at subendocardial level and becomes of importance if there is a blockage in an epicardial vessel. Patients with classic CAD are asymptomatic at rest. As the severity of the stenosis increases, coronary flow reserve declines, resting CBF is preserved by progressive vasodilation of the microcirculation, and the onset of angina of effort occurs with increased demand. Coronary artery bypass grafting aims to bypass epicardial blockages using either the internal mammary artery or with vein grafts taken from the leg and so increase myocardial blood flow and oxygen delivery.

General anaesthetic considerations

Preoperative assessment

This comprises history, examination and investigations. The history should concentrate on the symptoms of ischaemic heart disease, i.e. degree of angina pectoris (Canadian Heart Association Classification) and, when it occurs, previous infarction, exercise tolerance, shortness of breath and orthopnoea leading to functional debility (American Heart Association Classification). Diabetes mellitus, renal disease, hypertension, vascular disease and pulmonary disease are common associated problems. These are all added risk factors for patients undergoing CABG. Knowledge of perioperative medication is essential with antianginal agents and anticoagulant or platelet-inhibiting drugs being of particular importance. While the patient should continue with the usual antihypertensive and/or antidysrhythmic medication, platelet-inhibiting drugs, such as aspirin and clopidogrel, should be stopped 1 week prior to surgery to avoid antiplatelet effects at operation. Angiotensin-converting enzyme inhibitors have been associated with low SVR perioperatively and should, therefore, be omitted on the day of surgery.

On examination, physical findings are often few in this group of patients, but look for signs of right and left ventricular failure and check the arterial pulses. If there is a marked difference in right- and left-sided

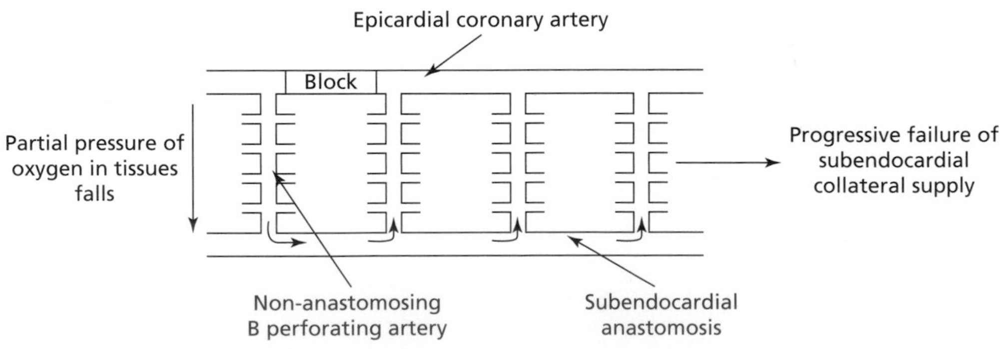

Figure 25.2 Perfusion of the left ventricular wall.

pulses one should monitor from the strongest, as this will be the better reflection of aortic root pressure. If carotid bruits or stenoses are present, make a note to avoid jugular lines on that side.

Investigations involve routine preoperative tests which include urea and electrolytes, haemoglobin, chest X-ray, ECG, as well as more invasive procedures, e.g. cardiac catheterization. The last can give information on left ventricular function and ejection fraction. A low ejection fraction, the presence of ventricular dys-synergy, high left ventricular end-diastolic pressure (LVEDP) or pulmonary hypertension suggest a strong possibility of post-CABG myocardial dysfunction. All patients must have a baseline 12 lead ECG for postoperative comparison.

Premedication

The purpose of premedication is to pharmacologically reduce apprehension, fear and the stress of painful events, e.g. insertion of an intra-arterial catheter prior to induction. Commonly used drugs include benzodiazepines (e.g. oral lorazepam, diazepam or temazepam) and intramuscular opiates (e.g. morphine). Metoclopramide, sucralfate and ranitidine may be used to reduce the volume and acidity of the gastric contents. Premedication should be supplemented with face-mask oxygen in a safe clinical environment.

Intraoperative management

Remember antibiotic prophylaxis.

Monitoring

Commence by establishing good peripheral venous access, an arterial line and a multilead ECG (leads II and V5). Following induction, additional monitoring will involve insertion of a central venous catheter, using the internal jugular or subclavian routes, temperature probes and urinary catheter. The use of a pulmonary artery catheter (PAC) varies from centre to centre, but one would be indicated in patients with abnormal left ventricular function, recent myocardial infarction or postinfarction sequelae, e.g. ventricular septal defect, left ventricular aneurysm, mitral regurgitation. In some patients who may or may not need a PAC it is sensible to insert a PAC sheath to facilitate easy insertion of a PAC postoperatively if required. Transoesphageal echocardiography use is increasing, is almost routine in some units and is mandatory for mitral valve repair surgery.

Anaesthesia

The fundamental principle of any anaesthetic technique is to minimize myocardial ischaemia and prevent awareness. It is probably the experience of use of the available drugs which is of greater importance than the particular agent itself. Prior to induction of anaesthesia, the patient should be preoxygenated. Induction of anaesthesia needs to be smooth with cardiovascular stability, but simultaneously adequate to prevent the sympathetic response to laryngoscopy and intubation. Agents which have been used successfully for induction with or without opioid supplementation include propofol, etomidate, thiopentone and ketamine. Some centres use high-dose opioid techniques (fentanyl 50 μg kg^{-1}) for the whole procedure, with very modest benzodiazepine supplementation.

Probably the most commonly used induction technique in UK practice is a slow bolus of opioid (fentanyl 10–15 μg kg^{-1}) followed by a small dose of induction agent. Maintenance is usually provided by an opioid infusion (e.g. remifentanil (1–3 μg kg^{-1} min^{-1}) or alfentanil 50 μg kg^{-1} h^{-1}), combined with a low dose of either a volatile or an intravenous agent. Propofol by infusion can be used for maintenance at a rate of 5–6 mg kg^{-1} h^{-1} or as target controlled infusions to achieve adequate serum levels during CPB. Of the volatile agents, isoflurane has received much attention because its known vasodilator properties have been implicated in causing myocardial ischaemia through the coronary steal mechanism. However, this has been shown not to be of relevance at concentrations less than 1.5% and may even provide protection against myocardial ischaemia. Both enflurane and halothane have been and are still used for maintenance in CABG anaesthesia. Isoflurane is probably the most commonly used volatile anaesthetic agent. If there is poor urine flow in the presence of an adequate circulating fluid volume and blood pressure consider furosemide (bolus or infusion). All the currently available muscle relaxants have been used to produce adequate intubating and maintenance conditions during anaesthesia for CABG. The cardiovascular side-effects of pancuronium are sometimes used therapeutically to counter the bradycardias caused by the fentanyl group of drugs.

During dissection of the internal mammary artery, one should observe the blood pressure during insertion of the Chevalier retractor. There can be a genuine fall owing to right ventricular compression or (if the arterial cannula is in the ipsilateral arm) an artefactual fall owing to stretching of the subclavian artery.

The management and sequelae of bypass are described in other sections. Adjust serum potassium to between 4.5 and 5.5 mmol L^{-1} prior to cessation of bypass.

In addition to the goals of providing anaesthesia and muscle relaxation, in the pre- and post-bypass periods myocardial ischaemia must be minimized by the anaesthetist, and this requires constant observation of the ECG. If ischaemic changes do occur (which can be manifested by dysrhythmias and low cardiac output as well as by ST segment changes),

in cardiac output. This dysrhythmia is often extremely resistant to both external and internal cardioversion, and inotropic support may be required to support systemic blood pressure. Inotropes may in turn cause tachycardia, thus worsening the situation, and should be administered with caution. These patients also have a relatively fixed cardiac output and severe reductions in SVR may be associated with a severe reduction in systemic blood pressure. Potent vasodilators including the nitrovasodilators should be used with extreme caution in this group.

Mitral incompetence

Physiological considerations

Mitral incompetence results in dilatation of both the left atrium and the left ventricle. During systole the regurgitant flow causes high pressure to be transmitted to the left atrium and increases left ventricular work. In contrast to mitral stenosis, there is no obstruction to forward flow through the valve, with the exception of a combined stenotic and regurgitative lesion. Any increase in SVR will limit left ventricular forward ejection and thus encourage retrograde flow into the more compliant atrium. An increased afterload causes decreased forward flow and increased regurgitant flow, and in this respect these patients are sensitive to peripheral vasoconstrictors. The magnitude of regurgitant flow is determined by the size of the regurgitant orifice and the pressure gradient across it; the orifice size tends to parallel ventricular size. Increased preload causes left atrial dilatation and further stretching of the mitral valve orifice, which may result in a decrease in ventricular forward flow owing to an increased regurgitant flow into the atrium. In common with mitral stenosis these patients may progress to pulmonary hypertension and cor pulmonale. It is important to realize that acute mitral incompetence may be due to posterior left ventricular papillary muscle damage induced by myocardial infarction. In this case, the left atrium may be small, making replacement of the valve technically difficult. This group are especially sensitive to increases in SVR. Patients with mitral regurgitation caused by coronary artery disease, including those with recent myocardial infarction, require extremely careful anaesthesia.

General anaesthetic principles

Anaesthetic technique is similar to that described for CABG and must include antibiotic prophylaxis. The anaesthetic aims for these patients are centred around the maintenance of forward flow through the left ventricle:

Systemic vascular resistance

- An increased SVR increases the tendency for regurgitative flow, and vasoconstrictors should be avoided.

Preload

- A large increase in preload causes atrial distension and the relatively rapid onset of pulmonary oedema.

Heart rate

- Bradycardia reduces ventricular filling and increases the degree of regurgitation; however, a moderate tachycardia increases forward flow, and is thus preferable.

Monitoring considerations

It has been suggested that faster, fuller and vasodilated are the principles on which forward flow in mitral regurgitation may be maintained. In these circumstances (especially when using potent vasodilators and with the dangers of vascular overfilling) a pulmonary artery catheter allows assessment of intravascular filling, measurement of cardiac output and evaluation of therapeutic intervention. In patients with high pulmonary artery pressures, evidence of tricuspid regurgitation should be looked for in the CVP trace. Passive tricuspid regurgitation results from right ventricle dilatation in the face of increased afterload from pulmonary hypertension (PHT). There are few attractive therapies for this combination of PHT and right ventricular failure and attention should be paid to basic principles, including the avoidance of hypoxia, hypercarbia and acidosis. One promising therapeutic strategy for the treatment of PHT is the use of prostaglandin E_1 (prostacyclin), a potent dilator of pulmonary arterial smooth muscle. It has been noted that prostacyclin is also a systemic vasodilator. However, it has the theoretical advantage of having pulmonary endothelial first-pass metabolism, and may be considered as a 'pulmonary-specific' vasodilator when given via the right atrium. Enoximone and milrinone may be used as they reduce systemic and pulmonary vascular resistance as well as improving inotropy.

Summary

Anaesthesia for replacement or repair of an incompetent mitral valve is dominated by the need for a relatively low SVR allowing the left ventricle to eject the majority of its output into the systemic circulation and reducing regurgitant flow into the left atrium. A high end-systolic LAP increases the incidence of pulmonary oedema and inhibits diastolic left atrial filling. Valve repair is becoming increasingly more common. TOE is vital in assessing the repair.

Bibliography

Braunwald E. Valvular heart disease. In: Braunwald E (ed.) *Heart Disease*, 5th edn. Philadelphia: W.B. Saunders, 1997, pp. 1007–76.

Chaffin JS, Dagget WM. Mitral valve replacement: a nine year follow up of risks and survivals. *Ann Thorac Surg* 1979; **27**: 3–12.

Cross-references

Cardiopulmonary bypass: principles, physiology and biochemistry, 568
Mitral valve disease, 156
Premedication, 619

Postoperative care of adult patients after cardiopulmonary bypass

Akbar Vohra

The increase in demand for cardiac surgery, caused mainly by coronary artery disease, has led to a marked rise in the number of patients presenting to postoperative ICUs. The trend has been towards the development of specialized postcardiac surgery units with protocol-based care becoming the norm. The protocols used and the duration of postoperative ventilation, etc., vary considerably from one unit to another. However, the basic principles of postoperative care are common to all patients and are summarized below. For convenience the postoperative period has been divided into transfer, early and late phases.

Transfer period

Following the completion of surgery, patients are usually transferred to their intensive care bed within theatre and transported on it to the ICU. The distances involved vary enormously from one hospital to another. This is a period of great potential instability and, unless the transfer distance is very short indeed, at the very least ECG and intra-arterial pressure monitoring should be continued. The development of modern transport monitors has made this a much easier task.

The early postoperative period (0–6 hours)

The essentials of the early postoperative care of these patients are summarized in Box 25.1.

Box 25.1 Care in the early postoperative period

- Analgesia and sedation
- Assisted ventilation with/without PEEP
- Measurement of arterial blood gases, potassium, haemoglobin, etc.
- Adjustment of inspired oxygen concentration
- Maintenance of cardiac rhythm; treatment of arrhythmias
- Control of postoperative hypertension
- Haemodynamic monitoring
- Manipulation of cardiac filling pressures
- Maintenance of adequate cardiac output
- Maintenance of adequate renal perfusion and urine output
- Fluid management; colloid replacement, crystalloids
- Monitoring and treatment of clotting/platelet abnormalities
- Reduction of heat loss; assisted rewarming

Analgesia and sedation

Adequate opioid analgesia is essential, but there is wide variability in the drugs and routes of administration used; fentanyl, alfentanil, pethidine and morphine are all popular. The use of high doses of fentanyl (40–60 mg kg^{-1}) intraoperatively provides analgesia well into the postoperative period; alfentanil is a potent short-acting agent and is given by continuous infusion. Remifentanil appears to be associated with an acute withdrawal syndrome sometimes requiring higher initial doses of opioid at the cessation of infusion. Morphine is widely available, cheap and has useful additional sedative properties, but care should be taken in patients with poor renal function due to the accumulation of active metabolites. Epidurals are used at some centres. The NSAIDs are now widely used after general surgery, but they all inhibit the renal protective actions of prostaglandins during hypotension and should be used with great caution in the early postoperative period. In some patients, despite adequate analgesia, additional sedation may be required; propofol, midazolam and isoflurane (0.4–0.6%) are popular and combine a short duration of action with acceptable haemodynamic stability. Shivering is an important complication in the early postoperative period as it markedly increases oxygen consumption and must be suppressed by adequate analgesia and sedation (e.g. pethidine 10–20 mg).

Assisted ventilation

The duration of mechanical ventilation after cardiac surgery is very variable even in routine patients, varying from none (extubation on the operating table) to several hours. Improvements in surgical and anaesthetic techniques with a reduction in CPB times, less hypothermia, epidurals, etc., have led to a trend towards earlier extubation in many centres. Safety is an important consideration and it seems prudent to continue mechanical ventilation until adequate rewarming (at the least to central normothermia), adequate analgesia, haemostasis and haemodynamic stability have been achieved.

A degree of atelectasis is common after cardiac surgery, especially if the pleura has been breached during internal mammary dissection. Low levels of positive end-expiratory pressure (PEEP; 2.5–5 cmH_2O) are widely used after cardiac surgery; they improve oxygenation in the presence of pulmonary oedema and may play a role in reversing atelectasis. The adverse haemodynamic effects of PEEP are exacerbated by hypovolaemia.

Most modern intensive care ventilators incorporate the facilities for weaning in the form of synchronized intermittent mandatory ventilation with inspiratory assist. Mandatory breaths are gradually reduced to zero and, if adequate ventilation is maintained, then the patient is extubated. Many factors may precipitate more prolonged periods of mechanical ventilation. These include previous lung pathology, haemodynamic instability, persistent pulmonary oedema, delayed neurological recovery and pulmonary infection.

Monitoring

Box 25.2 lists the basic monitoring required in the postoperative period.

Box 25.2 Basic monitoring after cardiopulmonary bypass

- ECG (rate, rhythm, ST changes)
- Intra-arterial blood pressure
- Central venous pressure
- $F_{I}O_2$, respiratory rate, airway pressures, tidal and minute volumes
- Arterial blood gases
- Pulse oximetry
- Serum potassium
- Blood loss
- Haemoglobin, clotting screen, platelet count
- Blood sugar
- Core and peripheral temperatures
- Chest X-ray
- Urine output

Haemodynamic manipulation

Skilled haemodynamic monitoring and manipulation are essential after CPB. In UK practice, most routine patients do not have pulmonary artery catheters inserted and the adequacy of cardiac output has to be estimated from a combination of arterial blood pressure, urine output, peripheral rewarming and the absence of a metabolic acidosis. Early hypotension is most commonly due to hypovolaemia exacerbated by the vasodilatation that occurs during the rewarming phase. CVPs should be maintained by the infusion of colloids, including blood, if indicated. The pressure required is variable, but, in the absence of significant ventricular dysfunction, pulmonary hypertension, etc., a level of 5–8 mmHg is a reasonable starting point. Hypertension after CPB is also common and should be treated to avoid excessive left ventricular workloads, suture-line disruption and bleeding. Having ensured adequate analgesia and sedation, nitrodilators (glyceryl trinitrate, sodium nitroprusside) form the mainstay of treatment.

Arrhythmias are common after cardiac surgery and require aggressive treatment because of their effects on cardiac output and blood pressure. When they occur, always quickly ensure that the patient has not become acutely hypoxic from a simple cause such as ventilator disconnection. Hypokalaemia is a common contributing factor and serum potassium should be maintained at 4.5–5.0 mmol L^{-1}. Following CPB, ventricular function is often impaired and many patients have relatively fixed stroke volumes. Persistent bradycardias should be avoided by making use of pacing, isoprenaline or dobutamine infusions, for example, to maintain the heart rate; rates of 60–100 beats min^{-1} are usually considered optimal.

The absolute indications for the instigation of more complex haemodynamic monitoring in the form of PAWP measurements and thermodilution cardiac output measurements are difficult to define. Failure to rewarm, oliguria, worsening metabolic acidosis and persistent hypotension despite apparently adequate filling pressures are all good indications. Pericardial tamponade should be high on the list of suspected causes if these conditions develop in the postoperative period. TOE should be considered at an early stage. Mixed venous oxygen saturation is also a good indicator of perfusion.

Inotropic agents, such as enoximone, dobutamine and epinephrine, are indicated if the cardiac index is low despite adequate filling. A low SVR occurring after prolonged bypass may require the use of norepinephrine.

Renal function

Although acute renal failure requiring dialysis is rare after uncomplicated cardiac surgery, degrees of oliguria are common. Although there is little scientific evidence, dopamine at 'renal' doses (e.g. 3 mg kg^{-1} h^{-1}) is still used both intra- and postoperatively. Dopexamine may be a suitable alternative. It is important to maintain a diuresis in the postoperative period so as to reverse the anaemia from haemodilution caused by the bypass prime and the cardioplegia. Good volume status, cardiac output and mean blood pressure are the mainstay for management. If oliguria persists despite an adequate cardiac output and blood pressure, small doses of a loop diuretic are indicated.

Fluid management

Cardiac filling pressures should be maintained by the infusion of colloid solutions, including the modified gelatins, albumin solutions and blood. Free water is required for the formation of urine, and in the absence of pulmonary oedema our routine practice is to give all patients 1 mL kg^{-1} h^{-1} of crystalloid (dextrose saline, saline or Hartmann's solution). Although circulating hypovolaemia is common, tissue dehydration is rare in the immediate postoperative period, the usual problem being an increase in total body water.

The late postoperative period (after 6 hours)

In a routine case, following extubation, the activities described above are continued, but the emphasis shifts towards preparing the patient for return to the high-dependency unit (HDU) or ward. Most patients require oxygen to be administered by face-mask to maintain arterial saturations above 95%. Oral, intramuscular or rectally administered analgesics may be prescribed and the patient undergoes regular chest physiotherapy. If postoperative complications develop, or if the patient's progress is slow, the intensive care administered during the first few hours is continued. In these circumstances, every effort must be made to look for correctable causes of the failure to progress. Observing the deterioration closely but without intervention achieves nothing.

Bibliography

Kaplan JA, Reich DL, Lake CL, Konstadt SN (eds) *Kaplan's Cardiac Anesthesia*, 5th edn. Philadelphia, PA: WB Saunders.

Rauf K, Vohra A, Fernandez-Jimenez P, *et al.* Remifentanil infusion in association with fentanyl/propofol anaesthesia in patients undergoing cardiac surgery. The effect on morphine requirement and postoperative analgesia. *Br J Anaesth* 2005; **95**(5): 611–15.

Cross-references

Cardiopulmonary bypass: principles, physiology and biochemistry, 568
Postoperative oliguria, 779
Postoperative pain management, 783

Postoperative care of paediatric patients after cardiopulmonary bypass

Sally Wilmshurst

After cardiac surgery, most children are kept sedated and ventilated on intensive care for a few hours to several days, the goal being to minimize cardiac work and oxygen requirements. In some circumstances, it is possible to expedite extubation and intensive care, especially after uncomplicated surgery. This process is called fast-tracking. Good analgesia is required. Sedation is usually achieved with a combination of opioid analgesia and midazolam infusions. Sometimes muscle relaxants are needed, especially if the chest remains open or if the patient is unstable. Organ dysfunction after cardiac surgery is not confined to the cardiovascular system, especially after surgery for complex lesions or when there has been a complication.

Cardiovascular system

Even in stable patients, careful attention to myocardial function is required and myocardial work should be kept to a minimum. Systemic blood pressure needs to be controlled to allow normal organ perfusion without hypertension, which can disrupt suture lines.

Low cardiac output syndrome is common after cardiac surgery and inotropes may be required, commonly a combination of milrinone and epinephrine is used. Milrinone is a phosphodiesterase inhibitor with venous, arterial and pulmonary artery dilating properties. As well as its inotropic action, it is also a lusitrope, promoting active diastolic relaxation without increasing myocardial oxygen demand. It is useful in fast heart rates, such as those seen in younger children, and is usually commenced in the operating theatre as a loading dose of 50 μg kg^{-1} followed by a maintenance infusion at 0.3–0.75 μg kg^{-1} min^{-1}.

MUF is a technique used after separation from CPB to remove water and inflammatory mediators in smaller patients. This reduces myocardial oedema and improves cardiac function.

Rhythm disturbances can be seen after cardiac surgery. Heart block can occur after trauma to the conducting tissue and may need pacing. Tachydysrhythmias also occur and can be managed with magnesium sulphate and antiarrhythmic therapy. Bleeding after cardiac surgery can lead to hypovolaemia, or to cardiac tamponade if concealed. Pulmonary hypertension is associated with some cardiac lesions and may require inhaled nitric oxide.

Respiratory system

A chest X-ray is performed soon after cardiac surgery to check the position of the endotracheal tube and chest drains, and to examine the lung fields. Pulmonary oedema and haemorrhage can occur in the early postoperative period and may need special ventilatory parameters. Bleeding and inflammation can lead to pleural effusions and a chylothorax can occur if there has been damage to lymphatic tissue in the chest. Damage to the phrenic nerve or recurrent laryngeal nerve can cause respiratory compromise.

Central nervous system

Rarely, brain injury can result from cardiac surgery, owing to low cardiac output states, emboli or bleeding. Deep hypothermic cardiac arrest states are a particular risk. The use of NIRS aims to warn of impending neurological injury and it is often continued into the postoperative period. After aortic cross-clamping for coarctation repair, there is a risk of spinal cord ischaemia.

Renal system

Urine output needs to be monitored throughout the case and in the postoperative period. Oliguria is common, particularly after MUF. If urine output falls below 0.5 mL kg^{-1} h^{-1} diuretic therapy can be used. Low cardiac output may lead to renal dysfunction, sometimes requiring renal replacement therapy, usually peritoneal dialysis or haemofiltration. Maintenance intravenous fluid is introduced slowly to avoid fluid overload. Electrolyte levels need monitoring.

Gastrointestinal system and nutrition

Gastrointestinal smooth muscle tone is reduced in the early postoperative period owing to anaesthesia, opiate therapy and cardiac bypass. A nasogastric tube is used to minimize gastric distension. Enteral nutrition is commenced as soon as reasonable. In neonates with low cardiac output syndrome, mesenteric ischaemia or necrotizing enterocolitis can occur.

Haematology

Chest drain output needs to be recorded and severe bleeding may require re-exploration of the chest either in the ICU or in theatre. Clotting factors and platelets are consumed on CPB and may require supplementation on ICU. Residual heparin may require protamine administration. TEG can guide coagulation management.

Infection

Routine antibiotics are continued in the postoperative period. Invasive lines and chest drain sites are monitored for infection and removed as soon as practical.

Extracorporeal life support

Occasionally, very sick patients require extracorporeal life support postoperatively while cardiac function recovers. This is undertaken at a few specialist centres.

Bibliography

Bingham R, Lloyd Thomas A, Sury M (eds). *Hatch & Sumner's Textbook of Paediatric Anaesthesia*, 3rd edn. London: Hodder Arnold, 2007.

Eliot May L. *Pediatric Heart Surgery: A Ready Reference for Professionals*. Milwaukee: Maxishare, 2008.

Lake CL, Booker PD. *Pediatric Cardiac Anesthesia*, 4th edn. Philadelphia: Lippincott, Williams & Wilkins, 2004.

Cross-references

Fluid and electrolyte balance, 754
Infants and children, 615
Postoperative oliguria, 779
Postoperative pain management, 783

Regional anaesthesia and cardiac surgery

Akbar Vohra

The clinical use of spinal opioids originated in the late 1970s when, following the description of opioid receptors in the spinal cord, various opioid drugs were administered both intrathecally and epidurally. The application of these techniques to cardiac surgery followed soon afterwards and, although the majority of the clinical experience to date in cardiac anaesthesia has been with intrathecal morphine, epidural opioids have also been used. Typically, 0.03 mg kg^{-1} morphine diluted with 10 mL normal saline administered to the lumbar cerebrospinal fluid using a 25 gauge bevelled or a 24 gauge Sprotte needle. Clonidine (50–100 μg mL^{-1}) may be added to the solution.

The advantages claimed for intrathecal morphine in cardiac surgery are:

- excellent analgesia, which can persist well into the postoperative period following ICU discharge
- reduced vasodilator use in the ICU
- less respiratory depression than with intravenous opioid use
- reduced hormonal stress response to surgery
- reduction in cardiac ischaemia and arrhythmias.

Epidural analgesia may be a better option than single-shot spinal anaesthesia because it may be continued for a number of days postoperatively. This varies between 2 and 5 days. These are inserted at the T1–T4 levels (usually (T2/3) in order to provide sympathetic blockade of the cardiac sympathetic fibres. The timing of the insertion is debatable. Some institutes insert them the day before in order to reduce the worries of bloody tap. Logistically, this is problematic because of the need for an appropriate sterile area and staffing during insertion. It is more logical to insert these on the day of the operation in the anaesthetic room in an adequately premedicated patient with full invasive monitoring. It also allows it to be used in the unstable patients in whom more time may be given to stop any preoperative anticoagulants. As heparin is not a fibrinolytic agent there should not be a problem giving it an hour after the epidural has been inserted. A 16 gauge Tuohy needle and catheter are inserted at the T2/3 level with the patient in the sitting position. We have used a combination of local anaesthetic (bupivacaine or ropivacaine) and opioid (diamorphine or fentanyl) to initiate and maintain the anaesthesia. With such high epidurals it is mandatory to monitor ascending blockade towards the phrenic nerve (C3–5). This may be performed with the Epidural Scoring Scale for Arm Movement (ESSAM) score. This utilizes the handgrip, wrist flexion and elbow flexion (C5–T1) to assess ascending motor blockade.

It should be noted that, although intrathecal morphine results in a reduction in the patient's demand for analgesia, there have been few controlled studies comparing this technique with other methods of analgesia and no studies have conclusively proven that intrathecal morphine provides better analgesia. Furthermore, although intrathecal morphine is associated with a modest improvement in respiratory parameters, such as peak expiratory flow rate and postoperative arterial carbon dioxide tension, it has not been shown to reduce time to extubation or ICU stay.

Many anaesthetists will not utilize regional anaesthesia because it is deemed to add a new potential for complications, ranging from the undesirable to the life threatening. Spinal and epidural anaesthesia are procedures that require a significant amount of skill, and should be associated with a small failure rate, particularly in the elderly, as well as the rare complications of infection and neurological sequelae. Post-spinal headache does not appear to be a problem in the cardiac surgical patient, urinary retention is not an issue owing to the necessity for catheterization, and backache attributable to dural puncture has not been reported. In common with intravenous opioids, up to 20% of patients will suffer from nausea and/or vomiting, and a much smaller number experience pruritus, which is often confined to the facial dermatomes and which may be severe.

The two most important problems associated with the use of spinal opioids in cardiac surgery are respiratory depression and the potential for spinal haematoma formation. Respiratory depression is characteristically delayed following the use of hydrophilic drugs such as morphine. It is believed to be due to slow rostral spread of the drug by bulk flow in the cerebrospinal fluid, which acts on the respiratory centre in the floor of the fourth ventricle many hours after administration. Several papers have attested to the fact that the phenomenon does not occur after the first 24 hours, during which time close respiratory monitoring is clearly required. This prerequisite is easily provided in the postcardiac surgery patient, as it is usual practice to nurse these patients in an ICU, HDU or step-down unit during this time. The respiratory depression associated with intrathecal morphine may be precipitated by the concomitant use of opioids by other routes (including premedication drugs), which should be given with caution, if at all. It is easily reversed with a carefully titrated dose of intravenous naloxone, which is insufficient to antagonize analgesia.

The controversy surrounding the use of spinal and epidural blocks in patients with abnormalities of coagulation reaches its zenith in cardiac surgery, as the patient is required to be fully anticoagulated. Spontaneous epidural haematomata in the presence of a coagulopathy, and haematomata following axial blocks, although rare, have been reported in the literature, and can lead to irreversible neurological damage. However, several large series from the 1980s have demonstrated the safety of axial blockade in patients who have subsequently been heparinized for vascular surgery. Indeed, there have been no reports of epidural haematoma following intrathecal morphine for cardiac surgery. Our own current practice is to insert epidurals on the day of surgery. We have had no problems in our patients over the past 13 years in over 2000 patients (unpublished data).

Notwithstanding the above argument, it is generally accepted that the pre-existence of an iatrogenic or other coagulopathy is an absolute contraindication to regional anaesthesia, although, if there were very strong indications, some anaesthetists might proceed in a patient receiving low-dose heparin or antiplatelet drugs. The other contraindications to spinal puncture – local infection, spinal deformity, neurological disease, raised intracranial pressure and patient refusal – also apply.

Bibliography

Aun C, Thomas D, St John-Jones L, *et al.* Intrathecal morphine in cardiac surgery. *Eur J Anaesthesiol* 1985; **2**: 426–9.

El-Baz N, Goldin M. Continuous epidural infusion of morphine for pain relief after cardiac operations. *J Thorac Cardiovasc Surg* 1987; **93**: 878–83.

Mathews ET, Abrams LD. Intrathecal morphine in open heart surgery. *Lancet* 1980; 2: 543.

Odoom JA, Sih IL. Epidural analgesia and anticoagulant therapy: experience with one thousand cases of continuous epidurals. *Anaesthesia* 1983; **38**: 254–9.

Razek E, Scott N, Vohra A. An Epidural Scoring Scale for Arm Movements (ESSAM) in patients receiving high thoracic epidural analgesia for coronary artery bypass grafting. *Anaesthesia* 1999; **54**: 1104–9.

Cross-references

Epidural and spinal anaesthesia, 707
Postoperative pain management, 783

Thoracic aorta surgery

Akbar Vohra

Physiological and pathological considerations

Aortic dissection

Aortic dissections are characterized by an intimal tear followed by a longitudinal separation within the media of the wall which extends parallel with the lumen. It usually presents acutely with severe anterior or posterior chest pain. Depending upon position and progression, dissections can cause aortic valve incompetence, interruption of the coronary, cerebral, spinal, subclavian, mesenteric, renal or femoral arteries. Clinical presentation may be related to these secondary effects. Young patients can have an associated connective tissue disorder such as Marfan syndrome. The major classification is into types A (involving the ascending aorta) and B (distal to the origin of the left subclavian), as shown in Fig. 25.3. The characteristics of type A and B dissections are shown in Table 25.2.

Aneurysmal dilatations

These are usually asymptomatic until they leak or produce symptoms owing to compression on surrounding structures such as the superior vena cava, left main bronchus or lung. Intimal deterioration can occlude smaller arteries; paraplegia, for example, may be the presenting symptom. There is often a history of hypertension and diabetes together with aneurysmal dilatation of the abdominal vessels.

Although clinical presentation and plain chest X-rays may suggest a diagnosis, accurate diagnosis depends upon special investigations such as aortography, CT scan, MRI scan and echocardiography.

Anaesthetic considerations

Preoperative

Perform a full neurological assessment and record any deficits. Reduce hypertension with the use of

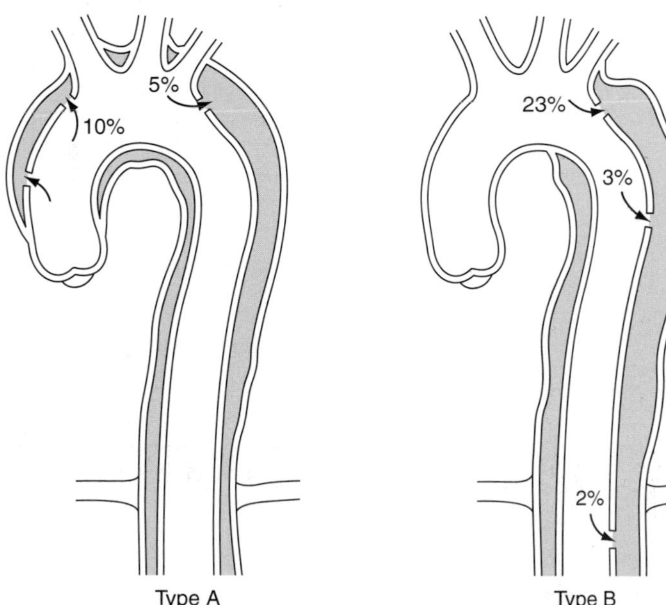

● **Figure 25.3** Type A and type B aortic dissections. Reproduced with permission from Ergin M A, Galla JD, Lansman S, et al. Acute dissections of the aorta; current surgical treatment. Surg Clin North Am 1985; 63: 721.

Table 25.2 Characteristics of type A and type B aortic dissections

	Type A	Type B
Frequency (%)	65–70	30–35
Male/female ratio	2:1	3:1
Average age	50–55	60–70
Associated hypertension (%)	50	80
Hypertension on admission	±	++
Associated atherosclerosis	±	++
Aortic regurgitation (%)	50	10
Intimal tear	Always present	Absent in 5–10%
Acute mortality (%)	90–95	40

Reproduced with permission from Ergin M A, Galla JD, Lansman S, *et al*. Acute dissections of the aorta; current surgical treatment. ***Surg Clin North Am*** 1985; **63**: 721.

vasodilators (e.g. sodium nitroprusside, nitrates and β-blockers). Catheterize and check renal function.

Insert two large-bore cannulae and an arterial line in the arm least affected by the lesion. Order at least 10 units of blood. Accompany patient to scan room, etc., and be prepared to resuscitate. Continued or suddenly increasing pain may indicate further dissection and the need for immediate surgery.

Perioperative

Antibiotic prophylaxis is essential. Provide renal protection with furosemide and mannitol. The anaesthetic technique is as for CABG.

Type A with involvement of ascending aorta only

- Full CPB is necessary with cardioplegia for myocardial protection. Replacement of the aortic valve and reimplantation of the coronary arteries may be required in addition to grafting of the ascending aorta.

Type A with involvement of aortic arch

- As above, but in addition the operation on the cerebral vessels requires total circulatory arrest at <18°C.

Type B with involvement of the descending aorta.

- Does not require CPB and is approached via a left thoracotomy. A double-lumen tube is preferred, to allow deflation of the left lung.

All of these operations necessitate cross-clamping of the aorta. When the clamp goes on there may be proximal hypertension, requiring the use of vasodilators. Unclamping produces a sudden fall in left ventricular afterload and systemic blood pressure. Fluid loading and/or vasoconstrictor agents will be required.

Some of the type B dissections may be corrected with the use of endoluminal stents. This involves an approach through the femoral or iliac arteries and therefore avoids the aforementioned problems leading to a reduction in perioperative morbidity. It involves an approach through the femoral artery with radiology for ensuring correct placement. It can be performed under local anaesthesia and sedation. Arterial monitoring is helpful.

Postoperative

Ensure stable haemodynamics. Monitor and preserve renal function wherever possible. The incidence of renal failure is 5% and is related to preoperative renal function and the cross-clamp ischaemic time. Central and peripheral neurological function need careful observation, although there is little that can be done to affect the course of intraoperative damage from ischaemia or embolization. The incidence of paraplegia is 5–10%. Postoperative hypotension should be avoided since it may contribute to the incidence of late-onset paraplegia.

Endoluminal stenting of aorta

This involves the use of stents specifically designed for each patient on the basis of spiral CT scans. Not all patients are suitable for this form of surgery. A stent is passed through the femoral route and placed in the aorta under X-ray control. It avoids the need for bypass or one-lung anaesthesia. It has minimal effect on the cardiovascular system because cross-clamping of the aorta is avoided. These are usually performed in theatre under general anaesthesia. However, some centres are performing these under sedation in the X-ray departments. These patients require direct arterial monitoring but central venous monitoring may not always be necessary. Occasionally, the left subclavian artery is occluded. This may, on rare occasions, necessitate carotid to axillary artery bypass surgery. Patients can be sent to the HDU.

Bibliography

Ergin M A, Galla JD, Lansman S, *et al.* Acute dissections of the aorta; current surgical treatment. *Surg Clin North Am* 1985; **63**: 721.

Cross-references

Blood transfusion, 735
Diabetes mellitus, 60
Hypertension, 151
One-lung anaesthesia, 714

Part 3

Anaesthetic Factors

Cardiopulmonary exercise testing

Dougal Atkinson and John A Moore

Accurate assessment of functional capacity is an integral part of preoperative assessment and cardiac risk stratification. Patients with limited cardiorespiratory reserve may be unable to meet the increased oxygen demand that surgery places upon the body, leading to both morbidity and mortality. A large retrospective analysis of patients undergoing non-cardiac surgery has identified heart failure as the most important cardiac determinant of postoperative mortality.

The identification of the high-risk patient with limited cardiorespiratory reserve enables the perioperative physician to make important decisions regarding patient care and the use of healthcare resources.

Cardiopulmonary exercise testing (CPET) is a safe, non-invasive test providing accurate and objective assessment of functional capacity. CPET has an established role both in diagnosis and in determining prognosis in heart failure. It is increasingly utilized in centres undertaking major surgery as a preoperative screening tool. Other objective measures of functional capacity are available (e.g. incremental shuttle walk test) in the preoperative setting, but CPET holds a number of advantages. These include:

- the ability to identify the potential cause(s) of any exercise limitation present and therefore the potential to modify this risk
- the identification of cardiac ischaemia.

Indications for preoperative CPET

Centres vary as to how they utilize preoperative CPET. The following indications incorporate current evidence:

- all patients ≥60 undergoing major abdominal (colorectal, upper gastrointestinal, major hepatobiliary, urology, gynae-oncology) and lung resection surgery
- any patient <60 undergoing major abdominal or lung resection surgery with known cardiorespiratory disease and/or estimated functional capacity <4 metabolic equivalents (METS).

Components of a CPET

A number of commercial CPET kits are available. The standard Wassermann protocol using a cycle ergometer is widely used for preoperative assessment. All tests utilize continuous $S_{p}O_2$ measurement, non-invasive blood pressure measurement and continuous 12-lead ECG monitoring. Each test has four key stages, as follows.

Static spirometry

- Forced expiratory volume in 1 second (FEV_1), forced vital capacity with/without slow vital capacity are performed.
- Maximum voluntary ventilation can be measured directly or more commonly estimated indirectly ($= FEV_1 \times 40$).

Unloaded exercise

- 3 minutes of unloaded exercise on a cycle ergometer with the patient maintaining a cadence of ~60 r.p.m.

Loaded exercise

- Resistance to pedalling is increased continuously in a ramp-like fashion at a rate of 10–25 W/min.
- A cadence of ~60 r.p.m. is maintained for as long as possible (ideally for 6–10 minutes) until the patient is symptom-limited or is unable to maintain the cadence.
- Variation exists between centres as to whether a patient is pushed to a submaximal or maximal point of exertion.

Recovery

- The patient remains monitored on the cycle until physiological parameters and any ECG changes have returned to normal.

CPET parameters

A number of CPET parameters are used in preoperative assessment.

Peak oxygen consumption (peak Vo_2)

This is the highest Vo_2 achieved by the patient during a test; 1 MET is equivalent to 3.5 mL kg^{-1} min^{-1} of Vo_2. Inability to achieve 4 METS is used to identify patients at increased cardiac risk in a number of preoperative guidelines.

Peak Vo_2 is widely used in thoracic surgery in the assessment of patients undergoing lung resection. The ability to achieve >20 mL kg^{-1} min^{-1} identifies patients at low risk of postoperative mortality. Patients unable to achieve 15 mL kg^{-1} min^{-1} should be considered carefully before proceeding to surgery.

Peak Vo_2 has limitations as a measure of functional capacity owing to its dependence on patient motivation. Results may not be reproducible and peak exercise may be neither achievable in the elderly comorbid population nor felt appropriate (e.g. a patient with a large abdominal aortic aneurysm).

Anaerobic or lactate threshold (AT)

This is defined as the upper intensity of exercise an individual can achieve using purely aerobic metabolism. Any further increase in exercise intensity beyond this point is achieved by a combination of aerobic and anaerobic metabolism. This marker of aerobic or functional capacity usually occurs at 50–60% of peak exercise capacity. It is achieved in the majority of preoperative patients undergoing CPET and is a reproducible measure of functional capacity. A number of validated methods for determining AT are available with the *V*-slope method the most widely used (Fig. 26.1). AT is recorded as the Vo_2 in mL min^{-1} or mL kg^{-1} min^{-1} at the point at which AT occurs.

There is an increasing evidence base supporting the use of AT in identifying patients at increased risk of both morbidity and mortality following major abdominal surgery (Table 26.1).

Ventilatory equivalent for carbon dioxide ($Eqco_2$ or V_E/Vco_2)

This provides a marker of V/Q matching within the lung. It defines the relationship between minute ventilation (V_E in L min^{-1}) and carbon dioxide production (Vco_2 in L min^{-1}) during exercise. Values are normally reported at the point

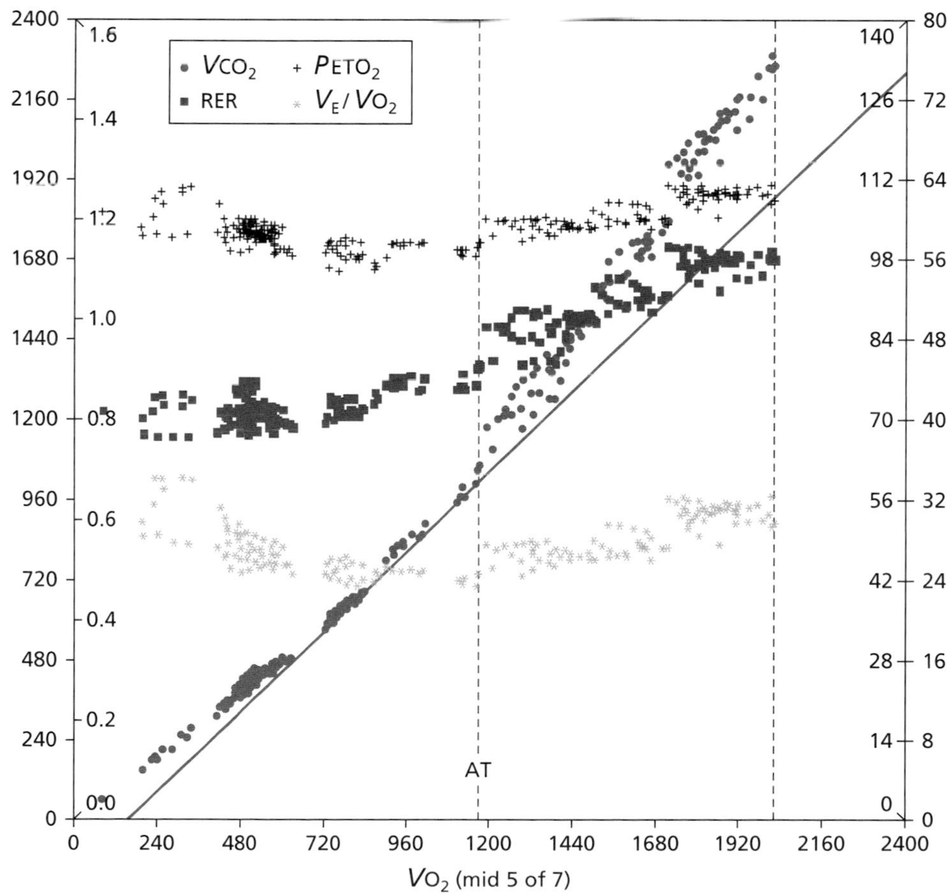

● **Figure 26.1** *V*-slope method to determine anaerobic threshold (AT). From the start of loaded exercise until AT, there is a linear relationship between increasing oxygen consumption (Vo_2) and carbon dioxide production (Vco_2) when plotted (filled circles); a 45° linear relationship is seen up until AT (solid line, *V*-slope); at AT, increasing lactic acid is buffered, leading to a disproportionate increase in Vco_2 compared with Vo_2 – upward deflection of the Vco_2/Vo_2 relationship is seen (upward displacement of filled circles); AT is the Vo_2 at which this upward deflection takes place in either mL min^{-1} or mL kg^{-1} min^{-1} (see dashed line). P_{ETO2}, .

- Dentures, contact lenses, prosthetic limbs, etc., should have been left on the ward. Headscarves, hairpieces, etc. may be retained in patients who request this.
- Patients who are deaf or who have impaired vision may benefit from retaining their hearing aid or glasses until the moment of induction of anaesthesia.
- All lipstick, nail varnish and cosmetics should have been removed.
- All jewellery should have been removed, or should be taped securely to the patient.
- Never remove the patient's identity badge unless absolutely essential, whereupon it must be immediately reattached to a different part of the patient.
- The site or side of the operation should have been marked with an indelible ink marker by the surgeon before leaving the ward. It is good practice to also ask the patient to identify the site and side of operation before inducing anaesthesia and to verify this with the operating list.

Cross-references

Acute kidney injury, 196
Chronic liver disease, 174
Diabetes mellitus, 60
Difficult airway: management, 651
Malignant hyperthermia, 770
Obesity, 189
Preoperative assessment of cardiovascular risk in non-cardiac surgery, 621
Preoperative assessment of pulmonary risk, 625
Sickle cell syndrome, 239
Smoking and anaesthesia, 120

Emergency surgery

Brian J Pollard

An emergency anaesthetic is one that is required as soon as possible. The implication is that there is not enough time available for the patient to be fully prepared for surgery. It is likely therefore that the patient's condition has not been fully optimized, there may be existing homeostatic disturbances and not all of the laboratory or other tests may be available before beginning.

Assessment

In the initial assessment of the patient, the first decision which must be taken relates to the urgency of the procedure. If the nature of the surgery is compelling and immediate, no time should be wasted. If it is possible to introduce some delay, however short, this should be done in order to allow the patient to be more fully assessed and for the patient's condition to be optimized.

Assessment should be the same as for elective procedures if time permits. Assess as fully as possible within the constraints of the degree of urgency. If the patient cannot give any history, look for warning cards and 'Medic-Alert' tags or bracelets. Look at any previous hospital notes and emergency department records. Ask friends or relatives if present. Perform appropriate investigations, depending upon available time. Obtain the results for those already instituted. Look for the presence of alcohol or drug intoxication, particularly in cases of trauma. Remember that in urgent procedures there is an increased chance of cardiac-related death in the presence of pre-existing cardiovascular disease. If the patient is of an ethnic origin where sickle disease is prevalent, treat as positive until proven to the contrary. If there is insufficient time to obtain the results of blood tests they should still be requested and then action taken if necessary when the results do become available.

Starvation

Assume that the patient has a full stomach. Even if the last food intake was over 6 hours ago the stomach may not be empty. In cases of trauma in particular, the stomach ceases to empty at the time of injury and may still contain partly digested food 12 or more hours later. Attempts at emptying the stomach using a nasogastric tube are not usually completely successful and should not be relied upon.

Preparation

Trained assistance must be available in the operating theatre. Make sure everything is prepared and ready before starting, including drawing up any drugs which you might want. If possible, check that blood has been cross-matched and is immediately available in theatre. Consider anaesthetizing the patient in the operating theatre and not in the anaesthetic room to minimize delays between induction and incision. Test all equipment before starting.

Insert at least one intravenous line (minimum size 16 G, preferably 14 G). If major blood loss is expected, or if the patient is markedly hypovolaemic, a second large peripheral line should be inserted and strong consideration given to inserting a central venous line.

Monitoring

Attach all monitors before starting and obtain baseline readings. Standard minimum monitoring should consist of pulse oximeter, electrocardiogram, non-invasive blood pressure and end-tidal carbon dioxide. Other monitors, e.g. nerve stimulator, should be added as necessary. Core temperature monitoring is advisable in all but the most minor emergencies. An arterial line should be considered for invasive arterial pressure monitoring. In general, time should not be wasted in securing additional monitoring lines (e.g. central line, pulmonary artery flotation catheter) unless this is deemed essential before starting. It is usually acceptable to establish these when the patient is anaesthetized and while preparation for surgery is progressing. A urinary catheter should be inserted in major cases. Oesophageal Doppler may be of value and should be considered in patients in whom there is likely to be marked cardiovascular instability.

Induction

Secure the airway as rapidly as possible. Use a rapid sequence induction technique with preoxygenation and cricoid pressure. Take a further blood sample if necessary for more tests, blood gases, cross-match, etc. Give drugs slowly, particularly in the hypotensive patient. Etomidate is a good choice in the high risk patient. It should not, however, be used as an alternative to adequate preoperative fluid replacement if there is time for the latter.

remains constant at around 7 mL kg^{-1}, the increased ventilation in younger patients is brought about by an increase in respiratory rate; this is approximately 30 breaths min^{-1} at birth, 24 breaths min^{-1} at 1 year and 12 breaths min^{-1} in the adult.

Lung compliance is reduced in infants and small airways tend to close at end-expiration. This tendency is increased during anaesthesia, thus increasing the risk of absorption atelectasis and hypoxaemia. To prevent these effects, most anaesthetic episodes in infants are managed with controlled ventilation and up to 5 cmH_2O positive end-expiratory pressure.

Ex-premature infants (gestation <37 weeks) with a postconceptual age of less than 60 weeks and a postnatal age of less than 4 months are at increased risk of apnoea following anaesthesia. These patients require careful monitoring for 24 hours postoperatively and should not be accepted as day-cases.

Cardiovascular system

Changes in the cardiovascular system mirror those in pulmonary ventilation (Fig. 26.3). The increased cardiac output in younger patients is brought about by an increase in heart rate; stroke volume remains constant at 1 mL kg^{-1} throughout life. Parasympathetic control is well developed at birth, but sympathetic control is incomplete. This may explain the normally reduced blood pressure in infants and their increased susceptibility to reflex bradycardia and hypotension. Bradycardia during anaesthesia can be prevented or treated with intravenous atropine (20 μg kg^{-1}).

Water and electrolytes

Approximately 1 mL of fluid is required per kilocalorie of energy expended; therefore, maintenance fluid rate and metabolic rate may be calculated using the same formula (Table 26.3). Maintenance requirements of sodium, chloride and potassium will be satisfied by administering a solution of 0.18% saline with 20 mmol potassium chloride per litre at the calculated fluid maintenance rate. However, 0.18% saline is a markedly hypotonic solution which, if used in large amounts, may result in hyponatraemia. Accordingly, it is currently recommended that a solution containing 0.45% saline be used for standard maintenance therapy. All intraoperative fluid requirements in children aged over 1 month should be managed initially by giving an isotonic fluid such as normal saline or Hartmann's solution (see p. 552).

Temperature maintenance

This is a problem in neonates and infants because of their small size, large surface area to body weight ratio and lack of subcutaneous fat. Hypothermia during anaesthesia can be prevented by monitoring the patient's temperature, increasing the temperature of the operating room and using heating devices such as warming mattresses and warm-air blowers.

Psychological factors

Childhood is a period of great emotional lability and impressionability. Stressful experiences in hospital make a more lasting impression on children, and behavioural disturbances frequently occur after they return home. The following may reduce the stress of hospitalization:

- age-appropriate psychological preparation with books, videos, play therapy and/or a preadmission visit to the hospital

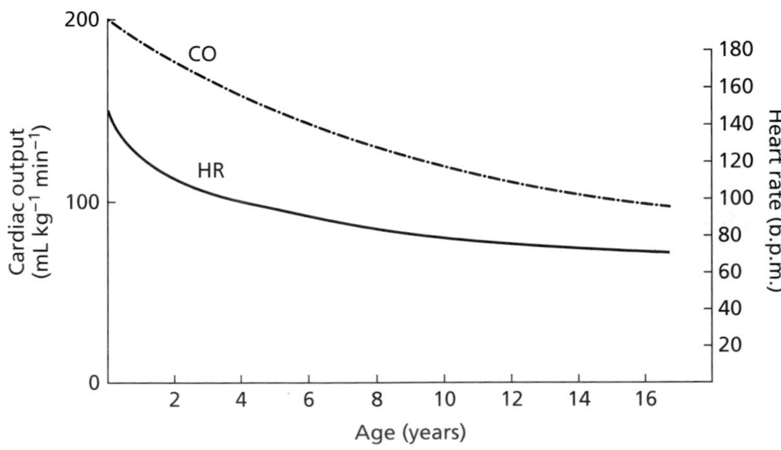

Figure 26.3 Variation cardiac output and (CO) and heart rate (HR) with age. Modified from Rudolph AM. *Congenital Diseases of the Heart*. Chicago: Year Book Medical Publishers, 1974.

Table 26.3 Maintenance fluid (and energy) requirements

Body weight (kg)	Amount and rate
0–10	4 mL kg^{-1} h^{-1}
10–20	40 mL + 2 mL kg^{-1} h^{-1} for each kilogram over 10
>20	60 mL + 1 mL kg^{-1} h^{-1} for each kilogram over 20

Modified from Holliday MA, Segar WE. The maintenance need for water in parenteral fluid therapy. *Pediatrics* 1957; **19**: 823–32.

- child-centred and family-friendly environments
- involvement of the child and parents in decisions about the proposed anaesthesia
- local anaesthetic cream or gel to venepuncture sites before surgery
- selective use of oral sedative premedication
- parental presence at induction.

Drug dosage

For many anaesthetic drugs, the distribution of per kilogram doses with age is biphasic with lower doses in neonates, reflecting immaturity of organ or enzyme systems, followed by higher doses in infants and children declining exponentially in line with normalized BMR towards the adult dose in adolescents However, there are notable exceptions to this general rule (e.g. succinylcholine, sevoflurane) and the available drug literature should always be consulted.

Thiopental

Neonates require 4–5 mg kg^{-1}, infants 7–8 mg kg^{-1} and children 5–6 mg kg^{-1} of thiopental for induction of anaesthesia. The reduced requirements in neonates can be explained by decreased plasma protein binding. The increased requirements in infants and children compared with adults (usual dose 4 mg kg^{-1}) may be due to their increased per kilogram cardiac output (a BMR-dependent function), as this would be expected to reduce the first-pass concentration of thiopental arriving at the brain.

Propofol

The use of propofol for induction and maintenance of anaesthesia is associated with rapid recovery and antiemesis. Average induction doses are 4 mg kg^{-1} for infants and 3–4 mg kg^{-1} for children. Pain on injection of propofol can be reduced by adding 20 mg of lidocaine to every 20 mL of 1% propofol.

Morphine

Neonates and infants aged less than 6 months appear sensitive to the respiratory depressant effects of morphine because of increased permeability of the blood–brain barrier and prolonged elimination times. Balanced anaesthesia in neonates may be supplemented with 25 µg kg^{-1} of morphine followed by maintenance doses of 5–10 µg kg^{-1} h^{-1}. Infants aged more than 6 months and children may be given a loading dose of 100 µg kg^{-1} with maintenance doses of 25 µg kg^{-1} h^{-1}. Neonates receiving morphine should be nursed in a high-dependency area with facilities for continuous monitoring of oxygen saturation and respiratory rate.

Atracurium

The neuromuscular junction of the neonate is three times more sensitive to the effects of non-depolarizing relaxants than that of the adult. However, because of the increased volume of ECF in younger patients, which approximates to the volume of distribution of muscle relaxants, dose does not vary significantly with age.

Atracurium 0.5 mg kg^{-1} produces about 30 minutes of neuromuscular blockade in children and adults. Recovery is slightly faster in neonates and infants owing to an increase in plasma clearance, which probably relates to the fact that 50% of the drug is eliminated by non-organ routes (e.g. Hofmann hydrolysis). Prompt recovery in patients of all ages makes atracurium an attractive drug for use in paediatric anaesthesia.

Succinylcholine

Succinylcholine doses of 3 mg kg^{-1} in infants and 2 mg kg^{-1} in children produce reliable intubating conditions within 60 seconds and the block resolves in 6–8 minutes. The increased dose requirement in younger patients reflects the greater volume of ECF into which the drug is distributed rather than any 'resistance' to the effects of the drug. In view of reports of succinylcholine-induced cardiac arrests in children with undiagnosed muscular dystrophy, it is recommended that the use of succinylcholine in children should be reserved for emergency intubation or instances when immediate securing of the airway is necessary.

Succinylcholine is effective when given intramuscularly in a dose of 4–5 mg kg^{-1}. This may be particularly helpful in the event of laryngospasm occurring during inhalation induction of anaesthesia, before intravenous access has been established. Control of the airway is usually gained within 60 seconds and the block resolves in about 20 minutes.

Neostigmine

Neostigmine antagonizes non-depolarizing neuromuscular blockade more rapidly in paediatric patients than in adults. The usual dose is 50 μg kg^{-1}. Increasing the dose does not increase the rate of reversal, which is unlikely to be satisfactory in the absence of a response to train-of-four stimulation.

Sevoflurane

Sevoflurane is the volatile anaesthetic agent of choice for infants and children owing to its relative lack of pungency and low blood solubility leading to rapid induction and recovery. In neonates and young infants, the MAC of sevoflurane is 3.3%, declining gradually throughout childhood to about 2.0% in the adult. Rapid emergence from sevoflurane anaesthesia may be associated with increased agitation in children who have not received adequate analgesia.

Bibliography

Anderson BJ, Meakin GH. Scaling for size: some implications for paediatric anaesthetic dosing. *Paediatr Anaesth* 2002; **12**: 205–9.

Meakin GH. Developmental pharmacology. In: Holzman RS, Mancuso TJ, Polander DM (eds) *A Practical Approach to Pediatric Anesthesia.* Philadelphia: Lippincott Williams & Wilkins, 2008, pp. 17–47.

Meakin GH, Welborn LG. Anaesthesia for infants and children. In: Healy TEJ, Knight P (eds) *Wylie and Churchill Davidson's A Practice of Anaesthesia,* 7th edn. London: Arnold, 2003, pp. 961–79.

Cross-reference

Paediatrics: overview, 552

Premedication

Brian J Pollard

Premedication is short for 'preoperative medication' or 'preliminary medication'. A drug, or a combination of drugs (the premed), is administered to the patient before anaesthesia and surgery.

A number of reasons exist for administering a premed, the commonest of which is patient anxiety. Reasons may also vary from patient to patient and within the same patient at different times. If a patient did not require a premed last time, it does not mean that he or she does not need one on this occasion. Circumstances also alter. The patient who did not require a premed on one occasion for a minor cosmetic procedure may be extremely anxious when facing a laparotomy for suspected malignancy. It must also be remembered that not every patient needs pharmacological premedication – a visit from the anaesthetist and an explanation of the procedure may be all that is required.

Sedative premedication is usually inadvisable in the old or frail patient. Profound sedation, confusion or disorientation may result.

The administration of a sedative premed will lead to a reduction in the requirements for anaesthetic agents, reduce the potential for awareness during tracheal intubation and surgery, assist in maintaining anaesthesia and reduce certain unwanted side-effects of anaesthesia.

Children require a premed more often than adults. Remember to scale the dose down. Some drugs are prepared in a flavoured liquid formulation for children; others may have to be mixed with a small quantity of juice. Older children may be better taking a tablet as a large volume of sweet syrup may be quite nauseating! Infants and neonates are special cases (see p. 615).

The factors that it may be necessary to consider in premedication are listed in Box 26.5.

Box 26.5 Potential factors which may be combined in the construction of an ideal premed for a particular patient

- Anxiolysis
- Amnesia
- Antiemesis
- Analgesia
- Antibiosis
- Antithrombosis
- Antisialagogue
- Antacid
- Antihistamine
- Antivagal

Anxiolysis

Many patients are apprehensive about forthcoming surgery and anxiolysis is welcome in such cases. Anxiety is a subjective sensation and it may be difficult to determine whether a patient is anxious or not. The patient who has had several previous anaesthetics may be more, not less, anxious. The severity and site of the surgery are poor indicators of potential for anxiety. An anxiolytic premed will lessen the normal stress response to surgery and anaesthesia. Benzodiazepines and opioids are the agents most commonly used to secure anxiolysis in the preoperative period.

Amnesia

Amnesia may be appropriate for a particularly traumatic occasion, especially if further procedures are planned. It is disliked by many patients, however, who are disturbed by the removal of part of a day of their life. Amnesic drugs will assist in reducing the incidence of awareness under general anaesthesia but they will not erase the memory of a period of awareness which has occurred. Amnesia may not be advantageous if it has been necessary to go to lengths to gain the patient's confidence for a procedure; the patient may also forget all of the positive points which have been emphasized on this occasion. The benzodiazepines are commonly used amnesics. Hyoscine is also a potent amnesic, although it may cause confusion in the elderly.

Antiemesis

This is useful for the patient who complains of previous sickness following surgery and is advisable if an opioid is used for premedication. The effect of an antiemetic given with the premed may be waning by the end of the procedure, however, requiring an additional dose to be administered. Prochlorperazine, metoclopramide, cyclizine and hyoscine are commonly used. The 5-HT_3 antagonists are usually reserved for situations when the simpler drugs do not work.

Analgesia

Analgesia is desirable if the patient has pain preoperatively. It also reduces the intraoperative requirements for anaesthetic agents and analgesics and improves comfort in the early postoperative period.

The opioids remain the most commonly used analgesics, although there is an increasing trend towards giving a dose of a non-steroidal anti-inflammatory drug (NSAID) as a part of the premed. NSAIDs lack the mild sedative and euphoric effect of the opioids which are useful as a part of the premed.

Antibiotics

These are used principally for prophylaxis against infection, particularly in patients who will have a foreign body (e.g. an artificial joint or a mesh hernia repair) inserted. Local hospital guidelines should be consulted. The antibiotic should be administered before the start of the surgical operation (i.e. before incision or insertion of any instrument).

Antithrombotic

This should always be considered in patients at risk from deep venous thrombosis. The newer low-molecular-weight heparins are regarded as more effective than unfractionated heparin. They are also more convenient as they only need to be given in a once daily dosage and the standard prophylactic regimen does not normally require monitoring.

Antisialagogue

This is essential for premedication in infants. It is useful when intraoral surgery is to be undertaken and also when fibreoptic intubation is planned. The principal disadvantage is the unpleasant dry mouth experienced by the patient. Atropine, hyoscine and glycopyrrolate are all potent drying agents.

Antacid

An antacid should be used if there is an increased risk of regurgitation of gastric contents. Particular risk factors include pregnancy, hiatus hernia with reflux and obesity. Sodium citrate is recommended because it is non-particulate. Ranitidine or another H_2 blocker needs to be given 1–2 hours preoperatively.

Antihistamine

This relatively unimportant consideration may be useful in atopic individuals. It may offer partial protection against endogenously released histamine.

Antivagal action

An antivagal action is important in ophthalmic surgery, although many anaesthetists administer the antivagal agent at the induction of anaesthesia rather than with the premed. It is indicated if repeated doses of succinylcholine are to be administered. It is not necessary in all cases; however, if not used, the potential for a profound bradycardia during surgery must always be remembered and atropine should be ready to hand at all times. Atropine and glycopyrrolate are the most effective antivagal agents for general use.

Cross-references

Awareness, 733
Difficult airway: management, 651
Paediatrics: overview, 552
Thrombosis and embolism, 793

Preoperative assessment of cardiovascular risk in non-cardiac surgery

Brian J Pollard

Perioperative cardiac morbidity (PCM) includes the occurrence of myocardial infarction (MI), unstable angina, congestive cardiac failure, serious arrhythmia or cardiac death during the perioperative period. In view of the stresses that anaesthesia and surgery impose upon the body it should be of no surprise that it is both a common and a major cause of death following these procedures.

The exact pathological mechanisms involved in perioperative MI are still not clear. In the usual setting of an MI, rupture of a coronary artery atherosclerotic plaque causes platelet aggregation and subsequent thrombus formation. During perioperative MI plaque rupture is seen in only 50% of cases. It is for this reason that many of these infarctions are thought to occur as a result of a prolonged imbalance between myocardial oxygen supply and demand in the presence of coronary artery disease (CAD). In those postoperative surgical patients who do suffer plaque rupture it is thought that an increased heart rate and contractility, induced by high circulating levels of catecholamines, cause shear stresses on the atherosclerotic plaques, predisposing them to rupture. Both of these observations help explain why perioperative MIs frequently do not occur intraoperatively, but typically peak at 1–3 days following surgery.

History, examination and clinical investigations have been used to identify individual patients at risk, often in the context of risk indices. A score is assigned to a specific clinical variable allowing a final total to stratify the patient's risk of suffering perioperative cardiac morbidity. In 1977 Goldman designed a risk index score which assigned patients to four classes from I (low risk) to IV (high risk). This risk index was modified in 1986 by Detsky, with the additional factors of unstable angina and remote MI, as well as the simplification of risk groups to three classes. Risk stratification is now used as a screening tool in order to decide which patients will benefit from further investigation of their cardiovascular system with advanced and more invasive investigations prior to surgery. Indeed, the whole focus of this process should be aimed at deciding on the optimal management of patients who are known to be at significant risk, instituting beneficial therapies (such as β-blockade when indicated) in the perioperative period and arranging a suitably safe environment for the patient postoperatively (e.g. critical care bed).

Preoperative assessment of cardiovascular disease

Routine

- Clinical history.
- Physical examination.
- Laboratory tests.
- Chest X-ray.
- 12-lead ECG.

Non-routine

- Exercise stress testing (cardiopulmonary exercise testing).
- Ambulatory ECG.
- Echocardiography.
- Nuclear imaging.
- Cardiac catheterization.

Proposed preoperative predictors of perioperative cardiac morbidity

Age

Increasing chronological age is widely recognized as a major risk factor in the development of CAD and is associated with a reduction in the cardiac response to stress. Age has been reported to be a predictor of morbidity only in the presence of other factors and hence may not be as important as overall physiological status.

Coronary artery disease

Patients with a documented previous MI have a greater risk of perioperative infarction (5–8%) which is associated with a high mortality (36–70%). The incidence of reinfarction has also been shown to reduce, with increasing time, in the 6 months following MI. If, for clinical reasons, surgery cannot be delayed following an MI, the reinfarction rate has been shown to be significantly reduced with the use of advanced haemodynamic monitoring techniques.

Angina is usually associated with angiographically significant (>70% stenosis) CAD. In these patients, 75% of ischaemic episodes are painless ('silent ischaemia'). Most perioperative ischaemia is silent and is more common during the first two postoperative days. Despite this, stable angina is felt to represent only an intermediate predictor of the risk for PCM. In contrast to this, patients with unstable coronary syndromes have a greatly increased risk of MI. These patients warrant urgent cardiological assessment, independent of their need for surgery.

Previous coronary artery bypass graft surgery

When undergoing major surgery, patients who have undergone a coronary artery bypass graft (CABG) are known to have a lower mortality than patients treated with purely medical therapy. For this reason, the current advice from the American College of Cardiology (ACC) and the American Heart Association (AHA) is that patients who have remained symptom-free within 5 years of a CABG do not require further invasive tests for risk stratification. Coronary artery bypass grafting does present its own risks of death, MI and stroke; therefore, it should only be performed if the patient has symptoms or coronary artery anatomy that mandate a CABG independent of planned non-cardiac surgery.

Percutaneous coronary intervention

There is very little hard evidence to prove that preoperative percutaneous coronary intervention is beneficial in patients undergoing non-cardiac surgery. Indeed, in one study of patients undergoing non-cardiac surgery within 6 weeks of coronary artery stent placement, 20% died, 18% had a non-fatal MI and 28% suffered major bleeding. For these reasons, it is suggested that percutaneous coronary interventions are performed purely on the grounds of clinical need, regardless of the patient's need for non-cardiac surgery.

Congestive cardiac failure

Congestive cardiac failure (CCF) is associated with a poor prognosis in CAD patients and is a predictor of cardiac mortality after acute MI. Although preoperative CCF is strongly predictive of PCM, the predictive value of specific signs seen in these patients is controversial.

Hypertension

Hypertension is known to be a risk factor for the development of CAD; however, mild to moderate hypertension is not an independent risk factor for PCM. Secondary causes of hypertension should be sought in the preoperative period. It is important to continue antihypertensive drugs into the perioperative period to prevent 'rebound hypertension' associated with sudden discontinuation of these drugs.

Diabetes mellitus

Diabetes mellitus is strongly associated with CAD. Although it is only a modest independent predictor of PCM, diabetes mellitus presents diagnostic difficulties because of the high incidence of 'silent ischaemia' and 'silent MI'. Autonomic neuropathy caused by diabetes mellitus confers greater risks of intraoperative blood pressure instability.

Dysrhythmias

The cardiac dysrhythmias associated with an increased PCM are symptomatic ventricular dysrhythmias associated with an underlying cardiac problem (e.g. CAD, cardiomyopathy) or atrial fibrillation. High-grade conduction abnormalities such as complete heart block, trifascicular block and bifascicular block all carry significant mortalities, independent of surgery.

Peripheral vascular disease

Significant coronary artery stenosis is present in 14–78% of patients with peripheral vascular disease (PVD) regardless of their CAD symptoms. Patients with PVD can present difficulties in assessing the severity of their CAD symptoms because their activities are limited by their PVD. Only 8% of patients with PVD have normal coronary angiograms. PVD patients undergoing vascular surgery have a high risk of PCM.

Renal failure

Chronic renal failure is an independent risk factor for PCM. Added to this, chronic renal failure is often associated with other risk factors for CAD (diabetes mellitus, hypertension).

Valvular heart disease

Patients with significant aortic stenosis have an increased incidence of sudden death owing to the potential for a severe decrease in cardiac output. The 1994/1995 Confidential Enquiry into Perioperative Deaths recommended preoperative cardiological assessment of the aortic valve in all patients with an ejection systolic murmur and evidence of left ventricular hypertrophy or myocardial ischaemia. The risks of PCM with other valvular lesions are less clearly defined and are probably related to the severity of the valvular defect and the presence of other cardiac abnormalities.

Cardiomyopathies

Cardiomyopathies may cause an increase in risk by decreasing ejection fraction and causing ventricular outlet obstruction. In addition to this, the cause of cardiomyopathy (e.g. alcohol, infiltration) may present a perioperative risk in its own right.

Cigarette smoking

Smokers are at a greatly increased risk of CAD; however, smoking has not been found to be an independent risk factor for PCM.

Cholesterol

Although there is a direct relationship between serum cholesterol and cardiovascular mortality, the risk of PCM is unknown.

Diagnostic tests

Biochemical data

Biochemical tests are useful in determining a patient's baseline renal function, which may be important in those who have hypertension, diabetes mellitus or who may be taking angiotensin-converting enzyme inhibitors. Serum potassium and magnesium should also be checked in those patients who are taking diuretics or who have a cardiac dysrhythmia.

12-lead electrocardiograph

A routine ECG is frequently performed in patients as part of a preoperative screening process. Despite this, they have not been found to be helpful in predicting patients likely to suffer PCM who have no cardiac risk factors. For these reasons, the suggested criteria for preoperative ECG are:

- age over 50 years
- risk factors for CAD
- clinical history suggesting cardiac dysrhythmias, CCF or other cardiac disease.

The abnormalities seen on a 12-lead ECG that are associated with an increased risk of PCM are:

- rhythm other than sinus
- ST-T wave abnormalities
- left ventricular hypertrophy
- pathological Q-waves
- conduction abnormalities.

The predictive values of the above ECG findings remain controversial.

Chest X-ray

Preoperative chest X-rays are useful to clarify clinical signs and to confirm the position of implanted devices such as a pacemaker. In over 70% of CAD patients, cardiomegaly is associated with a low ejection fraction (<40%) and may predict PCM.

Exercise stress testing

Exercise testing is used to cause an increase in heart rate to precipitate ECG evidence of myocardial ischaemia. Exercise testing also enables assessment of functional capacity. This form of testing has a sensitivity for detecting CAD of 68% and a specificity of 77%. A positive ischaemic response and a low exercise tolerance have been shown to be predictors of PCM in non-cardiac surgery. The main advantages of exercise testing are that it is usually locally available and is relatively inexpensive. The disadvantages of the test relate to exclusion factors, which include an abnormal baseline ECG and an inability to exercise (e.g. PVD).

Ambulatory ECG monitoring

This test is successful in detecting silent myocardial ischaemia. Of those patients with or at risk of CAD 18–40% have frequent ischaemic episodes (>75% are 'silent'). The usefulness of ambulatory ECG monitoring in assessing preoperative patients has not been defined.

Echocardiography

In the preoperative setting, echocardiography is used to assess valvular function, left ventricular function, the presence of left ventricular hypertrophy and the existence of pericardial effusions. Resting echo ejection fractions have not been found to correlate with PCM. Transthoracic echocardiography probably adds very little to the information acquired from routine clinical and electrocardiographic data in the majority of non-cardiac surgical patients.

Stress echocardiography involves imaging the heart at rest and under the influence of catecholamine stimulation, induced by either exercise or pharmacological agents, e.g. dobutamine. New areas of dyskinetic wall motion that develop during the test indicate the presence of myocardial ischaemia. Stress echocardiography has an excellent negative predictive value for PCM (93–100%) The test's relatively poor positive predictive value (7–30%) means that there is a high likelihood of a patient being subjected to further unnecessary evaluation prior to surgery. The other disadvantage is that local expertise, necessary for the test, may not be available.

Radionucleotide ventriculography

Multigated radionucleotide ventriculography (MUGA scan) is a test aimed at determining left ventricular ejection fraction. An ejection fraction of less than 35%, as assessed by MUGA scan, is associated with an increased risk of PCM. More recent studies have discovered that radionucleotide ventriculography adds very little to clinical assessment of patients and is probably not a cost-effective investigation.

Thallium scintigraphy

During this investigation, a radionucleotide agent is injected and then images of the myocardium obtained in the presence and absence of a coronary vasodilator (e.g. dipyridamole, adenosine). This illustrates reversible perfusion defects and indicates left ventricular function. Patients who demonstrate reversible or fixed perfusion defects probably have CAD, one of the main risk factors for PCM. A large study in 1994 confirmed previous evidence that thallium redistribution is not associated with perioperative MI, prolonged ischaemia or other adverse myocardial events. For this reason, thallium scintigraphy is not recommended as a routine test to assess preoperative patients.

Coronary angiography

This test is considered to be the 'gold standard' to assess coronary anatomy. Both the ACA and AHA recommend coronary angiography to investigate patients deemed to be at high risk with non-invasive testing. Coronary angiography carries its own risks; therefore, it is not indicated as a tool for stratifying PCM risk. Repeated coronary angiography is not indicated in patients who have had an adequate angiogram within the previous 2 years, with no worsening of symptoms.

Summary

The most important predictors of PCM are recent MI, severe or unstable angina, current CCF and critical aortic stenosis. These are all factors that can be determined by clinical history, examination and simple routine investigations. The use of non-routine, advanced tests, such as stress echocardiography and coronary angiography, should be restricted to patients in whom the additional information provided by the test will alter the management of the patient.

Bibliography

Detsky AS, Abrams HB, Forbath N, *et al.* Cardiac assessment in patients undergoing non-cardiac surgery. A multifactorial clinical risk index. *Arch Intern Med* 1986; **146**: 2131–5.

Gal J, Bogar L, Acsady G, Kertai MD. Cardiac risk reduction in non-cardiac surgery. The role of anaesthesia and monitoring techniques. *Eur J Anaesthesiol* 2006; **23**: 641–8.

Goldman L, Cardera DL, Nussbaum SR, *et al.* Multifactorial index of cardiac risk in non-cardiac surgical patients. *N Engl J Med* 1977; **297**: 845–50.

Grayburn PA, Hillis LD. Cardiac events in patients undergoing non-cardiac surgery: shifting the paradigm from non-invasive risk stratification to therapy. *Ann Intern Med* 2003; **138**: 506–12.

Hollenberg SM. Pre-operative cardiac risk assessment. *Chest* 1999; **115**: 51S–57S.

Juste RN, Lawson AD, Soni N. Minimising cardiac anaesthetic risk: the tortoise or the hare? *Anaesthesia* 1996; **51**: 255–62.

Kelion AD, Banning AP. Is simple assessment adequate for cardiac risk stratification before non-cardiac surgery? *Lancet* 1999; **354**: 1837–8.

Mangano DT. Peri-operative cardiac morbidity. *Anesthesiology* 1990; **70**: 153–84.

Mangano DT. Assessment of the patient with cardiac disease. *Anesthesiology* 1999; **91**: 1521–1526.

Nel L, Cone A. Cardiac assessment of patients undergoing non-cardiac surgery. In: Kaufman L, Ginsberg R (eds) *Anaesthesia Review*, 16. London: Churchill-Livingstone, 2001, pp. 29–51.

Cross-references

Cardiomyopathy, 136
Cardiopulmonary exercise testing, 600
Cardiovascular system: general considerations, 124
Coronary artery disease, 146

Preoperative assessment of pulmonary risk

Brian J Pollard

The development of postoperative pulmonary complications is determined principally by a number of risk factors:

- the severity of pre-existing pulmonary disease
- the patient's general state of health
- the nature and extent of surgery
- the anaesthetic technique
- preoperative and postoperative care.

It is difficult to assess the influence which individual variables may have on outcome, particularly with improvements in perioperative care and anaesthetic and surgical techniques, and in the health of the population as a whole. The risk from pre-existing pulmonary disease should be determined initially by history and examination. Additional risk factors (surgical, anaesthetic, age, etc.) can then be considered.

Pre-existing pulmonary disease

History

Dyspnoea

Dyspnoea is undue awareness of breathing or awareness of difficulty in breathing. Usually graded using Roizen's classification (Table 26.4). Dyspnoea at rest (grade IV) with low P_ao_2 (<7 kPa, 55 mmHg) is associated with an increased likelihood of requiring assisted ventilation after abdominal surgery. The aetiology should be sought (e.g. asthma, chronic bronchitis, emphysema, fibrosing alveolitis). Hypoventilation due to failure of neural input or muscle weakness may not cause dyspnoea.

Cough

Cough may indicate acute infection or, if productive of sputum on most days, suggests chronic bronchitis. Complications of excess sputum include airway plugging, atelectasis and respiratory infection. Loss of response to carbon dioxide and dependence on hypoxaemic respiratory drive need to be taken into account when planning the anaesthetic technique. Preoperative physiotherapy or bronchodilators may be required. Psychological preparation and training in breathing exercises can be invaluable. Sputum should be sent for culture.

Haemoptysis may be due to carcinoma, tuberculosis, pulmonary infarction or pneumonia, and must be distinguished from nasal bleeding.

Wheeze

Wheeze may indicate asthma, chronic bronchitis, emphysema or acute foreign body inhalation. Asthma should be assessed by frequency of attacks, current drug therapy, and history of hospitalization and ventilation. Steroid treatment contributes to muscle weakness and immunoincompetence, both of which may result in prolonged ventilation and respiratory colonization. Bronchospasm may occur with laryngoscopy, tracheal intubation and anaesthetic drugs that release histamine, particularly when given rapidly intravenously.

Table 26.4 Roizen's classification of dyspnoea

Grade 0	No dyspnoea while walking on the level at a normal pace
Grade I	Able to walk as far as desired provided the person takes their time
Grade II	Specific limitation: there is a need to stop and rest for a while after walking about 100–200 metres
Grade III	Dyspnoea on mild exertion: normal household tasks are limited by dyspnoeas
Grade IV	Dyspnoea at rest

Other factors

Cardiovascular disease, drugs, allergies, smoking.

Examination

Observation

- Rate and pattern of breathing.
- Ease of talking.
- Use of accessory muscles of respiration.
- Nicotine staining of hands.
- Finger clubbing (intrapulmonary shunting).
- Colour (cyanosis, anaemia).
- Deformity (kyphoscoliosis).
- Nutritional (obesity, malnutrition, muscle wasting).

Percussion

- Pleural effusion.
- Consolidation.

Auscultation

- Reduced breath sounds.
- Wheeze.
- Bronchial breathing.
- Pleural rub.

Investigation

Tests of pulmonary function will rarely be abnormal in the absence of physical symptoms and signs. They should be used to quantify risk.

Chest X-ray

Over 40 years of age, 4% of routine preoperative chest X-rays will detect an abnormality. The indications for a preoperative chest X-ray are:

- symptoms or signs of active lung disease
- patients with possible lung metastases
- symptoms and signs of heart disease
- recent immigrants from countries where tuberculosis is endemic and who have not had a chest X-ray in the previous year.

Emphysematous bullae increase the risk of pneumothorax with positive pressure ventilation. Collapse, consolidation, pleural effusion or pneumothorax require preoperative treatment. Cardiomegaly and pulmonary oedema also indicate high risk and require specialist management. Unstable patients should be transferred to an ITU or HDU for appropriate monitoring in order to maximize physiological reserve before surgery.

Spirometry

Although peak flow, FEV_1 and vital capacity may be useful to follow the progression of pulmonary dysfunction, numerous studies have failed to demonstrate their predictive value for individual patient outcome. Even patients with an FEV_1 of <0.5 litre may cope without requiring postoperative ventilation.

Maximum breathing capacity (MBC), calculated as $FEV_1 \times 35$ or peak flow × 0.25, may be used to assess respiratory reserve. MBC greater than 60 L min^{-1} is normal, and less than 25 L min^{-1} indicates severe pulmonary impairment.

Arterial blood gas tensions

A P_aO_2 of less than 7.1 kPa or less than 70% of normal for age, in combination with dyspnoea at rest, has been shown to predict dependence on postoperative respiratory support in patients undergoing upper abdominal surgery. P_aO_2 may be used with a graph of isoshunt lines to assess pulmonary shunting and to estimate oxygen requirements.

However, P_aCO_2 is of little predictive value for postoperative ventilation, but may be useful for detection of those with a hypoxic respiratory drive in whom postoperative administration of oxygen will need careful monitoring. Detection of metabolic acidosis in the critically ill patient may indicate demands on respiratory work which cannot be met by spontaneous ventilation.

Additional considerations

Surgical factors

Thoracic and upper abdominal surgery, by interfering with diaphragmatic movement, may both cause a reduction in functional residual capacity (FRC) postoperatively. In addition, as FRC falls below closing capacity, dependent airways close leading to increased ventilation–perfusion (V/Q) mismatch, shunt and atelectasis. Pain and the supine position further contribute to a reduction in FRC.

Anaesthetic factors

Anaesthesia causes a reduction in FRC and lung volume, leading to reduced compliance and increased shunting. Gas trapping of oxygen and nitrous oxide, which are soluble, may lead to alveolar collapse. General anaesthesia in excess of 2 hours increases risk of atelectasis and infection. The incidence of pneumonia in one study was 40% in patients following thoracic or abdominal surgery lasting >4 hours (8% when <2 hours).

Anaesthesia and surgery are associated with a reduced humoral immune response, impaired neutrophil chemotaxis and phagocytosis, and depressed mucociliary transport.

Age

Muscle weakness, a stiff rib cage and loss of elastic recoil in the elderly results in airway closure at higher lung volumes. After approximately 45 years of age closing capacity exceeds FRC when lying supine, which may contribute to risk of atelectasis. The incidence of pneumonia in one study was 18% over 30 years compared with 9% under 30 years, following thoracic or abdominal surgery.

Nutritional state

Obesity reduces chest compliance and FRC, and increases closing capacity. These are worsened by supine or head-down position. Postoperatively, the semierect position is preferred in order to limit hypoxaemia. Epidural analgesia reduces pulmonary complications, but the benefit is less in the very obese patient. In those heavier than 115 kg, the incidence of postoperative pneumonia was reported to be doubled. Systemic illness, chronic disease and steroids cause muscle weakness which may increase risk of pulmonary complications. Low serum albumin levels have been linked with increased risk of postoperative pneumonia.

Smoking

Smoking causes impaired mucociliary transport, reduced neutrophil activity, raised closing capacity and increased V/Q mismatch. The tracheobronchial tree is hyperactive and there is an increased risk of bronchospasm following airway manipulation. The risk of postoperative pneumonia is doubled in smokers. Carboxyhaemoglobin levels are reduced by stopping smoking for 12 hours, but 6 weeks is required for maximum benefit.

Sleep apnoea syndromes

Approximately 1 in 50 men develop obstructive sleep apnoea in the supine position, leading to hypoxaemia, hypercapnia and haemodynamic instability. Patients at risk may be identified by a history of snoring and daytime sleepiness. Sleep deprivation worsens the risk, as do hypnotic, analgesic and sedative drugs. Obstruction may occur following premedication, and airway maintenance may be difficult. Oxygen therapy alone may be inadequate, and nasal continuous positive airway pressure may be needed.

Upper respiratory tract infection

In a child with an upper respiratory tract infection (URTI) who receives a general anaesthetic, there is up to seven times the risk of a perioperative respiratory complication. Children under 1 year of age with an URTI should have elective surgery postponed. Risks increase if intubation is performed. In otherwise healthy children over 5 years and in adults, in whom there is no reduction in physical activity, no pyrexia and the chest examination is normal, there appears to be no increased risk from minor surgery of further respiratory complications. However, airways are often hyperactive with increased risk of bronchospasm, and lung defence mechanisms, particularly mucociliary clearance, may be impaired. For major surgery, few data are available of the effect on pulmonary risk, but, in combination with other risk factors, a cautious approach is wise.

Other factors

Other risk factors leading to respiratory failure should be identified. Prophylaxis may be needed for deep vein thrombosis leading to pulmonary embolus, particularly in the obese and in patients with prolonged immobilization. Preoperative hospitalization of more than 2 days doubles the risk of postoperative pneumonia.

Bibliography

Barrowcliffe MP, Jones JG. Respiratory function and the safety of anaesthesia. In: Taylor TH, Major E (eds) *Hazards and Complications of Anaesthesia*. Edinburgh: Churchill Livingstone, 1987, pp. 33–51.

Garibaldi RA, Britt MR, Coleman ML, *et al.* Risk factors of postoperative pneumonia. *Am J Med* 1981; **70**: 677–80.

Lawrence VA, Page CP, Harris GD. Preoperative spirometry before operations. A critical appraisal of its predictive value. *Arch Intern Med* 1989; **149**: 280–3.

Lumb AB. *Nunn's Applied Respiratory Physiology*, 5th edn. Oxford: Butterworth Heinemann, 2000.

Nunn JF, Milledge JS, Chen D, Dore C. Respiratory criteria of fitness for surgery and anaesthesia. *Anaesthesia* 1988; **43**: 543–51.

Zollinger A, Pasch T. The pulmonary risk patient. *Baillieres Clin Anaesthesiol* 1998; **12**: 391–403.

Cross-references

Anaesthesia and chronic obstructive pulmonary disease, 91
Asthma, 105
Failure to breathe or wake up postoperatively, 749
Obesity, 189
Smoking and anaesthesia, 120
The elderly patient, 607

Psychiatric disorders

Brian J Pollard

The incidence of psychiatric disorders within the general population is high. In general, the major relevance to anaesthesia is from the treatment and other patient comorbidities rather than from the psychiatric illness itself.

Anxiety disorders

Almost every patient suffers, or has suffered from, mild anxiety disorders at some time. It is only when it is particularly severe or does not spontaneously resolve that it requires treatment. The mainstay of treatment is members of the benzodiazepine family, although small doses of β-adrenergic blocking agents may be beneficial. There may be fear of anaesthesia and/or surgery present, and thoughtful preoperative counselling is valuable. The administration of a benzodiazepine premed is useful.

Depression

Depression is usually divided into two types – endogenous and reactive – although the distinction may not be very clear. Reactive depression is usually triggered by external events, e.g. bereavement. Symptoms include fatigue, mood disturbances, insomnia, loss of appetite, decreased ability to concentrate and a general feeling of loss of worth. Suicidal thoughts may also prevail. It is more common in women than in men and familial tendencies exist. The exact pathophysiology is not known but disturbances in central amine levels seem to be present. It may be difficult to distinguish from dementia in the elderly. Treatment of depression is with drugs and/or electroconvulsive therapy.

Tricyclic antidepressants

The original treatment, which has been mainly superseded by other drugs. Includes amitriptyline and imipramine. Side-effects include mild sedation, dry mouth, blurred vision, urinary retention (anticholinergic effects) and ECG changes (increased PR and QT intervals). An overdose may cause potentially fatal cardiac arrhythmias. Treatment with tricyclic antidepressants need not be interrupted during the operative period. An increased requirement for anaesthetic agents has been reported. Ephedrine should be given with care because there may be an exaggerated vasopressor response. A directly acting agent such as metaraminol may be preferable. Ketamine and pancuronium should be avoided or used with care. The injection of local anaesthetic containing epinephrine may result in increased blood pressure and cardiac rhythm disturbances.

Selective serotonin reuptake inhibitors

Members of this family (e.g. fluoxetine, paroxitine) are currently the most commonly prescribed drugs for depression. They are devoid of anticholinergic and cardiac side-effects. Fluoxetine in a potent inhibitor of the cytochrome P450 enzyme in the liver. This may affect the plasma levels and bioavailability of other coadministered drugs that rely on this pathway for metabolism. Selective serotonin reuptake inhibitors should not affect anaesthesia and may be safely continued throughout the perioperative period.

Monoamine oxidase inhibitors

These drugs tend not to be used as first-line treatment for depression. They do not have an anticholinergic effect nor a significant cardiac effect themselves. It is no longer recommended that monoamine oxidase inhibitors should be stopped 21 days before a general anaesthetic. The consideration with these drugs is the effect of inhibiting monoamine oxidase on the responses of other drugs and chemicals. Foods containing tyramine (e.g. cheese) should not be eaten. Care should be exercised in the choice of all drugs. Indirectly acting vasopressors (e.g. ephedrine) and pethidine should be avoided. Care should be exercised with other opioids as a hypertensive response has been reported. Ketamine, pancuronium and possibly halothane should be avoided. The use of epinephrine with the local anaesthetic in a regional block may be inadvisable. Vasoconstrictors should not be sprayed into the nose as an adjunct to surgery or nasotracheal intubation. Directly acting vasopressors, e.g. metaraminol, are recommended for the treatment of hypotension.

Manic disorders

The clinical presentation of mania is one of hyperactivity and heightened mood. It may progress to hallucinations and delusions. It appears to be inherited in an autosomal dominant manner and pathophysiological changes include abnormalities in central neurotransmitter regulation.

The routine treatment for manic disorders is lithium. Lithium has a very narrow therapeutic window. The therapeutic plasma level is 0.4–1 mmol L^{-1}; toxicity appears when the level is over 1.5 mmol L^{-1}; levels in excess of 2 mmol L^{-1} are potentially fatal. Signs of lithium toxicity include muscle weakness, sedation, ataxia, hypotension and ECG changes. Hypothyroidism, polyuria and polydipsia may occur with long-term treatment. Plasma lithium concentration must be measured before anaesthesia to ensure that it is not in the toxic range. There may be a reduced requirement for general anaesthetics. The action of neuromuscular blocking agents is prolonged. Exercise care if a dose of a loop diuretic, e.g. furosemide, is required as the plasma lithium concentration may be increased.

Schizophrenia

Patients with schizophrenia may exhibit a wide variety of symptoms including hallucinations, withdrawal from society, flat affect and disinterest in personal appearance. A wide variety of drugs are used in the treatment of schizophrenia, e.g. phenothiazines, haloperidol and clozapine. These drugs possess a wide variety of side-effects. These especially include extrapyramidal symptoms and signs, anticholinergic effects, sedation, dyskinesias and Parkinson disease-like symptoms. Postural hypotension may be present and there may be an exaggerated response to hypotensive drugs (including anaesthetic agents), fluid loss and intermittent positive pressure ventilation.

Bibliography

Anderson IM. The new antidepressants. *Curr Anaesth Critical Care* 1999; **10**: 3.

Miller RD, Way WL, Eger EI. The effects of alpha-methyl-dopa, reserpine, guanethidine and iproniazid on minimum alveolar anesthetic requirement (MAC). *Anesthesiology* 1968; 29: 1153–8.

Stack CJ, Rogers P, Linter SPK. Monoamine oxidase inhibitors and anaesthesia. *Br J Anaesth* 1988; **60**: 222–7.

Veenith T, Burnstein RM. Management of patients with neurological and psychiatric disorders. *Surgery* 2010; **28**: 441–5.

Marijuana

This agent is becoming more readily available and it is likely that its use may be legalized in some countries in the future. It is also increasingly being used for its medicinal purposes (antiemetic and claimed possible benefit in certain chronic neurological disorders). It is usually smoked and produces euphoria, drowsiness, tachycardia and postural hypotension. Long-term use may cause tar deposits in the lungs.

Anaesthesia

A reduced dose of anaesthetic agent may be required. Delayed recovery and respiratory depression are possible. There is otherwise little effect on anaesthesia.

Bibliography

Giuffrida JG, Bizzarri DV, Saurec AC, *et al.* Anesthetic management of drug abusers. *Anesth Analg* 1970; **49**: 273–82.

Kork F, Naumann T, Spiess C. Perioperative management of patients with alcohol tobacco and drug dependency. *Curr Opin Anaesthesiol* 2010; **23**: 384–90.

Lee PKY, Cho MH, Dobkin AB. Effects of alcoholism, morphinism and barbiturate resistance on induction and maintenance of general anesthesia. *Can Anaesth Soc J* 1974; **11**: 366–71.

May JA, White HC, Leonard-White A, *et al.* The patient recovering from alcohol or drug addiction: special issues for the anesthesiologist. *Anesth Analg* 2001; **92**: 1601–8.

Pleuvry BJ. CNS stimulants: basic pharmacology and relevance to anaesthesia. *Anaesth Intensive Care Med* 2006; **7**: 60–2.

Water and electrolyte disturbances

Brian J Pollard

The body is roughly 60% water, which is contained almost exclusively in lean tissue. Adipose tissue is virtually anhydrous. The approximate ratio of intracellular/interstitial/intravascular water is 10:3:1, or as a percentage of body weight 40:14:5.

Normal body water turnover is in the region of 2–3 L day^{-1}. Fluid intake is about 1200 mL, with an additional 1000 mL in solid food and about 400 mL day^{-1} is derived from oxidation of foodstuffs. Urine output amounts to 1500 mL, with 600–1000 mL insensible losses via the skin and respiratory tract, and 50 mL via the gut.

The principal extracellular ions are sodium and chloride, with a plasma osmolality of about 300 mOsm. Sodium and chloride ions permeate through the whole of the extracellular fluid.

The intra/extracellular fluid and electrolyte relationships are maintained via the relative permeabilities of sodium and potassium ions and the high protein content of the intracellular fluid with its negative charge. They are also maintained by activity of the Na^+ and K^+ pump.

Movement of fluid between the capillaries and the interstitial fluid is determined by the colloid oncotic and hydrostatic forces across the capillary wall.

Regulation of sodium and water balance

Total body sodium ion and water are controlled by a variety of mechanisms involving antidiuretic hormone (ADH) and atrial natriuretic peptide (ANP) – a 'hormone' released by the muscle cells of the heart (plasma levels correlate with right atrial pressures). ANP is thought to affect salt and water secretion via an effect on glomerular filtration and sodium absorption in the proximal tubule.

ADH is secreted in response to changes detected by osmoreceptors in the hypothalamus. An increase in osmolality stimulates ADH secretion and resorption of fluid in the collecting ducts owing to an increase in their permeability; less water is excreted and the urine is more concentrated.

The atrial receptors also have an effect on ADH secretion. Stretching, as in hypervolaemia, inhibits ADH secretion; loss of volume, such as following haemorrhage, stimulates it.

Renin–angiotensin system

Sodium and water balance are also controlled by the renin–angiotensin system. The juxtaglomerular cells are sensitive indicators of plasma sodium concentration and plasma volume by virtue of their sensitivity to:

- plasma sodium concentration
- blood pressure in afferent arterioles
- input from sympathetic nerves.

Renin secretion is stimulated by the three factors listed above. Renin cleaves angiotensin I from angiotensinogen in plasma, which is then converted to angiotensin II by converting enzyme and then to angiotensin III in the adrenal cortex, where it stimulates aldosterone secretion.

Aldosterone controls reabsorption of sodium from the distal tubule, but the system responds slowly and is the 'fine-tuning' of the sodium and water balance, controlling only the final 3% of the filtered load; its effect may take several days to become evident.

Disorders of the renin–angiotensin system may result in hypertension; failure of the aldosterone system results in sodium loss and hypotension.

ANP acts as a control both on the renin–angiotensin system and by inhibiting the reabsorption of sodium in the distal tubule; it is a vasodilator and thus also affects blood pressure directly.

Water homeostasis

The kidney, via the ADH response, has a huge reserve capacity to clear excess water, so excess intake normally only results in a transient decrease in osmolality. The sensation of thirst and the ADH, ANP and the renal–angiotensin system are all interlinked. Angiotensin II is a powerful thirst-causing substance, and ADH neurones and the thirst centre in the hypothalamus are closely associated.

Extracellular fluid homeostasis

This involves gain or loss of isotonic sodium chloride (NaCl), pure water or pure NaCl:

- cell membranes are effectively impermeable to sodium ions, so addition or loss of isotonic saline results in changes to only the extracellular fluid compartment (75% interstitial, 25% plasma)
- loss of extracellular water results in an increase in extracellular osmolality, which causes water to

move from the cells; with a gain in pure water the reverse is true

- changes in the extracellular fluid NaCl content alone are compensated for by movement of fluid into or from the intracellular fluid compartment.

Thus, a change in pure water or NaCl alone affects both intracellular as well as extracellular fluid, whereas isotonic changes affect only extracellular fluid.

Potassium homeostasis

The potential across cell membranes is largely controlled by the differential potassium ion concentrations. Changes in extracellular potassium have a disproportionately marked effect on the size of this potential. Potassium is lost from the cells in catabolic states and, in critical illness, this leads to disturbances in cell membrane function. Sodium leaks in and potassium leaches out, with a decrease in membrane potential. This can be restored with glucose and insulin and supplementary potassium. Recent work has shown that when insulin was used to aggressively control blood glucose levels, there was a significant improvement in mortality rates. This was ascribed to the tight control of blood glucose concentrations, but it could equally have been the result of a restoration of cell membrane function by the glucose and insulin.

Ninety per cent of potassium is reabsorbed from the kidney in the proximal tubule and the proximal part of the loop of Henle. The remaining 10% arrives in the distal tubule; it is via this 10% that all potassium regulation occurs. Reabsorption of potassium from the distal tubule is via an active pump in the tubular cells; in the presence of hyperkalaemia, aldosterone secretion increases in response to the direct effect of potassium on the adrenal cortex (a mechanism not involving the renin–angiotensin pathway). Sodium reabsorbed from this distal tubule is associated with secretion of potassium and hydrogen ions, the two cations being in competition with each other.

Calcium and phosphate homeostasis

The normal plasma concentration of calcium ions is 2.5 mM, but the physiologically important part is ionic calcium, which constitutes just under 50%: 46% of plasma calcium is protein bound and 6% is bound to phosphate.

Calcium ions are important in membrane excitability and are sensitive to pH changes, with alkalinity decreasing calcium ion concentration and acidosis increasing it (Table 26.5).

Metabolism and control of calcium ion concentration are inextricably bound up with phosphate metabolism; most calcium ions are contained in bone, which acts as a massive reserve in the control of calcium ion concentration. Intestinal uptake of calcium ions is in the range 20–70%, varying in response to changes in plasma concentration. Calcium and phosphate are excreted by the kidney – filtered out then absorbed under hormonal control (Table 26.6).

Table 26.5 Symptoms of changes in plasma calcium levels

Elevated [Ca^{2+}]	Decreased [Ca^{2+}]
Lethargy	Muscle cramps
Fatigue	Convulsions
Sensory loss	Increased neuromuscular excitability

Table 26.6 Hormonal control of calcium metabolism

Hormone	Source	Trigger to stimulation	Effect
Calcitonin	Parafollicular cells of thyroid		Stimulates bone deposition Decreases plasma Ca^{2+}
Parathormone	Parathyroid glands	Low plasma Ca^{2+}	Release of Ca^{2+} from bone Reabsorption from renal tubule Decreases renal reabsorption of phosphate
1,25-Dihydroxycholecalciferol	Derivative of vitamins D_2 and D_3 via metabolic pathways in liver and kidney		Ca^{2+} and phosphate absorption from the gut

Disturbances in fluid and electrolytes

Probably the commonest abnormality in clinical practice is hypovolaemia, i.e. loss of both fluid and electrolytes (Table 26.7), due either to blood loss or fluid loss, such as diarrhoea/vomiting, or to loss into the gastrointestinal tract in obstruction or burn injury. This is loss of both fluid and electrolytes and is best replaced by balanced salt solution, Ringer's lactate (Hartmann's solution) or 0.9% saline, although the last provides a large chloride load and tends to produce metabolic acidosis and lactate is metabolized in the liver to carbon dioxide and water and tends to produce alkalosis. If the hypovolaemia is severe enough to produce problems with cardiac output and peripheral perfusion, intravascular volume is more effectively repleted with colloidal solutions, such as albumin, or one of the synthetic colloids, or even blood.

The colloid versus crystalloid debate continues. The objection to the latter is that it takes, on average, three times as much crystalloid to produce a persistent

Table 26.7 Disturbances of water, sodium and potassium balance

Disorder	Causes	Clinical signs	Biochemical signs	Treatment
Water deficiency	Diabetes insipidus Hyperosmolar non-ketotic diabetic coma Nephrogenic diabetes insipidus Some types of chronic pyelonephritis	Loss of skin turgor Loss of eyeball tension Dry mucous membrane Low blood pressure Delirium Coma	Plasma Na^+ and Cl^- elevated Plasma hypertonic Na^+ conserved K^+ and H^+ excreted to produce hypokalaemic acidosis Haematocrit and plasma protein concentration increased Urine and plasma osmolality increased	Oral rehydration, if possible, or dextrose (5% i.v.)
Water excess	Heart failure Acute renal failure Iatrogenic(administration of 5% dextrose)	Abdominal and skeletal muscular twitching and cramps Stupor Convulsions In severe cases peripheral and pulmonary oedema	Low plasma Na^+ and Cl^- Increased blood and plasma volume Low osmolality Low plasma proteins and haematocrit	
Sodium chloride deficiency	Decreased intake unusual, but may occur in diarrhoea, malabsorption, severe vomiting Increased Na^+ loss in diabetic acidosis Chronic renal disease Excessive sweating Adrenal insufficiency	Symptoms develop as[Na^+] drops below 115 mmol L^{-1} Clouding of consciousness Convulsions Coma	Plasma Na^+ and Cl^- drop after 4 or 5 days Decrease in blood volume K^+ moves out of cells (to maintain tonicity) Na^+ conservation via renin–angiotensin–aldosterone system Metabolic alkalosis Haematocrit and plasma proteins increased (decreased in dilutional hyponatraemia)	
Sodium chloride excess	Iatrogenic (particularly intravenous nutrition) Primary aldosteronism	Oedema Congestive heart failure Fluid retained so osmolality and [Na^+] may be normal		

(continued)

Table 26.7 *(continued)*

Disorder	Causes	Clinical signs	Biochemical signs	Treatment
Potassium deficiency	Gastrointestinal losses Renal disease Diuretics Hormonal (aldosteronism) Cushing's disease Steroids Diabetic acidosis Trauma Burns Intravenous feeding with no added K^+	Drowsy Muscular weakness Paralytic ileus Bradycardia Heart block ST depression Inverted T waves Prolonged QT and PR intervals U waves		
Potassium excess	Renal failure Iatrogenic (administration of K^+) Na^+ conserving diuretics Adrenal insufficiency Acidosis Hypoxia	Anxiety Agitation Stupor Weakness Hyporeflexia Paralysis of extremities Peaked T waves Widened QRS and prolonged PR interval Arrhythmias Cardiac arrest		Acute treatment with Ca^{2+} salts Glucose/ insulin Ion exchange resins

increase in blood volume as it does colloid, because of rapid transfer of the former to the extracellular space. Colloid also eventually leaks into the extravascular space, but more slowly. The objection to colloid is that this type of problem is usually associated with an acute-phase response and an increase in capillary permeability, both generally and at the site of injury. Fluid that leaks from the intravascular space is sequestered in this 'third' or 'oedema' space, which may include the lung. When the patient recovers this fluid is remobilized and excreted. With colloid, this remobilization may be more protracted.

Fluid balance during surgery and anaesthesia

Patients arriving for surgery may have been starved for up to 12 hours and would be about 1 litre in deficit. This deficit is of both fluids and electrolytes, and so can be replaced with balanced salt solution. Fluid requirements during surgery depend on the extent of the surgery. It is conventional practice in the normal individual to transfuse blood when about 20% of the circulating blood volume has been lost. With blood loss, fluid requirements (in addition to blood replacement) are in the range 5–15 mL kg^{-1} h^{-1}, depending on the amount of blood loss and the extent of surgery. Hypotonic (glucose) solutions should not be given for volume replacement, as in the short term they produce significant hyperglycaemia (>20 mol L^{-1}) and in the longer term persistent hyponatraemia.

Too aggressive a use of fluids can cause problems in the postoperative period. Fluid retention of about 3 litres after abdominal surgery is not uncommon, but it has been demonstrated that if sodium and water is restricted postoperatively (2 litres per 24 hours and 70–80 mmol Na rather than the traditional 3 litres and 150 mmol Na) recovery is quicker and the incidence of postoperative complications lower.

Bibliography

Lobo DN, Bostock KA, Neal KR, *et al.* Effect of salt and water balance on recovery of gastrointestinal function after elective colonic resection: a randomised controlled trial. *Lancet* 2002; **359**: 1812–18.

Lobo DN, Macafee DAL, Allison SP. How perioperative fluid balance influences postoperative outcomes. *Best Pract Res Clin Anaesthesiol* 2006; **20**: 439–55.

Martinez-Riquelme AE, Allison SP. Insulin revisited. *Clin Nutr* 2002; **22**: 7–15.

Westphal M, Scholtz J, Van Aken H, Bein B. Infusion therapy in anaesthesia and intensive care: let's stop talking about 'wet' and 'dry'! *Best Pract Res Clin Anaesthesiol* 2009; **23**: vii–x.

Cross-references

Elective surgery, 610
Fluid and electrolyte balance, 754

27 Airway

Cyprian Mendonca

Airway and aspiration risk

Rajneesh Sachdeva

Inhalation of gastric contents into the tracheobronchial tree produces chemical pneumonia due to the acidic pH of the gastric contents. In 1946, Mendelson described the problems of gastric aspiration during obstetric anaesthesia. In the general population, the incidence of aspiration is low; however, during unexpected difficult intubation the risk is higher. Positive pressure ventilation through face-mask and supraglottic devices using a high peak pressure may lead to distension of the stomach and regurgitation of stomach contents.

Aspiration after tracheal intubation in elective patients has an incidence of 1.25 per 10 000 patients. In a report of difficult intubations from Australia, regurgitation occurred during one in seven cases of difficult intubation. In another prospective study involving 2833 emergency intubations outside the operating room, an aspiration risk of 13% was associated with difficult intubation involving more than two laryngoscopic attempts.

Risk factors for aspiration

- Full stomach.
- Raised intra-abdominal pressure.
- Gastrointestinal obstruction.
- Delayed gastric emptying due to drugs (opioids), pain and autonomic neuropathy.
- Gastro-oesophageal reflux.
- Hiatus hernia.
- Previous oesophageal surgery.
- Pregnancy.
- Difficult intubation.
- Straining or coughing during light plane of anaesthesia.
- Acute alcohol intoxication.

Prevention of aspiration

- Avoid general anaesthesia if possible.
- Delay non-emergency surgery (for 6 hours) to empty the stomach.
- Prophylactic drugs.
- Rapid sequence induction of general anaesthesia.
- Induction of anaesthesia in head-up position or left lateral head-down position.

Rapid sequence induction is a method of induction of a state of unconsciousness with complete neuromuscular paralysis to achieve rapid intubation without interposed mechanical ventilation in an effort to minimize risks of gastric aspiration.

The process of rapid sequence induction involves the following steps.

- Preparation of the patient, operating room and drugs. Patient assessment including airway evaluation and explanation of the procedure is essential. A trained anaesthetic assistant should be available.
- Patient positioning with pillow under the occiput.
- Preoxygenation of the patient with 100% oxygen through a tight-fitting face-mask, with eight vital capacity breaths or for 3–5 minutes of tidal volume breathing to denitrogenate the lungs.
- Paralysis after administration of a predetermined dose of intravenous induction agent. Neuromuscular blocking agent should only be administered after ensuring loss of consciousness to prevent awareness. To maintain cardiovascular stability, in some patients an opioid may be necessary to reduce the dose of induction agent.
- Protection of tracheobronchial tree by cricoid pressure (Sellick's manoeuvre).
- Placement of the tracheal tube under vision followed by auscultation, $ETco_2$ measurement and release of cricoid pressure after confirmation of correct placement of tracheal tube.

Succinylcholine is the muscle relaxant that is commonly used for rapid sequence induction owing to its rapid onset of action. Rocuronium also has a rapid onset of action and can be used as an alternative to succinylcholine. If there is difficulty in intubation, the action of rocuronium can be rapidly reversed using sugammadex.

Cricoid pressure

A properly trained assistant is mandatory. There are two approaches: single-handed and two-handed technique for performing cricoid pressure.

A bimanual technique is preferred by some – the neck support prevents the head from flexing on the neck. However, others prefer the single-handed technique that leaves the assistant's other hand free to help with intubation.

A nasogastric tube should be left in place, but it must be open to vent gas or liquid.

Cricoid pressure should be applied to the awake patient with a force of 10 N (1 kg), after preoxygenation but before intravenous induction.

If retching occurs after intravenous induction, the cricoid pressure should be released as oesophageal rupture may occur.

Cricoid pressure should be increased to a force of 30 N (3 kg) after loss of consciousness and before the onset of succinylcholine fasciculations. The assistant should practice the correct application of force on a weighing scale.

Sellick originally described a three-fingered technique, with the main force applied by the index finger; others have recommended two fingers. The assistant should try to keep the larynx in the midline.

Complications of cricoid pressure

In an awake patient, cricoid pressure can cause discomfort and anxiety. Cricoid pressure can distort the anatomy of the larynx either by displacing it laterally or by having too much force on the thyroid cartilage. This may worsen the laryngoscopic view. It can cause airway obstruction and restrict ventilation with a face-mask. Airway obstruction is directly related to the force applied: 40 N of cricoid pressure causes airway obstruction in about 35% of patients.

Prophylactic drugs

- H_2 receptor antagonist (ranitidine 150 mg orally or 50 mg intravenously): administered 30 minutes prior to induction of anaesthesia.
- Metoclopramide (10 mg by mouth): administered 30–60 minutes prior to induction of anaesthesia to stimulate gastric emptying.
- Non-particulate antacid (sodium citrate 30 mL): administered immediately prior to induction of anaesthesia.

Management of suspected aspiration

- Administer 100% O_2.
- Head-down tilt
- Oropharyngeal suction to clear the airway.
- Secure the airway with a tracheal tube.
- Immediate tracheal suction.
- Insert the nasogastric tube and empty the stomach.
- Mechanical ventilation and PEEP to treat hypoxaemia.
- Bronchodilators if needed.
- Chest X-ray to diagnose collapse or pneumonia.
- Supportive care includes fluid management and H_2 receptor antagonists for prophylaxis against stress ulcers.

Bibliography

Allman KG. The effect of cricoid pressure application on airway patency. *J Clin Anaesth* 1995; **7**: 197–9.

Georgescu A, Miller JN, Lecklitner ML. The Sellick maneuver causing complete airway obstruction. *Anesth Analg* 1992; **74**: 457–9.

Hartsilver EL, Vanner RG. Airway obstruction with cricoid pressure. *Anaesthesia* 2000; **55**: 208–11.

Hocking G, Roberts FL, Thew ME. Airway obstruction with cricoid pressure and lateral tilt. *Anaesthesia* 2001; **56**: 825–8.

Mort TC. Emergency tracheal intubation: complications associated with repeated laryngoscopic attempts. *Anesth Analg* 2004; **99**: 607–13

Shorten GD, Alfille PH, Gliklich RE. Airway obstruction following application of cricoid pressure. *J Clin Anaesth* 1991; **3**: 403–5.

Vanner RG. Tolerance of cricoid pressure by conscious volunteers. *Int J Obstet Anesthesiol* 1992; **1**: 195–8.

Vanner RG, Asai T. Safe use of cricoid pressure. *Anaesthesia* 1999; **54**: 1–3.

Warner ME, Warner ME. Clinical significance of pulmonary aspiration during the perioperative period. *Anesthesiology* 1993; **78**: 56–62.

Williamson JA, Webb RK, Szekely S, *et al.* The Australian Incident Monitoring Study. Difficult intubation: an analysis of 2000 incident reports. *Anaesth Intensive Care* 1993; **21**: 602–7.

Yentis SM. The effects of single-handed and bimanual cricoid pressure on the view at laryngoscopy. *Anaesthesia* 1997; **52**: 332–5.

Cross-reference

Hypoxaemia under anaesthesia, 670

such as bougie or uses an alternate device/technique following failed intubation with direct laryngoscopy.

In 2004, the Difficult Airway Society (DAS) of the UK developed guidelines for managing unanticipated difficult intubation in non-obstetric adult patients. The main emphasis is on avoiding airway trauma by multiple attempts at laryngoscopy and maintaining oxygenation. The basic structure of the DAS guideline (Fig. 27.3) includes four plans.

- Plan A: Initial tracheal intubation plan.
- Plan B: Secondary tracheal intubation plan.
- Plan C: Maintenance of oxygenation, ventilation and postponement of surgery.
- Plan D: Rescue technique for 'can't intubate, can't ventilate' scenario.

Bibliography

American Society of Anaesthesiologists Task Force on Difficult Airway Management. Practice guidelines for management of the difficult airway *Anesthesiology* 2003; **98**: 1269–77.

Benumof JL. ASA difficult airway algorithm: new thoughts and considerations. In: Hagberg CA (ed.) *Handbook of Difficult Airway Management.* Philadelphia: Churchill Livingstone, 2000, pp. 31–48.

Cook TM. A new practical classification of laryngeal view. *Anaesthesia* 2000; **55**: 274–9.

Cook TM, Scott S, Mihai R. Litigation related to airway and respiratory complications of anaesthesia: an analysis of claims against the NHS in England 1995–2007, *Anaesthesia* 2010; **65**: 556–63.

Cormack RS, Lehane J. Difficult intubation in obstetrics. *Anaesthesia* 1984; **39**: 1105–11.

El-Ganzouri AR, McCarthy RJ, Tuman KJ, *et al.* Preoperative airway assessment: predictive value of a multivariate risk index. *Anesth Analg* 1996; **82**: 1197–204.

Langeron O, Masso E, Huraux C, *et al.* Prediction of difficult mask ventilation. *Anaesthesiology* 2000; **92**: 1229–36.

Peterson GN, Domino KB, Caplan RA, *et al.* Management of the difficult airway. A closed claims analysis. *Anesthesiology* 2005; **103**: 33–9.

Rocke DA, Murray WB, Rout CC, Gouws E. Relative risk analysis of factors associated with difficult intubation in obstetric anaesthesia. *Anaesthesiology* 1992; **77**: 67–73.

Samson GL, Young JR. Difficult tracheal intubation: a retrospective study, *Anaesthesia* 1987; **42**: 487–90.

Yentis SM, Lee DJH. Evaluation of an improved scoring system for the grading of direct laryngoscopy. *Anaesthesia* 1998; **53**: 1041–4.

Cross-references

Difficult airway: management, 651
Hypoxaemia under anaesthesia, 670

Difficult airway: management

Cyprian Mendonca

A difficult airway generally means difficult tracheal intubation. But in clinical practice there may be difficulty with mask ventilation, difficulty with obtaining an adequate view of the larynx and difficulty in placing the tube in the trachea despite an adequate view of the larynx. The management of the difficult airway depends on whether the difficulty is anticipated or unanticipated. The management plan is also influenced by the degree of difficulty anticipated or encountered, location, availability of equipment and expertise. A structured approach to the management is more likely to result in a successful outcome. In 2004, The Difficult Airway Society in the UK produced guidelines for managing unanticipated difficult intubation.

The basic principles of airway management involves:

- preoperative assessment and anticipation
- preparation and choosing appropriate plans (primary plan and alternative plans)
- maintaining oxygenation throughout the procedure
- planning extubation
- maintaining records and communication.

Anticipated difficult airway

The management depends on:

- severity of difficulty expected
- presence or absence of upper airway obstruction.

Severe difficulty expected

Awake fibreoptic intubation (Fig. 27.4) is the method of choice, and is acceptable to most patients. Fibreoptic laryngoscopy can be regarded as a part of the preoperative examination and should be presented to the patient in that manner. The cardiovascular stability associated with fibreoptic intubation under topical anaesthesia is an attractive feature of the technique.

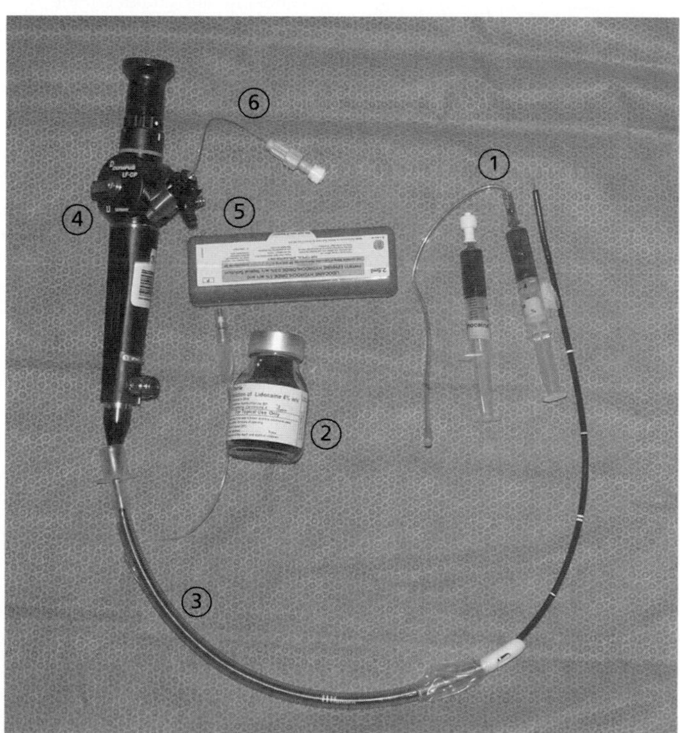

● **Figure 27.4** Equipment and drugs for awake fibreoptic intubation. 1, mucosal atomization device; 2, 4% lidocaine; 3, tracheal tube loaded on the fibreoptic scope; 4, fibreoptic scope; 5, 5% lidocaine with 0.5% phenylephrine; 6, epidural catheter (reproduced with permission from Mendonca C, Hillerman C, James J, Kumar A. *The Structured Oral Examination in Clinical Anaesthesia*. Shrewsbury: TFM Publishing, 2009).

Awake fibreoptic intubation

Nasal intubation is frequently easier in this group of patients, because of limited mouth opening, and the poor 'angle of attack' with the oral route.

Topical anaesthesia is more effective if glycopyrrolate is given to dry the mucosa. A vasoconstrictor should be applied to the nasal mucosa (xylometazoline or phenylephrine) before endoscopy.

Lidocaine is poorly absorbed from the nasopharynx; doses up to 10 mg kg^{-1} are acceptable. Lidocaine is irritant to the nasal and glottic mucosa. Initial application should be with a warm 1% solution or 2% gel or a small quantity of 4% solution; 10% lidocaine can then be applied to the pharyngeal mucosa. The epiglottis, glottis and trachea are liberally sprayed with 4% lidocaine through the endoscope (about 6 mL) using the 'spray as you go' (SAYGO) technique. An alternative is to inject 3–4 mL 4% lidocaine through the cricothyroid membrane. Coughing can be very vigorous, but will result in satisfactory anaesthesia. The glottis will not be anaesthetized if the patient does not cough.

It is foolish to attempt to pass a tube of greater than 7.0 mm ID over a fibreoptic endoscope. Flexible metal-reinforced tubes with short and soft bevel are recommended, and rotation of the tube as it is passed through the cords is helpful. The nasal tissues (or the shaft of the laryngeal mask) grip the tube and it is often necessary to apply several turns to the proximal end of the tube to produce one turn at the distal end. Severe laryngeal damage has been reported after awake fibreoptic intubation; the glottic reflexes must be obtunded, force should not be used and multiple attempts are not made.

It is sensible to administer some sedation as the tube is passed, as the passage of the tube through the nose is unpleasant. Target-controlled infusion of remifentanil (1–3 ng mL^{-1}) or propofol (0.5–1.5 μg mL^{-1}) is commonly used for providing conscious sedation.

Alternatively, if the mouth opening is about 20–25 mm or greater, awake tracheal intubation can also be performed using indirect laryngoscopes (Pentax Airway scope; Bullard laryngoscope). A supraglottic device such as the LMA can also be inserted under topical anaesthesia.

In certain scenarios, such as paediatric patients, patients with learning disabilities, hypersensitivity to local anaesthetics and uncooperative patients, it may not be possible to perform awake intubation.

Retrograde intubation is an alternative when fibreoptic technology and skill is not available. An epidural catheter or J-tipped wire is passed through a Tuohy needle into the pharynx, recovered in the pharynx and an introducer (a fibreoptic scope is ideal) or tracheal tube passed over it. If a fibreoptic scope is used, it should be preloaded with a tube and is advanced until it reaches the trachea and then the tube is railroaded over the scope.

Anticipated difficult airway with airway obstruction

The management depends on:

- urgency of action required (severity of airway obstruction and cause of airway obstruction)
- site of airway obstruction.

Acute airway obstruction can occur in patients with a previously normal airway owing to angioneurotic oedema, foreign body inhalation and postsurgery neck haematoma.

Chronic airway obstruction can occur with benign and malignant diseases involving the glottis and supraglottic regions, radiotherapy to the neck and previous surgery on the neck.

Stridor is the cardinal sign of a narrowed airway, which is said to occur at rest when the airway diameter is reduced by 50%. The diameter of the airway can be dangerously reduced without stridor being present. Complaints of awakening at night with sensations of choking are characteristic of glottic obstruction. Patients with airway obstruction should be allowed to adopt their preferred position and interfered with as little as possible. If the patient panics, the situation is likely to become truly dreadful.

Cervical haematomas (thyroid or anterior cervical surgery) produce oedema of the glottis and periglottic tissue. The swelling may be largely due to lymphatic obstruction and the haematoma may be small. The wound should be opened immediately to relieve lymphatic and venous obstruction.

When immediate intervention is required, a basic life support protocol including providing high-flow oxygen to the patient should be initiated. Inhalation of nebulized epinephrine (1 mL of 1:1000, in 10 mL of saline) may buy some time. In cases of anaphylaxis, epinephrine (0.5–1.0 mL of 1:10 000) should be given intravenously. Heliox may be beneficial in improving the turbulent flow across the obstruction.

- Recognition and evaluation of the critical airway obstruction is paramount.
- Team management in the form of senior anaesthetist, ENT surgeon and trained anaesthetic assistant is essential.

Patients with stridor can be divided into two groups:

- Severe stridor: nasendoscopy reveals intubation is impossible. In this group, the patient should have tracheostomy under local anaesthetic.

- Moderate stridor: nasendoscopy reveals intubation is possible. In this situation, inhalational induction should be performed with the ENT surgeon gowned and gloved, ready to perform tracheotomy or to perform rigid bronchoscopy with jet ventilation facility.

Patients may find it difficult to tolerate a supine position, so induction of anaesthesia and initial preparation of surgery should be performed in the head-up position.

There are two possible problems with awake fibreoptic intubation in these patients:

- local anaesthetic spray can lead to laryngospasm and complete airway obstruction
- advancement of the fibreoptic scope through the lesion can cause 'cork in the bottle' phenomenon leading to complete airway obstruction.

In some hands, fibreoptic intubation can be successful, but it is not a technique for the inexperienced. In patients with very swollen necks it may be the only sensible option.

Inhalational induction can only succeed if the airway is at least partially patent. The process is slow owing to increased collapsibility of the airway and reduced alveolar ventilation. After initial loss of consciousness, breathing becomes obstructed, and any airway manipulation and insertion of an oropharyngeal airway may lead to coughing and laryngospasm. The safety of inhalational induction is achieved only when spontaneous ventilation is maintained. Judicious use of an intravenous agent, such as propofol, and application of CPAP can be helpful. Intravenous glycopyrrolate may reduce troublesome secretions.

Oropharyngeal tumours

In patients with oropharyngeal tumours, awake fibreoptic intubation is a suitable option. The other possible option includes induction of anaesthesia following prophylactic placement of a cricothyroid cannula.

Subglottic or infraglottic tumours

The site and extent of the airway obstruction should be determined using CT/MRI scan. If assessment of the airway does not indicate difficult laryngoscopy, then conventional intubation can be done. Evaluation of the airway beyond the tube should be examined with the fibreoptic bronchoscope after the intubation.

Anterior mediastinal masses

Obstruction of the trachea or main bronchus can occur during anaesthesia in symptomless patients. In a patient with history suggestive of mediastinal mass, chest X-ray and CT scan can demonstrate the site of airway obstruction. Flow/volume loop studies are useful in quantifying the degree of airway obstruction and also in differentiating extrathoracic from intrathoracic airway obstruction. If the obstruction is likely to hamper the placement of a small tube and for lower tracheal and bronchial obstruction, cardiopulmonary bypass should be considered.

Extubation after intubation for airway obstruction

The minimum period of intubation should probably be 24 hours. Adequate sedation must be prescribed, to prevent accidental extubation. A small tube should have been passed, so that deflation of the cuff and blocking the tube can demonstrate a satisfactory airway.

Direct laryngoscopy and the unstable cervical spine

All airway manipulations will cause a degree of movement at the craniocervical junction and in the cervical spine. There is no evidence that direct laryngoscopy is more dangerous than any other method of intubation. Many patients with severe instability are in cervical fixation devices, which restrict mouth opening and cervical movements. In these circumstances, awake fibreoptic intubation is probably the method of choice. In trauma scenarios, manual in-line stabilization of the head and neck may reduce the quality of view when a direct laryngoscopy with Macintosh blade is used. Use of an alternative blade such as the McCoy or an indirect laryngoscope or intubating LM may have a role in these cases.

Blind nasal intubation

Skilful practitioners can achieve a remarkable degree of success. A combination of direct laryngoscopy and guiding a nasal tube towards the glottis with Magill's forceps is easier for most anaesthetists. Blind nasal intubation is a dying art owing to the availability of flexible fibreoptic systems.

Unanticipated difficult airway

This is a situation when a preoperative assessment reveals a normal airway but, following induction of anaesthesia, there is difficulty with mask ventilation or with tracheal intubation or with both. The scenario in which both mask ventilation and tracheal intubation is impossible (CICV) is very rare.

The principles of management involve:

- maintenance of oxygenation
- prevention of the airway trauma due to repeated attempts
- recognizing the difficulty and requesting help on time

- choosing an alternative technique/device rather than persistent attempts with the same technique/device.

The above principles can be implemented by adhering to a definitive, clear algorithm-based pre-existing plan. In the UK, guidelines published by the DAS are recommended. A flow chart, consisting of plans A, B, C and D, has been described for each of the following three scenarios.

- Unanticipated difficult tracheal intubation during routine induction of anaesthesia.
- Unanticipated difficult intubation during rapid sequence induction.
- Failed intubation, increasing hypoxaemia and difficult ventilation in a paralysed and anaesthetized patient.

Unanticipated difficult tracheal intubation during routine induction of anaesthesia (Fig. 27.5)

Plan A

Plan A is the primary tracheal intubation plan. The first attempt at the laryngoscopy should be performed in the best optimum condition. It includes an adequately anaesthetized/paralysed patient, optimum position of the head consisting of head extension and neck flexion (if not contraindicated). Anaesthesia should be induced following adequate preoxygenation.

In obese patients, ramping is used instead of 'sniffing the morning air' position. Ramping can be achieved by using pillows or blankets placed under the scapula, shoulders and nape of the neck, until the external auditory meatus and manubrium sternum are in a horizontal plane. Specially designed ramping devices are now available.

Optimum external laryngeal manipulation or a BURP (backward, upward and right-sided pressure on thyroid cartilage) manoeuvre should be applied to improve the laryngeal view. It is more successful when the laryngoscopist himself applies the pressure to determine the optimal direction, and then asks the assistant to perform the same manoeuvre.

If the best first attempt results in a poor view of larynx, then the decision should be made either to use a different blade/laryngoscope or bougie or to move on to plan B. Adequate mask ventilation should be ensured between the attempts at laryngoscopy.

The bougie is an outstandingly useful item and should always be ready for use. Disposable, single-use, tube introducers are much less effective than the classic gum elastic model.

Technique

- Continue exposure of the glottis with the laryngoscope throughout.
- Lubricate only the tip of the bougie.
- Pass the bougie, suitably bent, before loading a small (6.0–7.0 mm) tube.
- Lubricate the tip of the tube, and the bougie, as the tube enters the mouth.
- Rotate the tube 90° anticlockwise as it approaches the glottis.
- Remove the bougie and laryngoscope once the tube is positioned in the trachea.
- Confirm the position of the tube using an $ETco_2$ monitor, auscultation or oesophageal detector.

While passing the bougie, the correct position can be recognized by the clicks felt as it slides down the tracheal rings and by resistance for further advancement (distal hold up), once about 45 cm is advanced.

Alternative techniques such as fibreoptic intubation, optical stylets or optical/videolaryngoscopes can be used by those experienced in these techniques. But the maximum number of laryngoscope insertions should be limited to four and the same direct laryngoscope should not be used more than twice.

Plan B

Plan B is the secondary tracheal intubation plan. This is best achieved by using a 'dedicated airway device', defined as 'an upper airway device, which maintains airway patency while facilitating tracheal intubation'. The classic LMA and intubating LMA are the most commonly used rescue devices. It is recommended to perform fibreoptic-guided tracheal intubation through these devices.

Blind tracheal intubation through an LMA has a low success rate and can cause airway trauma. One-stage fibreoptic-guided intubation can be performed by directly loading a size 6 mm ID endotracheal tube over the fibreoptic scope. It requires a longer tube such as a microlaryngoscopy tube or a nasal RAE tube. Alternatively, an Aintree catheter can be passed over a fibreoptic laryngoscope and a tube rail-roaded over it after removal of the LMA.

Plan C

Plan C involves maintenance of oxygenation and ventilation, postponement of surgery and awakening the patient – if plans A and B have failed. If adequate oxygenation is achieved using dedicated airway devices, they should be left *in situ* until the patient is fully awake. The elective surgery should be postponed. If the dedicated airway device fails to maintain oxygenation, optimum bag-and-mask ventilation should be attempted. Two-person bag-and-mask

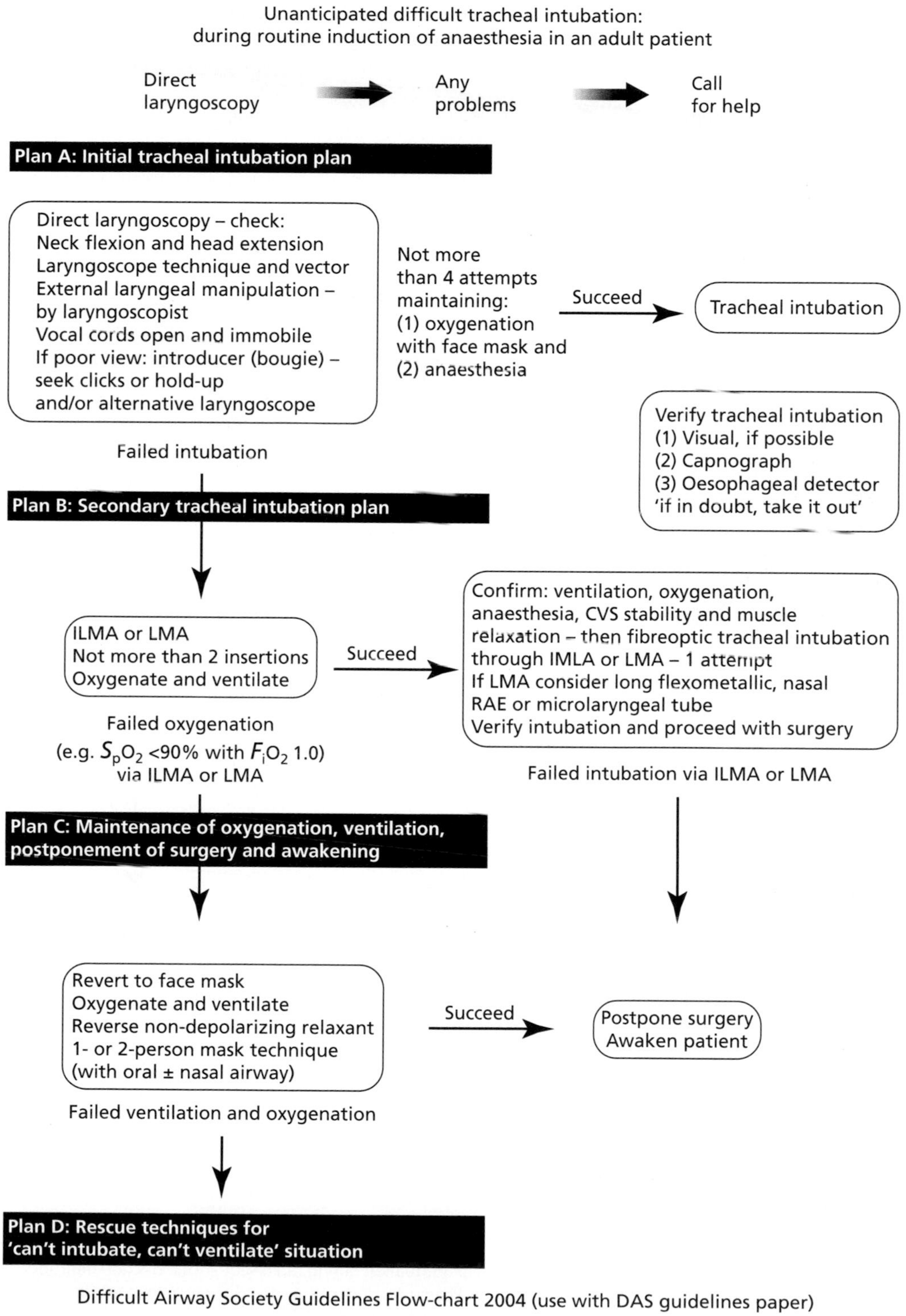

Unanticipated difficult tracheal intubation:
during routine induction of anaesthesia in an adult patient

Direct laryngoscopy → Any problems → Call for help

Plan A: Initial tracheal intubation plan

Direct laryngoscopy – check:
Neck flexion and head extension
Laryngoscope technique and vector
External laryngeal manipulation – by laryngoscopist
Vocal cords open and immobile
If poor view: introducer (bougie) – seek clicks or hold-up
and/or alternative laryngoscope

Not more than 4 attempts maintaining:
(1) oxygenation with face mask and
(2) anaesthesia

Succeed → Tracheal intubation

Verify tracheal intubation
(1) Visual, if possible
(2) Capnograph
(3) Oesophageal detector
'if in doubt, take it out'

Failed intubation

Plan B: Secondary tracheal intubation plan

ILMA or LMA
Not more than 2 insertions
Oxygenate and ventilate

Succeed →

Confirm: ventilation, oxygenation, anaesthesia, CVS stability and muscle relaxation – then fibreoptic tracheal intubation through IMLA or LMA – 1 attempt
If LMA consider long flexometallic, nasal RAE or microlaryngeal tube
Verify intubation and proceed with surgery

Failed oxygenation
(e.g. S_pO_2 <90% with F_iO_2 1.0)
via ILMA or LMA

Failed intubation via ILMA or LMA

Plan C: Maintenance of oxygenation, ventilation, postponement of surgery and awakening

Revert to face mask
Oxygenate and ventilate
Reverse non-depolarizing relaxant
1- or 2-person mask technique
(with oral ± nasal airway)

Succeed → Postpone surgery
Awaken patient

Failed ventilation and oxygenation

Plan D: Rescue techniques for 'can't intubate, can't ventilate' situation

Difficult Airway Society Guidelines Flow-chart 2004 (use with DAS guidelines paper)

● **Figure 27.5** Management of unanticipated difficult tracheal intubation during routine induction of anaesthesia (reproduced with permission from Henderson JJ, Popat MT, Latto IP, Pearce AC. Difficult Airway Society guidelines for management of the unanticipated difficult intubation. *Anaesthesia* 2004; **59**: 675–94).

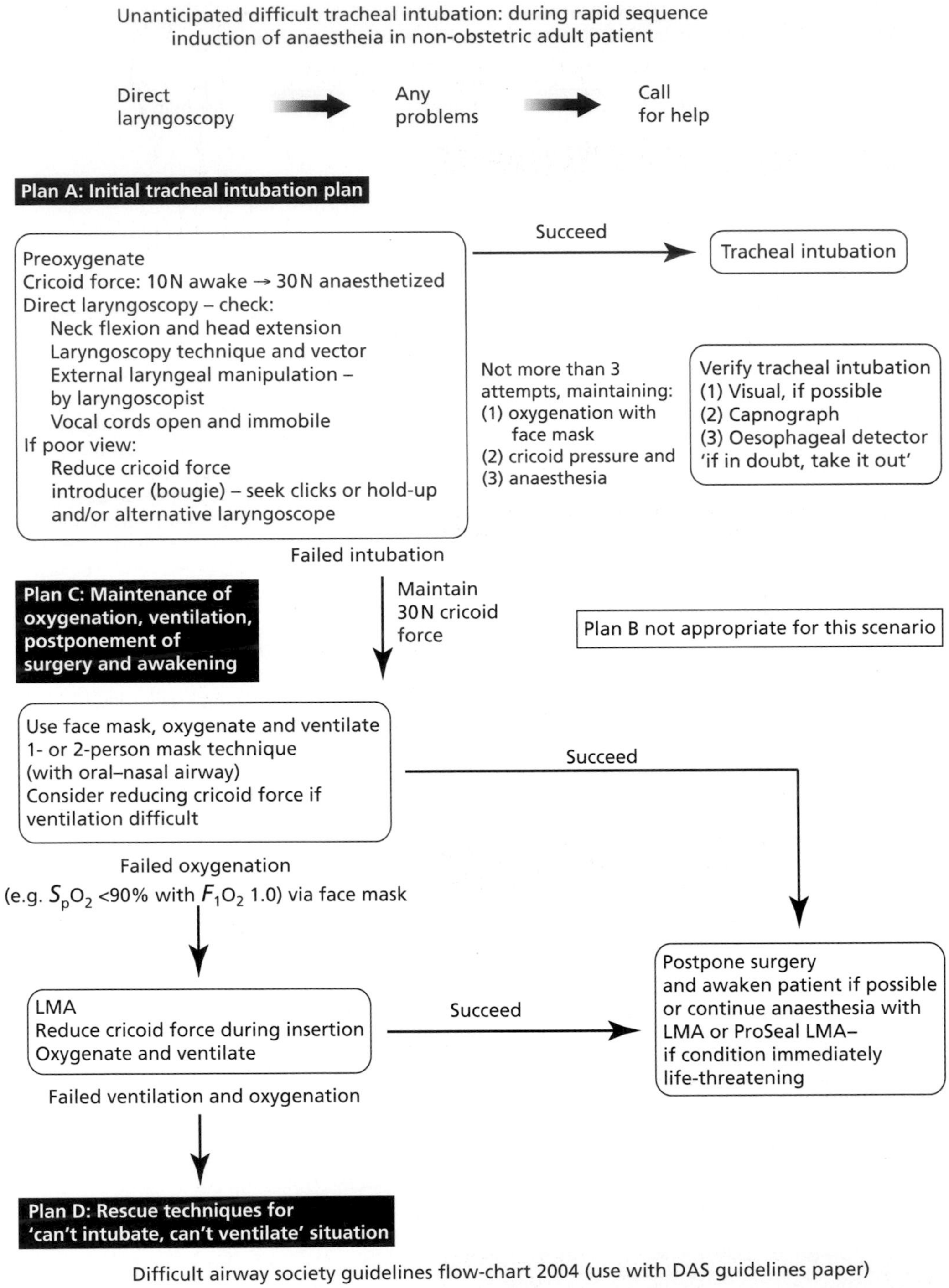

Unanticipated difficult tracheal intubation: during rapid sequence induction of anaesthesia in non-obstetric adult patient

Direct laryngoscopy → Any problems → Call for help

Plan A: Initial tracheal intubation plan

Preoxygenate
Cricoid force: 10 N awake → 30 N anaesthetized
Direct laryngoscopy – check:
Neck flexion and head extension
Laryngoscopy technique and vector
External laryngeal manipulation – by laryngoscopist
Vocal cords open and immobile
If poor view:
Reduce cricoid force
introducer (bougie) – seek clicks or hold-up
and/or alternative laryngoscope

Succeed → Tracheal intubation

Not more than 3 attempts, maintaining:
(1) oxygenation with face mask
(2) cricoid pressure and
(3) anaesthesia

Verify tracheal intubation
(1) Visual, if possible
(2) Capnograph
(3) Oesophageal detector
'if in doubt, take it out'

Failed intubation

Maintain 30 N cricoid force

Plan C: Maintenance of oxygenation, ventilation, postponement of surgery and awakening

Plan B not appropriate for this scenario

Use face mask, oxygenate and ventilate
1- or 2-person mask technique
(with oral–nasal airway)
Consider reducing cricoid force if ventilation difficult

Succeed → Postpone surgery and awaken patient if possible or continue anaesthesia with LMA or ProSeal LMA– if condition immediately life-threatening

Failed oxygenation
(e.g. S_pO_2 <90% with F_IO_2 1.0) via face mask

LMA
Reduce cricoid force during insertion
Oxygenate and ventilate

Succeed → Postpone surgery and awaken patient if possible or continue anaesthesia with LMA or ProSeal LMA– if condition immediately life-threatening

Failed ventilation and oxygenation

Plan D: Rescue techniques for 'can't intubate, can't ventilate' situation

Difficult airway society guidelines flow-chart 2004 (use with DAS guidelines paper)

Figure 27.6 Management of unanticipated difficult intubation during rapid sequence induction (reproduced with permission from Henderson JJ, Popat MT, Latto IP, Pearce AC. Difficult Airway Society guidelines for management of the unanticipated difficult intubation. *Anaesthesia* 2004; **59**: 675–94).

Failed intubation, increasing hypoxaemia and difficult ventilation in the paralysed anaesthetized patient: rescue techniques for the 'can't intubate, can't ventilate' situation

Failed intubation and difficult ventilation (other than laryngospasm)

Face mask
Oxygenate and ventilate patient
Maximum head extension
Maximum jaw thrust
Assistance with mask seal
Oral – 6 mm nasal airway
Reduce cricoid force – if necessary

Failed oxygenation with face mask (e.g. S_pO_2 <90% with F_iO_2 1.0)

Call for help

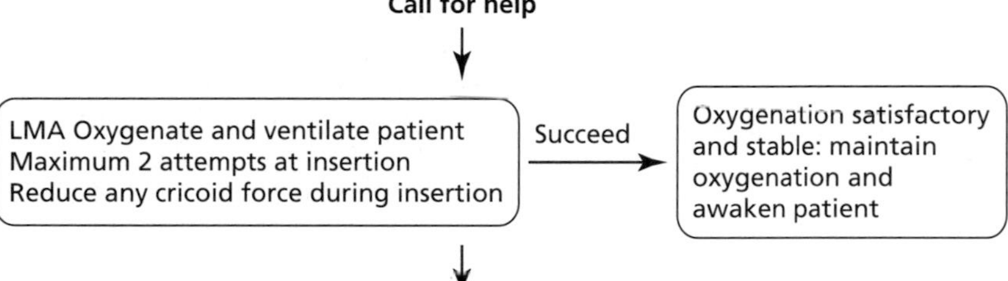

'Can't intubate, can't ventilate' situation with increasing hypoxaemia

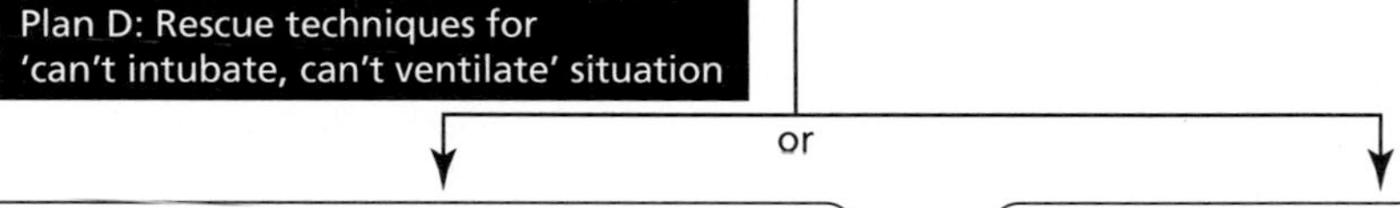

Cannula cricothyroidotomy

Equipment: kink-resistant cannuia, e.g. Patil (Cook) or Ravussin (VBM)
High-pressure ventilation system, e.g. Manujet III (VBM)

Technique:

1. Insert cannula through cricothyroid membrane
2. Maintain position of cannula – assistant's hand
3. Confirm tracheal position by air aspiration – 20 mL syringe
4. Attach ventilation system to cannula
5. Commence cautious ventilation
6. Confirm ventilation of lungs, and exhalation through upper airway
7. If ventilation fails, or surgical emphysema or any other complication develops – convert immediately to surgical cricothyroidotomy

Fail →

Surgical cricothyroidotomy

Equipment: scalpel – short and rounded (no. 20 or Minitrach scalpel)
Small (e.g. 6 or 7 mm) cuffed tracheal or tracheostomy tube.

4-step technique:

1. Identify cricothyroid membrane
2. Stab incision through skin and membrane
   Enlarge incision with blunt dissection (e.g. scalpel handle, forceps or dilator)
3. Caudal traction on cricoid cartilage with tracheal hook
4. Insert tube and inflate cuff

Ventilate with low-pressure source
Verify tube position and pulmonary ventilation

Notes:
1. These techniques can have serious complications–use only in life-threatening situations
2. Convert to definitive airway as soon as possible
3. Postoperative management – see other difficult airway guidelines and flow-charts
4. 4 mm cannula with low-pressure ventilation may be successful in patient breathing spontaneously

Diffcult airway society guidelines flow-chart 2004 (use with DAS guide lines paper)

● **Figure 27.7** Management of failed intubation, increasing hypoxaemia and difficult ventilation in a paralysed and anaesthetized patient (reproduced with permission from Henderson JJ, Popat MT, Latto IP, Pearce AC. Difficult Airway Society guidelines for management of the unanticipated difficult intubation. *Anaesthesia* 2004; **59**: 675–94).

ventilation and an oral or nasal airway should be considered. If plan C fails, then the decision should be made to move on to plan D.

Plan D

Plan D is a rescue technique of oxygenating for a CICV scenario. It consists of either cannula or surgical cricothyroidotomy.

Unanticipated difficult intubation during rapid sequence induction (Fig. 27.6)

In plan A, excessive cricoid pressure may lead to poor laryngoscopic view. Therefore, cricoid pressure should be limited to 30 N. If required, pressure should be reduced with suction in hand. Plan B is not appropriate in this situation when succinylcholine has been used as the muscle relaxant. If intubation is attempted while the muscle relaxant is wearing off, there is an increased risk of laryngospasm and failure of the technique. In plan C, if surgery needs to continue, the airway can be maintained with an LMA ProSeal or classic LMA. If plan C fails, plan D should be implemented.

Failed intubation, increasing hypoxaemia and difficult ventilation in a paralysed and anaesthetized patient (CICV scenario) (Fig. 27.7)

Fortunately, this scenario is very rare. Persistent attempts at laryngoscopy and tracheal intubation can lead to airway oedema and change a 'can't intubate, can ventilate' situation into a CICV scenario. It is essential to recognize this and implement immediate action to oxygenate the patient. If the optimum bag-and-mask ventilation and a supraglottic airway device fail to oxygenate the patient, the decision should be made to perform cricothyroidotomy. The available methods of cricothyroidotomy have been briefly described in the previous section (see Artificial airways, p. 642).

Bibliography

Barker P, Mason RA, Thorpe MH. Computerised axial tomography of the trachea. A useful investigation when a retrosternal goitre causes symptoms. *Anaesthesia* 1991; **46**: 195–8.

Benham SW. Management of the anticipated difficult airway. In: Popat M (ed.) *Difficult Airway Management*. Oxford: Oxford University Press, 2009, pp. 55–64.

Calder I, Koh KF. Cervical haematoma and airway obstruction. *Br J Anaesth* 1996; **76**: 887–8.

Calder I, Calder J, Crockard HA. Difficult direct laryngoscopy in patients with cervical spine disease. *Anaesthesia* 1995; **50**: 756–63.

Caponas G. Intubating laryngeal mask airway. *Anaesth Intensive Care* 2002; **30**: 551–69.

Charters P, O'Sullivan E. The 'dedicated airway': a review of the concept and update of current practice. *Anaesthesia* 1999; **54**: 778–86.

Cohn AI, McGraw SR, King WH. Awake intubation of the adult trachea using the Bullard laryngoscope. *Can J Anaesth* 1995; **42**: 246–8.

Crosby ET. Airway management in adults after cervical spine trauma. *Anesthesiology* 2006; **104**: 1293–318.

Goh MH, Liu XY, Goh YS. Anterior mediastinal masses: an anaesthetic challenge. *Anaesthesia* 1999; **54**: 670–4.

Henderson JJ. The use of paraglossal straight blade laryngoscopy in difficult tracheal intubation. *Anaesthesia* 1997; **52**: 552–60.

Henderson JJ. Development of the 'gum-elastic bougie'. *Anaesthesia* 2003; **58**: 103–4.

Henderson JJ, Popat MT, Latto IP, Pearce AC. Difficult Airway Society guidelines for management of the unanticipated difficult intubation. *Anaesthesia* 2004; **59**: 675–94.

Ho AMH, Chung DC, To EW, Karmakar MK. Total airway obstruction during local anaesthesia in a nonsedated patient with compromised airway. *Can J Anaesth* 2004; **51**: 838–41.

Joo HS, Kapoor S, Rose DK, Naik VN. The intubating laryngeal mask airway after induction of general anesthesia versus awake fibreoptic intubation in patients with difficult airways. *Anesth Analg* 2001; **92**: 1342–6.

Lee BJ, Kang JM, Kim DO. Laryngeal exposure during laryngoscopy is better in the 25 degree back up position than the supine position. *Br J Anaesth* 2007; **99**: 581–6.

Maktabi MA, Hoffman H, Funk G, From RP. Laryngeal trauma during awake fibreoptic intubation. *Anesth Analg* 2002; **95**: 1112–14.

Mason RA. Fielder CP. The obstructed airway in head and neck surgery. *Anaesthesia* 1999; **54**: 625–8.

McCleod ADM, Calder I. Direct laryngoscopy and cervical cord damage: the legend lives on. *Br J Anaesth* 2000; **84**: 705–9.

Moore EW, Davies MW. Inhalational versus intravenous induction. A survey of emergency anaesthetic practice in United kingdom. *Eur J Anaesthesiol* 2000; **17**: 33–7.

Nolan JP, Wilson ME. An evaluation of the gum elastic bougie. Intubation times and incidence of sore throat. *Anaesthesia* 1992; **47**: 878–81.

Popat M. *Practical Fibreoptic Intubation*. Oxford: Butterworth-Heinemann, 2001.

Rao SL, Kunselman AR, Schuler HG, DesHarnais S. Laryngoscopy and tracheal intubation in head elevated position in obese patients: a randomized, controlled, equivalence trial. *Anesth Analg* 2008; **107**: 1912–18.

Shaw IC, Welchew EA, Harrison BJ, Michael S. Complete airway obstruction during awake fibreoptic intubation. *Anaesthesia* 1997; **52**: 582–5.

Sidhu VS, Whitehead EM, Ainsworth QP, *et al.* A technique of awake fibreoptic intubation. Experience in patients with cervical spine disease. *Anaesthesia* 1993; **48**: 910–13.

Silk JM, Hill HM, Calder I. Difficult intubation and the laryngeal mask airway. *Eur J Anaesthesiol* 1991; **Suppl. 4**: 47–51.

Cross-references

Artificial airways, 642
Difficult airway: management, 651
Difficult airway: overview, 647

Difficult airway: new devices

Cyprian Mendonca

Many new devices, based on the principle of indirect laryngoscopy and developed for the management of the difficult airway, have been introduced into clinical practice. An ideal device intended for use in a difficult airway scenario should be easy to use, simple and quick to set up, suitable for both paediatric and adult use, suitable for both nasal and oral route, portable and reliable.

Direct laryngoscopy

A 'line of sight' must be established from eye to glottis by aligning the oral, pharyngeal and laryngeal axes (Fig. 27.8). This requires:

- Extension of the head at atlanto-occipital joint, combined with a slightly flexed cervical spine – the 'sniffing the morning air' position, described by Magill.
- Artificial protrusion of the mandible, tongue and hyoid bone with the blade of the laryngoscope. The pattern of blade designed by Robert Macintosh is almost universally employed in the UK. However, there is renewed interest in straight laryngoscope blades, such as the pattern introduced by Henderson, since a line of vision can be established in cases resistant to the Macintosh.

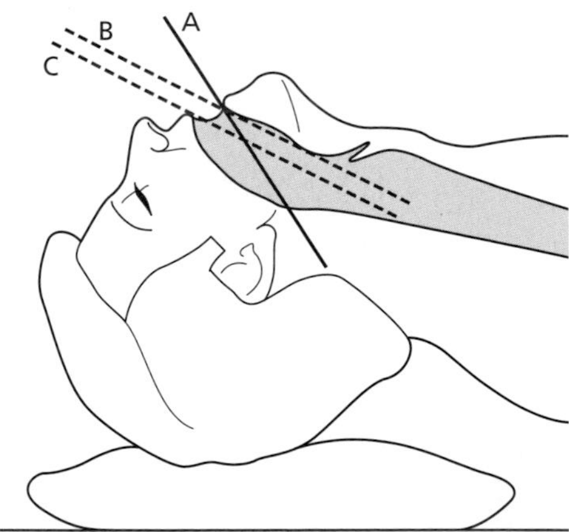

Figure 27.8 Head in neutral position, none of the axes are aligned. A, oral axis; B, pharyngeal axis; C, laryngeal axis. All three axes can be aligned by flexion of the cervical spine (elevation of head) and extension at the atlanto-occipital joint.

It is not always possible to achieve a line of sight; an inadequate view of the larynx is the result. A poor laryngoscopic view using direct laryngoscopy necessitates additional force, external laryngeal manipulation, use of a gum elastic bougie or stylet or an alternate technique to achieve success.

Indirect laryngoscopy

A simple example of indirect laryngoscopy is visualizing the image of the larynx using an otolaryngoscopic mirror illuminated with light, placed in the patient's mouth. Indirect laryngoscopy does not require the alignment of oral, pharyngeal and laryngeal axes. Therefore, it requires less force to be applied and comparatively fewer haemodynamic changes. In recent years, as a result of advances in fibreoptic systems and video technology, there have been several new airway devices (Fig. 27.9), based on indirect laryngoscopy that have emerged into clinical practice. A classification of indirect laryngoscopes is shown in Table 27.1.

Bullard laryngoscope

The Bullard laryngoscope (Circon) was the first indirect rigid fibreoptic laryngoscope, introduced in the late 1980s. It consists of a rigid blade with a fibreoptic system and a dedicated rigid stylet to facilitate insertion of the tracheal tube. A light bundle transmits the light to the distal end of the blade and an image bundle transmits the image to the eyepiece. Using a video camera system the image can be viewed on an external monitor. It also consists of a working channel, which allows suctioning of secretions, administration of oxygen or application

Table 27.1 Classification of indirect laryngoscopes

Optical stylets		Bonfils	Shikani		
Rigid laryngoscopes	With tube channel	Airtraq	Pentax Airway Scope	CTrach	
	Without tube channel	Bullard	C-Mac	Glidescope	McGrath

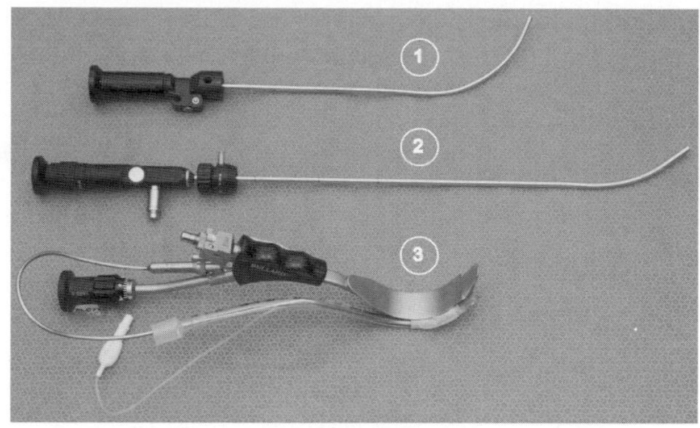

● **Figure 27.9** Rigid fibreoptic laryngoscope and optical stylets. 1, Shikani optical stylet; 2, Bonfils fibreoptic stylet; 3, Bullard laryngoscope.

of local anaesthetics. It can be used in patients with reduced mouth opening and with minimal head and neck manipulation.

Optical stylets

The Bonfils (Karl Storz Endoscopy Ltd) is a rigid fibreoptic stylet, of 40 cm in length and 5 mm in outer diameter, with an angulated distal end. It can be used in patients with limited mouth opening. It has a success rate of 96.8% in patients with a normal airway, on the first attempt.

The Shikani optical stylet (Clarus Medical) is a high-resolution endoscope and has a malleable stainless steel sheath. It is available in two different sizes (adult and paediatric). It can be used in conjunction with a Macintosh laryngoscope.

Both of the above devices can be used with an eyepiece or can be connected to a video camera system. Both have been shown to cause less movement of the upper cervical spine than the Macintosh laryngoscope.

Videolaryngoscopes

Videolaryngoscopes transmit the image to an external monitor, from a miniature video camera placed at the distal end, via a fibreoptic bundle or a system of prisms. Some of them have an inbuilt tube channel that directs the tracheal tube into the larynx. Others require a stylet to direct the tracheal tube into the larynx.

C-Mac video laryngoscope

The C-Mac video laryngoscope (Karl Storz Endoscopy Ltd) consists of a reusable blade which is similar to the Macintosh blade. It exhibits a curvature of 60° with a digital camera view of 80°. A small digital camera and a high-power light-emitting diode are located at the distal third of the blade. The camera is connected to a high-resolution, 18 cm thin-film transistor monitor with a single cable. The blade is available in three different sizes (2, 3 and 4). Recently, a more curved version of the blade was introduced as an aid to difficult intubation

Glidescope videolaryngoscope

The Glidescope (Verathon Medical) consists of a video baton that incorporates a high-resolution camera, a light-emitting diode and a portable liquid crystal display (LCD) monitor. The disposable plastic blades are available in different sizes that need to be mounted on the video baton. A paediatric version of the video baton is also available. Successful placement of the tracheal tube requires an angulated stylet. There have been reports of successful use in both anticipated and unanticipated difficult intubations.

McGrath videolaryngoscope

The McGrath (Aircraft Medical Ltd) is a battery-powered portable laryngoscope with a 33 by 22.5 mm LCD screen mounted on top of the laryngoscope handle. The camera stick incorporates a miniature camera and light source. A disposable, clear acrylic, curved blade (13 mm in thickness) covers the camera stick. An angulated stylet is required for facilitating the tube placement.

Pentax Airway Scope (AWS) videolaryngoscope

The Pentax AWS (Hoya Corporation) is also a battery-powered laryngoscope consisting of a handle with a built-in 6 cm LCD screen and a 12 cm cable with a miniature video camera. The disposable polycarbonate blade (PBLADE) incorporates a tube channel, which guides the tube into the glottic opening when the image is correctly aligned on the monitor.

Airtraq optical laryngoscope

The Airtraq (Prodol Meditec) is a single-use device which consists of an anatomically shaped laryngoscope with a built-in tube channel. A battery-operated light-emitting diode is present at the tip and provides the illumination. The image of the larynx is transmitted to the proximal viewfinder through a combination of lenses and prisms. The image can also be transmitted to an external wireless monitor. It is available in various sizes, including sizes for use in infants.

LMA-CTrach

The CTrach (LMA-CTrach; Intavent Orthofix Ltd) is a modification of the intubating LMA. It comprises an in-built integrated fibreoptic system and a detachable LCD colour viewer. At the distal end, there is a lens, situated behind the epiglottic elevating bar, which captures the image and transmits it to the viewer. It enables visualization of the larynx and facilitates intubation under direct vision.

Advantages of videolaryngoscopes

- Easy to learn the skill.
- Useful as a teaching aid.
- Causes fewer haemodynamic changes.
- Useful in patients with reduced cervical spine mobility.
- Useful in patients with limited mouth opening.
- Possible role in the difficult airway.

The main disadvantage is the cost, which needs to be justified to support routine clinical use.

Laryngoscopy versus tracheal intubation

The process of tracheal intubation can be divided into two steps:

- visualization of the larynx.
- placement of the tube in the trachea.

In general, visualization of the larynx is easy with most indirect laryngoscopes, but further skill is required for placing the tube in the trachea. The success rate and learning curve for correct tube placement can be variable among the different indirect laryngoscopes. When using the devices without a tube channel, tracheal tube placement can be difficult despite having a very good view of the larynx. This is because oral, pharyngeal and tracheal axes are not aligned and therefore the tube must be inserted around a curvature, without direct vision. Therefore, an angulated stylet or tube introducer is required. Most studies report that the indirect laryngoscopy skill is easy to learn.

There are several additional benefits and roles for videolaryngoscopes:

- Videolaryngoscopes have a role in teaching and evaluating the laryngoscopy procedure.
- Videolaryngoscopes enable an anaesthetic assistant to be more effective in assisting intubation. Assistants can perform the external laryngeal manoeuvres and cricoid pressure more effectively as they can observe the laryngeal view on the monitor.
- Videolaryngoscopes can contribute to better record-keeping, guarding against claims of airway injuries, through recording images and videoclips.
- They can be used as an alternative laryngoscope in the plan A (DAS guidelines) of managing an unanticipated difficult airway. The currently published literature is inadequate to support the role of videolaryngoscopes in difficult intubation. However, large multicentre trials, comparing the various videolaryngoscopes with direct laryngoscopy, should determine the role for videolaryngoscopes in difficult intubation.

Bibliography

Adnet F, Racine SX, Borron SW, *et al.* A survey of tracheal intubation difficulty in the operating room: a prospective observational study. *Acta Anaesthesiol Scand* 2001: **45**; 327–32.

Cohn AI, McGraw SR, King WH. Awake intubation of the adult trachea using the Bullard laryngoscope. *Can J Anaesth* 1995; **42**: 246–8.

Cooper RM, Pacy JA, Bishop MJ, McCluskey SA. Early experience with a new videolaryngoscope (Glidescope) in 728 patients. *Can J Anaesth* 2005; **52**: 191–8.

Hastings RH, Vigil AC, Hanna R, *et al.* Cervical spine movement during laryngoscopy with the Bullard, Macintosh, and Miller laryngoscopes. *Anesthesiology* 1995; **82**: 859–69.

Howard-Quijano KJ, Huang YM, Matevosian R. Video-assisted instruction improves the success rate for tracheal intubation by novices. *Br J Anaesth* 2008; **101**: 568–72.

Jungbauer A, Schumann M, Brunkhorst V, *et al.* Expected difficult tracheal intubation: a prospective comparison of direct laryngoscopy and video laryngoscopy in 200 patients. *Br J Anaesth* 2009; **102**: 546–50.

Kaplan MB, Hagberg CA, Ward DS, *et al.* Comparison of direct and video-assisted views of the larynx during routine intubation. *J Clin Anaesth* 2006; **18**: 357–62.

Maharaj CH, Costello JF, Harte BH, Laffey JG. Evaluation of the Airtraq and Macintosh laryngoscopes in patients at increased risk of difficult tracheal intubation. *Anaesthesia* 2007; **63**: 182–8.

Malin E, Montblanc J, Ynineb Y, *et al.* Performance of the Airtraq laryngoscope after failed conventional tracheal intubation: a case series. *Acta Anaesthesiol Scand* 2009; **53**: 858–63.

Maruyama K, Yamada T, Kawakami R, *et al.* Upper cervical spine movement during intubation: fluoroscopic comparison of the Air Way Scope, McCoy laryngoscope, and Macintosh laryngoscope. *Br J Anaesth* 2008; **100**: 120–4.

Mihai R, Blair E, Kay H, Cook TM. A quantitative review and meta-analysis of performance of non-standard laryngoscopes and rigid fibreoptic intubation aids. *Anaesthesia* 2008; **63**: 745–60.

Pott LM, Murray WB. Review of video laryngoscopy and rigid fibreoptic laryngoscopy. *Curr Opin Anaesthesiol* 2008; **21**: 750–8.

Rudolph C, Schneider JP, Wallenborn J, Schaffranietz L. Movement of the upper cervical spine during laryngoscopy: a comparison of the Bonfils intubation fibrescope and the Macintosh laryngoscope. *Anaesthesia* 2005; **60**: 668–72.

Sharma DJ, Weightman WM, Travis A. Comparison of the Pentax Airway Scope and McGrath videolaryngoscope with the Macintosh laryngoscope in tracheal intubation by anaesthetists unfamiliar with videolaryngoscopes: a manikin study. *Anaesth Intensive Care* 2010; **38**: 39–42.

Suzuki A, Toyama Y, Katsumi N, *et al.* The Pentax-AWS clinical assessment of performance in 320 cases. *Anaesthesia* 2008; **63**: 641–7.

Thong SY, Lim Y. Video and optic laryngoscopy assisted tracheal intubation: the new era. *Anaesthesia Intensive Care* 2009; **37**: 219–33.

Watts AD, Gelb AW, Bach DB, Pelz DM. Comparison of the Bullard and Macintosh laryngoscopes for endotracheal intubation of patients with a potential cervical spine injury. *Anesthesiology* 1997; **87**: 1335–42.

Cross-references

Artificial airways, 642
Difficult airway: management, 651

Difficult airway: prediction

Cyprian Mendonca

The prediction of difficult airway is based on history, clinical examination and investigations. Previous 'difficult airway alerts', surgeries or injuries in the head and neck region, radiotherapy, snoring and obstructive sleep apnoea can suggest possible difficult airway. A detailed clinical examination involves various predictive tests. In certain cases, further investigations such as X-rays of the neck, CT scans and nasendoscopy may provide useful information.

In clinical practice despite full airway assessment, many of us have experienced the scenarios where a predicted difficult intubation turns out to be easy and a predicted easy intubation unexpectedly turns out be the most difficult one. On a similar basis, predicting difficult intubation has been described as a pointless ritual.

Airway assessment forms an essential component of preoperative assessment. Predicting a difficult airway should be focused on predicting difficult mask ventilation (DMV) and predicting difficult tracheal intubation.

Predicting difficult mask ventilation

Predictors of DMV include full beard, Mallampati grade 3 or 4, age more than 55 years, BMI >30 kg m^{-2}, limited jaw protrusion, edentulous, history of snoring and sleep apnoea. These can be remembered using the mnemonic 'OBESE' (obese, bearded, elderly, snorers and edentulous).

Obesity is associated with increased perioperative mortality. In obese patients the airway space behind the base of the tongue is reduced. Obesity is also associated with impaired airway patency during sleep and obstructive sleep apnoea. Owing to reduced oxygen reserve, despite preoxygenation, patients can desaturate quickly during induction of anaesthesia.

Predicting difficult intubation

Cases with readily identifiable problems, such as facial injuries, can be predicted. However, serious difficulty is, fortunately, very rare in apparently normal people. It is therefore unlikely that any single predictive method will be successful.

Various tests have been described (Mallampati, Patil), which appear to perform well when applied retrospectively to difficult patients. However, prospective trials have shown that the false-positive rate associated with prediction in a general population is very high. It is also unfortunately the case that the available tests have sensitivities of about 50% (i.e. half the cases are missed).

The current position is somewhat difficult, as is the case in all programmes where symptomless populations are 'screened' for diseases such as cervical, breast or prostate cancer. The screening may not be effective in reducing mortality and may actually increase morbidity, but practitioners may be criticized for not attempting to predict problems.

Available tests

Mallampati test (with Sampson and Young's modification)

The patient sits opposite the anaesthetist with mouth wide open and tongue protruded. Depending on the view of the pharynx, four classes have been described.

- Class 1: Faucial pillars, soft palate, posterior pharyngeal wall and uvula are seen.
- Class 2: Soft palate, part of posterior pharyngeal wall and base of uvula are seen.
- Class 3: Only soft palate visible.
- Class 4: Even soft palate is not visible.

It estimates the size of the tongue in relation to the oral cavity. Classes 1 and 2 indicate that displacement of the tongue by the laryngoscope is likely to be easy. Classes 3 and 4 are associated with difficult laryngoscopy using a Macintosh laryngoscope. There is interobserver variation and it has been found to have poor sensitivity and poor positive predictive values in general surgical patients (approximately 50% and 10–25%, respectively).

Tests of cervical movement appear to be difficult to apply successfully, but the only series in which the Mallampati performed well was in a cervical spine disease population, and the Mallampati appears to be as good as any test in cervical spine problems, probably because craniocervical extension is required for normal mouth opening.

Interincisor gap

With the mouth maximally open, the gap between the incisors is measured. If <3 cm, difficult laryngoscopy is likely.

Mandibular protrusion

Mandibular protrusion can be assessed on an ABC basis:

- Class A: able to protrude the lower incisors anterior to the upper incisors.
- Class B: lower incisors reach just the margin of the upper incisors.
- Class C: lower incisors cannot protrude to the upper incisors.

Direct laryngoscopy is always difficult in patients with grade C protrusion, but it is a rare finding, largely confined to patients with rheumatoid arthritis.

Thyromental distance (Patil's test)

Thyromental distance is an indicator of mandibular space. It is the distance between the uppermost part of the thyroid cartilage to the tip of the chin (mentum), with the neck fully extended and mouth closed. If <6 cm, predicts difficult laryngoscopy.

Sternomental distance

In 1994, Savva described the concept of sternomental distance. It is the distance between the sternal notch to the tip of the chin with the neck fully extended and mouth closed. If <12.5 cm, predicts difficult laryngoscopy.

Movement of cervical spine

Flexion and extension movements of the cervical spine and atlanto-occipital movements are important for direct laryngoscopy. Cervical spine movement can be assessed as follows.

With a finger on the patient's chin and the other one on the occipital protuberance, the head is extended maximally and the position of the chin in relation to the occipital protuberance is noted.

- If the chin is higher than the occipital protuberance, normal cervical spine mobility.
- If the two fingers are at the same level, moderate limitation of cervical spine mobility,
- If the chin is lower than the occipital protuberance, severe limitation of cervical spine mobility.

Wilson risk score

The five risk factors included are:

1 weight
2 head and neck movement
3 jaw movement
4 receding mandible
5 buck teeth.

Each factor can score 0–2 points, to give a maximum of 10 points. A total score of ≥2 is associated with increased risk of difficult intubation.

A combination of the above tests has a better predictive value than any single test. The Mallampati test, thyromental distance, ability to protrude the mandible and movement of the cervical spine are commonly used. A meta-analysis by Shiga *et al.* has shown that a combination of the Mallampati test and thyromental distance is a better predictor of difficult laryngoscopy.

Bibliography

Calder I. Difficult airways: causation and prediction. In: Calder I, Pearce A (eds) *Core Topics in Airway Management*. Cambridge: Cambridge University Press, 2005, pp. 113–22.

El-Ganzouri AR, McCarthy RJ, Tuman KJ, *et al.* Preoperative airway assessment: predictive value of a multivariate risk index. *Anesth Analg* 1996; **82**: 1197–204.

Frerk CM. Predicting difficult intubation. *Anaesthesia* 1991; **46**: 1005–8.

Hiremath AS, Hillman DR, James AL, *et al.* Relationship between difficult tracheal intubation and obstructive sleep apnoea. *Br J Anaesth* 1998; **80**: 606–11.

Kheterpal S, Han R, Tremper KK, *et al.* Incidence and predictors of difficult and impossible mask ventilation. *Anesthesiology* 2006; **105**: 885–91.

Langeron O, Masso E, Huraux C, *et al.* Prediction of difficult mask ventilation. *Anesthesiology* 2000; **92**: 1229–36.

Mallampati SR, Gugino LD, Desai SP, Freiberger D. A clinical sign to predict difficult tracheal intubation: a prospective study. *Can Anaesth Soc J* 1985; **32**: 429–34.

Nichol HC, Zuck D. Difficult laryngoscopy: the anterior larynx and the atlanto-occipital gap. *Br J Anaesth* 1983; **55**: 141–3.

Reed AP. Evaluation and recognition of the difficult airway. In: Hegberg A (ed.) *Benumof's Airway Management: Principles and Practice*, 2nd edn. St Louis: Mosby, 2007, pp. 221–35.

Savva D. Prediction of difficult tracheal intubation. *Br J Anaesth* 1994; **73**: 149–53.

Sampson GLT, Young JRB. Difficult tracheal intubation: a retrospective study. *Anaesthesia* 1987; **42**: 487–90.

Shiga T, Wajima Z, Inoue T, Sakamoto A. Predicting difficult intubation in apparently normal patients. A meta-analysis of bedside screening test performance. *Anesthesiology* 2005; **103**: 429–37.

Vaughan RS. Predicting difficult airways. *Br J Anaesth CEPD Rev* 2001; **1**: 44–7.

Wilson ME. Predicting difficult intubation. *Br J Anaesth* 1993; **71**: 333–4.

Wilson ME, Spiegelhalter D, Robertson JA, Lesser P. Predicting difficult intubation. *Br J Anaesth* 1988; **61**: 211–16.

Williamson JA, Webb RK, Szekely S, *et al.* Difficult intubation: an analysis of 2000 incident reports. *Anaesth Intensive Care* 1993; **21**: 602–67.

Yentis SM. Predicting difficult intubation: worthwhile exercise or pointless ritual? *Anaesthesia* 2002; **57**: 105–9.

Cross-reference

Difficult airway: management, 651

Effect of general anaesthesia on the airway/upper alimentary canal

Cyprian Mendonca

A 'submarine' analogy can be made regarding safety during anaesthesia – depth is safety. Most of the troublesome phenomena we experience, such as coughing, biting, breath-holding, laryngospasm and regurgitation, occur during light planes of anaesthesia.

Effect on oropharyngeal and glottic structures

Induction of anaesthesia usually causes obstruction of the upper airway. Alterations in the tone of the skeletal muscles of the pharynx and neck are thought to be responsible. Recent radiographic and MRI studies have shown that, at induction of anaesthesia, the most important cause of obstruction is approximation of the soft palate to the posterior pharyngeal wall.

Increasing depth of propofol anaesthesia is associated with increased collapsibility of the upper airway, which is associated with profound inhibition of genioglossus muscle activity. This dose-related inhibition seems to be the combined result of depression of central respiratory output to upper airway dilator muscles and of upper airway reflexes.

The standard manoeuvres employed to clear an obstructed airway – head tilt, chin lift and jaw thrust – stretch the anterior neck tissues, which lifts the glottic opening from the posterior pharyngeal wall. A nasopharyngeal airway can be useful at this stage, whereas insertion of an oropharyngeal airway in light planes of anaesthesia may induce coughing and laryngospasm. CPAP is often effective in relieving airway obstruction, particularly in children.

Recognition of an obstructed airway

Patients with a tendency to upper airway obstruction during sleep are vulnerable during anaesthesia and sedation. These include obesity, maxillary hypoplasia, mandibular retrusion, bulbar muscle weakness and specific obstructive lesions, such as nasal obstruction adenotonsillar hypertrophy. Such abnormalities not only increase vulnerability to upper airway obstruction during sleep or anaesthesia, but also make intubation difficult. While problems with airway maintenance may be obviated during anaesthesia by the use of aids such as the laryngeal mask airway, identification of risk and caution are keys to management.

Recognizing an obstructed airway is equally important. The hallmark of upper airway obstruction is diminished or absent air flow in the presence of continued respiratory effort. A conscious patient will complain of difficulty in breathing. The patient may be restless, agitated, dysphonic, aphonic, anxious, unwilling to be supine and, ultimately, exhausted. Patients' complaints have sometimes been ignored on the grounds that an oximeter showed near normal readings.

A spontaneously breathing patient will generate large negative intrathoracic pressures (but not if there is also respiratory depression), which will cause:

- noisy inspiration, owing to turbulent gas flow (a completely obstructed airway is silent)
- signs of respiratory distress including tracheal tug and intercostal recession
- paradoxical respiratory movements
- negative pressure pulmonary oedema can develop if the obstruction continues.

A ventilated patient will have high inflation pressures.

In both spontaneous and ventilated patients:

- carbon dioxide excretion may be impaired – capnometer traces may be flattened or absent
- arterial blood gases may show a respiratory acidosis
- desaturation may be late and sudden, if the $F_{I}O_2$ is high
- oximetry is not a good monitor of airway patency.

Pulmonary oedema following relief of airway obstruction

The large transpulmonary pressure gradients during obstruction may cause alveolar fluid collection. This presents as pulmonary oedema when the obstruction is relieved. Positive pressure ventilation may be required and an adult respiratory distress syndrome-like picture may result.

Glottic reflexes

The minimum alveolar concentration of volatile anaesthetic (MAC) for glottic stimulation is 30% higher than for surgical incision. Tachycardia and hypertension follow laryngoscopy and intubation, unless adequate depth of anaesthesia is achieved.

Laryngospasm

Glottic closure reflexes are hyperexcitable during light anaesthesia. Laryngospasm may complicate induction of anaesthesia, surgical stimulation, extubation and recovery. It is probably the most frequent serious airway complication. The incidence is reduced if propofol is used for the induction of anaesthesia. Desaturation can often be avoided by giving 100% oxygen. Deepening the level of anaesthesia with intravenous propofol is usually effective. Muscle relaxants may be required to relieve laryngospasm and succinylcholine remains popular for this indication, owing to its rapid onset; even a small dose will usually suffice. The intense stimulation caused by bilateral digital pressure in 'the laryngospasm notch' (the posterior temporomandibular joint) has been claimed to be an effective treatment for laryngospasm and breath-holding (Larson's manoeuvre).

Oesophageal sphincter function and anaesthesia

The lower oesophageal sphincter

The intraluminal pressure at the gastro-oesophageal junction is 15–25 mmHg above gastric pressure, which normally prevents gastro-oesophageal reflux. The pressure is produced by smooth muscle cells of the lower oesophageal sphincter. Contraction of the surrounding skeletal muscle of the diaphragmatic crura increases the intraluminal pressure during inspiration, and also during straining. Straining does not cause gastro-oesophageal reflux in normal conscious patients. Reflux does not occur spontaneously during anaesthesia, but diaphragmatic tone decreases and thus its protective effect may be lost. Reflux is associated with hiccough, straining, deep inspiration with surgical stimulus and bucking on the tracheal tube, all features of light anaesthesia.

A sudden, brief rise in lower oesophageal sphincter pressure (LOSP) is seen at the same time as the onset of fasciculation after succinylcholine, probably as a result of diaphragmatic contraction. Studies have shown that cricoid pressure can significantly decrease LOSP especially in awake volunteers, probably induced by mechanical discomfort. These effects could be blocked by the use of an infusion of remifentanil. Remifentanil abolishes spontaneous oesophageal motility and completely eliminates the experience of discomfort induced by cricoid pressure. The opioids morphine and pethidine decrease LOSP when given intravenously and hence have been used with caution when there has been an increased risk of regurgitation.

Intravenous atropine and other cholinergics can cause a decrease in LOSP sufficient to permit free reflux. Sphincter pressure is unaffected when atropine is combined with neostigmine.

Very small, and probably clinically insignificant, decreases in sphincter pressure are caused by intravenous and inhalational anaesthetic agents, the laryngeal mask airway and the lithotomy position. The steep Trendelenburg position used during pelvic laparoscopy does not cause gastro-oesophageal reflux.

The oesophagus

The oesophagus is a muscular tube about 25 cm in length, which begins at the caudal border of the cricoid cartilage and ends at the cardiac orifice of the stomach, usually about 1.5 cm below the diaphragm. The upper quarter is composed of skeletal muscle only; the lower third is smooth muscle only; and the middle is a mixture of the two types. The oesophagus can contain large volumes of fluid (up to 200 mL). Refluxed gastric contents are cleared by oesophageal peristalsis, which is initiated by swallowing or local reflexes.

Both general anaesthesia and intravenous atropine inhibit oesophageal motility. Oesophageal clearance may not occur during general anaesthesia. The refluxed contents will remain in the oesophagus, increasing the risk of regurgitation into the pharynx, until swallowing recommences as the patient awakes.

The upper oesophageal sphincter

The upper oesophageal sphincter is formed by the lamina of the cricoid cartilage anteriorly and the striated muscle cricopharyngeus posteriorly. Resting upper oesophageal sphincter pressure is about 40 mmHg. Relaxation of the upper oesophageal sphincter at induction of anaesthesia can precipitate regurgitation.

Both intravenous thiopentone and succinylcholine decrease upper oesophageal sphincter pressure to less than 10 mmHg, a pressure low enough to allow regurgitation of oesophageal contents. The low upper oesophageal sphincter pressure caused by succinylcholine is not further reduced by laryngoscopy. With thiopentone, the fall in sphincter pressure starts before loss of consciousness.

Intravenous induction with ketamine or inhalational induction with halothane maintains upper oesophageal sphincter pressure, in the absence of neuromuscular blockade. Upper oesophageal sphincter pressure may rise to over 100 mmHg during coughing and straining under light anaesthesia, and prevent regurgitation.

Intravenous benzodiazepines, such as midazolam, reduce upper sphincter pressure. They also depress laryngeal reflexes. Heavy sedation may allow aspiration.

There have been case reports of regurgitation during anaesthesia when a laryngeal mask has been in use. This is probably no more frequent than when an oral Guedel airway and face-mask are used.

Bibliography

Chung DC, Rowbotham SJ. A very small dose of suxamethonium relieves laryngospasm. *Anaesthesia* 1993; **48**: 229–30.

Drummond GB. Keep a clear airway (editorial). *Br J Anaesth* 1991; **66**: 153–6.

Eastwood PR, Platt PR, Shepherd K, *et al.* Collapsibility of the upper airway at different concentrations of propofol anaesthesia. *Anaesthesiology* 2005; **103**: 470–7.

Herrick IA, Mahendran B, Penny FJ. Postobstructive pulmonary edema following anaesthesia. *J Clin Anaesth* 1990; **2**: 116–20.

Hillman DR, Platt PR, Eastwood. PR. The upper airway during anaesthesia. *Br J Anaesth* 2003; **91**: 31–9.

Larsen CP. Laryngospasm: the best treatment. *Anesthesiology* 1998; **89**: 1293–4.

Mathru M, Esch O, Lang J, *et al.* Magnetic resonance imaging of the upper airway. Effects of propofol anesthesia and nasal continuous positive airway pressure in humans. *Anesthesiology* 1996; **84**: 253–5.

Nandi PR, Charlesworth CH, Taylor SJ, *et al.* Effect of general anaesthesia on the pharynx. *Br J Anaesth* 1991; **66**: 157–62.

Nawfal M, Baraka A. Propofol for relief of extubation laryngospasm. *Anaesthesia* 2002; **57**: 1036.

Thorn K, Thorn S, Wattwil M. The effects of cricoid pressure, remifentanil, and propofol on esophageal motility and the lower esophageal sphincter. *Anesth Analg* 2005; **100**: 1200–3.

Vanner RG. Oesophageal sphincter function. In: Prys-Roberts C, Brown BR (eds) *International Practice of Anaesthesia.* Oxford: Butterworth-Heinemann, 1996, pp. 1–11.

Cross-references

Difficult airway: overview, 647

Hypoxaemia under anaesthesia, 670

Hypoxaemia under anaesthesia

Payal Kajekar

Hypoxaemia is defined as a decrease in the partial pressure of the oxygen in blood and is considered to be severe when oxygen saturation falls below 90%. Acute hypoxaemia will eventually cause circulatory arrest owing to myocardial hypoxia and, at some time around the point of arrest, irreversible cardiac damage occurs. Following cardiac arrest, consciousness is lost within 10 seconds and irreversible brain damage can occur within 4–5 minutes. The period of anoxia necessary to produce circulatory arrest will depend on cardiovascular status, the oxygen content of the body prior to the anoxic episode and the oxygen consumption.

The oxygen content of the blood depends on oxygen saturation and haemoglobin in the blood and can be calculated from the equation

$$\text{Arterial oxygen content (ml dL}^{-1}) = [(\text{Hb} \times 1.34 \times S_ao_2)] / 100\ (\%) + (0.003 \times P_ao_2)$$

where Hb is the haemoglobin, S_ao_2 is the percentage of haemoglobin saturated with oxygen and P_ao_2 is the partial pressure of arterial oxygen in mmHg.

The oxygen delivery (oxygen flux) to the tissues is calculated by multiplying cardiac output (CO) and arterial oxygen content (C_ao_2) of the blood.

The term 'hypoxia', on the other hand, is used to define deficiency of oxygen at tissue level. There are several types of hypoxia, including anaemic hypoxia, hypoxaemic hypoxia, stagnant hypoxia and tissue hypoxia. Hypoxaemic hypoxia is due to reduced oxygen saturation in arterial blood.

Perioperative causes of hypoxaemia

Equipment failure

A rapid check of the equipment is always the first step in correcting any hypoxaemic episode. In particular, the inspired oxygen concentration, the patency and correct connection of the anaesthetic circuit and any artificial airway should be checked.

Low inspired oxygen concentration

This can be due to an accidental decrease in F_io_2 owing to equipment failure, misconnections or low-flow anaesthesia.

Hypoventilation

Hypoventilation results from central or peripheral depression of ventilation, and/or an obstructed airway. The effect of hypoventilation on oxygen saturation is complex. Oxygen absorption depends more on the F_io_2 than on alveolar ventilation. At a given inspired oxygen concentration, reducing alveolar ventilation makes little difference to oxygenation, until a 'critical' level is reached (Fig. 27.10).

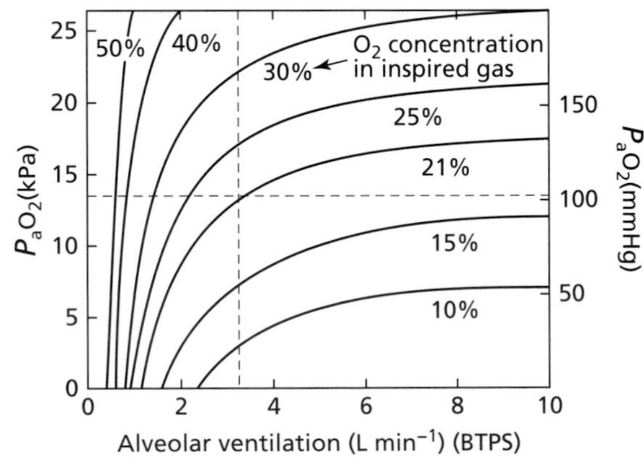

Figure 27.10 Effect of ventilation on alveolar gas tensions (P_aO_2, F_IO_2 and alveolar ventilation). BTPS, body temperature and pressure saturated. Reproduced with permission from Benumof JL. Respiratory physiology and respiratory function during anesthesia. In: Miller RD (ed.) Anesthesia, 3rd edn. New York: Churchill Livingstone, 1990, 504–49. Note that at high levels of F_IO_2, the critical level of ventilation is reduced, but when reached the P_aO_2 may fall suddenly. P_aO_2 depends on F_IO_2 and P_aO_2. The relationship is described by the alveolar air equation, which in its simplest form (applicable only to a patient breathing 100% oxygen) is: $P_{alv}O_2 = P_IO_2 - P_aCO_2$. Corrections have to be introduced if there are other components to the inspired gas.

Apnoeic oxygenation

Provided the airway is at least partially open, passive entrainment of high oxygen concentrations can prevent desaturation during lengthy periods of apnoea, since the P_aco_2 rises by only about 0.5 kPa min^{-1} (see the alveolar air equation in the legend to Fig. 27.10).

Practical points

- Hypoxaemia due to hypoventilation will respond rapidly to an increase in F_Io_2.
- S_po_2 readings are not a reliable guide to the adequacy of ventilation; when the F_Io_2 is high, oximeters measure saturation not ventilation.

Shunt

The term 'shunt' is used here to mean failure of oxygenation of blood during passage through the pulmonary circulation ('venous admixture'). In most cases, this is due to ventilation/perfusion mismatch. The normal shunt fraction is about 2% and is due to the bronchial and thebesian veins draining directly into the left atrium without being oxygenated. Anatomic shunts are caused by right-to-left intracardiac shunts (tetralogy of Fallot or reverse flow through an atrial septal defect or a ventricular septal defect) and intrapulmonary fistulae (connection between branches of pulmonary artery and vein). The other causes of shunt include general anaesthesia, intermittent positive pressure ventilation (IPPV), bronchial intubation, aspiration, oesophageal intubation and pulmonary oedema.

Low cardiac output and hypoxia

A reduced cardiac output may result in low mixed venous oxygen content, because more oxygen is extracted in the tissues. In many circumstances, increased venous admixture causes a decrease in shunt fraction, so that P_ao_2 is not decreased. However, anaesthesia may interfere with this useful adaptation, and desaturation results. Reductions in cardiac output may result in areas of ventilated lung being underperfused and increases in output may improve the ventilation/perfusion profile. In any case, a fall in cardiac output will decrease the oxygen flux to the tissues (Fig. 27.11). It is, therefore, necessary to ensure that cardiac output is adequate, particularly when the patient has pulmonary pathology.

Deadspace

The term 'deadspace' is used to describe the part of inspired air that fails to take part in gas exchange. The volume of conducting airways leading up to the alveoli constitute the anatomical deadspace. The part of the alveolar air that does not take part in gas exchange accounts for alveolar deadspace. The alveolar deadspace increases in pulmonary embolism and in conditions with reduced cardiac output.

Hypoxia during airway management

Failed airway management

The importance of ventilation when unable to intubate and awareness of the difficult intubation/ventilation algorithm is essential. Repeated attempts at intubation may make mask ventilation more and more difficult owing to trauma, tissue swelling and inadequate depth of anaesthesia. Studies have shown that the rate of hypoxaemia, oesophageal intubation, regurgitation and aspiration are all accelerated beyond two attempts.

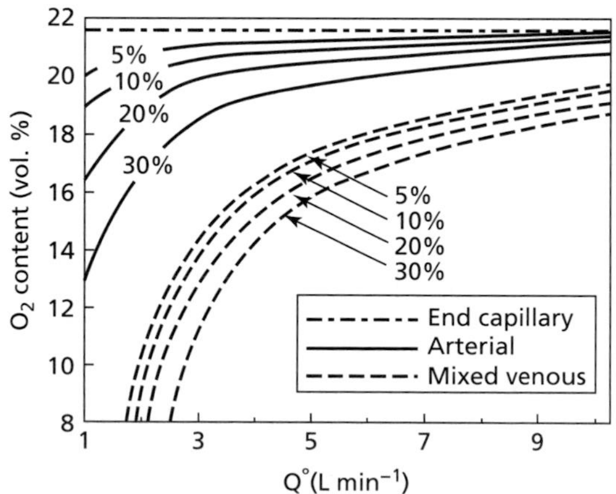

Figure 27.11 Oxygen content, cardiac output and 'shunt'. At higher levels of shunt, a drop in cardiac output may be associated with a substantial fall in saturation. Reproduced with permission from Kelman GR, Nunn JF, Prys Roberts C, Greenbaum R. The influence of cardiac output on arterial oxygenation: a theoretical study. *Br J Anaesth* 1967; 39: 450–8.

Bronchial intubation

Bronchial intubation is usually suspected when desaturation occurs following a successful tracheal intubation. This is supplemented by clinical findings, such as unilateral chest movement and unilateral breath sounds. Endoscopy using a fibreoptic scope can confirm the placement of tracheal tube in the trachea or in main bronchus. Once confirmed, the tube should be gradually withdrawn, under direct vision and reassessed. Failure to recognize and correct an endobronchial intubation may lead to hypoxaemia, lung or lobar collapse and barotrauma.

Oesophageal intubation

Oesophageal intubation is a complication that can result in hypoxic brain damage and death if unrecognized. The risk of hypoxaemia, regurgitation and aspiration increases significantly with multiple oesophageal intubations when compared with single oesophageal intubation. Oesophageal intubation can be minimized by auscultation of chest and abdomen, monitoring end-tidal CO_2 ($ETco_2$), oesophageal detector device and ultrasonography. It is vital to appreciate that no one method is completely reliable, and this includes capnometry.

Upper airway obstruction

Upper airway obstruction is one of the common causes of hypoxaemia under anaesthesia. There are several reasons including artificial airway kinking, failure to maintain the upper airway or laryngospasm. Laryngospasm is essentially closure of the true vocal cords resulting in complete or partial obstruction of the airway. The incidence of laryngospasm can be as much as 5%, especially in higher risk surgeries such as paediatrics and ENT. Fatalities have also resulted because of negative pressure pulmonary oedema following airway obstruction due to laryngospasm. Postoperative nocturnal airway obstruction in patients with obstructive sleep apnoea is an increasing problem, owing to the prevalence of obesity. Opiate drugs will increase the tendency to obstruction, both while they are administered and for some nights after cessation of treatment, because of a rebound increase in REM sleep. Patients known to suffer from obstructive sleep apnoea should be nursed in high-dependency unit environments, while suspected cases and obese patients should receive nocturnal oxygen.

Aspiration

Aspiration can also be potentially fatal, it can cause acute desaturation and hence hypoxaemia can lead to chronic problems as well. Severe forms may require mechanical ventilation.

Effects of hypoxaemia

Hypoxaemia and cardiac effects

Acute hypoxaemia can present as bradycardia or the catecholamine effects can cause tachycardia and hypertension followed by other arrhythmias. Continued hypoxia will eventually cause acute ischaemia of the heart leading to myocardial infarction and cardiac arrest. The period of anoxia necessary to produce circulatory arrest will depend on cardiovascular status, the oxygen content of the body prior to the anoxic episode and the oxygen consumption.

Hypoxaemia and central nervous system effects

The neurological symptoms of hypoxaemia depend on the severity and the speed of onset. Mild hypoxaemia can cause restlessness, anxiety, headaches, disorientation and confusion. Continued further hypoxia can cause seizures, Cheyne–Stokes respiration, apnoea and coma. Severe cerebral damage is invariable, but it is sometimes possible to restore circulatory function. Many survivors die later as a result of the complications of coma.

Preoxygenation

Desaturation (S_ao_2 less than 90%) is common during induction of (and emergence from) anaesthesia. This can be prevented in most cases by allowing the patient to breathe high concentrations of oxygen before induction and emergence. Farmery and Roe have developed a computer model which predicts the effect on S_ao_2 of increasing durations of apnoea occurring after breathing varying fractions of inspired oxygen. Their model predicts that the S_ao_2 will decline to 60% after 9.9 minutes if the subject was breathing 100% oxygen before the apnoea, and in 2.8 minutes after breathing air.

Some of the factors affecting desaturation are oxygen consumption, oxygen content and alveolar partial pressure of oxygen. In the anaesthetized patient, the oxygen consumption (Vo_2) remains fairly constant at around 250 mL min^{-1}. Although the arterial partial pressure of oxygen (P_ao_2) decreases in direct relation to the P_Ao_2, the arterial haemoglobin oxygen saturation (S_ao_2) remains around 90% owing to the shape of the oxygen dissociation curve. The S_ao_2 only starts to decrease when the store of oxygen in the lungs is depleted and the P_ao_2 is of the order of 6–7 kPa. Its subsequent decline is of a constant and rapid nature, about 30% every minute. At the start of this rapid decline, the S_ao_2 is still 90–95% and this inflection point is defined as 'critical hypoxaemia'. It is for this reason that oximetry is not a good tool for predicting impending severe hypoxaemia. However, because oximetry detects the decrease in S_ao_2 before any clinical signs are apparent, it has proved invaluable in detecting critical situations and has helped improve clinical practice to avoid these situations.

Various factors significantly influence the time period from the onset of apnoea to critical hypoxaemia. These are functional residual capacity (FRC), preoxygenation, maintenance of a patent airway, metabolic rate, physiological shunt and deadspace. The FRC is the most important store of oxygen in the body. The greater the FRC, the longer apnoea can be tolerated before critical hypoxaemia develops. Patients with reduced FRC (e.g. lung disease, kyphoscoliosis, pregnancy and obesity) reach critical hypoxaemia more rapidly.

Preoxygenation aims to replace nitrogen in the FRC with oxygen and hence is also referred to as 'denitrogenation'. This causes a significant increase in body oxygen store and therefore increases tolerance to apnoea substantially. For an adult with a normal FRC and Vo_2, if the F_Eo_2 is 0.9 (i.e. as would be found after effective preoxygenation), the lungs would contain about 2000 mL of oxygen (i.e. 10 times Vo_2). Clinically relevant situations where preoxygenation is extremely beneficial are pregnancy, critical illness, obesity and even in children because of increased oxygen consumption and decreased FRC.

Since accurate identification of difficult mask ventilation remains elusive, it is good practice to preoxygenate all patients. About 3–5 minutes of ventilation is required to wash out the nitrogen in the lungs, blood and tissues. A non-rebreathing circuit must be used for this purpose, such as a Mapleson A circuit with an 8 L min^{-1} fresh gas flow, and the efficacy of the system will be substantially reduced if there is any leak around the face-mask. The most efficient method of preoxygenation appears to be to allow the patient to take eight deep breaths of oxygen in 1 minute. Less complete, but clinically valuable, preoxygenation can be accomplished by applying a standard recovery pattern oxygen mask to all patients on arrival in the anaesthetic room.

Obesity and hypoxaemia

An obese patient has multiple pulmonary abnormalities, including decreased vital capacity, expiratory reserve volume, inspiratory capacity and FRC. The supine positioning of such a patient further decreases expiratory reserve volume and FRC owing to small airways collapse, cephalad displacement of diaphragm and increased thoracic blood volume. FRC declines steeply with increasing BMI and reaches values of around 1 litre or less in subjects whose BMI exceeds 40 kg m^{-2}. The time to develop hypoxaemia is significantly shorter in obese patients. In addition, there are several other problems during airway management, such as difficult mask ventilation, difficult tracheal intubation and increased risk of aspiration. For morbidly obese patients (BMI of 40 kg m^{-2}), preoxygenation in the head-up position increases FRC and achieves better oxygenation.

With increasing BMI, closing volume can encroach on FRC during normal tidal ventilation, leading to airway closure and ventilation/perfusion (V/Q) mismatch. A modest preoperative (A–a) O_2 gradient and shunt fraction can deteriorate markedly on induction of anaesthesia requiring high F_Io_2 and positive end expiratory pressure (PEEP) to maintain an adequate arterial Po_2. The incidence of obstructive sleep apnoea increases with obesity and increasing age. Depressant drugs, including many anaesthetic agents and analgesics, accentuate this. The combination of reduced chest wall and diaphragmatic tone during general anaesthesia, the increased incidence of atelectasis and secretion retention render the morbidly obese patient at risk of rapid desaturation during periods of hypoventilation or apnoea. These problems persist into the postoperative period. In addition to supplemental oxygen, a multimodal approach, involving breathing exercises, physiotherapy, and in some cases continuous positive airway pressure (CPAP), may be necessary in the immediate postoperative period.

Bibliography

Baraka AS, Taha SK, Aouad MT, *et al.* Pre-oxygenation: comparison of maximal breathing and tidal volume breathing techniques. *Anesthesiology* 1999; **91**: 612–16.

Benumof JL. Preoxygenation. Best method for both efficacy and efficiency? *Anesthesiology* 1999; **91**: 603–5.

Caplan RA, Posner KL, Ward RJ, Cheney FW. Adverse respiratory events in anaesthesia: a closed claims analysis. *Anesthesiology* 1990; **72**: 828–33.

Domino KB, Posner KL, Caplan RA, *et al.* Airway injury during anesthesia: a closed claims analysis. *Anesthesiology* 1999; **91**: 1703–11.

Farmery AD, Roe PG. A model to describe the rate of oxyhaemoglobin desaturation during apnoea. *Br J Anaesth* 1996; **76**: 284–91.

Gallagher SF, Haines KL, Osterlund LG, *et al.* Postoperative hypoxemia: common, undetected, and unsuspected after bariatric surgery. *J Surg Res* 2010; **159**: 622–6.

Henig NR, Pierson DJ. Mechanisms of hypoxemia. *Resp Care Clin North Am* 2000; **6**: 501–21.

Bibliography

Adewale L. Anatomy and assessment of the pediatric airway. *Pediatr Anesth* 2009; **19**: 1–8.

Ahmed I, Russell W. Jaw thrust: are we applying it correctly? *Pediatr Anesth* 2009; **20**: 107–8.

Cote CJ, Hartnick CJ. Pediatric transtracheal and cricothyrotomy airway devices for emergency use: which are appropriate for infants and children? *Pediatr Anesth* 2009; **19**: 66–7.

Mason D, McDouall S. Management of paediatric difficult airway. In: Popat M (ed.) *Difficult Airway Management.* Oxford: Oxford University Press, 2009, pp. 115–29.

Morgan GA, Steward DJ. Linear airway dimensions in children: including those from cleft palate. *Can Anaesth Soc J* 1982; **29**: 1–8.

Peterson J, Johnson N, Deakins K, *et al.* Accuracy of the 7–8–9 rule for endotracheal tube placement in the neonate. *J Perinatol* 2006; **26**: 333–6.

Robb PJ, Bew S, Kubba H, *et al.* Tonsillectomy and adenoidectomy in children with sleep-related breathing disorders: consensus statement of a UK multidisciplinary working party. *Ann R Coll Surg Engl* 2009; **91**: 371–3.

Walker RWM, Ellwood J. The management of difficult intubation in children. *Pediatr Anesth* 2009; **19**: 77–87.

Weber T, Salvi N, Orliaguet G, Wolf A. Cuffed vs non-cuffed endotracheal tubes for pediatric anesthesia. *Pediatr Anesth* 2009; **19**: 46–54.

White MC, Cook TM, Stoddart PA. A critique of elective pediatric supraglottic airway devices. *Pediatr Anesth* 2009; **19**: 55–65.

Cross-references

Artificial airways, 642
Difficult airway: management, 651
Difficult airway: new devices, 660

28 Equipment and monitoring

Baha Al-Shaikh

Compressed oxygen outlets

One or more compressed oxygen outlets are usually present and allow oxygen at pipeline pressure (400 kPa) to be utilized for various other functions, e.g. driving ventilators or a Sanders-type jet ventilator device.

In some AWSs, it may not always be possible to identify the individual components listed above. It is important to obtain specific training before using an unfamiliar anaesthetic machine or AWS. A back-up system to maintain anaesthesia (e.g. intravenous anaesthetic agent) as well as an independent means of ventilation with oxygen (self-inflating bag) must always be present in case of unexpected problems. Electrically powered anaesthetic workstations should always be plugged directly into a wall-mounted mains socket, and never via a multisocket extension lead. The majority of AWSs include an integral battery that provides power in the event of electrical supply failure; however, this frequently will provide only a short respite. The integral battery may be augmented by a uninterruptible power supply to provide additional longevity or power to the monitoring system.

Bibliography

Al-Shaikh B, Stacey S. *Essentials of Anaesthetic Equipment*, 3rd edn. Edinburgh: Elsevier, 2007.

British Standards Institution. *European Standard BS EN 740: 1998 Anaesthetic Workstations and Their Modules: Particular Requirements.* London: British Standards Institution, 1998.

British Standards Institution. *International Standard IEC 60601: Medical Electrical Equipment Part 2-13 (ISO 8835-Part 1), Particular Requirements for the Safety of Anaesthetic Workstations*, 2nd edn. London: British Standards Institution, 1998.

Davey A, Diba A (eds). *Ward's Anaesthetic Equipment*, 5th edn. Philadelphia: Elsevier, 2005.

Cross-references

Breathing systems, 683
Ventilators, 696

Breathing systems

James DA Wood and Baha Al-Shaikh

Breathing systems deliver anaesthetic gas mixtures to the patient. Several classification systems have been described: those that classify them as 'open', 'semi-open', 'semi-closed' or 'closed' (Table 28.1); whether they allow rebreathing or not; and whether they have an 'adequate' or 'inadequate' fresh gas flow to meet the patient's minute volume, e.g. the Mapleson systems (adequate) or the circle system (inadequate).

The most common classification used is that derived by the physicist Mapleson, who classified breathing systems, excluding the open ones and those with non-rebreathing valves, according to their configuration and functional performance with respect to fresh gas flow (FGF) requirements for spontaneous ventilation (Table 28.2). His classification of five systems has since been expanded to six systems labelled A–F.

Systems with inadequate fresh gas flow

Systems that allow the use of 'inadequate FGF' reduce the amount of volatile anaesthetic agent required, so reducing costs and pollution, and they also allow for effective warming and humidification of the gases. However, with inadequate FGF, the composition of gases at the patient end of a system can be very different from those of the FGF. They should, therefore, always be used with monitoring of the inspired gases.

For systems using an 'inadequate' gas flow, a method must be used to remove the CO_2, which would otherwise build up. This is normally achieved by the use of chemical CO_2 absorption. Several versions are available:

- soda lime: 94% $Ca(OH)_2$, 5% NaOH, 1% KOH with silicates to make granules
- Baralyme: 80% $Ca(OH)_2$, 20% $Ba(OH)_2$
- Amsorb: $CaCl_2$, $Ca(OH)_2$.

The chemical absorbers include indicator dyes which change colour when the absorbent is exhausted. Certain volatile anaesthetic agents cannot be used with such absorbers. Moisture is required for efficient CO_2 absorption as well as to prevent CO formation (and compound A formation with sevoflurane).

Other substances that can potentially accumulate in such systems include CO, methane, acetone, ethanol, hydrogen and substance A. However, they do not generally become clinically significant. CO accumulation and subsequent carboxyhaemoglobin formation is said to occur at less than 0.1% per hour, so may become significant in smokers when ultralow flows are used; oxygen flushes of the system (e.g. once an hour) will prevent this. For substance A, Baralyme is worse than soda lime, and Amsorb is the safest.

Waters' canister (bidirectional flow)

- An obsolete system with a cylinder containing soda lime with a reservoir at one end and a face-mask, fresh gas inlet and expiratory valve at the other.
- Its usefulness is limited by its cumbersome size, while its efficiency is limited by the rapid exhaustion of soda lime nearest to the patient (results in increasing deadspace) and channelling of gas flow.

Circle system (unidirectional flow)

- The lower the FGF entering the circle, the longer the time constant for the system to reach steady state and the less control there is over the concentrations within the system.

Time constant = Volume of circle/(FGF – uptake)

- In the absence of monitoring, low-flow use with the circle system can result in the delivery of hypoxic mixtures. In addition, there may be inadvertent wrong dosage of inhalational agent

Table 28.1 A classification of breathing systems

	Definition	Examples
Open	Entirely open to the atmosphere, ambient air is the fresh gas supply	Rag and bottle
Semi-open	Mainly open to atmosphere with some restriction to ambient air, which acts as the fresh gas supply	Schimmelbusch mask
Semi-closed	Air intake prevented but venting of excess gas to the atmosphere	Mapleson systems
Closed	No air intake or venting of exhaust gases	Totally closed circle system

● **Table 28.2** Mapleson breathing systems.

Name	Alternative names	Diagram	FGF requirements for	
			Spontaneous ventilation	Controlled ventilation
Mapleson A	Magill system	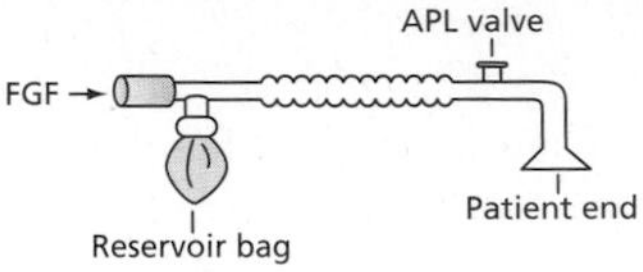 APL valve; FGF; Patient end; Reservoir bag	1 × MV	3 × MV
	Lack system	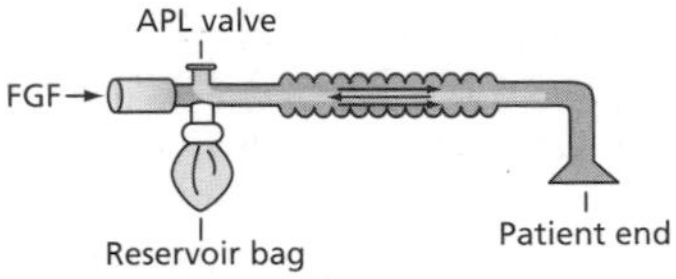 APL valve; FGF; Reservoir bag; Patient end		
Mapleson B		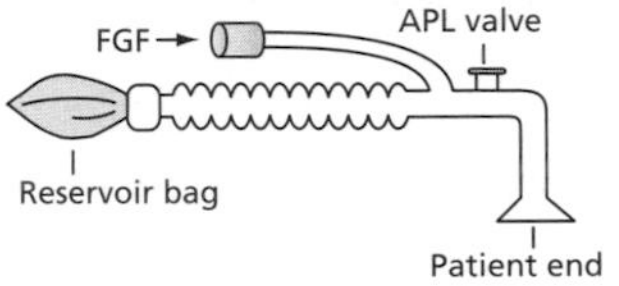 FGF; APL valve; Reservoir bag; Patient end	1.5 × MV	1 × MV
Mapleson C	Waters' system	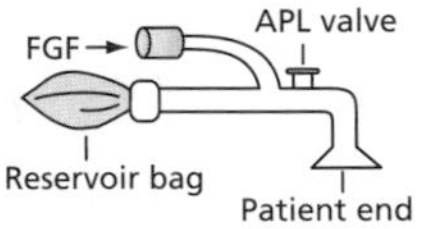 APL valve; FGF; Reservoir bag; Patient end	1.5 × MV	1 × MV
Mapleson D		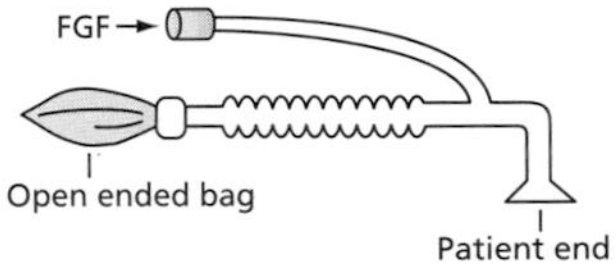 FGF; Open ended bag; Patient end	2 × MV	1 × MV
	Bain system	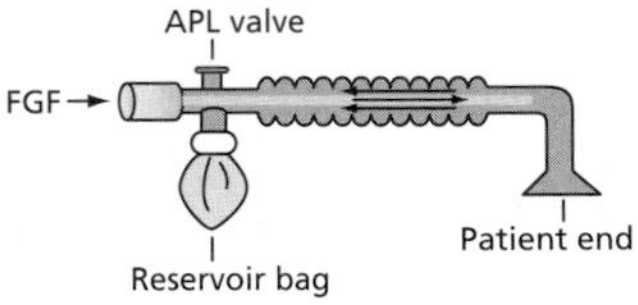 APL valve; FGF; Patient end; Reservoir bag		
Mapleson E	Ayre's T-piece	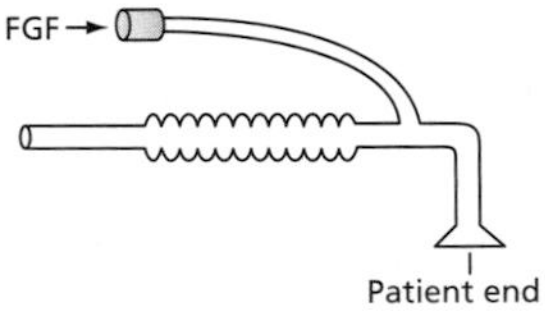 FGF; Patient end	3 × MV	3 × MV
Mapleson F	Jackson-Rees	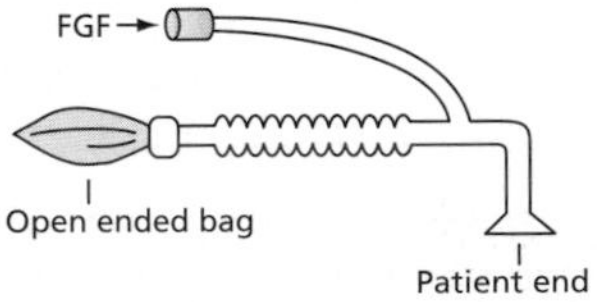 FGF; Open ended bag; Patient end	3 × MV	3 × MV

APL, adjustable pressure-limiting; FGF, fresh gas flow; MV, minute resting ventilation of an anaesthetized patient (approximately 70 mL kg^{-1} min^{-1}).

and rebreathing owing to unrecognized exhaustion of CO_2 absorbent.

- Monitoring minimizes these risks and should be essential with the circle system. Oxygen concentration, volatile agent concentration, capnography and circulating gas volume (e.g. by rising of ventilator bellows) should be monitored.

Systems with adequate fresh gas flow

Non-rebreathing valve systems (unidirectional flow)

Require the FGF to match the patient's minute ventilation exactly. Too high a flow may result in the valve jamming in inspiration, causing barotrauma, hypoventilation and falling cardiac output. For this reason, they are not used in practice.

Reservoir systems (bidirectional flow)

The reservoir in these systems refers to the site where bidirectional flow and storage of gases occur (Fig. 28.1). The reservoir portion of the system should be approximately equal to the patient's tidal volume; it may be situated in the exhaust limb in *efferent* reservoir systems, the supply limb in *afferent* reservoir systems or at the junction of the supply and exhaust limb in *junctional* reservoir systems.

Mapleson A

Also known as the Magill system, while its coaxial variant is known as Lack system. It is an *afferent* reservoir system.

Advantages

- Maximal efficiency in spontaneous ventilation.
- Good heat and moisture exchange.

Disadvantages

- Very inefficient in controlled ventilation.
- Cannot be used with a ventilator.
- The adjustable pressure-limiting (APL) valve at the patient end places weight and bulk near the patient, making adjustment and scavenging difficult.

Mapleson B and C systems

Junctional reservoir systems that, although differing in their length of tubing to the reservoir, act in an equivalent fashion. The Mapleson C system is also known as a Waters' circuit.

Advantage

- Reservoir bag close at hand for monitoring respiration and controlling ventilation with simple interchange between spontaneous and controlled ventilation.

Disadvantages

- Intermediate efficiency in all modes of ventilation.
- APL valve at the patient end makes scavenging and adjustment difficult and results in weight and bulk near the patient.

Mapleson D

Its coaxial form is known as the Bain system. It is an *efferent* reservoir system.

Advantages

- Minimal deadspace, so may be used for children and adults.
- Simple interchange between spontaneous and controlled ventilation.
- Useful for limited access to head and neck.
- Efficient in controlled ventilation.
- Scavenging convenient.

Disadvantages

- Inefficient in spontaneous ventilation.
- Bain system inner tube disconnection results in a very large deadspace.

Mapleson E

Also known as the Ayre T-piece. It is an *efferent* reservoir system.

Advantages

- Its low resistance to breathing makes it useful for spontaneous ventilation in small children.
- Minimal deadspace, so may be used for children.

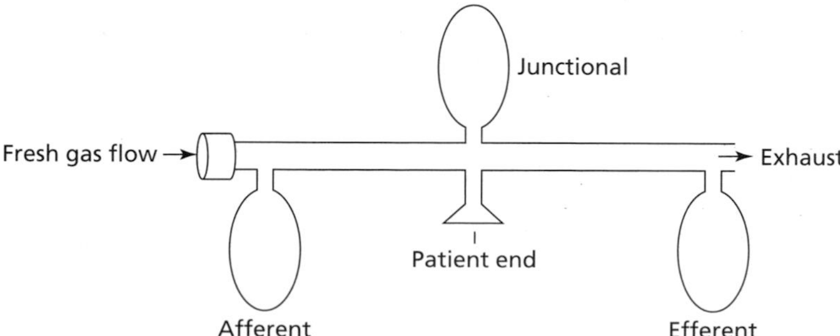

Figure 28.1 The reservoir is where storage of gases occurs. It may be situated in the exhaust limb in efferent reservoir systems (Mapleson D, E, F), the supply limb in afferent reservoir systems (Mapleson A) or at the junction of the supply and exhaust limb in junctional reservoir systems (Mapleson BC).

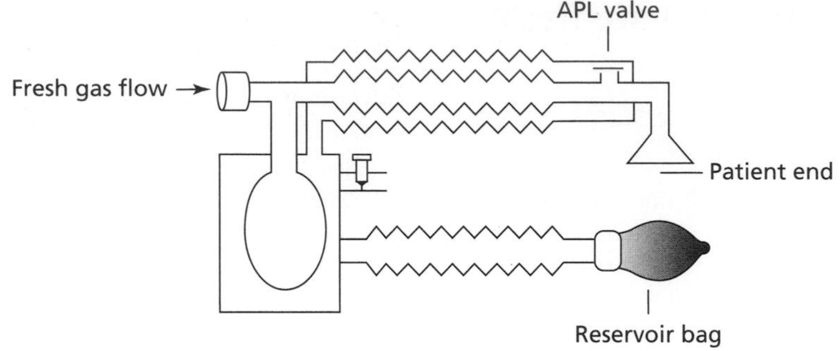

Figure 28.2 Enclosed afferent reservoir (EAR) system. APL, adjustable pressure-limiting; FGF, fresh gas flow.

Disadvantages

- Inefficient in spontaneous and controlled ventilation.
- Difficult to scavenge.
- Difficult to apply continuous positive airway pressure (CPAP).

Mapleson F

Also known as the Jackson Rees modification of the Ayre T-piece or the Rees T-piece, it was added to Mapleson's classification by Jackson Rees. The design adds an open-ended bag to the T-piece. Versions with an integrated APL valve and closed reservoir bag are available. It is an *efferent* reservoir system.

Advantages

- Minimal deadspace, so may be used for children.
- Reservoir bag close at hand for monitoring respiration and controlling ventilation with simple interchange between spontaneous and controlled ventilation.

Disadvantages

- Scavenging difficult (unless an APL valve is included).
- Inefficient in spontaneous ventilation.

Combination systems

Combination systems attempt to combine the advantages of efferent and afferent reservoir systems. For example, the Humphrey ADE system combines the Mapleson A, D and E systems in one unit with interchange enabled by use of the Humphrey block valve assembly.

Enclosed afferent reservoir systems

These systems are similar to the Mapleson D but have an additional reservoir on the FGF limb enclosed within a chamber connected to the main limb (Fig. 28.2). Despite their advantages, such systems are not widely used. A further variation – the enclosed efferent afferent reservoir system – has also been described which is more efficient still.

Advantages

- Efficient for spontaneous and controlled ventilation.
- Convenient interchange between modes of ventilation.
- Satisfactory humidity even without a heat moisture exchanger.
- Easy scavenging.
- Low deadspace, so suitable for children.

Disadvantages

- Difficult to understand how it works.
- Internal leak results in large deadspace.

Bibliography

Al-Shaikh B, Stacey S. *Essentials of Anaesthetic Equipment*, 3rd edn. Edinburgh: Elsevier, 2007.

Davey A, Diba A (eds). *Ward's Anaesthetic Equipment*, 5th edn. Philadelphia: Elsevier, 2005.

Miller DM. Breathing systems reclassified. *Anaesth Intensive Care* 1995; **23**: 281–3.

Miller DM, Miller JC. Enclosed afferent reservoir breathing systems. *Br J Anaesth* 1988; **60**: 469–75.

Cross-references

The anaesthetic machine, 680
Ventilators, 696

Depth of anaesthesia

Sarath Varghese and Baha Al-Shaikh

Anaesthesia is a balance between the amount of the anaesthetic given and the varying state of arousal, which is affected by the changeable intensity of surgical stimulation. It is vital to get this balance right as, if too little anaesthetic is administered, patients risk awareness during surgery.

Depth of anaesthesia can be represented as a balance between the factors causing hypnosis and the stimulating factors which lighten anaesthesia. To measure the depth of anaesthesia, the following can be used.

Non-specific techniques

- Clinical signs (PRST: blood *p*ressure, heart *r*ate, *s*weating, *t*ears). These are unreliable indices of awareness. They can be influenced by other factors such as inadequate analgesia or drugs that affect the autonomic nervous system (e.g. atropine, atenolol).
- End-expiratory volatile agent concentration, so estimating minimal alveolar concentration.
- Estimated plasma concentration (Cp_{50}) from target controlled infusion.

Specific techniques

- Non-EEG: e.g. the isolated forearm technique, lower oesophageal contractility, frontalis muscle activity (partly used in entropy; see below) and heart rate/ECG variability.
- EEG: the brain activity (measured as EEG) can form the basis of depth of anaesthesia measurement as it is the end-organ for anaesthetic effect:
  - raw EEG changes with depth of anaesthesia, but this requires specialist interpretation and is not readily quantifiable
  - processed EEG is commonly used. Early methods looked at spectral analysis. More recently, more complex methods have evolved, all of which use advanced analysis and processing of the EEG.

The following discussion looks at the processed EEG techniques.

Table 28.3 The range of the BIS values in relation to the clinical state

BIS index	Clinical state
100	Awake
>70	Light sedation
60–70	Deep sedation
60	General anaesthesia
40–60	Moderate hypnotic state
40	Deep hypnotic state (burst suppression)
0	No cortical electrical activity

Bispectral index monitors

Bispectral index (BIS) is the most established of the commercially available monitors in which the changes to the EEG waveform that occur during anaesthesia are analysed. A complex mathematical algorithm is used to analyse the data, producing a simplified, easy to interpret output variable that is generated in real time with a range between 0 and 100 to denote depth of anaesthesia; 100 represents the fully awake patient and 0 represents cortical electrical silence (Table 28.3). The BIS monitor uses a frontotemporal electrode connected to a microprocessor.

Bispectral analysis is a technique used for analysing complex waves. Originally it was used to analyse complex oceanographic waves in several dimensions; a similar process can be used to analyse the EEG.

In order to calculate the BIS, the following techniques are used:

- Fourier transformation in which the signal is processed using a mathematical algorithm to decompose the complex EEG signal into separate functions based on the frequency, phase (time) and power of each constituent sine wave.
- Power spectrum in which each of the constituent waves of the EEG with different frequencies can be represented on a two-dimensional graph.
- Phase spectrum is the function of the phase relationships of component sine waves, so quantifying synchronization of the EEG signal.
- Artefact detection that can be classified into two types:
  - artefacts caused by electromyographic (EMG) activity, ECG signals, diathermy or pacemaker spikes
  - artefacts caused by more insidious changes in the EEG signal over time. A system of comparing

Ventilators

Mark Snazelle and Baha Al-Shaikh

Ventilators can be divided according to their functions (Table 28.5).

Three common types of ventilator

Volume preset, time cycled, flow generator

- Used in adult theatre and ICU ventilators.
- A preset tidal volume is delivered despite changes in lung compliance.
- Inflation pressure depends on lung compliance and is limited by a safety blow-off valve (usually 60 cmH_2O).
- Time cycling.
- Powerful machines powered by a high-pressure driving gas (400 kPa) or substantial electric motors.

Pressure preset, time cycled, flow generator

- Used in paediatric ventilators.
- Set airway pressure (usually 15–20 cmH_2O) not exceeded during inspiration.
- Cycles to expiration at the end of a set time, even if the desired inflation pressure is not reached.
- Inspiratory flow rate must be set at high enough level to reach the desired pressure in the time allowed for inspiration.
- Tidal volume delivered is affected by changes in lung compliance.
- Compensates to a degree for leaks, e.g. uncuffed paediatric tracheal tube or laryngeal mask.

Time cycled, pressure generator

- Weighted bellows apply constant set pressure during inspiration.
- Inspiratory flow is high initially and then declines (characteristic of a pressure generator).
- Delivered tidal volume will depend on the pressure in the bellows and the lung compliance.
- Possible to set a desired tidal volume only if there is sufficient weight on bellows.

Other ventilators

Ventilators can also be classified by how they work. The commonest types used in operating theatres are:

- Minute volume dividers: these use the power of the FGF from the anaesthetic machine and divide the delivered minute volume into preset tidal volumes.
- T-tube occluders: these occlude intermittently the expiratory limb of a T-piece; the constant gas flow into the circuit then inflates the patient's lungs
- Bag squeezers: these compress a bellows in the breathing system, usually by means of high-pressure gas or an electric motor
- Intermittent blowers: these are powered by a high-pressure driving gas which enters the breathing system in controlled 'bursts'.

Checking and setting

Checking and setting the ventilator and its breathing system before use is vital:

- connect to electricity supply, high-pressure gas, low-pressure gas, etc.

Table 28.5 Classification of ventilators according to their functions

Inspiratory phase gas control	Volume: a preset volume is delivered Pressure: a preset pressure is not exceeded
Cycling (inspiration–expiration)	Volume Pressure Time Flow
Inspiratory flow characteristic	Flow generator: the inspiratory flow pattern predetermined by ventilator settings Pressure generator: the inspiratory pressure applied to the patient's airway is determined by ventilator settings

- set tidal volume to 10 mL kg^{-1} or inflation pressure to 15 cmH_2O
- set respiratory rate to 12 breaths min^{-1}
- set the inspiration/expiration (I/E) ratio to 1:2, with an inspiratory time of not less than 1 second
- switch on and see if pressure develops in the system
- check that the pressure relief valve is functioning at the correct value
- check that gas monitoring is present and working
- check that airway pressure monitor is working
- check manual mode functioning (if fitted)
- check that the emergency air intake is patent (if appropriate).

Many modern anaesthetic and ICU ventilators now have automated programmes for checking the ventilatory breathing system.

Modes of ventilation

Sophisticated ventilators may function in a number of modes, some of which provide mandatory ventilation and others which provide some form of respiratory support when triggered by the patient. Triggered modes (see below) can be safely used only when there are spontaneous patient breaths.

- IPPV: generic term used for all forms of positive pressure ventilation.
- Controlled mandatory ventilation: mandatory mode where a preset minute volume is delivered, usually to a paralysed or apnoeic patient as any patient respiratory efforts are ignored.
- Triggering indicates the ability of the ventilator to detect the initiation of a spontaneous breath by the patient, usually by detecting a set negative pressure in the breathing system. The patient triggers the onset of the inspiratory phase.
- Pressure support ventilation (PSV) is one commonly used mode in which the patient triggers the inspiratory phase. The adjustable level of pressure support (often 5–20 cmH_2O) determines the degree of respiratory support provided by the ventilator. Often the inspiratory phase during pressure support is terminated when the inspiratory flow rate decreases below a critical value.
- Assist control (AC): the ventilator provides a breath with a preset tidal volume (or preset peak pressure) each time the patient initiates a breath. Back-up rate of mandatory breaths in case of apnoea.
- Synchronized intermittent mandatory ventilation (SIMV): similar to AC but ventilator provides a preset mechanical breath (the mandatory breath) every specified number of seconds (e.g. for 12 breaths per minute this is a 5 second cycle). Ventilation is synchronized to the first patient breath in the set cycle. Additional patient breaths after the first in the cycle are not supported, though PSV is commonly added to support these breaths (PSIMV).
- PSIMV is therefore a mode in which a mandatory number of breaths is delivered; breaths are synchronized to the first breath of a set time cycle, and further spontaneous breaths are supplemented by pressure support.
- Pressure-regulated volume control: under dual control of pressure and volume. Tidal volume is preset, then the ventilator delivers pressure-controlled breath until the tidal volume is achieved. Designed to optimize peak inspiratory pressures.
- Airway pressure release ventilation (APRV): the ventilator cycles between two pressure levels (upper and lower pressure levels). Baseline airway pressure is the upper level, with pressure intermittently being released to allow removal of waste gases.
- Biphasic positive airway pressure (BIPAP): single ventilation mode (on Drager machines) which can be used throughout weaning. Uses the principle of APRV, but also with spontaneous breathing. Flow is generated mechanically by alternating between the two pressure levels, and also by patient triggering. Can deliver mandatory ventilation alone, SIMV ventilation or purely spontaneous ventilation. When the upper level is weaned to the same as the lower one, this is CPAP, and the patient takes over ventilation.

Note that this is not to be confused with BiPAP (bilevel positive airway pressure), which is a non-invasive, pressure support ventilatory system.

- Proportional assist ventilation (PAV): form of synchronized ventilation in which the ventilator generates pressure in proportion to the patient's effort and responds to changes in lung dynamics. No target tidal volume, pressure or flow is needed. The level of support given is dialled up as the percentage of patient work of breathing to be overcome (usually started at 80%).
- Adaptive support ventilation: similar to PAV, but a different algorithm (Hamilton Medical). Meant to optimize breathing pattern, promote spontaneous breathing and reduce weaning time.
- Neurally adjusted ventilatory assist: novel mode of positive pressure ventilation in which the ventilator is controlled by the patient's own neural control of breathing. Electrodes on a nasogastric tube monitor electrical impulses from the phrenic nerve at the level of the diaphragm, and adjust ventilatory parameters accordingly.
- Positive end-expiratory pressure (PEEP), which is during controlled ventilation.
- CPAP is continuous positive airway pressure during spontaneous respiration and is functionally

the same as PEEP. It can be used both in invasive ventilation and non-invasively.

High-frequency ventilation

This refers to ventilation occurring at rates well in excess of those in normal breathing.

- High-frequency jet ventilation: gas is passed by a small-bore catheter, placed either sub- or supraglottically. Ventilation rate can be from 4 to 11 Hz. Exhalation is passive. Uses include glottic/laryngeal surgery, bronchopleural fistula and adult respiratory distress syndrome (ARDS); thought to reduce ventilator-induced lung injury (VILI).
- High-frequency oscillatory ventilation: pressure wave is generated by a moving diaphragm controlled electromagnetically. Respiratory rates of up to 15 Hz are achieved. Pressure oscillates about the distending pressure (analogous to PEEP). Tidal volumes are less than deadspace. Multiple mechanisms of gas transfer have been proposed but the exact mechanism is yet to be fully understood. Can produce pressures less than ambient pressure; hence, gas is pushed in during inspiration and actively 'pulled out' during expiration. Uses include severe ARDS and neonatal ventilation. Also thought to reduce VILI.

The ideal ventilatory breathing system

The ideal ventilatory breathing system should have the following characteristics:

- wide range of tidal volumes and respiratory rates to encompass paediatric and adult use
- pressure- or volume-controlled modes
- adjustable inspiratory/expiratory timing (I/E ratio)
- airway pressure display, with alarm limits
- expired minute volume display, with alarm limits
- adjustable, monitored inspired oxygen concentration
- provision of PEEP/CPAP
- sophisticated ventilatory modes
- humidification
- adjustable inspiratory waveforms
- adjustable pressure relief valve
- facility for drug administration into breathing system (nitric oxide, inhaled bronchodilator).

Complications of prolonged ventilation

- VILI: direct lung injury caused by a combination of barotrauma, volutrauma, atelectrauma and biotrauma.
- Ventilator-associated pneumonia: greater than 48 hours of ventilation. Symptoms and signs include fever, increasing purulent secretions, hypoxia, new X-ray changes.

Bibliography

Davey A, Moyle J, Ward C (eds). *Ward's Anaesthetic Equipment*, 3rd edn. Philadelphia: WB Saunders, 1992, pp. 197–241.

Ehrenwerth J, Eisenkraft JB. *Anesthesia Equipment, Principles and Applications*. St Louis: Mosby, 1993.

Dräger Medical. BIPAP – Two steps forward in intensive-care ventilation. An introductory guide to Evita ventilation. Available from www.frca.co.uk/documents/BIPAP-Booklet.pdf.

Hayes B. Ventilators: a current assessment. In: Adams AP, Atkinson RS (eds) *Recent Advances in Anaesthesia and Analgesia*, vol. 18. Edinburgh: Churchill Livingstone, 1993, pp. 83–102.

Singer BD, Corbridge TC. Basic invasive mechanical ventilation. *South Med J* 2009; **102**: 1238–45.

Slutsky AS, Brochard L, Vincent JL. *Update in Intensive Care Medicine: Mechanical Ventilation*. Berlin: Springer-Verlag, 2005, pp. 63, 83, 125.

Ward NS, Dushay KM. Clinical concise review: mechanical ventilation of patients with chronic obstructive pulmonary disease. *Crit Care Med* 2008; **36**: 1614–19.

Cross-references

Breathing systems, 683

The anaesthetic machine, 680

29 Techniques

Baha Al-Shaikh

Blind nasal intubation

Mark Snazelle and Baha Al-Shaikh

Blind nasotracheal intubation (Box 29.1) is a useful technique in the anaesthetist's armamentarium in dealing with difficult airway patients, especially when a fibreoptic scope is not available. It can be used for intubating spontaneously breathing patients with or without sedation, or under general anaesthesia. This method has the advantage of being independent from visualization of the glottis and has a good chance of success in a variety of patients of different ages and body sizes, in both elective as well as selected emergency situations. However, it can cause upper airway bleeding in approximately 20% of patients that can compromise subsequent fibreoptic efforts. With the advent of readily available fibreoptic scopes, this technique has all but been superseded by awake fibreoptic intubation, where the glottis can be visualized, reducing the risks of both failure and trauma.

Box 29.1 Blind nasal intubation; indications and contraindications

- Indications (similar to fibreoptic-assisted intubation)
  - Difficult laryngoscopy due to limited mouth opening, mandibular agenesis, buck teeth
  - History and/or anticipated difficulty with other techniques of intubation
  - Severe risk of aspiration
  - Inability to apply a face-mask
  - Cervical injuries limiting neck movement
  - Severe risk of haemodynamic/respiratory instability on induction of general anaesthesia/paralysis
- Contraindications
  - Airway tumours, abscesses or trauma
  - Recent nasal surgery
  - Coagulopathy
  - Basal skull fracture and unstable mid-face injuries

Sedation for awake blind nasal intubation

As with awake fibreoptic intubation, it is essential that the patient cooperates with the technique and is able to speak and respond to commands. Providing suitable sedation to the patient may improve the chances of a successful intubation. This can easily be achieved using intravenous propofol by target-controlled infusion (TCI) 0.5–1 µg mL^{-1} target plasma concentration combined with opioids (e.g. fentanyl), which offer analgesia. Benzodiazepines such as midazolam can be used as alternatives when titrated carefully. Remifentanil TCI has been increasingly being used as a sole means of analgesia and sedation in awake intubation.

Airway anaesthesia

Local anaesthesia of the airway is used in awake or sedated patients. Careful explanation is given to the patient before sedation and local anaesthetic administration. Nebulized lidocaine 4% (4–10 mL) can be used and acts within 10 minutes. This achieves global mucosal coverage and is a good starting point in anaesthetizing the airway, but is rarely sufficient as a sole technique, so some supplemental form of local anaesthesia is usually required.

It should be remembered that the effect of local anaesthesia may worsen the upper airway obstruction. Furthermore, in patients with a full stomach, local anaesthesia should not extend beyond the glottis.

- An anticholinergic/antisialagogue is usually given, such as glycopyrrolate 0.2 mg intravenously, to reduce secretions and improve the contact of topical anaesthesia.
- *Nose*: in addition to the local anaesthetic, the nasal mucosa should be gently prepared with a vasoconstrictor to reduce bleeding and oedema. Phenylephrine 1%, xylometazoline (Otrivin) or cocaine 4% can be used. Full effectiveness requires application for 2–5 minutes, with a duration of action of 30–45 minutes. Phenylephrine 0.5% is also available in a combined preparation with lidocaine 5% (co-phenylcaine).
- *Mouth, pharynx/larynx*: amethocaine lozenges and nebulized lidocaine can be used. The superior laryngeal nerves can be blocked bilaterally: 3 mL of 2% lidocaine is injected inferomedial to the greater cornu of the hyoid on both sides providing a 20–30 minute block.

Alternatively, 4% lidocaine may be gargled or sprayed to the tonsillar pillars; 10% lidocaine is very irritant to mucosal membranes and, although very effective, should only be used where topicalization with a weaker local anaesthetic solution has been performed beforehand.

- *Trachea*: the mucosa below the larynx can be blocked by a midline transtracheal injection of local

Table 29.1 Tube placement

Position	Confirmation	Response
Trachea	Breath sounds continue through tube with its advance, coughing through tube	Secure tube, auscultate bilaterally, confirm $ETco_2$
Anterior	Breath sounds continue through the tube, but unable to advance further, coughing mostly through the tube	Slightly withdraw and readvance tube while the patient's head and neck are gradually flexed
Left/right piriform fossa	No breath sounds, tube unable to advance, no cough, tube may be palpable on one side of the neck	Slightly withdraw until breath sounds through tube resume, slowly rotate (back toward midline) and readvance
Oesophagus	No breath sounds, tube continues to advance, no cough	Withdraw tube until breath sounds through tube resume, then (separately or together): *Extend* patient's head and readvance *Inflate cuff* (e.g. 15 mL of air) so directing the tip anteriorly, advance until resistance is felt, maintain some advancing pressure on tube while cuff is *slowly deflated* Apply posterior pressure on the larynx and readvance tube

$ETco_2$, end-tidal CO_2.

anaesthetic through the cricothyroid membrane: 3 mL of 2–4% lidocaine is injected using a 23G needle with its bevel directed downwards. On penetration of the trachea the patient exhales as deeply as possible so that the subsequent deep inspiration (and cough) will result in maximal distribution of lidocaine.

It is important to note that great care must be taken to remain vigilant regarding total dosage of local anaesthetic, as exceeding recommended dosages is easy, and side-effects become more prevalent at higher doses.

Intubation

The patient is positioned with the neck flexed and the head extended at the atlantoaxial joint (sniffing position) if the cervical spine is stable. A prewarmed, well-lubricated, curved, nasal tracheal tube (7.0–7.5 mm internal diameter) is gently passed perpendicularly through the more patent nostril into the hypopharynx. With the other nostril and the mouth occluded, the tube is advanced in midline listening for the breath sounds. The tube is passed into the larynx during inspiration. The CO_2 concentration in the exhaled air can be used to monitor the progress and to confirm tube position.

The tube is advanced until one of the five positions shown in Table 29.1 is reached.

Movement of the breathing system reservoir bag, condensation on the tracheal tube/catheter mount and audiocapnography can provide further confirmation of the position of the tube.

Bibliography

Latto IP. Management of difficult intubation. In: Latto IP, Vaughan RS (eds) *Difficulties in Tracheal Intubation*, 2nd edn. London: W.B. Saunders, 1997, pp. 140–3.

Murrin KR. Awake intubation. In: Latto IP, Vaughan RS (eds) *Difficulties in Tracheal Intubation*, 2nd edn. London: W.B. Saunders, 1997, pp. 161–71.

Stone DJ, Gal TJ. Airway management. In: Miller RD (ed.) *Anesthesia*, 4th edn. Edinburgh: Churchill Livingstone, 1994, pp. 1423–6.

Williams KA, Barker GL, Harwood RJ, Woodall NM. Combined nebulization and spray-as-you-go topical local anaesthesia of the airway. *Br J Anaesth* 2005; **95**: 549–53.

Woodall NM, Harwood RJ, Barker GL. Complications of awake fibreoptic intubation without sedation in 200 healthy anaesthetists attending a training course. *Br J Anaesth* 2008; **100**: 850–5.

Cross-references

Artificial airways, 642
Difficult airway: overview, 647
Local anaesthetic toxicity, 767

$$\text{Ventilation-priming dose} = 1.3\ \text{MAC} \times (\text{volume of system} + \text{volume of lungs})/100 = \text{mL of anaesthetic vapour}$$

Table 29.3 Volumes of system and lungs

Components	Volume (mL)
Absorber (2 kg)	2000
Breathing tubing (1 m)	1000
FRC	3000

FRC, functional residual capacity.

Uptake and elimination of gases/vapours

Uptake of inhalation agent

The uptake into the circulation and tissues can be calculated using Lowe's formula:

$$V_{an}\ (\text{arterial prime})\ (\text{mL min}^{-1}) = f\text{MAC} \times \lambda_{B/G} \times Q \times t^{-1/2}$$

where f MAC is the target concentration (1.3 MAC), $\lambda_{B/G}$ is the blood/gas solubility coefficient of the agent, Q is the cardiac output and t is the time constant.

This arterial prime dose equilibrates initially with the blood. Owing to the continuous uptake of agent into the tissues, further anaesthetic agent is required to provide for this uptake into the tissues.

Tissue uptake

The amount of anaesthetic agent taken up by the tissues decreases with time. This affects the rate of uptake of the agent into the circulation, which decreases inversely with the square root of elapsed time.

The amount of anaesthetic vapour uptake in the first minute is shown in Table 29.4.

Uptake of oxygen

Oxygen uptake during anaesthesia is generally lowered by 10–30%. This is due to the metabolic depression caused by the anaesthetic agents leading to decreased consumption. This uptake is almost stable throughout the entire duration of anaesthesia. For clinical purposes, oxygen consumption can easily be estimated as:

$$V_{O_2}\ (\text{mL min}^{-1}) = 3.5 \times \text{body weight (kg)}$$

Uptake of N_2O

The uptake of N_2O (Table 29.5), like volatile anaesthetic, follows a power function. As it is not metabolized, its uptake is determined solely by the alveolar-arterial partial pressure difference. This is high at the beginning of anaesthesia but reduces with time as the tissues become progressively more saturated with N_2O. The uptake of N_2O by a normal adult patient can be roughly estimated by:

$$V_{N2O}\ (\text{mL min}^{-1}) = 1000 \times t^{1/2}$$

Table 29.5 Tissue uptake of nitous oxide

Time (min)	N_2O uptake (mL min^{-1})
1	1000
25	200
50	140
>120	90

CO_2 output

CO_2 output can be estimated by:

$$V_{CO2}\ (\text{mL min}^{-1}) = 3 \times \text{body weight}$$

However, during anaesthesia, output is lowered by the effects of anaesthetic agent on metabolism. For example, during deep inhalation anaesthesia with sevoflurane or isoflurane, the output of CO_2 in a 70 kg patient will typically be around 150 mL min^{-1}.

Inhalational agents elimination

To lower the inhalational agent concentration rapidly, the vaporizer is set at zero and FGF is increased. Leaving a low FGF leads to a slow decrease in the agent's concentration as the vapour must leave the system through the APL valve, and during low-flow anaesthesia very little vapour is actually vented. The

Table 29.4 Tissue uptake of inhalational agents in first minute

	Halothane	Enflurane	Isoflurane	Sevoflurane	Desflurane
MAC (% v/v)	0.75	1.68	1.2	2.1	6.1
$\lambda_{B/G}$	2.3	1.8	1.4	0.65	0.42
Uptake in first minute (mL min^{-1})	69	121	67.2	54.6	120

MAC, minimum alveolar concentration; $\lambda_{B/G}$, the blood/gas solubility coefficient of the agent.

lower the solubility of the anaesthetic agent used, the more rapidly the concentration decreases.

Denitrogenation

- In closed circle anaesthesia, using oxygen and N_2O as the carrier gases, an initial period of high FGF is needed to denitrogenate the circle system and FRC. This is important to avoid the build-up of an unacceptable level of nitrogen in the system.
- A 70 kg adult has approximately 2500–3000 mL of nitrogen, of which 1300 mL is dissolved in the body (450 mL in the blood and 850 mL in the fat). The remaining 1200–1700 mL is contained in the FRC.
- With a high initial FGF of 10 L min^{-1}, more than 95% of nitrogen is usually washed out of the FRC and circle in approximately 5 minutes. Thereafter, nitrogen build-up occurs slowly owing to release by tissues.

CO_2 absorption

- CO_2 absorption is achieved by the use of soda lime (more common in UK) or Baralyme (more common in the USA).
- Soda lime consists of 94% calcium hydroxide, 2–5% sodium hydroxide, 0.2% silica (to prevent disintegration of the granules), an indicator dye and a zeolite, which is added to maintain a higher pH for longer. Older variants also contained 1% potassium hydroxide, which acted as a catalyst for the reaction.
- Soda lime is capable of absorbing 25 litres of CO_2 per 100 g. However, in practice, small canisters containing 500 g of soda lime appear exhausted with a CO_2 load of 10–12 litres 100 g^{-1} and jumbo absorbers containing 2 kg of soda lime appear exhausted with a CO_2 load of 17 litres 100 g^{-1}.
- Soda lime and its additives are made into granules to increase the surface area for absorption and to minimize resistance to gas flow. The granule size is measured in 'mesh'. The usual size is 4–8 mesh.
- Baralyme consists of 80% barium hydroxide and 20% barium octahydrate. It is less efficient than soda lime, but is more stable in dry environments, and produces less heat.
- The absorber granules are consumed more rapidly the lower the FGF used. This is because most of the exhaled gases pass through the absorber with very little being discarded through the APL valve.
- CO_2 absorption by soda lime or Baralyme is an exothermic reaction resulting in heat and water vapour formation. The humidity generated by the reaction makes the use of a heat and moisture exchanger unnecessary.
- Sevoflurane is partly degraded by soda lime forming a vinyl ether (compound A), which is nephrotoxic in rats. The amount produced is proportional to the sevoflurane concentration and the temperature of the absorber. The latter is higher with lower FGF. Sevoflurane use in humans is safe, although it is advisable that it should not be used with a FGF of less than 1.5 L min^{-1} for more than 3–4 hours.
- Anaesthetic agents with the CHF_2 side-chain (enflurane, isoflurane and desflurane) can react with soda lime or Baralyme to form carbon monoxide. This is only significant when the water content is less than 1.5% in soda lime or less than 5% in Baralyme. Carbon monoxide is produced when the absorber has been flushed with dry fresh gas for a considerable period of time without being attached to a patient before the agent is used (i.e. dry absorber). Humidity prevents its production.
- The CO_2 absorbent Amsorb does not contain a strong base (sodium or potassium hydroxide) and does not produce compound A or carbon monoxide when used with sevoflurane or desflurane.

Control of moisture

Prolonged use of the circle system results in significant condensation of water vapour. This can result in sticking of the one-way valves owing to surface tension, potentially turning the entire volume of the system into deadspace. This complication can be reduced by using a hydrophobic filter (i.e. heat and moisture exchanger) at the end of the expiratory limb before the CO_2 absorber, or by changing the breathing tubing between patients.

Monitoring

The following monitoring is recommended for the use of closed circle, ultra-low-flow and low-flow anaesthesia, owing to the possible variations between FGF composition and inspired and expired gas compositions:

- inspired and end-tidal oxygen
- inspired and end-tidal CO_2 ($ETco_2$).
- inspired and end-tidal N_2O
- inspired and end-tidal agent
- tidal volume
- standard monitoring.

Bibliography

Baum JA. *Low Flow Anaesthesia*, 2nd edn. Oxford: Butterworth-Heinemann, 2000.

Baum JA. Aitkenhead AR. Low flow anaesthesia. *Anaesthesia* 1995; **50**: 37–42.

Baxter AD. Low and minimal flow inhalation anaesthesia. *Can J Anaesth* 1995; **44**: 643–52.

Anaesthesia UK. *Circle System*, 2010. See www.frca.co.uk/article.aspx?articleid=100143.

Mapleson WW. The theoretical ideal fresh-gas flow sequence at the start of low-flow anaesthesia. *Anaesthesia* 1998; **53**: 264–72.

White DC. Closed and low flow system anaesthesia. *Curr Anaesth Critical Care* 1992; **3**: 98–107.

Cross-references

The anaesthetic machine, 680
Breathing systems, 683
Ventilators, 696

Epidural and spinal anaesthesia

Baha Al-Shaikh

Indications

- *Surgery*: axial blocks can be used alone for surgery below the level of T6 when it may be preferable if there is a risk of aspiration or difficult intubation. When compared with general anaesthesia, postoperative mortality and morbidity are reduced with increased mental alertness and responsiveness. The latter is of a particular importance in pregnant women.
- *Postoperative*: in addition to the superior analgesia, there is a significant reduction in the incidence of respiratory depression, pneumonia, deep vein thrombosis (DVT), pulmonary embolus and ileus leading to shorter hospital stay.
- *Pre-emptive analgesia*: this has been shown in animal studies but not in human surgery. However, it has been shown that its use can influence the development of chronic pain syndromes after surgery.
- *Modification of the perioperative stress response*: axial blockade reduces the hormonal and metabolic response to surgery. This may be of benefit in the management of high-risk surgical patients.

Contraindications

- Patient refusal.
- Coagulopathy or full therapeutic anticoagulation.
- Sepsis at site.
- Hypovolaemia.
- Anaphylaxis to drugs used.
- Fixed cardiac output.
- Raised intracranial pressure.

Differential blockade

Small-diameter fibres (sensory and autonomic) are more easily blocked than large motor fibres as local anaesthetic penetrates them more easily. Thus autonomic function, temperature and pain sensation are lost before loss of motor function. The concentration of local anaesthetic agent used similarly influences the type of block produced. Low concentrations produce analgesia with minimum motor blockade. High concentrations produce profound motor blockade in addition to analgesia. Sympathetic block is usually two levels above the sensory block, which in turn is two levels higher than the motor block.

Controversies

Epidural haematoma

- *Antiplatelets*: it is suggested that clopidogrel should be stopped 7–10 days before an epidural block and catheter insertion owing to the increased risk. The use of other antiplatelets such as aspirin and non-steroidal anti-inflammatory drugs (NSAIDs) does not appear to be associated with an increased risk of epidural haematoma formation.
- *Low-dose heparin and low-molecular-weight heparin (LMWH)*: in the absence of other risk factors, there is no evidence of an increased risk. The risk of a haematoma formation is 1:150 000 following an epidural block and 1:220 000 following a spinal block. To reduce risk, block should be sited at least 4 hours after low-dose heparin and 12 hours following LMWH. A similar guideline applies to removal of an epidural catheter.
- *Low platelet count*: although a count of less than 100×10^9 L^{-1} is generally regarded as a contraindication to an epidural, thromboelastography has been found to be normal with counts as low as 50×10^9 L^{-1}.
- *Temporary intraoperative anticoagulation*: this is safe as long as the anticoagulation is delayed an hour after siting the block and the epidural catheter is removed only after clotting has returned to normal.

Serious long-term neurological sequelae

This appears to be extremely rare. Possible causes include trauma, infection, chemical irritation, compression and ischaemia of the spinal cord.

Pre-existing neurological deficit

Although this is not a specific contraindication, a detailed history, clinical examination, documentation and counselling are essential.

Pre-existing systemic infection

There is an increased risk of meningitis and epidural abscess following an axial block. Risk may be reduced with prophylactic antibiotics.

Epidural and spinal opioids

Opioids provide analgesia by binding to receptors in the dorsal horn of the spinal cord. They lack sensory, motor or autonomic effects and have a synergistic effect when used with local anaesthetic. This allows the use of low-concentration local anaesthetic solutions with low opioid doses. Highly lipid-soluble drugs, such as fentanyl or sufentanil, may also have some systemic action. Opioids containing preservative are neurotoxic and should be avoided. Commonly used opioids include fentanyl, sufentanil, diamorphine, morphine and pethidine.

Side-effects

Side-effects may occur with any opioids or either route but tend to be more common following morphine and intrathecal administration. Naloxone is effective in the treatment.

- *Pruritus*: the most common side-effect, often minor but may be severe in 1% of patients. It is often localized to the head, face, neck or upper chest but can occasionally be generalized. Incidence is unrelated to dose. Pruritus is thought to result from interaction of opioid with opioid receptors in the trigeminal nucleus or nerve root.
- *Nausea and vomiting:* may result from interaction with opioid receptors in the area postrema. Incidence (30%) is higher in females and is similar with opioids given parenterally.
- *Urinary retention*: is not dose related and thought to result from binding with opioid receptors in the sacral spinal cord, inhibiting parasympathetic outflow with relaxation of detrusor muscle.
- *Respiratory depression*: the incidence of respiratory depression requiring intervention is 1% and is similar to that of parenteral opioids. It may present within minutes or after several hours. Early respiratory depression results from systemic absorption and is commonly associated with highly lipid-soluble drugs. Late respiratory depression results from cephalad migration and interaction with opioid receptors in the medullary centre and is more commonly associated with water-soluble drugs such as morphine. The risk is increased in the elderly, children, concomitant use of parenteral opioids or respiratory depressant drugs and pre-existing respiratory impairment.

Other reported rare side-effects include muscle rigidity, sexual dysfunction, reduced gastric emptying, hair loss, water retention and reactivation of herpes simplex labialis virus.

Epidural anaesthesia

Anatomy

- The epidural space lies between the dural sac and the periosteum lining the vertebral bodies, extending from the foramen magnum to the sacral hiatus.
- Anteriorly, it is bounded by the posterior longitudinal ligament; posteriorly, by the ligamentum flavum; and, laterally, by the vertebral pedicles and intervertebral foramina.
- It communicates freely with the paravertebral space via the intervertebral foramina.
- It contains nerve roots, venous plexuses, fat and lymphatics.

Technique

- Access can be gained through the ligamentum flavum via a median or paramedian approach with a loss of resistance technique using saline or air or through the sacrococcygeal membrane as a caudal block.
- Lumbar or thoracic regions are commonly used in adults while the caudal route is most common in children.
- Local anaesthetic solution injected into the epidural space acts on nerve roots or the spinal cord.
- As epidural local anaesthetic provides segmental analgesia, it should be sited at the level where anaesthesia is required. Epidural opioids act at spinal cord level so the site of insertion is less important.
- The incidence of dural tap is 1–3% depending on the experience of the operator and patient anatomy.

Advantages

- Level of block can be controlled with titrated doses of local anaesthetic and site of epidural cannulation.
- Greater cardiovascular stability owing to slow onset of block and the ability to titrate local anaesthetic via an epidural catheter.
- Block can be maintained and extended via an epidural catheter.

Disadvantages

- Slow onset.
- Use of large volume of local anaesthetic increases the risk of toxicity.
- Risk of catheter migration, knotting or fragmentation.
- Risk of dural puncture with postdural puncture headache.
- Subjective end-point may result in higher failure rate.

Spinal anaesthesia

Anatomy

- Cerebrospinal fluid is located within the subarachnoid space.
- The spinal cord ends at the lower border of L1 in adults and L3 in children. Lumbar puncture above these levels increases the risk of spinal cord damage and should therefore be avoided.

Technique

- A line joining the upper part of the iliac crests is at L4 or the L4–L5 interspace and serves as a useful landmark for lumbar puncture.
- Dural puncture may be done via a median or paramedian approach. The spinal needle passes through skin, subcutaneous tissue, supraspinous ligament, interspinous ligament, ligamentum flavum, epidural space, dura and into the subarachnoid space where cerebrospinal fluid (CSF) is obtained.
- Local anaesthetic solution injected mixes with the CSF and acts on nerve roots and dorsal root ganglia.
- The extent of the block obtained is mainly determined by the baricity of the local anaesthetic agent, position of the patient and the concentration and volume of local anaesthetic injected.
- Hyperbaric solutions such as heavy bupivacaine, which contains 8% glucose, have a higher specific gravity than the CSF and therefore tend to move downwards following injection. A small volume (1 mL) of hyperbaric solution injected in the sitting position and the patient left sitting for at least 5 minutes produces a 'saddle' block suitable for perineal operations. A unilateral block may similarly be produced with hyperbaric solution in the lateral position, but the block becomes bilateral when the patient is turned supine.
- Hypobaric solutions, such as plain L-bupivacaine, have a lower specific gravity than CSF and tend to rise following injection; therefore, they produce an unpredictable level of block.
- The density and duration of the block is influenced by the dose, while the height of the block is also influenced by the volume and the speed of injection. Large volumes of concentrated solutions produce motor blockade over a large area, whereas low doses block sensory and sympathetic fibres with preservation of motor function.

Advantages

- Clear end-point of technique, thus low failure rate.
- Rapid onset of block.
- Use of a small non-toxic dose of local anaesthetic.
- Rapid sacral block.
- Posture with heavy bupivacaine produces a reliable low haemodynamically stable block.
- Good muscle relaxation.

Disadvantages

- Difficulty in controlling height of block above T10.
- Greater haemodynamic instability resulting from higher denser block.
- Risk of postdural puncture headache.
- Single-shot technique limits the ability to extend anaesthesia or analgesia intraoperatively.

Postdural puncture headache

The incidence is increased in young patients, females, obstetric patients, the larger the size of the spinal needle and with the use of cutting (Quincke) rather than pencil-point (Whiteacre or Sprotte) needles. An incidence of 1% is reported with the use of 26 or 27G spinal needles, and of 15 and 75% with 20 and 16G needles, respectively.

Spinal catheters

They are introduced into the CSF through spinal needles, providing flexibility as anaesthesia can be extended with titrated boluses of local anaesthetic. Their use has been limited by a high incidence of postdural headache, risk of infection and reports of cauda equina syndrome following continuous spinal anaesthesia. The introduction of a 32G microcatheter may reduce the incidence of headache, although difficulty may be experienced on advancing the catheter.

Combined spinal–epidural anaesthesia

This offers greater flexibility, the spinal block providing rapid onset while the epidural catheter can be used to extend the block.

- *Single-space technique*: the epidural space is located with a Tuohy needle and a long spinal needle passed through it into the CSF. The spinal needle is withdrawn following injection and a catheter is passed into the epidural space. The risk of the epidural catheter migrating through the hole made in the dura into the CSF is low as very small gauge spinal needles (e.g. 26G) are used.
- *Double-space technique*: spinal injection is performed and an epidural catheter inserted in an intervertebral space above.

Bibliography

Barreiro G, van Zundert A, Al-Shaikh B Unexpected cardiac arrest in spinal anaesthesia. *Acta Anaesthesiol Belg* 2006: **57**: 365–70.

One-lung anaesthesia

R Kadayam Sreenivasan and Simon Stacey

One-lung anaesthesia involves deliberate and complete functional separation of the two lungs with specially designed endotracheal tubes. It provides special advantages for certain types of thoracic surgery but also causes significant physiological disturbances in pulmonary gas exchange.

Indications

Absolute

- To prevent contamination or spillage: pus, secretions or blood from the contralateral lung.
- To control the distribution of ventilation between the two lungs in the presence of, for example, a bronchopleural fistula, giant unilateral cyst/bulla, surgical opening of a major airway, tracheobronchial tree disruption.
- Unilateral bronchopulmonary lavage, e.g. for alveolar proteinosis.

Relative

- To facilitate surgical exposure, e.g. for pulmonary surgery (pneumonectomy, lobectomy or thoracoscopy) or non-pulmonary surgery (oesophageal surgery, descending thoracic aneurysm, thoracic spinal surgery). Many thoracic procedures can be accomplished with a normal tracheal tube.

Techniques of lung separation

- Double-lumen tube, e.g. Robertshaw (red rubber), Bronchocath (PVC). Allows rapid transition between one-lung ventilation and two-lung ventilation; either lung can be suctioned and continuous positive airway pressure (CPAP) can be applied to the non-ventilated lung.
- Bronchial blockers, e.g. Cook Arndt endobronchial blocker, Cohen Flexitip, Phycon blocker, Univent tube. Cannot ventilate or suction distal to the blocker.
- Uncut tracheal tube. This can be advanced into the relevant main bronchus. Not ideal, but useful in an emergency situation.
- Papworth BiVent tube. A new double-lumen endotracheal tube designed to enable rapid and reliable lung isolation using a bronchus blocker without endoscopic guidance. Allows suctioning of the collapsed lung through a central opening in the bronchial blocker but not ventilation.

Physiological effects of the lateral decubitus position

Awake, closed-chest, lateral decubitus position

Gravity causes a vertical gradient in the distribution of pulmonary blood flow with the dependent lung better perfused. The dome of the lower diaphragm is pushed higher into the chest and hence can contract more efficiently. Thus, the better perfused dependent lung is better ventilated regardless of the side on which the patient is lying.

Anaesthetized, closed-chest, lateral decubitus position

There is no difference in the distribution of pulmonary blood flow between the dependent and non-dependent lung when compared with an awake patient. But ventilation is now switched from the dependent to the non-dependent lung for a number of reasons. First, loss of FRC with induction of anaesthesia leads to the dependent lung moving to a less favourable portion and the non-dependent lung moves to a more favourable portion of the pressure–volume curve. Second, the high curved lower diaphragm no longer confers any advantage in ventilation. Third, weight of the mediastinum, abdominal contents and the chest wall all impede lower lung ventilation

Anaesthetized, open-chest, paralysed, lateral decubitus position

The dependent lung is less compliant, poorly ventilated and overperfused, whereas the non-dependent lung is overventilated and underperfused, resulting in a considerable degree of V/Q mismatch.

With the onset of one-lung ventilation the preferential distribution of ventilation to the upper lung is completely eliminated. Perfusion to this lung continues and this results in increased shunt. At this stage, the dependent lung receives the entire minute volume and a high proportion (about 60%) of the cardiac output.

Hypoxic pulmonary vasoconstriction increases the pulmonary vascular resistance of the collapsed lung.

However, its effects and the effects of anaesthetic agents on it are usually of little clinical importance in routine thoracic practice.

Preoperative assessment and investigations

- Full blood count; urea and electrolytes, e.g. ↓Na^+ with the syndrome of inappropriate antidiuretic hormone secretion (SIADH).
- Chest X-ray: it is important to assess the anatomy of the airways to see if endobronchial intubation is possible. Often a CT of the thorax is also available.
- Arterial blood gases.
- Pulmonary function tests and cardiopulmonary exercise testing.
- ECG.

Perioperative management

Monitoring

- ECG.
- S_aO_2.
- F_iO_2, $ETCO_2$, end-tidal for agent.
- Airway inflation pressure, flow–volume loops are also useful.
- Blood pressure: this should be measured ideally via arterial cannulation on the dependent side, which also allows for sampling for arterial blood gas analysis.
- Fluid balance and blood loss.
- Core temperature.
- Central venous pressure.
- Nerve stimulator to assess neuromuscular function.
- Central venous cannulation should ideally be performed on the same side as the thoracotomy in order to minimize the risk of pneumothorax to the dependent lung.

Anaesthetic technique

- Premedication is not mandatory and the type, if any, will largely depend on the patient and the mode of postoperative analgesia chosen.
- Give general anaesthesia (total intravenous anaesthesia (TIVA) or inhalational agent) with muscle relaxation and controlled ventilation, usually through a double-lumen tube.

Double-lumen tubes

Usually Robertshaw double-lumen endobronchial tubes are available in three sizes (small, medium and large). The PVC derivative (Bronchocath) is more malleable but more likely to migrate peroperatively and suffer cuff damage by teeth during insertion. They are available in a wide range of right and left sizes: Ch 41, 39, 37, 35 (32 and 28 are left only). Care must be taken not to overdistend the bronchial cuff since bronchial rupture may be catastrophic.

The right main bronchus gives rise to the right upper lobe bronchus after 2.5 cm. Right-sided endobronchial tube placement should be avoided when possible because of the high risk of right upper lobe occlusion.

The correct positioning of a double-lumen tube is traditionally confirmed by observation of chest expansion and auscultation while each lumen in turn is occluded. However, reliance on clinical signs alone will miss a significant number of malpositioned tubes. The National Confidential Enquiry into Perioperative Deaths (1998) highlighted the morbidity and mortality associated with malpositioned double-lumen tubes. The use of a flexible fibreoptic bronchoscope allows direct visual confirmation of tube position and is now the method of choice.

Arterial hypoxaemia

This is one of the most important problems encountered during one-lung anaesthesia. The elimination of CO_2 during one-lung ventilation is not a problem if the minute volume is maintained at the amount previously delivered to the two lungs. Two-lung anaesthesia should be maintained for as long as possible.

Management of hypoxaemia during one-lung ventilation

- Increase inspired oxygen up to 100%.
- Check position of double-lumen tube with fibreoptic bronchoscope. Suctioning of secretions may be required.
- Ensure adequate blood pressure and cardiac output.
- Positive end-expiratory pressure (PEEP) 5–10 cmH_2O to the dependent lung to decrease atelectasis and increase FRC. Excessive PEEP increases pulmonary vascular resistance and may increase shunt.
- CPAP 5–10 cmH_2O with 100% oxygen to the non-ventilated lung to facilitate oxygen uptake in this lung while not adversely affecting the surgical conditions.
- Abandon one-lung ventilation and intermittently ventilate the collapsed lung after warning the surgeon.
- Early clamping of the appropriate pulmonary artery will stop the shunt.

Postoperative period

Adequate pain relief, physiotherapy and high-dependency care are important factors for reducing the incidence of postoperative complications and hospital stay.

Bibliography

Eastwood J, Mahajan R. One-lung anaesthesia. *Br J Anaesth CEPD Rev* 2002; **2**: 83–7.

Ghosh S, Falter F, Goldsmith K, Arrowsmith JE. The Papworth BiVent tube: a new device for lung isolation. *Anaesthesia* 2008; **63**: 996–1000.

National Confidential Enquiry into Perioperative Deaths. *The Report of the National Confidential Enquiry into Perioperative Deaths 1996/1997.* London: NCEPOD, 1998, pp. 57–61.

Pennefather SH, Russell GN. Placement of double lumen tubes: time to shed light on an old problem (editorial). *Br J Anaesth* 2000; **84**: 308–11.

Vaughan RS. Double-lumen tubes (editorial). *Br J Anaesth* 1993; **70**: 497–8.

Wilson WC, Benumof JL. Anaesthesia for thoracic surgery. In: Miller RD (ed.) *Miller's Anesthesia*, 6th edn, vol. 2. Edinburgh: Elsevier, 2006, pp. 1847–939.

Cross-references

Complications of position, 743
Hypoxaemia under anaesthesia, 670
Thoracic surgery: overview, 408

Prolonged anaesthesia

Rajesh Pattanayak and Baha Al-Shaikh

Various problems are associated with prolonged anaesthesia. Adequate preparation, good management and close attention to detail may reduce the associated risks. Prolonged anaesthesia contributes to perioperative complications, which in turn may lead to delayed hospital discharge.

Problems associated with prolonged anaesthesia

- Accumulation of anaesthetic agents leading to delayed emergence. This depends on the drug's total tissue uptake, which is related to drug solubility and the average concentration used.
- Potential toxicity of administered agents:
  - Inhalational agents: degradation of inhalational agents by CO_2 absorber may lead to accumulation of toxins. Sevoflurane is partly degraded by soda lime forming a vinyl ether (compound A), which is nephrotoxic in rats. Although problems have not been noted in clinical practice, the United States Food and Drug Administration recommends the use of sevoflurane with FGF rates of at least 2 L min^{-1} for procedures lasting more than 1 hour.
  - Inorganic fluoride production due to the hepatic metabolism of sevoflurane and enflurane can be nephrotoxic in patients with chronic renal impairment.
  - Nitrous oxide: prolonged exposure to N_2O may result in acute vitamin B_{12} deficiency with megaloblastic anaemia and neurological deficit. N_2O oxidizes cobalamin, which inactivates methionine synthetase resulting in decreased methionine production. Toxic manifestations may occur in susceptible individuals after shorter exposures. Risk of nitrous oxide toxicity is increased in pernicious anaemia, exposure to DNA synthesis inhibitors (e.g. methotrexate), pre-existing bone marrow depression, folate deficiency, diseases of the ileum and malabsorption (e.g. Crohn disease).
  - N_2O also causes expansion of air spaces, e.g. pneumothorax.
- Impairment of gas exchange and respiratory mechanics, notably development of hypoxaemia and hypercarbia secondary to dependent atelectasis.
- The influence of anaesthetic agents on renal function can lead to water and salt retention. Disturbances in intermediary carbohydrate metabolism affected by anaesthetic agents aids in the development of metabolic acidosis.
- Although anaesthetic agents alter the physiology intraoperatively, their retention in the body can extend untoward effects into the postoperative period.
- Decreased carbohydrate metabolism also results in intraoperative hyperglycaemia.
- Problems with accurate management of fluid and electrolyte balance.
- Inadvertent perioperative hypothermia, defined as a core body temperature below 36°C, can lead to increased wound infection, surgical bleeding, impaired immune function and increased incidence of myocardial ischaemia and infarction, malignant arrhythmias and postoperative shivering.
- Prolonged immobility can lead to:
  - increased risk of DVT
  - nerve damage and pressure sores
  - bilateral compartment syndrome
  - rhabdomyolysis
  - corneal damage if eyes are left open.
- Postoperative delirium.
- Immunosuppression and increased susceptibility to infections.
- Increased opportunity for human error due to fatigue.

Preparation

- Manpower, patient supports and padding for pressure areas.
- Adequate scavenging: in the UK, recommended maximum accepted concentrations over an 8 hour time-weighted period are:
  - 100 parts per million (p.p.m.) for N_2O
  - 50 p.p.m. for enflurane and isoflurane
  - 10 p.p.m. for halothane.
- Low-flow circuit system.
- Maintenance of body temperature (appropriate selection of theatre temperature, forced air warmer, warming blanket, fluid warmers, humidification of inspired gases, clothing/limb wrapping, hat). Forced air warmers have been found to be the most effective, even when applied to a limited surface area of body.

Monitoring

- ECG.
- S_aO_2.
- Direct blood pressure.
- Core and skin temperature.
- Blood loss.
- Bispectral index analysis.
- Tracheal tube cuff pressure.
- Peripheral nerve stimulator.
- Blood gases (temperature corrected), electrolytes, glucose, coagulation.
- Pressure–volume loop and lung compliance.
- Inspiratory and expired concentration of oxygen, nitrous oxide, anaesthetic vapour and CO_2 concentration.
- Fluid balance (central venous pressure, hourly urine output via urinary catheter).
- Cardiac output.

Anaesthetic technique

The technique chosen is dependent on the surgery proposed, anticipated blood loss and the chronic health status of the patient. Controlled ventilation provides the ability to manipulate oxygenation and CO_2. There have been case reports of healthy patients having prolonged surgery on the extremities breathing spontaneously via a laryngeal mask for 8 hours with no adverse effect. Regional anaesthesia may be used as the sole anaesthetic technique for surgery on the lower extremities, but the prolonged immobilization often necessitates light general anaesthesia or sedation for patient comfort.

- Consider using oxygen/air technique, omitting nitrous oxide with minimum F_iO_2 to achieve an acceptable oxygen saturation or tension
- Consider TIVA/TCI.
- Give muscle relaxants by infusion (e.g. atracurium) with guidance from train-of-four.
- Use high-volume/low-pressure cuff with regular tracheal tube suctioning.
- Pay careful attention to body positioning with frequent repositioning of the head.
- Cover exposed body surfaces.
- Eye protection (lubrication, tapes, padding or eye shields).
- DVT prophylaxis (thromboembolism deterrent stockings/heparin/mechanical calf compression).
- Use a team of staff to avoid fatigue.

Postoperative care

Consider:

- ICU/high-dependency unit stay for continued ventilation until warm and stable; awaken slowly
- regular physiotherapy
- maintenance of DVT prophylaxis
- ensure adequate fluid input and output.

Bibliography

Brimacombe J, Shorney N. The laryngeal mask airway and prolonged balanced regional anaesthesia. *Can J Anaesth* 1993; **40**: 360–4.

Dodds C. Prolonged anaesthesia for plastic and reconstructive surgery. *Curr Anaesth Crit Care* 1996; **7**: 20–4.

Girgis Y, Broome IJ. Monitoring failure and awareness hazard during prolonged surgery. *Anaesthesia* 1997; **52**: 504–5.

Higuchi H, Sumikura H, Sumita S, *et al.* Renal function in patients with high serum fluoride concentration after prolonged sevoflurane anesthesia. *Anesthesiology* 1995; **83**: 449–58.

Cross-references

Monitoring, 690

Water and electrolyte disturbances, 633

Regional anaesthesia techniques

Baha Al-Shaikh

The use of regional anaesthesia is spreading with improved understanding of pain physiology, better technical skills, the development of new devices, such as new and better needles and catheters, more reliable nerve stimulators, stimulating catheters, sophisticated infusion pumps, percutaneous electrode guidance, and the widespread development of ultrasound nerve localization. Regional anaesthetic techniques are used to block nerve(s)/plexuses. Spinal/epidural blocks are discussed under Epidural and spinal anaesthesia, p. 707.

Indications

- As the sole anaesthetic technique.
- With sedation or general anaesthesia.
- To provide analgesia (e.g. postoperative, following fractures, etc.).

Absolute contraindications

- Patient refusal.
- Infections at the site of needle insertion.
- Allergy to local anaesthetics (rare with the amides; common with the esters).

Relative contraindications

- Coagulopathy.
- Pre-existent unstable neurological deficit.
- Lack of patient cooperation.

Preoperative preparations

- Full patient assessment with informed consent.
- Resuscitation facilities must be available owing to the risk of local anaesthetic toxicity.
- The patient is starved, consented and prepared for general anaesthesia conversion in the event of failure of the local anaesthetic technique.
- Intravenous access is established and monitoring is connected.
- If combined with general anaesthesia, the block can be done either before or after the induction. However, if possible, it may be advisable to do the block before induction to reduce the risk of undetected direct trauma to the nerve tissues.
- Accurate positioning of the patient.
- A sterile technique is used.
- Sound knowledge of the potential side-effects of the blocks is essential, e.g. interscalene blocks have an almost 100% incidence of phrenic nerve palsy on the affected side. Thus, bilateral interscalene blocks are contraindicated.

Nerve block needles

- Short bevelled blunt needles with a side port for injecting the local anaesthetic solution are used. The bluntness gives a better feedback feel as the needle passes through the different layers of tissues and minimizes the potential trauma to the nerve tissues.
- Teflon-coated insulated needles with an exposed tip are used. The electric current passes through to the tip, allowing easier identification of the nerve(s)/plexus.
- 22G size needles are optimal for the vast majority of blocks. The lengths can vary (e.g. 50, 100 and 150 mm) depending on the depth of the nerve/plexus.
- The immobile needle technique is used when large volumes of local anaesthetic solutions are injected. One operator maintains the needle in position, while the second operator, after aspiration, injects the local anaesthetic solution through the side port. This reduces the possibility of accidental misplacement and intravascular injection.

Nerve stimulators

Linear and constant-output battery-operated stimulators designed to produce visible muscular contractions at a predetermined current and voltage once a nerve/plexus has been located. Their use can increase the success rate of nerve blocks.

- The stimulator has two leads: one is connected to an ECG skin electrode and the other to the locating needle. The polarities of the leads are clearly indicated and colour coded with the negative lead being attached to the needle. Less current is needed if the needle is connected to the negative lead.
- A small current is used to stimulate the nerve fibres, causing the motor fibres to contract with a frequency of 1–2 Hz. The stimulus has a short duration (1–2 ms) to generate painless motor

contraction. The low currents used stimulate the larger Aα motor fibres more than C pain fibres.

- An initial high current (e.g. 2–3 mA) is used until nerve stimulation is noticed. Then the current is reduced until a maximal stimulation is obtained with minimal output (e.g. 0.5 mA), indicating that the tip of the needle is very close to the nerve.
- The stimulation is markedly reduced after a small volume (about 2 mL) of local anaesthetic solution is injected. This is due to displacement of the nerve from the needle tip.
- Using the nerve stimulator is not an excuse for not having a sound knowledge of the anatomy required to perform a block.

Nerve mapping pens

- Nerve mapping is transcutaneous nerve stimulation to locate superficial nerves to a maximum depth of approximately 3 cm.
- Can be used to help to identify the best site for needle puncture especially if anatomical conditions and landmarks are difficult to identify.
- Pen-shaped atraumatic electrodes are used with a conductive tip giving 1 ms duration stimuli. Different kinds of sensation (tingling, pin-prick or a slight burning sensation) due to the stimulation of various sensory cells in the skin can be caused.

Stimulating catheters

- These function in principle like insulated needles but can be inserted to provide a continuous block.
- The catheter is made from insulating plastic material with a metallic wire inside, which conducts the current to its exposed tip electrode.
- Usually, a nerve block needle is placed close to the nerve then the stimulating catheter is introduced through it and the nerve stimulator is connected to the catheter. Stimulation through the catheter should reconfirm the catheter tip position in close proximity to the target nerve(s). The threshold currents needed with stimulating catheters may be considerably higher.

Ultrasound

- Ultrasound – longitudinal high-frequency waves – travels through a medium by causing local displacement of particles so causing changes in pressures with no overall movement of the medium.
- Recently, electrical peripheral nerve stimulators have been used under ultrasound guidance (dual guidance technique). Ultrasound provides additional information through visual feedback, which may make peripheral nerve block procedures safer and even more reliable. Ultrasound is created by converting electrical energy into mechanical vibration utilizing the piezoelectric (PE) effect. The PE materials vibrate when a varying voltage is applied.
- The basic components of an ultrasound machine are the pulser (transmitter), transducer, receiver, display and memory. An image is generated when the pulse wave emitted from the transducer is transmitted into the body, reflected off the tissue interface and returned to the transducer. Returning ultrasound waves cause PE crystals within the transducer to vibrate, generating a voltage. Therefore, the same crystals can be used to send and receive sound waves.
- Transducer probes have many shapes and sizes that determine their field of view. The frequency of emitted sound waves determines how deep the sound waves penetrate and the resolution of the image. The linear probes are most often used for the majority of peripheral blocks. The curved arrays are used for deep nerve structures (lower frequency is required). Smaller footprint probes are useful for children and for certain uses such as very superficial blocks (e.g. ankle blocks).
- It is important to remember that the use of ultrasound does not eliminate the risk of intraneural injection.

Local anaesthetic drugs

The choice of local anaesthetic drugs depends on:

- speed of onset
- potency
- duration of action
- sensory–motor differentiation
- potential toxicity.

Lidocaine, prilocaine, ropivacaine, bupivacaine, L-bupivacaine and etidocaine are some of the amide local anaesthetics that are currently available (Table 29.6).

- Lidocaine and bupivacaine have been used extensively in various regional blocks.
- Prilocaine is the agent of choice for intravenous regional anaesthesia. Its metabolite, *o*-toluidine, may cause methaemoglobinaemia, appearing as cyanosis, when 1.5 g 100 mL^{-1} of haemoglobin is in the reduced state. This is rapidly reversed with the intravenous injection of 1 mg kg^{-1} of methylthioninium (methylene blue).
- L-bupivacaine is a single *S*(−)-isomer of bupivacaine with a similar clinical profile but less systemic toxicity.

Table 29.6 Local anaesthetic drugs

Local anaesthetic	Onset	Duration	Relative potency	Toxicity
Lidocaine	Fast	++	++	++
Prilocaine	Fast	++	++	+
Bupivacaine	Moderate	+++	++++	+++
L-Bupivacaine	Moderate	+++	++++	++
Ropivacaine	Moderate	+++	++++	++
Etidocaine	Fast	++++	+++	+++

- Ropivacaine has a better sensory–motor differentiation than bupivacaine, mainly affecting the sensory fibres. This makes it ideal for postoperative analgesia.
- Etidocaine has a rapid onset and very prolonged duration of action. The motor fibres are mainly affected.

Vasoconstrictors

These are added to the local anaesthetic solution. They cause vasoconstriction at the site of injection and slow the rate of absorption, thus prolonging the duration of action and reducing systemic toxicity. Vasoconstrictors are absolutely contraindicated in blocks near end-arteries, such as ring blocks and penile blocks, and intravenous regional anaesthesia due to the risk of ischaemia.

- Epinephrine 1:200 000 concentration is used. This low concentration is to reduce the systemic side-effects of epinephrine, which are particularly undesirable in patients with cardiovascular disease. If given intravenously, 15 µg (3 mL of 1:200 000) of epinephrine will increase the heart rate by at least 30% within 1 minute; 1:200 000 epinephrine is useful in combination with lidocaine, reducing the peak concentration in the blood and causing a 50% decrease in the peak plasma concentration when used for subcutaneous infiltration, but a 20–30% decrease when used for intercostal or brachial plexus blocks. Epinephrine decreases the blood concentration of bupivacaine significantly less than that of lidocaine, so that it is not usually worth using bupivacaine with epinephrine.
- Felypressin is a vasoconstrictor with fewer systemic side-effects than epinephrine. It is mainly used in dental and ENT surgery.

Bibliography

Al-Shaikh B, Stacey S. *Essentials of Anaesthetic Equipment*, 3rd edn. Edinburgh: Elsevier Churchill Livingstone, 2007.

Fredrickson MJ, Ball CM, Dalgleish AJ. Prospective randomized comparison of ultrasound guidance versus neurostimulation for interscalene catheter placement. *Reg Anesth Pain Med* 2009; **34**: 590–4.

Sites BD, Neal JM, Chan V. Ultrasound in regional anesthesia: where should the 'focus' be set? *Reg Anesth Pain Med* 2009; **34**: 531–3.

Urmey WF, Grossi P. Percutaneous electrode guidance: a noninvasive technique for prelocation of peripheral nerves to facilitate peripheral plexus or nerve block. *Reg Anesth Pain Med* 2002; **27**: 261–7.

Cross-reference

Local anaesthetic toxicity, 767

Total intravenous anaesthesia

Mark Snazelle and Baha Al-Shaikh

Total intravenous anaesthesia (TIVA) is a technique in which general anaesthesia is induced and maintained using one (or more) drugs administered intravenously. A continuous intravenous infusion is used most commonly in the form of a TCI pump. Inhalational anaesthetic agents are not required.

Characteristics of the ideal agent

- Rapid onset (mainly un-ionized at physiological pH).
- High lipid solubility.
- Rapid metabolism and elimination, through different pathways to ameliorate accumulation of drug or metabolites.
- Analgesic properties at subanaesthetic concentrations.
- No adverse effects on major organ systems.
- No emetic effects.
- No pain on injection and not irritant if injected extravascularly.
- Safe following inadvertent intra-arterial injection.
- No epileptiform movements, excitation or emergence phenomena.
- No interaction with other anaesthetic drugs.
- No toxic effects.
- No histamine release or hypersensitivity reactions.
- Water-soluble formulation.
- Stable for the duration of the infusion with no deterioration on exposure to light.
- Long shelf-life.
- No absorption into plastic.

Both hypnosis and analgesia can be achieved using an intravenous technique. At the present time, propofol is the hypnotic of choice for TIVA. Analgesia can be achieved using the newer short-acting opioids, such as alfentanil and remifentanil. More recently, TCI has been widely used, although TIVA can also be achieved using intermittent bolus injection or manual infusion techniques.

TIVA must achieve the following goals: smooth induction, reliable and titratable maintenance and rapid emergence. Achieving these has been possible with TCI.

Propofol

Propofol is highly lipid soluble and is available as either a 1 or 2% lipid–water emulsion (with soya bean oil and egg phosphatide), as its water solubility is low. It is cleared from the body mainly by hepatic metabolism. It has, however, been successfully used in patients with liver cirrhosis, and the pharmacokinetics are not significantly affected.

The pharmacokinetics of propofol may be influenced by age. Values for clearance and plasma concentration on awakening are higher in children than in adults. Children require significantly higher doses of propofol than do adults. The rapid recovery from propofol is owing to its short distribution phase, high clearance rate and short elimination half-life.

Dose–response relationship

In order to compare TIVA with inhalational anaesthesia, $CP50_m$ has been used. This is the plasma concentration required to prevent 50% of patients from responding to painful stimuli – similar to MAC. It is important to note, however, that, at present, no method for measuring propofol concentration directly in the plasma is commercially available and so $CP50_m$ values are based on calculated data only. As there is considerable variation in the uptake and effect of propofol between individual patients, it has been proposed by many that depth of anaesthesia monitoring (such as bispectral index analysis) be used during TIVA on paralysed patients.

Target-controlled infusion

As there is no 'patient-end' measurement available for intravenous agents comparable to end-tidal monitoring of volatile agents, sophisticated TCI syringe drivers are used. These incorporate real-time pharmacokinetic models that deliver the appropriate dose of the drug to achieve and maintain the requested target concentration. For this to be achieved, the appropriate infusion rates needed to produce the required target concentration are continuously calculated by the microprocessor within the syringe driver.

Anaesthesia is induced by the syringe driver infusing propofol rapidly, giving a bolus calculated to achieve the required plasma concentration. This is followed by a progressively decreasing infusion rate calculated to match the transfer of drug in and out of the peripheral compartments (and therefore maintain the required plasma concentration).

To increase the target plasma concentration further, the syringe driver delivers another bolus to achieve the desired concentration and then maintains this higher concentration with a higher infusion rate. To decrease the target plasma concentration, the syringe driver stops infusing until the microprocessor calculates that the new target has been achieved. The new, lower level is then maintained.

The predicted concentration in the brain, which is displayed as the effect site concentration, increases slower than that of the plasma (plasma site concentration). Modern TCI pumps, such as the Asena PK or Frenenius Base Primea, now have software allowing titration to a choice of either plasma site or effect site concentrations, depending on the mathematical pharmacological model used.

The Marsh model (used in pumps such as the Diprifusor) requires age to be input into the pump but does not incorporate it into its calculations. The Schnider model has been developed more recently, and requires age, height and body weight to be input so the pump can calculate lean body mass, and calculate dosages accordingly. The Schnider model allows for effect site concentration to be targeted specifically, whereas the Marsh model was designed primarily for targeting plasma site concentration (although effect site concentration is also calculated).

Propofol TCI allows easy control and rapid change of the target propofol concentration. In adult patients under the age of 55 years, a target propofol concentration of 4–8 μg mL^{-1} is usually adequate for the induction of anaesthesia. Induction is smooth and usually takes 60–120 seconds. When coadministering an analgesic, anaesthesia can be maintained using propofol concentrations of approximately 3–6 μg mL^{-1}. Lower target concentrations are used in elderly patients, reducing the risks of side-effects. Owing to the differing pharmacokinetic profile in children, propofol TCI has not been used extensively in the paediatric population. Considerable interest in potential pharmacokinetic modelling in this field does currently exist, however.

Manual infusion and manual intermittent bolus techniques

Manual infusion can be achieved by a bolus dose for induction using a syringe driver with a rapid bolus facility. Anaesthesia is maintained using a step-down sequence of infusion rates. Before the advent of TCI, a popular method was to administer a 1 mg kg^{-1} propofol bolus followed by 10 mg kg^{-1} h^{-1} for 10 minutes, 8 mg kg^{-1} h^{-1} for 10 minutes, and 6 mg kg^{-1} h^{-1} thereafter – the Bristol model. This model was originally described, however, to include premedication with fentanyl and coadministration of nitrous oxide. A manual intermittent bolus technique has also been used but leads to wide variations and fluctuations in the plasma concentrations and the anaesthetic effects. The majority of anaesthetists now prefer to use a TCI system because of their simplicity and reliability.

Analgesia

Since propofol has no analgesic properties, TIVA is generally achieved by combining a propofol infusion with a regional local anaesthetic block or supplemental opioids. The shorter acting opioids are often suggested as an ideal complement to propofol. Of these, alfentanil and remifentanil are widely used.

When propofol and alfentanil are administered together, alfentanil can increase the concentration of propofol by up to 20% because of its effect on clearance and redistribution. Alfentanil concentration can be increased by propofol, possibly because of the inhibition of oxidative phosphorylation of alfentanil via cytochrome P450. Similar interaction can happen with other opioids.

Remifentanil

Remifentanil (a fentanyl derivative and pure μ agonist) has a unique metabolic and pharmacokinetic profile. It undergoes rapid methyl esterase hydrolysis by tissue and plasma esterases to relatively inactive metabolites. Its effect is terminated by rapid metabolic clearance (elimination half time is 3–10 minutes) rather than redistribution, unlike fentanyl and alfentanil, resulting in rapid reduction in plasma concentration even after prolonged infusion. It does not accumulate in either hepatic or renal failure.

The time required for the drug concentration to fall by 50% (context-sensitive half-time) is always the same at about 3 minutes, leading it to be described as context *insensitive*. This is independent of age, weight, sex, or hepatic and renal function, making it ideal for a continuous intravenous technique.

Remifentanil can be given via TCI using the Minto pharmacokinetic model. This is easy to use and allows easy titration based on the patient's age, weight and height. Remifentanil has become the opioid of choice in TIVA for many anaesthetists, certainly in longer or more stimulating procedures. Care must be taken, however, to ensure adequate analgesia after remifentanil has worn off. This can be ensured either by local/regional techniques or by judicious administration of an alternative opioid toward the end of the case.

Uses of TIVA

TIVA has been used successfully in a wide range of surgical procedures, including cardiac and intracranial ones (propofol increases cerebral compliance). TIVA is potentially useful when inhalational anaesthesia is difficult or contraindicated, e.g. rigid bronchoscopy, malignant hyperpyrexia susceptibility. TCI has also been successfully used for sedation in a variety of procedures.

Advantages of TIVA

- Avoiding the use of nitrous oxide with its potential effects on air emboli, pneumothoraces and bone marrow suppression.
- Elimination of volatile agents and their possible toxicity to the liver and kidney and their effect on the uterus, as well as possible environmental effects.
- Elimination of the need for accurately calibrated vaporizers.
- Superior quality recovery with less hangover.
- Propofol is a powerful antiemetic.

Disadvantages

- Pharmacokinetic and pharmacodynamic variability of response to the injected drug.
- Lack of ability to accurately assess actual blood levels.
- Variations in the haemodynamic state of the patient.
- Requirement for dedicated intravenous access, and risk of disconnection.

Bibliography

Campbell L, Engbers FH, Kenny GNC. Total intravenous anaesthesia. *CPD Anaesth* 2001; **3**: 109–19.

Peck TE, Hill SA. *Pharmacology for Anaesthesia and Intensive Care*, 3rd edn. Cambridge: Cambridge University Press, 2008, Section 1, pp. 81–4, and Section 2, pp. 102–3.

Petrie J, Glass P. Intravenous anaesthetics. *Curr Opin Anaesthesiol* 2001; **14**: 393–7.

Sivasubramaniam S. *Target Controlled Infusions in Anaesthetic Practice*. World Anaesthesia Archive, 2007. See www.frca.co.uk

Cross-references

Awareness, 733

Malignant hyperpyrexia: clinical presentation, 770

30 Management problems

Brian J Pollard

- Total spinal anaesthesia — *Brian J Pollard*
- Transport of the critically ill — *Brian J Pollard*
- Trauma — *Brian J Pollard*
- Transurethral resection of the prostate syndrome — *Brian J Pollard*

Allergic reactions

Brian J Pollard

Allergic reactions are unpredictable and may be potentially life-threatening. Prompt recognition and treatment are essential. The incidence of anaphylactic reactions is between 1:10 000 and 1:20 000 anaesthetics. The estimated mortality is 5–10%.

When associated with anaesthesia, the causative agents are commonly:

- neuromuscular blockers, especially succinylcholine (50–70%)
- latex (notably risen in recent years) (>10%)
- antibiotics
- induction agents
- colloids
- opioids
- radiocontrast media.

Pathophysiology

Anaphylactic and anaphylactoid reactions are clinically indistinguishable (Fig. 30.1). The terms refer to the triggering pathway responsible for the final common end-point, i.e. the release of potent circulating inflammatory mediators from degranulated mast cells.

Anaphylactic reactions involve cross-linking of two adjacent IgE antigen-specific antibodies to the mast-cell surface causing a type I hypersensitivity reaction.

Reactions caused by any other triggering pathways are, therefore, anaphylactoid. The majority of the reactions caused by anaesthetic drug mixtures are anaphylactoid, causing 'aggregate anaphylaxis'.

In many cases, previous sensitization to the antigen or similar compound cannot be demonstrated.

Significant clinical features

When associated with anaesthesia, symptoms often occur rapidly but may not manifest until after 30 minutes in the case of anaphylaxis to latex.

- Profound hypotension or cardiac arrest may be seen in over 80% of cases.
- Hypoxia may be present due to:
  - inability to ventilate
  - bronchospasm
  - laryngeal oedema.
- Urticarial or erythematous rashes feature more prominently in the out-of-hospital setting.

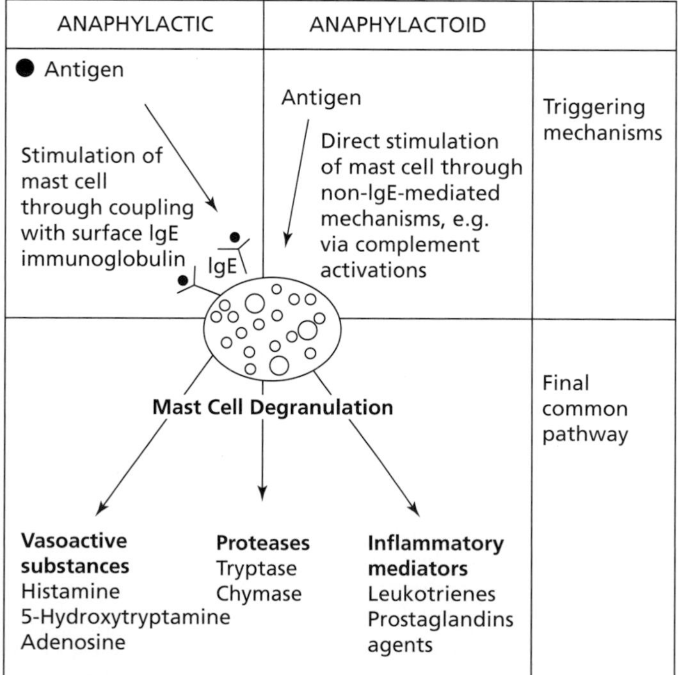

Figure 30.1 Immune mechanisms of anaphylactic and anaphylactoid reactions. The 'antigen' refers to the drug or substance responsible for activating the triggering mechanism. In some cases, for example penicillin, binding to a hapten (carrier protein) is necessary prior to coupling with surface membrane IgE antibody.

Primary treatment (from AAGBI guidelines)

- Discontinue administration of suspected agent.
- Assess and maintain airway, check breathing, check circulation (ABC guidelines).
- Give 100% oxygen.
- Call for help.
- Elevate legs to increase venous return.
- If necessary begin cardiopulmonary resuscitation.
- Give epinephrine:
  - intravenously 0.5 mL of 1:10 000, repeat as necessary
  - or intramuscularly 1 mL of 1:1000 (1 mg) repeat as necessary.
- Start intravenous fluid resuscitation with colloid or crystalloid.

Secondary treatment

- Chlorpheniramine 10 mg intravenously.
- Hydrocortisone 200 mg intravenously.
- Epinephrine infusion (0.05–0.1 μg kg^{-1} min^{-1}), i.e. 10–20 mL h^{-1} of 1 mg in 50 mL solution for a 70 kg man.
- Consider sodium bicarbonate
- Consider bronchodilators (aminophylline, salbutamol).
- Airway evaluation (before extubation).
- Arrange transfer to a critical care area if necessary.

Further investigation

- Investigations should not be undertaken at the expense of resuscitation.
- A detailed written record of events is important in establishing the diagnosis.
- As soon as possible, take 10 mL venous blood and store at −20°C.
- Repeat blood sample 1–2 hours later.
- Repeat blood sample after 24 hours.
- Released mast cell tryptase indicates a reaction has taken place: elevated up to 6 hours after cell degranulation in 70% of cases.
- The anaesthetist is responsible for providing advice for the patient and for ensuring appropriate follow-up takes place.
- Seek advice from a specialist in allergy and clinical immunology as further investigation is required.
- See useful addresses for the Committee on Safety of Medicines (CSM), Medic-Alert and British Society of Allergy and Clinical Immunology websites.
- Commonly skin prick tests are performed with a range of drugs at concentrations of 1 in 10–1000 several weeks after the acute episode and after discontinuation of antihistamines (false negatives occur).
- Radioallergosorbent tests are available for succinylcholine, latex and penicillins. A morphine-based solid immunoassay has been developed to act as a highly sensitive generic marker for non-depolarizing muscle relaxant allergy. As yet, screening is not advised by the Association of Anaesthetists of Great Britain and Ireland (AAGBI).

Latex allergy

There has been an increasing incidence of latex allergy over the last 20 years, especially in certain population groups with previous repeated exposure to latex. This is particularly prevalent in patients with a history of numerous surgical procedures; for example, in patients with spina bifida, the incidence may be in excess of 60%, mainly because of the repeated urethral catheterizations required. The incidence in healthcare workers is about 10%, and in the general population about 0.7%.

Other important associations:

- reactivity to party balloons, barrier contraceptives, dentists' gloves
- cross-reactivity to certain foods (banana, kiwi, chestnut, avocado)
- positive investigation (serological tests, skin prick, intradermal testing).

Sensitivity to latex may vary from contact dermatitis to anaphylaxis. Anaphylaxis may occur via any route, but is more likely after intravenous or direct mucosal exposure.

Management of the patient with latex allergy

- Providing a latex-free environment is the most important management strategy.
- Preoperative immunological testing may be helpful in selected cases, but false negatives occur.
- Consider premedication with chlorpheniramine, ranitidine, hydrocortisone.
- Put the patient first on the morning operating list to minimize exposure to airborne antigens.
- Communicate risks to other anaesthetic, nursing and surgical staff.
- Check ALL equipment is latex free, especially gloves (all staff), face-masks, reservoir bag, syringes and drip injection ports.
- Departments should have a management protocol and a designated box of latex-free equipment available.
- Monitor postoperatively for delayed reactions for up to 1 hour.
- Vigilance and full resuscitation resources are essential.

Bibliography

Association of Anaesthetists of Great Britain and Ireland and British Society of Allergy and Clinical Immunology. *Suspected Anaphylactic Reactions Associated with Anaesthesia.* London: AAGBI, 2009.

Clarke RSJ, Watkins J. Drugs responsible for anaphylactic reactions in anaesthesia in the United Kingdom. *Ann Fr Anesth Reanim* 1993; **12**: 105–8.

Dakin MJ, Yentis SM. Latex allergy: a strategy for management. *Anaesthesia* 1998; **53**: 774–81.

Farley CA, Jones HM. Latex allergy. *Br J Anaesth CEPD Rev* 2002; **2**(1).

Fisher M. Anaphylaxis to anaesthetic drugs: aetiology, recognition and management. *Curr Anaesth Crit Care* 1991; **2**: 182–6.

Lieberman P. Anaphylactic reactions during surgical and medical procedures. *J Allergy Clin Immunol* 2002; **110**: S64–9.

Poley GE Jr, Slater JE. Latex allergy. *J Allergy Clin Immunol* 2000; **105**: 1054–62.

Useful websites

Association of Anaesthetists. See aagbi.org/publications/guidelines.htm

British Society of Allergy and Clinical Immunology. See www.bsaci.org

Committee on Safety of Medicines (CSM). Yellow card reporting scheme. See www.mhra.gov.uk

Medic-Alert Foundation. See www.medicalert.org.uk

Cross-references

Cardiopulmonary resuscitation, 738
Intraoperative bronchospasm, 762

Amniotic fluid embolism

Brian J Pollard

Amniotic fluid embolism (AFE) is the syndrome that occurs when amniotic fluid gains entry into the maternal circulation. It may be the composition of the amniotic fluid that determines the severity of the pathological events constituting the syndrome. The syndrome has similarities to anaphylaxis and septic shock and the same mediators may be involved. Interestingly, in primate models, clear autologous amniotic fluid produced no clinical effect when injected into the maternal circulation.

AFE has an incidence of about 1:50 000 pregnancies. Approximately 20% of women who develop AFE do not survive. AFE occurs most commonly during labour, but has been associated with the list of events shown in Box 30.1.

Box 30.1 Aetiological factors in amniotic fluid embolism

- Dilatation and curettage
- Termination of pregnancy
- Intra-amniotic saline infusion
- Amniocentesis
- Amniotomy
- Induction of labour
- Insertion of prostaglandin gel
- Lower uterine segment, cervical and vaginal tears
- Caesarean section
- Uterine rupture

Morgan, in his 1979 review of AFE, effectively refuted the association between AFE and tumultuous labour, oxytocin augmentation of labour, traumatic delivery, large babies and fetal death preceding AFE. Recently, it has been suggested that amniotic fluid containing meconium and the presence of a male fetus influence the severity of the response to AFE.

Clinical presentation

The three main maternal features of AFE are:

1 cardiorespiratory problems
2 convulsions
3 haematological problems.

These may be accompanied by fetal distress.

Cardiorespiratory problems

The classical presentation is at or around delivery, with the symptoms and signs of severe cardiorespiratory collapse (Box 30.2). From case reports in which patients have survived long enough to have a pulmonary flotation catheter inserted, the picture has been one of left ventricular heart failure with elevated left ventricular end-diastolic pressure and elevated pulmonary capillary wedge pressure. These measurements validate the clinical and radiographic picture of pulmonary oedema, which occurs in many of the 50–75% of patients who survive the initial cardiopulmonary collapse. Whether, as previously thought, severe intrapulmonary shunting, pulmonary hypertension and right heart failure precede, or even precipitate, the documented left heart failure is unproven. There is evidence of release of a potent vasoconstrictor in AFE that may be responsible for pulmonary, coronary and even systemic vasoconstriction. It has been suggested that endothelin may be the vasoconstrictor.

Box 30.2 Cardiorespiratory symptoms and signs

- Dyspnoea
- Hypoxia
- Hypotension
- Convulsions
- Bronchospasm
- Arrhythmias
- Cardiac arrest
- Fetal bradycardia

Convulsions

Convulsions due to cerebral hypoxaemia or hypotension may delay the diagnosis of AFE by confusion with eclampsia.

Haematological problems

Coagulopathy accompanying cardiorespiratory collapse, following cardiorespiratory collapse or occurring without cardiorespiratory symptoms or signs is the other main feature of AFE. The coagulopathy may be obvious as severe vaginal haemorrhage or as severe haemorrhage during caesarean section and may be compounded by uterine atony. Activation of the extrinsic pathway of the clotting cascade by fetal antigens or trophoblastic tissue exerting a thromboplastin-like effect may possibly be the trigger. Occasionally, AFE has to be included in the differential diagnosis when abnormal bleeding occurs from wounds or intravenous access sites without preceding evidence of AFE. In 40% of cases of AFE there is evidence of coagulopathy, and this should be anticipated if the diagnosis of AFE has been made.

Treatment

Cardiac arrest

Commence cardiac arrest algorithm with lateral tilt where appropriate.

Hypoxia or hypotension without cardiac arrest

- Avoid aortocaval compression by lateral tilt when appropriate.
- Administer 100% oxygen; when appropriate intubate and ventilate.
- Site a large-bore cannula. If the patient is hypotensive, give colloid rapidly and inotropes (dopamine) and/or vasoconstrictors (phenylephrine) as indicated depending on availability.
- Full monitoring including, if possible, an arterial line.
- Site a central venous pressure (CVP) cannula or a pulmonary flotation catheter if available.
- Manipulate fluids and cardiovascular drugs according to haemodynamic measurements, including diuretics if there is evidence of pulmonary oedema; an oesophageal Doppler probe may be useful.
- Deliver the fetus if still *in utero*. Although a 79% fetal survival has been reported, survival of a neurologically intact infant is around 39%.
- Transfer to the ITU.

Coagulopathy

- Take blood for a full coagulation screen, including platelets.
- Inform the haematology laboratory of the problem.
- Give fresh-frozen plasma (FFP), platelets, cryoprecipitate and concentrated red cells, depending on clotting results and blood loss. Haematological advice should be sought before the use of serine protease inhibitors or heparin.
- Give oxytocics if uterine atony is present, syntocinon intravenously, ergometrine intravenously, or prostaglandin $E_1\alpha$ by intramuscular or intrauterine injection.

Other reported treatments

- Cardiopulmonary bypass and pulmonary thrombectomy may be required.
- Nitric oxide and inhaled aerosol prostacyclin may be needed to treat refractory hypoxaemia.
- Extracorporeal membrane oxygenation and intra-aortic balloon counterpulsation may be needed.

Confirmation of diagnosis

Antemortem laboratory diagnosis of AFE

In 1947, Gross and Benz reported that centrifuged blood obtained from the right heart of patients with AFE showed three strata rather than two, and that this was pathognomonic of AFE. They also advocated looking at sections of smears of this 'flocculent' layer for mucous and squames. In 1985, Masson and Ruggieri described a new diagnostic application of the pulmonary artery catheter to obtain microvascular blood and demonstrated the presence of fetal squames in suspected AFE. However, Clark *et al.* advocated caution in 1986 when they showed that squames could be demonstrated in both pregnant and non-pregnant patients. Meticulous technique using the correct stain and evidence of other amniotic fluid debris, such as mucin, hair and fat droplets, should be obtained to validate the diagnosis of AFE. Other methods are based on the estimation of plasma zinc coproporphyrin, a component of meconium, and a monoclonal antibody technique to detect mucin-like glycoproteins in maternal serum.

Postmortem diagnosis of AFE

The presence of amniotic fluid debris, squames, lanugo hair and mucin on sectioning of lung specimens is the cornerstone of the diagnosis of AFE.

Differential diagnosis

- Local anaesthetic toxicity.
- Transfusion reaction.
- Other emboli.
- Septic shock.
- Myocardial infarction.
- Anaphylaxis.
- Eclampsia.
- Placental abruption.
- Uterine rupture.

Bibliography

Clark SL. New concepts of amniotic fluid embolism: a review. *Obstet Gynaecol Surv* 1990; **45**: 360–8.

Clark SL, Pavlova Z, Greenspoon J. Squamous cells in the maternal pulmonary circulation. *Am J Obstet Gynecol* 1986; **154**: 104–6.

Clark SL, Hankins GDV, Dudley DA, *et al.* Amniotic fluid embolism: analysis of the national registry. *Am J Obstet Gynecol* 1995; **172**. 1158–69.

Davies S. Amniotic fluid embolism: a review of the literature. *Can J Anesth* 2001; **48**: 88–98.

Gross P, Benz EJ. Pulmonary embolism by amniotic fluid. *Gynecol Obstet 1947*; **85**: 315–20.

Kanayama N, Ohi H, Tereo T. Determining zinc coproporphyrin in maternal plasma: a new method for diagnosing amniotic fluid embolism. *Clin Chem* 1992; **38**: 526–9.

Knight M, Tuffnell D, Brocklehurst P, *et al.* Incidence and risk factors for amniotic fluid embolism. *Obstet Gynaecol* 2010; **115**: 910–17.

Kobayashi H, Yamazaki T, Naruse H, *et al.* A simple non-invasive sensitive method for diagnosis of amniotic fluid embolism by monoclonal antibody TKH-2. *Am J Obstet Gynecol* 1993; **168**: 848–53.

Masson RG, Ruggieri J. Pulmonary microvascular cytology. A new diagnostic application of the pulmonary artery catheter. *Chest* 1985; **88**: 908–14.

Morgan M. Amniotic fluid embolism. *Anaesthesia* 1979; **34**: 20–32.

Tuffnell DJ, Johnson H. Amniotic fluid embolism: the UK register. *Hosp Med* 2000; **61**: 532–4.

Cross-references

Anaesthesia for elective caesarean section, 472
Cardiopulmonary resuscitation, 738
Disseminated intravascular coagulation, 219
Intraoperative bronchospasm, 762

Awareness

Chris JD Pomfrett

Definition

- The patient remembers part or all of the anaesthetic or surgical procedure.
- Recall of specific words or sounds in the operating room will distinguish awareness from hallucination or dreaming.
- A clinically relevant proportion (e.g. 21%) of awareness is accompanied by pain, and may give rise to postoperative psychological trauma and litigation.
- Recall may be explicit, when the patient is capable of unprompted speaking of the event, or implicit, when subconscious learning during anaesthesia surfaces as a behavioural change, sometimes after a considerable time delay. Implicit recall has been studied using postoperative hypnosis of the patient or recall of key words or phrases.

Recollection

Events recalled may be many if the patient is aware (Table 30.1). Auditory stimuli are most frequently recalled, especially negative comments regarding the patient's condition or appearance.

Table 30.1 Events recalled and sequelae following awareness*

	%	Sample size
Event		
Sounds	30	18
Surgery without pain	25	15
Pain	21	13
Paralysis	20	12
Intubation	15	9
Anxiety or panic	11	7
Sequelae		
Temporary distress	84	51
Recurrent nightmares	16	10
Psychotherapy	13	8
Post-traumatic stress disorder	10	6

*From Domino *et al.* (1999).

Incidence

The widely reported incidence of awareness is around 0.2%, whereby 1:500 patients will be aware (Table 30.2).

Identification

- Increased blood pressure (BP), heart rate, sweating, tear formation.
- Advanced monitoring using electroencephalograph (EEG)-based technology, e.g. bispectral index in which numbers above 60 on a 0–99 scale indicate increased probability of awareness.
- Structured postoperative interview, avoiding leading questions.
- The hand-written anaesthetic record is limited as a method of determining why awareness and recall have occurred.

Sequelae

- Sleep disturbances, e.g. nightmares.
- Flashbacks.
- Anxiety, possibly bordering on psychosis.
- Increased fear of anaesthesia.

Causes

Induction

- Intubation immediately after induction with an intravenous agent (i.e. too early) may lead to awareness of intubation.
- Any delay before intubation (e.g. waiting for the relaxant to take effect, problems with intubation) may mean that the action of the intravenous induction agent will be wearing off.

Between induction and surgery

Any delay between induction and transfer into the operating room may allow the blood concentration of the intravenous agent to decay before an inhalational agent has reached anaesthetic levels, leading to awareness of incision.

During surgery

- Anaesthetic machine incorrectly maintained.
- Low minute-volume settings on some electrically driven ventilators may lead to dilution of the

Table 30.2 Incidence of awareness

Date of study	% Awareness	% Dreaming	Sample size
Structured interview			
1960	1.2	3	656
1971	1.6	26	120
1973	1.5	–	200
1975	0.8	7.7	490
1990	0.2	0.9	1000
2004	0.18	–	7826
No structured interview			
1983	13	–	91 (caesarean)
1984	11	–	37 (casualty)
1986	8	11	36 (caesarean)
1988	0	19	120 (paediatric)
1990	0	3	200 (caesarean)

anaesthetic with air, leading to awareness during surgery.
- Oxygen bypass tap left on.
- Exhausted vaporizer.
- Failure to eliminate air from a closed circuit.
- Exhausted, disconnected or malfunctioning syringe driver.

Prevention

- Know exactly how your anaesthetic machine and associated equipment works and check it all before use.
- Periodically check vaporizer levels and use an agent meter.
- Flush circles with a high flow for the first 5 minutes.
- Consider use of a commercial depth-of-anaesthesia monitor, especially if the patient is suspected of being at risk of awareness, e.g. a history of possible past awareness.
- Remember that patients differ considerably in their anaesthetic requirements.

Treatment

- Postoperative interview.
- Referral to a psychologist for counselling.

Bibliography

Couture LJ, Edmonds HL. Monitoring responsiveness during anaesthesia. *Baillieres Clin Anaesthesiol* 1989; **3**: 547–58.

Domino K, Posner K, Caplan R, Cheney F. Awareness during anesthesia: a closed claims analysis. *Anesthesiology* 1999; **90**: 1053–61.

Ekman A, Lindholm ML, Lennmarken C, Sandin R. Reduction in the incidence of awareness using BIS monitoring. *Acta Anaesthesiol Scand* 2004; **48**: 20–6.

Liu WHD, Thorp TAS, Graham SG, Aitkenhead AR. Incidence of awareness with recall during general anaesthesia. *Anaesthesia* 1991; **46**: 435–7.

Moerman N, Bonke B, Oosting J. Awareness and recall during general anaesthesia. *Anesthesiology* 1993; **79**: 454–64.

Blood transfusion

Niall O'Keeffe

Concerns about disease transmission and potential shortages in a safe supply have led to a more critical approach to the use of blood and blood products. Two-thirds of all transfusions are given during the perioperative period. Commonly used blood products are listed in Table 30.3.

Massive transfusion

Blood transfusion remains the treatment of choice when there is severe acute blood loss, e.g. major trauma, ruptured aortic aneurysm, obstetric haemorrhage. In an emergency, group O rhesus-negative or type-specific packed cells may be given. Haemolysis will occur in 3% of these 'transfusion episodes'. The use of FFP (15 mL kg^{-1}) and platelets (target platelet count 75 × 10^9 L^{-1}) should be considered early in the management of a patient with massive haemorrhage. Optimal use of blood products is guided by a combination of laboratory tests and the use of near patient testing devices such as the thromboelastograph. Continuing blood loss will be exacerbated by hypotension, hypocalcaemia, acidosis and hypothermia.

When bleeding is controlled and the patient stable, consideration should be given to starting prophylaxis against venous thrombosis, as these patients subsequently become hypercoagulable, and are therefore at risk of thromboembolism.

Risks of transfusion

The overall morbidity of blood transfusion is 1 in 30 transfusion episodes. There are risks associated with all homologous transfusions.

Acute life threatening complications

These are due to:

- red cell incompatibility
- transfusion-related acute lung injury (TRALI)
- anaphylaxis.

Table 30.3 Commonly used blood products

Product	Use
Red cells	Increase oxygen-delivering capacity of the blood: acute or chronic anaemia
Platelets	Prevention or treatment of haemorrhage in patients with thrombocytopenia
Fresh-frozen plasma	Replacement of coagulation factors Thrombotic thrombocytopenia Reversal of warfarin when prothrombin complex concentrate not available
Cryoprecipitate	Hypofibrinogenaemia (as can occur in massive transfusions) Haemophilia: when factor concentrates not available
Fibrinogen concentrate	Hypofibrinogenaemia: fibrinogen can be replaced more rapidly and reliably using fibrinogen concentrate; unfortunately, it is not yet licensed in the UK
Prothrombin complex concentrate	Product of choice for reversal of the effect of warfarin (contains factors II, VII, IX and X)
Factor VIII and IX*	Haemophilia
Factor VIIa*	Management of haemophilia patients with inhibitors Management of major haemorrhage: unlicensed for this use

*Recombinant factor VIIa, VIII and IX are now available and avoid the risks of transmission of virus infections.

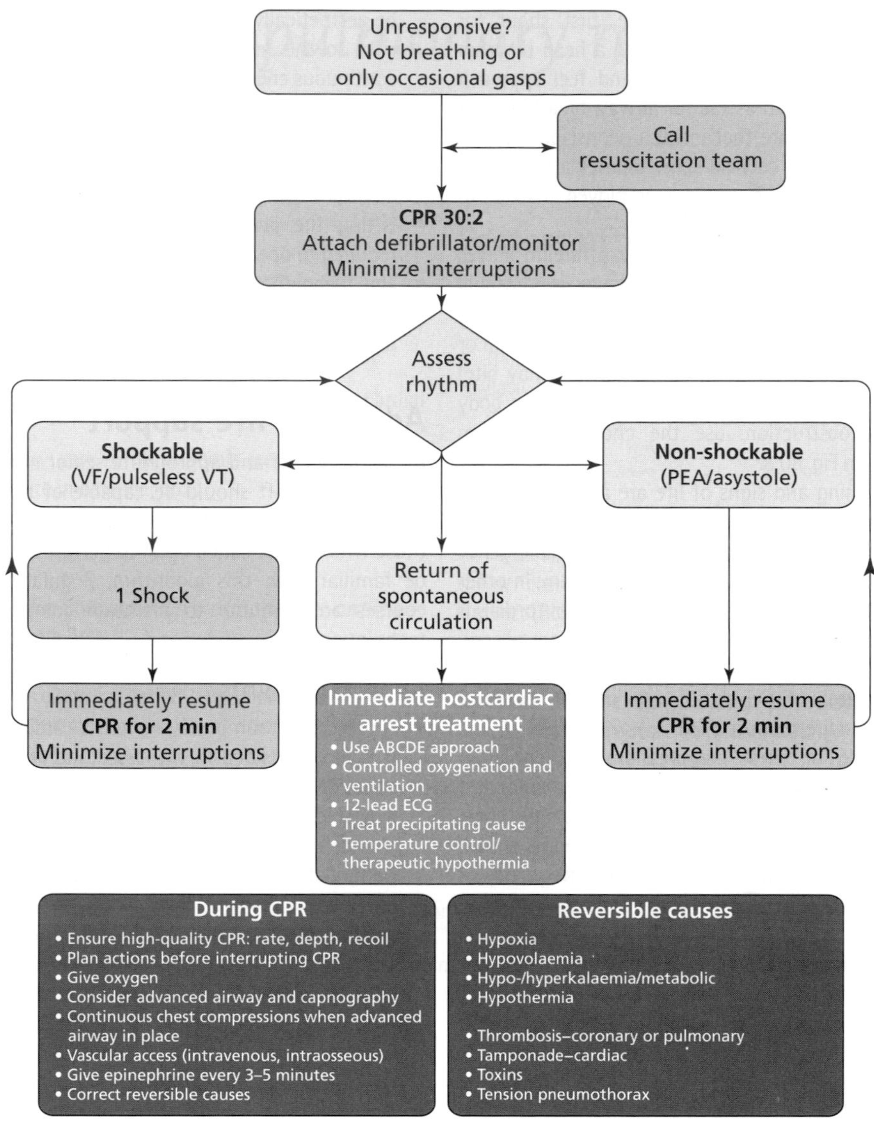

Figure 30.4 Adult life support algorithm. Reproduced from Resuscitation Council (UK). *Adult Basic Life Support*. Resuscitation Guidelines 2010. London: Resuscitation Council (UK), 2010.

ECG rhythm from being a perfusing one, and the coronary and cerebral perfusion pressure (CPP) must be preserved until the rhythm is associated with a palpable circulation. Furthermore, a 2 minute cycle of CPR should not be interrupted to analyse rhythms or to undertake pulse checks, unless the patient shows an obvious sign of life. Following 2 minutes of CPR, pause briefly to assess the rhythm (palpate for a pulse if a change in rhythm is observed that could provide a perfusing rhythm) and administer a further single defibrillation at the same energy level. Epinephrine 1 mg (1:10 000 concentration) should be administered after the third shock but should not delay defibrillation if it is not immediately available; defibrillation and effective chest compressions are the primary treatment. Epinephrine should be given every alternative 2 minute cycle of CPR (every 3–5 minutes) thereafter. Advanced airway interventions should be considered. However, only intubate the patient if sufficiently competent and trained to do so. Prolonged attempts at tracheal intubation may adversely affect the quality of chest compressions, through cessation of chest compressions, and will

compromise coronary and cerebral perfusion. Supraglottic airway devices are easier to use and can be inserted without interrupting chest compressions. Once the airway is secured, chest compressions may be continued uninterrupted at a rate of 100 per minute. Ventilations should continue at 10 per minute. If VF or VT persists after 2 minutes of CPR, a further shock at 150–360 J biphasic (or as manufacturer's guidelines) or 360 J monophasic should be delivered without delay.
- Fine VF may masquerade as asystole on the ECG; if there is any uncertainty, do not delay chest compressions. Fine VF is very unlikely to be defibrillated into a perfusing rhythm and will increase myocardial injury directly via the electrical current and through interruptions in coronary blood flow. The treatment is CPR for another 2 minutes to reoxygenate the myocardium.
- Epinephrine is given to improve cerebral and coronary blood flow, not to terminate VF or asystole.
- Epinephrine 1 mg (1:10 000 concentration) is indicated immediately in PEA and then every alternative cycle (3–5 minutes).
- Amiodarone 300 mg should be considered in refractory VF or VT (when the rhythm does not respond to the first three shocks).
- Sodium bicarbonate is no longer recommended at an early stage, as it may worsen intracellular acidosis. It may be given for severe metabolic acidosis later in the process of resuscitation, preferably guided by arterial blood gases.
- PEA is usually secondary, and CPR is unlikely to be successful unless the underlying cause is treated.
- In PEA, calcium chloride 10 mL of 10% may be useful in hypocalcaemia, hyperkalaemia or after use of calcium channel blockers.
- Central line insertion during CPR is hazardous and should only be attempted by the experienced; it should be undertaken with minimal interruptions to chest compressions. Intravenous access is quicker, easier to perform and safer. Any intravenous drug administration during cardiac arrest should be followed with at least a 20 mL flush to expedite entry into the circulation. If intravenous access cannot be established, the intraosseous route should be used. Intracardiac injection and endotracheal route of drugs is not recommended.

Postresuscitation care

The patient should be nursed in an ITU or high-dependency unit (HDU) following successful resuscitation. The return of spontaneous circulation is just the first step in recovery in which ALS aims to stabilize the patient, minimize any cerebral and cardiac injury which has occurred and protect against systemic ischaemic-reperfusion injury.

The following points should be considered.

History

- Previous medical history.
- Events preceding the arrest.
- Cause of the arrest.

Examination

Airway

- Maintain an open airway as dictated by the patient's condition.
- Consider tracheal intubation, sedation and controlled ventilation in any patient with obtunded cerebral function. Check endotracheal tube position.
- Obtain an arterial blood gas and adjust ventilation and inspired oxygen to maintain oxygenation between 94 and 98%.

Breathing

- Respiratory rate/work or breathing and support with ventilation as necessary.
- Observe chest movements, symmetry and auscultate for pneumothorax.
- Consider fractured ribs or sternum.

Circulation

- Pulse.
- BP.
- Adequacy of perfusion.
- Jugular venous pressure.
- Urine output. Catheterize the patient to ensure effective monitoring.

Patients who have ST segment elevation myocardial infarction should be considered for coronary angiography and percutaneous coronary intervention.

Disability

- Neurological
  - Glasgow Coma Score
  - pupil size and reactivity
  - neurological deficit.
- Capillary or central blood glucose monitoring.
- Observe for risk of fitting.

Exposure

Full body assessment to ascertain any further issues such as injuries, signs of bleeding, allergic or septic rashes, etc. Monitor temperature – hyperthermia is common in the first 48 hours after cardiac arrest.

Investigations

- Arterial blood gases.
- Chest X-ray.

appears to have minimal effect on the therapeutic effectiveness of ECT in clinical practice. Etomidate is another alternative, but the increased muscle tone and pain on injection have limited its use for ECT.

Muscle relaxation is used to reduce the incidence of fractures related to ECT. Succinylcholine (0.5 mg kg^{-1}) is the drug of choice. Following modified ECT, only 2% of patients suffer muscle pain.

Intubation is not normally necessary and the airway can be maintained by correct head position and an oral airway. Assisted ventilation with 100% oxygen is mandatory until spontaneous respiration returns. Because of the seizure and clamping of jaws that occurs with ECT, it is advisable to insert a mouth gag to prevent damage to the teeth and injury to lips and the tongue.

Following administration of ECT, bradycardia and even asystole may occur, and atropine or glycopyrrolate may be required. These drugs may accentuate the sympathetic response that invariably follows, putting undue stress on the myocardium. The use of a short-acting β-blocker, such as esmolol, has been advocated to attenuate the sympathetic response to ECT, and should be available to treat arrhythmias and hypertension that persist into the recovery period. Prolonged seizure following ECT is uncommon and can easily be aborted with diazepam.

Post-electroconvulsive therapy management

Patients having had ECT should be closely monitored until fully recovered.

Outcome

Mortality following ECT is 0.02–0.04%. Arrhythmias, myocardial infarction, congestive cardiac failure and sudden cardiac arrest are the commonest causes of death, nearly always occurring during the recovery period.

Morbidity following ECT includes memory loss, confusion, drowsiness, muscular aches, weakness, anorexia and amenorrhoea.

Bibliography

Gaines GY, Rees DI. Anaesthetic consideration for electroconvulsive therapy. *South Med J* 1992; **85**: 469–82.

Matters RM, Beckett WG, Kirkby KC, King TE. Recovery after electroconvulsive therapy: comparison of propofol with methohexitone. *Br J Anaesth* 1995; **75**: 297–300.

Mayur PM, Shree RS, Gangadhar BN, *et al.* Atropine premedication and the cardiovascular response to electroconvulsive therapy. *Br J Anaesth* 1998; **81**: 466–70.

O'Flaherty D, Giesecke AH. Electroconvulsive therapy and anaesthesia. *Curr Opin Anaesthesiol* 1991; **4**: 436–440.

O'Flaherty D, Husain MM, Moore M, *et al.* Circulatory responses during electroconvulsive therapy. The comparative effect of placebo, esmolol, and nitroglycerine. *Anaesthesia* 1992; **47**: 563–7.

Simpson KH, Lynch L. Anaesthesia and electroconvulsive therapy (editorial). *Anaesthesia* 1998; **53**: 615–17.

Failure to breathe or wake up postoperatively

Brian J Pollard

All anaesthetic agents and opioids are respiratory depressants and may cause apnoea. Failure to breathe postoperatively may also follow the use of intraoperative muscular relaxation. Remember that there may be more than one cause operating simultaneously and causes may be cumulative.

Failure to breathe postoperatively

Non-depolarizing agents

- Inadequate antagonism of neuromuscular block is less common with the newer neuromuscular blocking agents. The effects of non-depolarizing muscle relaxants are usually antagonized with neostigmine (50 µg kg^{-1}) (together with atropine (20 µg kg^{-1}) or glycopyrrolate (10 µg kg^{-1})), and this should have been given before 'failure to breathe' is noted. Sugammadex will only antagonize a block resulting from an aminosteroid agent (rocuronium and, to a lesser extent, vecuronium).
- Look for concomitant drugs which themselves depress neuromuscular function or potentiate a neuromuscular blocking agent, e.g.
  - aminoglycoside antibiotics
  - verapamil
  - phenytoin
  - ciclosporin A.
- Cholinergic crisis secondary to excessive neostigmine (rare).

Depolarizing agents

- Pseudocholinesterase deficiency (genetic or acquired).
- Dual block (type II block).

Other factors

- Respiratory depressants.
- Opioids.
- Volatile anaesthetic agents.
- Benzodiazepines.
- Pain, especially if thoracic or abdominal in origin.
- Hypocapnia.
- Severe hypercapnia.
- Hypothermia, especially in children.
- Metabolic disturbance.
- Acidosis.
- Hypokalaemia.
- Hypomagnesaemia.
- Coexisting neuromuscular disease.
- Intraoperative cerebral event.

Management

The patient may be pink and display an acceptable S_pO_2.

- Ensure the patient's safety.
- Ensure that the airway is protected and that adequate ventilation is maintained, by hand if necessary.
- If the patient is conscious, reassure them and consider sedation.
- Monitor vital signs:
  - ECG
  - S_pO_2
  - non-invasive BP
  - end-tidal CO_2 ($ETCO_2$), if possible.
- Determine cause:
  - monitor neuromuscular function
  - review dose of muscle relaxant
  - review dose of reversal
  - check if other agents which may affect a block have been given
  - check whether all anaesthetic agents are turned off
  - consider the patient's metabolic status
  - measure the patient's temperature.
- If residual paralysis is present and the post-tetanic count is 12 or more, a further dose of neostigmine and an anticholinergic (up to 100 µg kg^{-1} total dose of neostigmine) may help.
- If excessive narcotic is present, give increments of 0.1 mg naloxone.
- If central respiratory depression is present, consider titrated doses of doxapram (1–1.5 mg kg^{-1} over 30 seconds).
- If excessive benzodiazepines have been used, give flumazenil (200 µg over 15 seconds, then 100 µg every 60 seconds, as required).
- Control pain with local techniques or carefully titrated doses of opioids.

- Optimize the patient's metabolic condition.
- Wait.
- If ventilation is still not adequate, transfer the patient to the ITU.

Normal awakening

Awakening occurs when the concentration of anaesthetic agent in the brain falls to a level insufficient to maintain unconsciousness. This occurs as a result of the redistribution (usually) or metabolism of intravenous agents and the elimination of volatile agents. It is therefore a passive process, with specific antagonists existing only for opioids and benzodiazepines.

Failure to wake up

Causes

There may be more than one reason present, and effects are cumulative:

- overdose (absolute or relative) of anaesthetic agent, premedication (including benzodiazepines), or opioid
- hypothermia, particularly in children
- hypercapnia
- hypothyroidism
- severe liver disease, in which anaesthesia may precipitate encephalopathy
- cerebral hypoxia.

Management

- Ensure the patient's safety.
- Ensure that the airway is protected and that ventilation is adequate.
- Continue monitoring:
  - ECG
  - non-invasive BP
  - $S_{p}O_2$.
- Assess cause:
  - arterial blood gas analysis
  - core temperature
  - coexisting disease.
- Treat any treatable causes:
  - correct any abnormalities in acid–base status
  - rewarm if necessary
  - administer a cautious dose of antagonists, if appropriate.
- Wait.
- Consider transfer to the ITU if awakening continues to be delayed.

The only cause of prolonged (hours or days) failure to recover from anaesthesia is a cardiorespiratory or cerebrovascular disaster with cerebral hypoxia. Thankfully, this is rare.

Bibliography

Fuchs-Buder T. *Neuromuscular Monitoring in Clinical Practice and Research*. Heidelberg: Springer, 2010.

Morris RW. Desaturation. *Baillieres Best Pract Res Clin Anaesthesiol* 1993; **7**: 215–35.

Pollard BJ. *Applied Neuromuscular Pharmacology*. Oxford: Oxford University Press, 1994.

Ward DS, Temp JA. The role of hypoxia in the control of breathing. In: Kauffman L (ed.) *Anaesthesia Review*, vol. 8. London: Churchill Livingstone, 1991, pp. 89–102.

Fat embolism

Arabella P Stevens

Definition

Fat embolism is defined as the presence of fat globules within the lung parenchyma or peripheral microcirculation. The fat embolism syndrome (FES) is defined as fat in the circulation associated with a clinical pattern of symptoms and signs. It is associated with:

- fractures of long bones and pelvis
- prosthetic joint replacement
- liposuction
- bone marrow harvest or transplant
- acute pancreatitis
- hepatic necrosis and fatty liver
- acute sickle cell crisis (bone marrow necrosis)
- altitude illness
- following extracorporeal circulation
- major soft-tissue injury
- severe burns.

The commonest group is patients with long-bone fractures and in this situation fat embolism can be demonstrated to be present in over 90% of patients. FES is seen in only 1–10%. Those at highest risk include young adult males and those with closed or multiple fractures.

Three clinical forms of FES are described.

Subclinical fat embolism syndrome

Frequently seen in patients with long-bone fractures. Mild hypoxaemia and minor haematological abnormalities develop up to 3 days after injury.

Non-fulminant (subacute) fat embolism syndrome

Seen in up to 5% of major trauma patients. Onset may be delayed by 12–36 hours after injury. Classical syndrome of hypoxaemia and respiratory failure, petechial rash, fever, tachycardia, neurological symptoms and associated haematological abnormalities.

Fulminant fat embolism syndrome

Sudden onset, within a few hours of injury. Pulmonary and systemic embolization of fat, right ventricular failure and cardiovascular collapse. This can occur intraoperatively. Progresses rapidly, often with a fatal outcome.

Pathophysiology

Two theories have gained acceptance, a mechanical and a biochemical model. Fat emboli are thought to originate from exposed marrow at the site of injury. Fat globules enter the circulation, facilitated by movement of the fracture site. Subsequent pulmonary and neurological damage is thought to be partly due to vascular occlusion (mechanical theory), and partly due to local effects of free fatty acids released from fat emboli (biochemical theory).

Respiratory insufficiency results from emboli entering the venous circulation and lodging in the pulmonary circulation. The free fatty acids released are toxic to pneumocytes and capillary endothelium, causing intra-alveolar haemorrhage, oedema and a chemical pneumonitis. Cerebral involvement and a petechial rash result from fat emboli entering the arterial circulation, either via the pulmonary alveolar capillaries or via precapillary pulmonary shunts which have opened as a result of pulmonary hypertension.

Diagnosis

Respiratory insufficiency

- Occurs in 75% of patients with FES.
- Dyspnoea, tachypnoea and hypoxaemia are associated with fine inspiratory crackles on auscultation, 12–36 hours following injury.
- Chest X-ray is normal at first, and then shows bilateral evenly distributed fleck-like pulmonary shadows. Classically described as a 'snow storm' appearance.
- In 10% of cases respiratory failure develops and progresses to the adult respiratory distress syndrome.

Cerebral features

Neurological signs exist in up to 80% of patients with FES, and can precede respiratory signs. Encephalopathy produces drowsiness, confusion and/or coma. A subgroup develops focal neurological signs such as decerebrate posturing, hemiparesis or tonic–clonic seizures. The severe neurological symptoms of FES usually resolve. A CT scan may show generalized cerebral oedema or high-density spots but is non-specific and usually unhelpful. MRI may detect specific lesions in the presence of a normal CT scan.

Dermatological features

These occur in 60% of cases.

A petechial rash develops within 36 hours of the event. Found in conjunctivae, oral mucous membrane, neck and axillae. This distribution may be explained by fat droplets accumulating in the aortic arch prior to embolization to non-dependent skin via the subclavian and carotid vessels. Factors contributing to the rash may be stasis, loss of clotting factors and platelets, and endothelial damage from free fatty acids leading to rupture of thin-walled capillaries. It is self-limiting, usually resolving within 7 days.

Other features

- Pyrexia and tachycardia are common non-specific findings.
- ECG may show signs of right ventricular strain.
- Retinal haemorrhages and exudates can occur.
- Renal emboli may result in oliguria, lipuria, proteinuria or haematuria; these changes are short-lived and unrelated to any subsequent renal impairment.
- Jaundice is rare and self-limiting.

Laboratory findings

- A decrease in haematocrit seen at 24–48 hours is thought to be secondary to intra-alveolar haemorrhage. Thrombocytopenia (platelet count $<150 \times 10^9$) and other coagulation abnormalities may be seen.
- Blood and urine may show fat globules (non-specific signs). Fat macroglobulinaemia and elevated free fatty acids and triglyceride levels in serum. High free fatty acid levels may result in hypocalcaemia because of their affinity for calcium.

Other investigations

A pulmonary artery catheter may be useful in detecting a rise in mean pulmonary artery pressure or in sampling pulmonary artery blood for fat.

Bronchoscopy and bronchoalveolar lavage in trauma patients have been used to provide samples containing macrophages, which act as lung scavengers and may contain fat in FES. This may be used to aid diagnosis but is not an adequately specific test in isolation for FES.

Management

Treatment is supportive:

- Early resuscitation and stabilization to minimize the stress response and hypovolaemia
- Maintain adequate oxygenation and ventilation.
- Indications for respiratory support:
  - sustained S_aO_2 <90% and P_aO_2 <8 kPa on oxygen
  - respiratory rate of >35 breaths min^{-1}.
- Avoid hypovolaemia:
  - systolic blood pressure <90 mmHg is associated with adverse outcomes
  - fluid resuscitation with balanced electrolyte solutions and albumin is recommended
  - albumin use is considered potentially therapeutic in its ability to bind free fatty acids.

Surgical management

- There is level 1 evidence that early (within 24 hours) surgical stabilization of long-bone fractures reduces the risk of pulmonary complications.
- Intramedullary nail insertion and reaming is recognized to cause increased fat embolization. The method of fracture stabilization chosen should take into account the physiological state of the patient and concomitant injuries.
- Adequate analgesia should be maintained to limit the sympathomimetic response to injury.

A number of specific therapies have been tried:

- Corticosteroids (methylprednisolone) used as prophylactic treatment have been shown to reduce the risk of FES and hypoxaemia in patients with long-bone fractures of the lower limbs. Optimal timings and doses are unclear.
- Heparin is known to clear lipaemic serum by stimulating lipase activity and, in experimental models, has been shown to reduce pulmonary complications. Despite its associated bleeding risks, it has been used clinically but has not shown consistent benefits in reducing lung injury.
- Alcohol, which decreases serum lipase activity, and dextrose, which decreases free fatty acid mobilization, have both been used empirically but there is little evidence to support these treatments.
- Aspirin has previously been recommended as a prophylactic agent as it blocks the production of thromboxane, which occurs in animal models of FES. However, current evidence does not support its use.

Outcome

The overall mortality of FES is 5–15%. The condition is usually self-limiting with adequate supportive therapy. Long-term morbidity is related to focal neurological lesions.

Bibliography

Bannier B, Poirier T, Viaud JY, *et al.* Bronchoalveolar lavage in fat embolism. *Intensive Care Med* 1992; **18**: 59–60.

Cavallazzi R, Cavallazzi AC. The effect of corticosteroid on the prevention of fat embolism syndrome after long bone fracture of the lower limbs: a systematic review and met-analysis. *J Bras Pneumol* 2008; **34**: 34–41.

Gurd AR. Fat embolism, an aid to diagnosis. *J Bone Joint Surg* 1970; **52B**: 732–7.

Mellor A, Soni N. Fat embolism. *Anaesthesia* 2001; **56**: 145–54.

Robert JH, Hoffmeyer P, Broquet PE, *et al.* Fat embolism syndrome. *Orthop Rev* 1993; **22**: 567–71.

Talbot M, Schemitsch EH. Fat embolism syndrome: history, definition, epidemiology. *Injury* 2006; **37**S, S3–7.

Van Besouw JP, Hinds CJ. Fat embolism syndrome. *Br J Hosp Med* 1989; **42**: 304–11.

White T, Petrisor BA, Bhandari M. Prevention of fat embolism syndrome. *Injury* 2006; **37**S: S59–67.

Fluid and electrolyte balance

Simon Varley

Introduction

Both coexisting disease and the surgical pathology can impair the complex homeostatic mechanisms which safeguard normal physiological function. Normal cellular function during the perioperative period requires a stable chemical environment.

Perioperative fluids and electrolytes are required for maintenance and the replacement of abnormal losses. Where possible they should be given orally or enterally.

Inappropriate fluid administration can result in harmful water overload and disordered electrolyte and acid–base balance (including hyponatraemia, hypernatraemia and hyperchloraemic metabolic acidosis). Fluid management is a contributory factor in postoperative morbidity, mortality and length of stay.

The pathophysiological response to surgery increases the risk of complications from inappropriate perioperative fluid management.

Physiology

Body water content varies with age and sex as a percentage of body weight (Table 30.4).

Approximately two-thirds of the total body water (TBW) is intracellular fluid (ICF) and one-third is extracellular fluid (ECF). The ECF is further subdivided into interstitial fluid and plasma.

The TBW and electrolytes in a 70 kg man are distributed between the various compartments, as shown in Table 30.5.

Osmotic activity

Water moves between compartments from areas of low solute concentration to areas of high concentration by osmosis. The number of osmotically active particles in solution is expressed in osmoles (Osm). Osmolarity is the number of particles per litre of solvent (Osm L^{-1}), and osmolality is the number of particles per kilogram of solvent (Osm kg^{-1}). The density of water is 1 kg L^{-1}; osmolality and osmolarity are therefore equivalent in the body.

Osmolality can be estimated by adding the concentrations of osmotically active particles within compartments. ECF osmolality is usually calculated by adding the plasma concentrations (mmol L^{-1}) of sodium, potassium, chloride, urea and glucose. An alternative commonly used rule of thumb is to add twice the sodium plus urea plus glucose.

Osmotic pressure is calculated by multiplying osmolalities by 19.3 to give pressures (mmHg). Thus, ICF has an osmolality of 281 mOsm L^{-1} and an osmotic pressure of 5430 mmHg, but plasma has an osmolality of 281 mOsm L^{-1} and an osmotic pressure of 5453 mmHg. This difference of 23 mmHg is due to the presence of plasma proteins.

The redistribution of infused fluid within the body will depend on its composition relative to that of each compartment, as shown in Table 30.6. Salt solutions are excluded from the ICF by the cell membrane Na^+/K^+ pump. Dextrose (5%) behaves like water and is distributed throughout the TBW.

Normal homeostasis

Humans have evolved to retain water and sodium efficiently. Even healthy individuals are slow to excrete a sodium load. Sodium excretion is not active and probably occurs by suppression of the renin–angiotensin–aldosterone system.

Blood volume is maintained at the expense of serum osmolality in hypovolaemia. If hypotonic solutions are administered, this may exacerbate hyponatraemia and water overload.

Table 30.4 Body water composition in health as a percentage of body weight

	Total body water (%)	Intracellular fluid (%)	Extracellular fluid (%)
Neonate	75	40	35
Infant	70	40	30
Adult male	60	40	20
Adult female	55	35	20
Elderly female	45	30	15

Table 30.5 Distribution of water (L) and electrolytes (mmol L^{-1}) in a normal 70 kg man

	Intracellular fluid	Extracellular fluid	
		Interstitial fluid	Plasma
Water (L)	28	11	3
% of total body weight	40	16	4
Na^+	10	140	140
K^+	150	4	4
Ca^{2+}	–	2.5	2.5
Mg^{2+}	26	1.5	1.5
Cl^-	–	114	114
HCO_3^-	10	25	25
Cl^-	–	114	114
HCO_3^-	10	25	25
HPO_4^{2-}	38	1	1
SO_4^{2-}	–	0.5	0.5
Protein$^-$	74	2	16

Table 30.6 Approximate percentage distribution of infusions within compartments*

	Intracellular fluid (%)	Extracellular fluid	
		Interstitial fluid (%)	Plasma (%)
Saline (0.9%)	0	79	21
Dextrose (5%)	67	26	7

*These figures demonstrate why large volumes of crystalloids are required to expand plasma volume.

Water

A normothermic 70 kg man with a normal metabolic rate loses approximately 2500 mL of water per day or 35 mL kg^{-1} h^{-1} (urine, 1500 mL; faeces, 100 mL; sweat, 500 mL; lungs, 400 mL). Insensible loss increases by 10% for each 1°C rise in body temperature. Water is gained from ingested fluid (1300 mL), food (800 mL) and metabolism (400 mL). Maintenance requirements are therefore approximately 1.25 mL kg^{-1} h^{-1} for adult surgical patients.

Sodium

Loss in faeces and sweat is about 10 mmol day^{-1}, renal excretion being mainly dependent on dietary intake. Average requirements are 1 mmol kg^{-1} day^{-1}.

This could be provided by:

- 2500 mL of 4% dextrose/0.18% saline over 24 hours
- 2000 mL of 5% dextrose and 500 mL of 0.9% saline over 24 hours.

Potassium

Loss is via the same routes as sodium, but renal retention is less efficient. The average requirement is 1 mmol kg^{-1} day^{-1}. This should be added to the infusion regime.

Perioperative fluid management

Assessment

The fluid status of a patient undergoing surgery will depend on the presenting complaint (including the severity of physiological derangement), the previous health of the individual and whether surgery is elective or urgent.

Fluid and electrolyte balance should be determined by repeated clinical assessment throughout the perioperative period and should include an estimate of total balance and intravascular volume (vascular filling).

Total balance

The history will point to decreased intake or increased loss:

- note the duration of preoperative fasting
- review the ability of the patient to maintain fluid balance during illness

- consider normal variations in fluid balance at extremes of age
- identify increased losses: pyrexia, diarrhoea, vomiting and haemorrhage
- an acute abdomen may result in large volumes of fluid sequestered in the abdominal compartment.

Examination should include mucous membranes, skin turgor, sensorium, heart rate, blood pressure, respiratory rate and urine output.

- Up to 15% deficit in TBW:
  - stuporose
  - parched mouth
  - sunken eyes
  - fast and thready pulse
  - respiratory distress
  - hypotension
  - extreme oliguria.
- Body weight should be monitored regularly following admission.
- Charts should be regularly reviewed to identify urine output and losses via nasogastric tubes and drains.
- Fluid prescription charts should be analysed to identify the volume and type of fluid administered.
- Investigations including simple blood tests supply additional information:
  - elevated urea or creatinine
  - elevated haematocrit
  - check plasma levels of sodium and potassium.

Intravascular volume

Assessment is by pulse, blood pressure, capillary refill, jugular venous pressure.

Invasive and non-invasive measures of intravascular volume can include:

- central venous catheters (CVP)
- arterial catheters (arterial pressure and pulse pressure variation)
- pulmonary artery catheters (central and pulmonary capillary wedge pressure and cardiac output)
- transoesophageal Doppler monitoring (stroke volume, flow time corrected)
- devices utilizing arterial pressure waveform to calculate haemodynamic parameters (stroke volume, stroke volume variation).

The goal of clinical assessment is to determine the fluid and electrolyte balance of each compartment.

Perioperative fluid therapy

Patients should commence surgery in a state of normal and stable fluid and electrolyte balance.

In general, healthy patients undergoing elective minor surgery do not need perioperative fluid replacement unless they are unable to drink normally in the early postoperative period.

In other patients, the following should be considered.

Preventing and replacing preoperative deficits

Correction of a deficit in maintenance (normal daily intake) fluids should be with the equivalent of 1.25 mL kg^{-1} h^{-1} of dextrose (4%)/saline (0.18%) in proportion to the oral intake of the patient.

Patients presenting as an emergency may have had significantly reduced intake over several days. This may continue while they are an inpatient and is exacerbated by repeated periods of nil by mouth.

Abnormal losses and redistribution is common in surgical patients and includes:

- bowel preparation
- sequestration (bowel obstruction or ileus)
- vomiting and diarrhoea
- enterocutaneous fistulae
- stoma
- wounds
- haemorrhage.

Significant hypovolaemia may occur with inflammatory conditions, including severe infections (sepsis), peritonitis and pancreatitis.

All routes by which fluid and electrolytes can be lost from the appropriate compartments should be considered.

Replacement is based on an estimate of the composition and volume of loss. Losses from the gut are particularly important, and although the compositions of the various gastrointestinal secretions differ they are adequately replaced with equal volumes of saline (0.9%) and potassium chloride (10–20 mmol L^{-1}) or Hartmann's solution.

In severe hypovolaemia with signs of shock, give colloid (10 mL kg^{-1}) as a bolus, with additional fluid given according to the patient's response.

The properties of intravenous fluids are shown in Table 30.7.

Intraoperative management

The goal is to maintain ideal tissue perfusion (oxygen delivery) while avoiding fluid compartments becoming overloaded. Inappropriate administration of unbalanced colloids can result in salt overload (hypernatraemia and hyperchloraemic metabolic acidosis) and can precipitate a hyperoncotic state.

Fluid management is complicated by the dynamic interaction between anaesthesia and surgical insult (including the stress response). Intravascular hypovolaemia can be relative (vasodilatation) and absolute (reduction in blood volume).

Maintenance fluid can be provided by dextrose (4%) with saline (0.18%) at 1.25 mL kg^{-1} h^{-1}.

Table 30.7 Properties of intravenous fluids in comparison with plasma

	Sodium (mmol L^{-1})	Potassium (mmol L^{-1})	Chloride (mmol L^{-1})	Duration of plasma volume expansion
Plasma	136–145	3.5–5.0	98–105	–
5% dextrose	0	0	0	Not applicable
0.9% saline	154	0	154	<30 minutes
Hartmann's solution	131	5	111	<30 minutes
4% gelatin	145	0	145	1–2 hours
6% HES 130/0.4	154	0	154	4–8 hours

HES, hydroxyethyl starch.

Additional fluids should be administered based on continuous clinical assessment and the physiological goals for the individual patient. This should be judged according to the patient's response, including heart rate, blood pressure, tissue perfusion, CVP if necessary, and urine output (not less than 0.5 mL kg^{-1} h^{-1}).

Vascular filling can be guided by measures of stroke volume (flow) and cardiac output. Flow can be measured continuously using transoesophageal Doppler and devices which derive calculations of stroke volume from the arterial pressure waveform. Applying the Frank–Starling curve, small (250 mL) boluses of colloid are infused to maximize stroke volume early in the intraoperative, thereby maintaining 'optimal' tissue perfusion throughout surgery. Cardiac output is also dependent on contractility, which can be increased with cautious use of inotropes.

There is evidence that such 'flow-guided' therapy reduces complications and length of stay in major surgery. When fluid therapy is given by rote or based on routine clinical observations (including CVP and urine output), patients are more likely to receive either inadequate or excessive amounts of fluid intraoperatively.

Goal-directed haemodynamic therapy targets oxygen delivery (600 mL min^{-1} m^{-2}) with intravenous fluids (colloids) and, if necessary, inotropes and blood transfusion. This strategy has been shown to reduce morbidity and mortality in surgical patients with a predicted risk of mortality in excess of 20%.

Postoperative requirements

- Maintenance: 1.5 mL kg^{-1} h^{-1} of 4% dextrose with 0.18% saline.
- Estimate and replace other fluid and electrolyte losses.

Opinions about the electrolyte requirements of postoperative patients differ widely in clinical practice. Although the stress response to surgery increases renal excretion of potassium, tissue trauma and catabolism release intracellular potassium, which helps to maintain plasma levels. Potassium is not required for the first 24–48 hours in most patients.

Whatever fluid composition is chosen, all fluid replacement should be regularly reviewed according to the patient's response: heart rate, blood pressure, respiratory rate, tissue perfusion, plasma electrolytes, urine output (at least 0.5 mL kg^{-1} h^{-1}) and body weight.

Blood loss

Blood should be given to maintain a reasonable haematocrit for the individual patient. Transfusion will be guided by clinical assessment of the patient, the pattern of bleeding and measures of haemoglobin and haematocrit.

Consider transfusion when 10% of estimated blood volume has been lost (Table 30.8). Give blood when 15% or more has been lost.

Table 30.8 Estimated blood volumes

	Volume (mL kg^{-1})
Infant	90
Child	80
Adult male	70
Adult female	60

FFP and platelets given to correct coagulopathy also replace blood volume.

Bibliography

Ganong WF. *Review of Medical Physiology*, 13th edn. San Francisco: Lange, 1985.

Guyton AC. *Textbook of Medical Physiology*, 6th edn. Philadelphia: W.B. Saunders, 1981.

Shearer ES, Hunter JM. Perioperative fluid and electrolyte balance. *Curr Anaesth Crit Care* 1992; **3**: 71–7.

Powell-Tuck J, Gosling P, Lobo DN, *et al.* on behalf of BAPEN Medical, The Association for Clinical Biochemistry, The Association of Surgeons of Great Britain and Ireland, The Society of Academic and Research Surgery, The Renal Association and The Intensive Care Society. *British Consensus Guidelines on Intravenous Fluid Therapy for Adult Surgical Patients*. London: NHS National Library of Health.

Cross-reference

Water and electrolyte disturbances, 633

Intraoperative arrhythmias

Brian J Pollard

Over 60% of patients may experience some form of arrhythmias perioperatively. The majority are benign. This must not, however, obscure the association of rhythm disturbance with potential serious adverse outcomes. The significance of the arrhythmia has to be evaluated in the context of:

- preoperative coexisting medical problems and drug treatment
- the surgical condition
- the operative procedure
- anaesthetic drugs and technique
- haemodynamic effect of the arrhythmias, and the risk of progression to a more serious arrhythmia.

For example, in a fit patient having an anaesthetic for minor surgery, a nodal rhythm producing negligible fall in blood pressure is unlikely to require treatment. The same rhythm in a patient with aortic stenosis, or in a fit patient about to have squint surgery, is likely to require intervention.

Preoperative evaluation

Conditions associated with arrhythmias are given in Box 30.4.

Box 30.4 Preoperative conditions associated with arrhythmias

- Ischaemic heart disease
- Pre-existing arrhythmias
- Hypertension
- Congestive heart failure
- Electrolyte disorders
- Valvular heart disease
- Medications:
  - β_2-agonists
  - Theophylline
  - Tricyclic antidepressants
- Less common causes:
  - Thyrotoxicosis
  - Cardiomyopathies (including alcoholic)
  - Myocarditis
  - Trauma (myocardial or intracranial)
  - Connective tissue disorders
- Drug and solvent abuse

The following symptoms and signs may indicate an arrhythmia in a conscious patient:

- paroxysmal dyspnoea
- palpitations
- dizziness
- syncope.

Physical examination and a 12-lead ECG with rhythm strip may not help. Further evaluation requires 24 hour ECG monitoring. The diagnosis and management of arrhythmias can be complex, particularly with the proarrhythmic potential of antiarrhythmic drugs. A cardiological opinion may be required.

Hypokalaemia

Hypokalaemia is a common electrolyte disturbance. It prolongs repolarization non-uniformly, which predisposes to arrhythmias. While a serum potassium as low as 3.0 mmol L^{-1} is usually acceptable, this may not be so in the presence of other risk factors (e.g. digoxin). The effect of ventilation should be remembered. A pH change of 0.1 will change the serum potassium 1.0 mmol L^{-1} in the opposite direction.

Hyperkalaemia, hypomagnesaemia and hypercalcaemia

These changes can all provoke arrhythmias. In contrast, extremes of sodium seem to have little effect.

Monitoring

V1 is the lead of choice for rhythm monitoring. In a three-lead system, MCLI or -II is best.

Anaesthetic factors

See Box 30.5.

Box 30.5 Anaesthetic factors which may induce arrhythmias

- Hypotension or hypertension (e.g. inadequate anaesthesia)
- Hypoxia
- Hypercarbia
- Laryngoscopy
- Central venous pressure lines (irritation by line tip; microshock hazard)
- Drugs:
  - Volatile anaesthetic agents
  - Succinylcholine
  - Pancuronium

Certain anaesthetic agents, in particular the volatile agents, may specifically induce arrhythmias. The development of arrhythmias, however, may indicate an adverse change to myocardial oxygen balance. The relationship between volatile agents and arrhythmias involves effects on:

- action potential duration
- automaticity
- calcium flux
- interactions with epinephrine
- myocardial oxygen balance.

Atrioventricular conduction is prolonged least with isoflurane and sevoflurane. The direct volatile agent effect of decreased automaticity is countered by the potentiation of catecholamine arrhythmias. The significance of coronary steal in clinical practice is doubted.

Surgical factors

See Box 30.6.

Box 30.6 Surgical factors which may induce arrhythmias

- Catecholamines
  - Endogenous: from any surgical stimulus
  - Exogenous: topical or infiltrated epinephrine
- Autonomic stimulation
  - Peritoneal and visceral traction
  - Peritoneal insufflation
  - Trigeminovagal reflexes (most notably the oculocardiac reflex, but seen throughout the trigeminal nerve distribution)
  - Laryngoscopy, bronchoscopy, oesophagoscopy
  - Carotid artery and thyroid surgery
- Direct stimulation of the heart
- During cardiac or thoracic surgery
- Embolism
  - Thrombus
  - Fat
  - Bone cement
  - Air
  - Carbon dioxide
  - Amniotic fluid
- Other
  - Aortic cross-clamping
  - Limb reperfusion
  - Glycine intoxication

Assessment

Intraoperatively, more than one factor is likely to be contributing to a new arrhythmia:

- identify the rhythm and evaluate its significance
- identify and remove any precipitating factors
- optimize myocardial oxygen balance
- if the arrhythmia persists, consider specific treatment.

Management

- Correct factors which may be contributing to the development of the arrhythmia, e.g. hypoxia, hypercapnia, hypokalaemia, hypomagnesaemia, inadequate anaesthesia.
- Treat the whole patient and not just the ECG.
- If the circulation is inadequate, external cardiac massage will be needed.
- Synchronized cardioversion is often a more attractive treatment option in the already anaesthetized patient.
- Consider an antiarrhythmic drug.

The negative inotropic effect of many antiarrhythmic drugs should be remembered. Adenosine is a useful agent for supraventricular tachycardias. Its value in slowing supraventricular tachycardia but not ventricular tachycardia (Box 30.7) is particularly valuable intraoperatively when a 12-lead ECG is difficult to record. Adenosine will also be effective in Wolff–Parkinson–White tachycardia. Alternatively, disopyramide or propranolol may be used, but verapamil and digoxin are contraindicated.

Box 30.7 Distinguishing broad complex tachycardias*

- Supraventricular tachycardia (SVT)
  - No axis change and same pattern of bundle branch block as pre-SVT ECG
  - Conforms to right or left bundle branch block pattern
  - Dominant R in V1 and Q in V6
- Ventricular tachycardia (VT)
  - Axis change from previous ECG
  - Deep S wave in V6
  - Fusion beats
  - Capture beats

*Haemodynamic stability is not a distinguishing factor. VT is much commoner than broad complex SVT, especially if a previous ECG shows narrow complexes.

Bibliography

Atlee JL, Bosnjck ZJ. Mechanisms for cardiac dysrhythmias during anaesthesia. *Anesthesiology* 1990; **72**: 347–74.

Gleva MJ, Hogue CW. Antiarrhythmic agents. In: Evers AS, Maze M (eds) *Anesthetic Pharmacology*. Edinburgh: Churchill Livingstone, 2004, pp. 621–40.

Singh BN, Opie LH, Marcus FI. Antiarrhythmic agents. In: Opie LH (ed.) *Drugs for the Heart*, 3rd edn. Philadelphia: W.B. Saunders, 1991, Ch. 8.

Cross-references

Cardiac conduction defects, 132
Coronary artery disease, 146
Fluid and electrolyte balance, 754
Pacing and anaesthesia, 777
Water and electrolyte disturbances, 633

Intraoperative bronchospasm

Brian J Pollard

Bronchospasm is caused by constriction of bronchiolar smooth muscle within the airways. It is characterized by an expiratory wheeze and elevated airway pressures. Many patients suffer from mild bronchospasm as a part of the conditions of asthma, chronic obstructive chest disease and allergic reactions. It is usually benign, can be severe, is occasionally life-threatening and, on rare occasions, it can be fatal. During anaesthesia it is rare in comparison with upper airway obstruction and occlusion of the breathing circuit, both of which should be excluded before the diagnosis of bronchospasm is made.

Asthma, coronary artery disease, smoking and respiratory infection are recognized as risk factors. A significant number of cases, however, including those leading to adverse outcomes (brain damage, death), will occur in those without such factors.

One study revealed an overall incidence of 1.7 per 1000 anaesthetics, with a higher incidence at ages 0–9 years (4.0 per 1000) and 50–69 years (1.8 per 1000). These subgroups were analysed according to a number of variables (Table 30.9). Interestingly, cardiac disease is associated with an increased frequency of bronchospasm. This may be due to abnormal cardiopulmonary reflexes.

Causes of bronchospasm

Airway instrumentation

- Instrumentation and irritation of the airway may produce reflex bronchospasm.
- Tracheal intubation is the commonest trigger.
- Carinal stimulation, e.g. by a tracheal tube or suction catheter.
- More likely under light anaesthesia.

Surgical stimulation

- Any surgical stimulation can trigger reflex bronchoconstriction.
- Patients undergoing upper abdominal, intraoral, anal and cervical procedures are more prone to this reflex.
- Inadequate anaesthesia may be a predisposing factor.

Bronchial aspiration

- May present with unilateral bronchospasm.
- Could account for the higher incidence in children and during abdominal surgery.

Anaphylactic and anaphylactoid reactions

- Bronchospasm is the first sign in 25% of reactions.
- Bronchospasm is the sole feature in 8% of reactions.

Drugs

- β-adrenergic blockers: inhibition of β_2-mediated bronchodilatation.
- Neostigmine: muscarinic effect if inadequately blocked by anticholinergic drugs.
- Non-steroidal anti-inflammatory drugs (NSAIDs): contraindicated in patients with aspirin-induced asthma (beware of the 'aspirin triad' of asthma, nasal polyps and aspirin intolerance).

Table 30.9 Incidence of bronchospasm

Age group (years)	Studied variable	Incidence of bronchospasm (per 1000 cases)
0–9	Organic heart disease	15.3
	Abnormal ECG	24.3
	Respiratory infection	41.1
	Obstructive lung disease	21.9
	Tracheal intubation	9.1
50–69	Previous myocardial infarction	5.4
	Obstructive lung disease	7.7

- Overall, up to 1 in 10 adult asthmatics will react adversely to various drugs.

Regional techniques

- Bronchospasm has been reported during solely regional techniques.
- Reports of bronchospasm occurring during spinal and epidural anaesthesia exist.
- Psychological factors may trigger bronchospasm in asthmatics.

Clinical features

- Tachypnoea or laboured respiration.
- Intercostal recession.
- Expiratory wheeze.
- Increased airway pressure.
- Decreased compliance.
- Ventilation and oxygenation become increasingly difficult.
- Hypoxia and cyanosis.
- Air trapping with hyperinflation of the chest.
- Acute pulmonary hypertension and reduced venous return due to elevated intrathoracic pressure result in a fall in cardiac output in the severest cases.
- Pneumothorax due to barotrauma (suspect pneumothorax if there is a sudden deterioration).

Management

The action to be taken depends on the severity of the bronchospasm and the availability of equipment and agents. The majority of cases occur as a reflex response to airway instrumentation or surgery and are relatively mild. They are managed simply by temporarily interrupting surgery and deepening anaesthesia. Further methods are indicated if there is an inadequate response.

General management

- Give 100% oxygen and summon help if required.
- Exclude upper airway and breathing and circuit problems.
- Exclude other important differential diagnoses (Table 30.10).

Specific management

Volatile agents

- All are effective bronchodilators.
- Many patients respond to an increase in the inspired concentration.
- Isoflurane is the least arrhythmogenic and is the agent of choice if using epinephrine.

β_2-adrenoreceptor agonists

- Salbutamol
  - 250 μg i.v. (4 μg kg^{-1})
  - intravenous infusion (5–20 μg min^{-1})
  - nebulized in circuit (2.5–5 mg).
- Terbutaline (250–500 μg i.v.).

Aminophylline

- May not give additional bronchodilatation if volatile agents are being used.
- Inferior to β_2-adrenoreceptor agonists.
- Administer 5 mg kg^{-1} slowly intravenously.

Corticosteroids

- Of benefit in acute bronchospasm, although the mechanism of action is unclear.
- Onset of action not as rapid as other agents.
- Hydrocortisone (200–500 mg i.v.) or methylprednisolone (1 g i.v.) single dose.

Epinephrine

- First-line agent in severe reactions and in anaphylaxis.
- Give 3–5 mL of 1:10 000 intravenously (adult).

Table 30.10 Differential diagnosis of bronchospasm

Diagnosis	Notes
Upper airway obstruction	Chin lift, jaw thrust, insert airway
Obstructed laryngeal mask	Reposition – if in doubt, remove
Obstructed tracheal tube	Verify patency – pass suction catheter, pass bronchoscope. If in doubt, remove
Breathing circuit malfunction	Check equipment
Breathing circuit obstruction	Check equipment
Tension pneumothorax	Airway pressure, auscultate chest
Oesophageal intubation	Observe capnograph trace

Ketamine

- Powerful bronchodilator.
- Consider if there is a poor response to other agents.

Ventilation

- Give 100% oxygen.

Aim to reduce any risk of barotrauma and maintain oxygenation:

- use a low frequency of ventilation with a long expiratory time (minimizes pulmonary distension)
- use low tidal volumes to limit airway pressures.

A degree of hypercapnia is acceptable, provided that oxygenation is maintained. The minute volume can be increased as the bronchospasm resolves.

'Educated-hand' manual ventilation may produce better oxygenation with higher minute volumes and lower airway pressures than mechanical ventilation.

In the most severe cases, expiration due to passive recoil of lung and thorax cannot occur – manual deflation of the chest may buy time (best with two people):

- inflate with 100% oxygen
- disconnect tracheal tube
- squeeze lateral aspects of chest for 10–15 seconds
- repeat this cycle.

Worst-case scenario: catastrophic bronchospasm with the risk of severe barotrauma – cardiac arrest is imminent. Consider cardiopulmonary bypass, if available.

Bibliography

Entrup MH, Davis FG. Perioperative complications of anaesthesia. *Surg Clin North Am* 1991; **71**: 1151–73.

Grover A, Canavan C. Critical incidents: the respiratory system. *Anaesth Intensive Care Med* 2007; **8**: 352–7.

Olsson GL. Bronchospasm during anaesthesia. A computer-aided incidence study of 136,929 patients. *Acta Anaesthesiol Scand* 1987; **31**: 244–52.

Cross-reference

Asthma, 105

Intraoperative hypertension

Brian J Pollard

Episodes of hypertension are relatively common during anaesthesia. Whether it is ultimately harmful to the patient depends on its degree, cause and duration, and on the condition of the patient. These factors also govern how actively it is treated.

The definition of an episode of hypertension is generally defined as an elevation of blood pressure over 15% of the patient's baseline (the baseline being determined by a series of recordings) or a systolic BP greater than 160 mmHg and/or a diastolic BP greater than 95 mmHg.

The blood pressure (mean arterial blood pressure (MAP)) is determined by the systemic vascular resistance (SVR) and cardiac output (CO) according to the equation (after Ohm's law)

$$MAP = SVR \times CO$$

The commonest cause of an increase in MAP is a raised SVR as a result of vasoconstriction. A raised BP does not imply a raised CO. Indeed, the increased afterload due to vasoconstriction often causes a reduced CO.

Complications of intraoperative hypertension

- Myocardial ischaemia (especially subendocardial), myocardial infarction or heart failure.
- Haemorrhage from the operation site.
- Rupture of an existing aneurysm.
- Encephalopathy, cerebral oedema or cerebral haemorrhage.
- Severe hypertension may precipitate acute renal failure.

Management

If severe and life-threatening (e.g. MAP >150 mmHg with signs of myocardial ischaemia), immediate therapy is warranted. Otherwise the cause should be sought and treated if possible. Confirmation of the diagnosis may require a trial of one therapy. If there is no definite diagnosis, non-specific therapy may need to be instituted.

Causes

Inadequate anaesthesia/analgesia

- This is the commonest cause. It usually accompanies a change in level of stimulation (e.g. movement of endotracheal tube) or a waning of drug effect. It is usually associated with tachycardia (bradycardia if vagal tone increased), lacrimation, tachypnoea, movement or laryngospasm.
- Treatment may include increasing anaesthesia and/or analgesia (e.g. remifentanil) or consider reducing stimulation.

Anxiety during local anaesthetic techniques

Reassure the patient and give sedation, if necessary.

Inadequate ventilation

Carbon dioxide retention causing catecholamine release.

Treatment

- Check equipment and correct fault.
- Optimize airway/ventilation.
- Consider instituting intermittent positive pressure ventilation (IPPV).

Omission of regular antihypertensive medicine

- This may cause rebound hypertension (particularly clonidine).
- Assess preoperative therapy and administer appropriate drug, or use non-specific therapy.

Drug interaction

- For example, monoamine oxygenase inhibitors plus vasopressors or opioids (especially pethidine).
- May require drug therapy (e.g. β-blockers or sodium nitroprusside).

Drugs given by surgeon (e.g. for haemostasis)

- For example, epinephrine infiltration.
- A β-blocker may be indicated

Drug error/side-effect

The wrong drug, dose or mode of administration. Ketamine, ergotamine, desflurane anaesthesia (greater than 1.0 MAC), etc. may cause hypertension.

Treatment

- Careful handling and labelling of all drugs.
- Use dedicated intravenous lines or locate connection close to patient to reduce the risk of variable administration rate.

Artefact

- Use of the wrong size BP cuff.
- Resonance in the arterial catheter.
- Incorrect zero point.

Management

- Use appropriate cuff.
- Calibrate arterial line and compare with cuff BP.
- Use correct tubing or clamping device.
- Check zero point.

Tourniquet pain

- Slow onset, often after 1 hour.
- Bilateral tourniquets with exsanguination may cause sufficient fluid shift to increase blood pressure.

Treatment

- Consult with surgeon.
- May need drug therapy.

Pre-eclampsia

- Treat with a non-specific hypotensive agent.
- See Induced hypotension during anaesthesia, p. 711.

Phaeochromocytoma

- A rare but important cause.
- Undiagnosed phaeochromocytoma is associated with a high perioperative mortality (c. 50%).

Treatment

- If suspected, a small bolus dose of phentolamine (2.5–5 mg) usually gives a significant fall in BP (if systolic BP falls more than 35 mmHg, phaeochromocytoma is likely).
- Give α-blockers in addition to β-blockade (β-blockade alone may worsen vasoconstriction).
- Remifentanil may be useful.

Rare causes

- Fluid overload.
- Aortic cross-clamping.
- Hyperthyroid storm.
- Malignant hyperthermia.
- Raised intracranial pressure.
- Interference with carotid body or brainstem or spinal cord.
- Bladder distension (especially postoperatively).
- Alcohol or addictive drug withdrawal.
- Autonomic hyper-reflexia.

Non-specific treatment

If the cause of hypertension cannot be removed or diagnosed, the following may be useful.

Vasodilators

- Anaesthetic agents (e.g. isoflurane, sevoflurane, propofol): easy to control.
- Hydralazine: arteriolar dilator, peak action after about 20 minutes following 5–10 mg i.v.
- Glyceryl trinitrate: arterial and venous dilator; dose 10–200 μg min^{-1}.
- Nifedipine: sublingual or intranasal; onset 1–5 min following a 10 mg dose.
- Labetalol: combined α- and β-blockade; dose 5–20 mg i.v.
- Sodium nitroprusside: arteriolar dilator; very rapid response; administer by continuous intravenous infusion (0.5 mg kg^{-1} min^{-1} starting dose); larger doses may cause cyanide poisoning.

β-blockers

- Propranolol: non-selective; dose 0.5–1 mg i.v.
- Esmolol: rapid onset; short half-life (9 minutes); 500 μg kg^{-1} loading dose; 50–780 μg kg^{-1} min^{-1} infusion.
- Metoprolol: cardioselective (β_1); 5–15 mg i.v.

α-blockers

- Phentolamine (0.2–2 mg i.v.).

Analgesics

- Remifentanil.

Ganglionic blockers

- Trimetaphan (1–5 mg i.v.).

Postoperative care

- Continue to monitor patient.
- Provide adequate analgesia.
- Administer face-mask oxygen (reduce myocardial ischaemia).
- May need continuing therapy.
- May need investigations to exclude complications (e.g. myocardial infarctions) or to identify cause of hypertension.

Cross-reference

Hypertension, 151

Local anaesthetic toxicity

Brian J Pollard

Considering the large numbers of local anaesthetics administered, the frequency of toxic reactions is very small. The most important considerations are central nervous system (CNS) and cardiac toxicity. Causes of such toxicity are related to elevated plasma drug levels. This is the result of:

- accidental (or misinformed) overdose
- inadvertent intravenous injection.

There is a general relationship between plasma levels of local anaesthetics and symptoms and signs of toxicity (Table 30.11).

Initial excitation is due to selective inhibition of inhibitory pathways in the CNS. With increasing blood levels, there is an inhibition of both inhibitory and facilitatory pathways, leading to generalized CNS depression.

However, although a general relationship between blood levels and toxicity exists, the rate of injection (if intravenous) or uptake also influences the chance of toxicity; for example, a faster rate of injection produces signs of toxicity at lower venous plasma levels.

Methods of reducing plasma levels

Uptake is highest with concentrated solutions:

- saturation of local binding sites
- greater intrinsic vasodilating effects.

Uptake is highest from vascular sites, such as the epidural and intercostal spaces, and least from subcutaneous tissues.

The principal technique for minimizing plasma levels is to reduce vascular uptake by the addition of epinephrine.

Pharmacology of local anaesthetic toxicity

- Potency varies directly with lipid solubility.
- Cardiac depression and CNS excitability varies directly with potency.

The mechanism for cardiac depression is unclear, but some experiments suggest that it may be related to decreased intracellular calcium. In addition, at high plasma levels, there will be generalized vasodilatation compounding the vascular collapse.

The relative potencies of bupivacaine and lidocaine are about 4:1, which is similar to their relative CNS toxicities. Both the blood levels required for cardiac toxicity and the ratio of the doses required for cardiac toxicity compared with doses required for CNS toxicity suggest that bupivacaine is considerably more cardiotoxic than lidocaine, ropivacaine or levobupivacaine.

Influence of acidosis

- The convulsive threshold is decreased.
- An increase in P_aco_2 leads to an increase in cerebral blood flow (CBF), thus allowing more drug to enter the brain.

Table 30.11 The effect of increasing plasma drug levels

Symptom/sign	Drug level
Tingling in tongue and perioral region	Low
Dizziness	↓
Blurred vision	↓
Tinnitus	↓
Twitching and signs of CNS excitation	Intermediate
Loss of consciousness	↓
Convulsions	↓
Deep coma	↓
Respiratory and cardiac arrest	High

- A decrease in intracellular pH will increase the amount of ionized drug; this limits diffusion and prevents drug leaving the cell.
- Decreased plasma protein binding results in more free drug.

Thus, acidosis increases the chances of developing CNS toxicity and also prolongs the toxicity.

Clinical aspects of local anaesthetic toxicity

Sensible precautions

- All resuscitation facilities and drugs must be available.
- Access to circulation should be secured before initiation of the procedure.
- Trained assistance should be available.
- Maintain dialogue with the patient during performance of the block.

Prevention

- Careful technique.
- Aspirate before injection and intermittently aspirate during prolonged injection if large volumes are used.
- Choice of drug, e.g. do not use bupivacaine for intravenous regional anaesthesia.

Ester local anaesthetics are metabolized by plasma cholinesterase. Thus, if toxic plasma levels are achieved, the toxic reaction should be short lived (except in the rare case of atypical cholinesterase).

Recognizing toxicity

- CNS: sudden alteration in mental state (agitation, loss of consciousness, convulsion).
- Cardiovascular system: cardiovascular collapse (bradycardia, tachycardia, asystole, VF).

Treatment

Minor reactions

- Stop the injection.
- Observe the patient.

Major reactions

- Stop the injection.
- Give 100% oxygen.
- Call for help if necessary.
- Resuscitate according to standard guidelines (airway, breathing, circulation).
- Treat convulsions (e.g. thiopental, propofol, diazepam).
- Intravenous fluids, inotropes and vasopressors may be needed.
- If a cardiac arrest occurs then proceed to ALS protocol.
- Prolonged CPR and resuscitation may be required.
- Give an immediate intravenous bolus of 20% lipid emulsion 1.5 mg kg^{-1}.
- Start an intravenous infusion of 20% lipid emulsion at 15 mL kg^{-1} h^{-1}.
- If cardiovascular instability continues the intravenous bolus of lipid emulsion may be repeated twice at 5 minute intervals. The infusion rate may be increased to 30 mL kg^{-1} h^{-1}.
- Do not exceed a maximum dose of 12 mL kg^{-1} of 20% lipid emulsion.

Lidocaine

- Is a potent antiarrhythmic agent.
- Arrhythmias are uncommon after overdosage.
- At high plasma levels, decreased cardiac conduction may be seen.

Bupivacaine

- *S* isomer of bupivacaine is less toxic than the *R* isomer of bupivacaine.
- May potentiate arrhythmias.
- Exact mechanism is unknown.
- Markedly depresses the rapid phase of depolarization of the cardiac action potential and prolongs the refractory period.
- May cause one-way block leading to re-entrant arrhythmias.
- Ventricular fibrillation is common in severe toxicity.
- Pregnant women are more sensitive to cardiotoxicity.

Bupivacaine seems to be significantly associated with cardiac toxicity compared with other local anaesthetics. CPR is very difficult in bupivacaine-induced cardiotoxicity because the drug binds to cardiac muscle (exacerbated by acidosis).

Ropivacaine

This amide drug is intermediate in structure and potency to mepivacaine and bupivacaine. It is represented as the S isomer rather than a racemic mixture.

- Aggressive CPR may be successful with ropivacaine cardiotoxicity.
- Larger doses are required to produce early features of CNS toxicity and cardiotoxicity.
- Animal studies show a similar cardiotoxicity profile in both the pregnant and non-pregnant state.
- Produces greater differential block with the motor block being less intense and of shorter duration.

Levobupivacaine

- Single *S* isomer of bupivacaine.
- Long acting.
- Intermediate in toxicity.
- Human volunteer studies suggest lesser cardiac depression with smaller changes in the indices of cardiac contractility than bupivacaine.
- Human studies also suggest lesser CNS depression than bupivacaine.
- Lethal dose is higher than bupivacaine.

Bibliography

Association of Anaesthetists of Great Britain and Ireland. *Management of Severe Local Anaesthetic Toxicity*. London: AAGBI, 2010. See aagbi.org/publications/guidelines.htm

Gristwood RW. Cardiac and CNS toxicity of levobupivacaine. *Drug Saf* 2002; **25**(3): 153–63.

Moore DC. Administer oxygen first in the treatment of local anaesthesia induced convulsions. *Anesthesiology* 1980; **53**: 346–7.

Richards A, McConachie I. The pharmacology of local anaesthetic drugs. *Curr Anaesth Crit Care* 1995; **6**: 41–7.

Scott DB. Maximum recommended doses of local anaesthetic drugs. *Br J Anaesth* 1989; **63**: 373–4.

Whiteside JB, Wildsmith JAW. Developments in local anaesthetic drugs. *Br J Anaesth* 2001; **87**: 27–35.

Cross-reference

Regional anaesthetic techniques, 719

Malignant hyperthermia: clinical presentation

Philip M Hopkins

Because of the reduction in major morbidity and mortality from other causes, malignant hyperthermia (MH) is now one of the major potential anaesthetic hazards for the otherwise healthy individual. This is despite the mortality from MH declining from above 70% prior to 1980 to below 4% currently. It is argued by some that, with the use of modern monitoring equipment and the mandatory availability of intravenous dantrolene, mortality from MH should be zero.

The key to prevention of death from an MH reaction undoubtedly is recognition by the attending anaesthetist of the early signs of the reaction followed by an appropriate therapeutic response. It is interesting to note that the rapid decline in mortality in the UK began before the introduction of intravenous dantrolene: this is attributed to increasing awareness of the condition among UK anaesthetists.

MH is now known to be a genetically heterogeneous disorder. More than 30 different mutations of the major gene implicated in MH susceptibility (*RYR1* – the sarcoplasmic reticulum calcium release channel gene) have been reported, but in many MH families the precise molecular defect is yet to be determined. The result of each defect is, however, the same and that is to cause an uncontrollable rise in intracellular calcium ion concentration in skeletal muscle cells in the presence of the triggering drugs (any potent inhalation anaesthetic drug or succinylcholine). This rise in myoplasmic calcium ion concentration is sufficient to explain all the clinical and biochemical features of MH, knowledge of which is so crucial if an anaesthetist is to have the best chance of successfully managing a MH reaction.

The nature and course of MH reactions show considerable variation. The components of a reaction can be very crudely divided into metabolic and muscle activity, both of which lead to rhabdomyolysis. The balance and severity of metabolic and muscle activity components generally varies according to which triggering drugs have been used. This is assumed to be a reflection of the dynamics of the rise in intracellular calcium ion concentration.

The response to succinylcholine

Succinylcholine is thought to produce a rapid and marked rise in intracellular calcium, but its duration of effect is limited. The predominant feature is thus increased muscle activity evident as rigidity. This muscle rigidity is sometimes generalized, but may be limited to the jaw muscles (see Masseter muscle spasm, p. 772). Because of the limited duration of effect of succinylcholine, homeostatic mechanisms restore the intracellular calcium towards resting levels, usually within 10 minutes. The muscle activity leads to extrusion of potassium ions, creatine kinase and myoglobin. The hyperkalaemia due to succinylcholine alone usually is not life-threatening (unlike with the muscular dystrophies in which succinylcholine can cause grossly elevated serum potassium concentration), but the myoglobinaemia may be sufficient to cause acute renal failure. Indeed, postoperative renal failure has been the only presenting feature in some MH-susceptible patients. Serum creatine kinase is an indicator of the degree of muscle damage, reaching a maximum (often >20 000 units) after about 24 hours. Although metabolic processes will have been stimulated, the duration of the stimulus is so short that the resulting clinical features are mild and usually not noticed.

The response to potent inhalation anaesthetics

The nature of the response to potent inhalation anaesthetics suggests that they cause a steadily increasing intracellular calcium ion concentration. Calcium, at concentrations lower than those required to activate the contractile apparatus, has other important intracellular functions. One of these is the regulation of the phosphorylation, and hence the activity, of various enzymes, including rate-limiting enzymes of the glycolytic pathway. During a gradually increasing intracellular calcium ion concentration, the first detectable features result from this metabolic stimulation: the earliest clinical signs are caused by increased carbon dioxide and lactate production. In the spontaneously breathing patient, there will be an increasing respiratory rate, while where a circle system is in use the soda lime will be rapidly exhausted. Whatever mode of ventilation and breathing system is being used, the increased carbon dioxide production will be detected as an increasing end-tidal partial pressure of carbon dioxide by capnography. Either simultaneously with, or shortly following, the hypercapnoea, a tachycardia develops secondary to the effects of acidaemia on the cardiovascular regulatory centre of the midbrain. By the same mechanism there is a tendency for the blood pressure to rise, although in some cases the blood pressure falls, presumably because of a predominant effect of local metabolites on the vascular smooth muscle. As well as an increase in lactate and carbon dioxide as by-products of metabolism, there is an increase in oxygen consumption that may lead to a fall in the saturation of haemoglobin with oxygen, detectable with pulse oximetry. Arterial blood gases taken at this stage will show acidaemia, hypercarbia, a base deficit and, usually, mild hypoxaemia.

The name, malignant hyperthermia, was originally coined because the most obvious clinical feature was that patients would become excessively hot and then they invariably died. This was, of course, at a time when monitoring during routine anaesthesia was purely clinical. We now know that hyperthermia resulting from the hypermetabolic state is a relatively late manifestation and, whereas during the 1970s and early 1980s monitoring of body temperature was advised for every anaesthetic, capnography has now superseded it. However, when some doubt exists as to whether some metabolic signs are due to MH, the finding of a rapidly rising body temperature is very persuasive, although, as indicated above, in some cases there is a delay before the rate of temperature rise becomes remarkable.

It is commonly considered that there is a stage of a MH reaction beyond which death is almost inevitable: this is likely to relate to the integrity of the mitochondria. In the early stages of the reaction, mitochondria respond to the increased production of pyruvate by increasing its utilization to produce more ATP. This is important in limiting the intracellular calcium ion concentration as ATP is required for the normal functioning of two of the most important mechanisms for removing calcium from the myoplasm: the calcium pumps of the sarcolemma, and the sarcoplasmic reticulum. The mitochondria themselves, however, also sequester calcium ions, the rate being entirely dependent on the myoplasmic calcium ion concentration. In the presence of continued release or influx of calcium into the myoplasm the intramitochondrial calcium ion concentration will continue to increase until the accumulated calcium disrupts the mitochondria. A situation is thus reached where glycolysis is stimulated and the only route for further metabolism of pyruvate is to lactate. Simultaneously, there is a rapid decline in ATP production, leading to a reduced rate of calcium removal from the myoplasm, and hence setting up a vicious cycle. It is at this stage that muscle rigidity will become apparent. Muscle rigidity itself restricts microvascular perfusion of the tissue, in which case dantrolene administered intravenously will not reach its site of action. The perfusion of the muscle will also be compromised as muscles swell within their fascial compartments as a result of the oedema associated with mitochondrial failure and cell death.

Calcium ions also stimulate activity of some intracellular phospholipases, leading to increased turnover of sarcolemmal phospholipid. Under these circumstances, maintenance of the integrity of the sarcolemma is an ATP-dependent process, and when the demand for ATP exceeds the supply, the membrane permeability increases. This will result in increased leakage of calcium into the cell and also leakage out of intracellular constituents such as potassium ions, creatine kinase and myoglobin. The resulting hyperkalaemia at this stage can be sufficient to cause cardiac arrest while, if the acute reaction is survived, the myoglobinaemia can result in renal failure.

A further feature of an advanced MH reaction is DIC. Heat itself and/or procoagulant proteins that leak from dying muscle cells can cause DIC.

The response to the potent inhalation anaesthetics tends to be more rapid following succinylcholine, with some florid reactions occurring within 15 minutes. In the laboratory setting, halothane certainly seems to be the most potent trigger of the potent inhalation anaesthetics, but clinical responses to enflurane, isoflurane and sevoflurane can be indistinguishable from those caused by halothane. Cases of human MH have been triggered by desflurane, but these are too few to comment on this drug's comparative potency or efficacy as an MH trigger.

Bibliography

Glahn KPE, Ellis FR, Halsall PJ, *et al.* Recognising and managing a malignant hyperthermia crisis: Guidelines from the European Malignant Hyperthermia Group. *Br J Anaesth* 2010; **105**: 417–20.

Hopkins PM. Malignant hyperthermia: advances in clinical management and diagnosis. *Br J Anaesth* 2000; **85**: 118–28.

Cross-reference

Masseter muscle spasm, 772

Masseter muscle spasm

Philip M Hopkins

The major problem with masseter muscle spasm (MMS) is in defining what it means. The first common usage of the term arose when MH reactions subsequently occurred in patients whose mouths had been difficult to open following the use of succinylcholine. This association was apparent in 70% of patients given succinylcholine who went on to develop MH. Awareness of this association between MMS and MH led to referral of many patients who developed MMS for investigation of their MH status. Of those with MMS as the only abnormal feature, 28% have proven to be susceptible to MH. This figure rises to 57% if there were accompanying metabolic features, or 76% if the MMS was followed by other features of muscle damage, such as myoglobinuria or severe incapacity from muscle pains. From this experience, which is similar among MH investigation centres, it seemed clear that patients developing MMS were at high risk from MH until proven otherwise. However, at that stage there was no definition of what was meant by MMS.

The situation really started to become confusing in the late 1980s with the publication of studies in which the tension developed by the jaw muscles following succinylcholine was found to rise in virtually all children and in a large proportion of adults. The unfortunate outcome of these studies was that some interpreted the results as meaning that most patients develop MMS following succinylcholine. The next stage in this trail of false logic was to extrapolate this interpretation for comparison with the incidence of MH in patients referred because of MMS. The result of this erroneous comparison could only be that the incidence of MH in the population was much higher than previously thought, or that the *in vitro* contracture tests used for MH diagnosis had a very high false-positive response rate.

A more consistent explanation can be realized by examining how patients came to be investigated for their MH status following an episode of 'MMS'. These cases were not those in which there was a measured increase in jaw muscle tension, rather they were cases in which the attending anaesthetist experienced a clinical problem in opening the mouth in order to achieve tracheal intubation. Prior to the publications by van der Spek *et al.* (1987) and Leary and Ellis (1990), the commonly encountered mild and transient resistance to mouth opening following injection of succinylcholine was probably attributed to a failure of relaxation rather than to muscle tension development. The cases referred for MH investigation were therefore outside the normal experience of the attending anaesthetist in terms of the severity and duration of the difficulty in mouth opening.

The term 'MMS' is therefore of practical and clinical significance only if its use is restricted to severe and, perhaps more importantly, prolonged (more than 2 minutes) episodes of resistance to mouth opening following succinylcholine.

Another misleading feature of the relationship between MMS and MH is the lack of metabolic response following MMS. This is a reflection of the disproportionate effect of succinylcholine as an MH triggering drug in terms of the balance between increased muscle activity and increased metabolic activity (see Malignant hyperthermia: clinical presentation, p. 770). Also, a metabolic response may not be observed even if the anaesthetic is continued with volatile drugs, as we know that patients susceptible to MH do not have a reaction with every exposure to triggering drugs. The reasons for this are not clear.

Management of masseter muscle spasm

Immediate

The patient who has been given succinylcholine will obviously be paralysed, so the first priority is ventilation of the lungs. Fortunately, upper airway muscle tone seems to be maintained, thereby making ventilation with a face-mask via the nose a viable proposition.

Differential diagnosis

Establish that the correct dose of succinylcholine has been given, intravenously; check the ampoule, syringe and injection site. It is, however, unusual for mouth opening to be a major problem even when no neuromuscular blocking drug has been given, unless the dose of induction agent was also inadequate: this would of course occur if a cannula had become dislodged from its intravenous site during induction.

Further anaesthetic management

This will depend on the urgency of the surgery and the feasibility of continuing non-urgent surgery without the use of volatile anaesthetic drugs. If the surgery is not urgent and continuation with a volatile-free technique potentially compromising, the patient should be allowed to wake up. Should the surgery need to proceed, then ventilation should continue via the face-mask until the spasm has eased, when a non-depolarizing neuromuscular blocker can be given and intubation subsequently achieved. Anaesthesia should be maintained with intravenous drugs.

Recording of diagnostic predictors

Although the patient who develops MMS must be considered to be potentially susceptible to MH until proven otherwise, evidence of metabolic stimulation and other indicators of increased muscle activity increase the likelihood of MH. Therefore, the patient should be immediately observed for the presence of generalized muscle rigidity and the duration of MMS should be recorded. An accurate chart of heart rate, blood pressure, pulse oximeter, capnograph and central temperature readings should be made. Blood for arterial blood gas and serum potassium analysis should be sent. In the postoperative period, the first voided urine should be analysed for the presence of myoglobin and the serum creatine kinase should be estimated at 12 and 24 hours.

Further investigations

Patients should be referred for determination of their MH status by muscle biopsy and *in vitro* contracture testing. They should be advised that they and all members of the family should be treated as potentially susceptible to MH until proven otherwise. In the interim, the reactor should undergo electromyographic studies to exclude congenital myotonia, some variants of which can be asymptomatic.

Bibliography

Christian AS, Halsall PJ, Ellis FR. Is there a relationship between masseter muscle spasm and malignant hyperthermia? *Br J Anaesth* 1989; **62**: 540–4.

Leary NP, Ellis FR. Masseteric muscle spasm as a normal response to suxamethonium. *Br J Anaesth* 1990; **64**: 488–92.

van der Spek AFL, Fang WB, Ashton-Miller JA, *et al.* The effect of succinylcholine on mouth opening. *Anesthesiology* 1987; **67**: 459–65.

Cross-reference

Malignant hyperthermia: clinical presentation, 770

Neuroleptic malignant syndrome

Brian J Pollard

Neuroleptic malignant syndrome (NMS) was first described in 1960 by Delay. It is a rare, potentially fatal condition caused either by treatment with dopamine receptor antagonists or by withdrawal of dopamine receptor agonists.

Pathogenesis

Central mechanisms

There is acute dopaminergic transmission block in the:

- nigrostriatum, which produces rigidity
- hypothalamus, which produces hyperthermia
- corticolimbic system, which produces an altered mental state.

Peripheral mechanisms

The clinical similarities between NMS and MH suggest a common pathophysiological element. *In vitro* halothane-caffeine contracture tests carried out on NMS and MH patients have not, however, supported any intracellular association between the two syndromes.

The pathophysiological mechanism underlying the skeletal muscle rigidity in NMS is controversial. The current view leans towards this being central in origin. This is supported by the observation that neuromuscular blocking drugs produce flaccid paralysis in NMS, whereas in MH they have no effect.

Excitatory amino acids

There is now believed to be a relative glutaminergic transmission excess as a consequence of a dopaminergic block and it may be that drugs which antagonize glutamate have beneficial effects.

Incidence

Approximately 0.5–1%.

Clinical features and diagnosis

NMS usually develops over a period of 24–72 hours following exposure to neuroleptic agents. This exposure can have been over a period of days or months and may even follow a low dose of a neuroleptic agent. The features may continue for up to 10 days, even after stopping the triggering agent (Table 30.12).

Mortality

Figures of 8–30% are frequently quoted, but the number of deaths has declined since 1984 (less than 11% now, versus 25% before 1984). These figures are apparently independent of the use of dopamine agonists and dantrolene.

Mortality from NMS is due to:

- respiratory failure (commonest cause)
- renal failure secondary to myoglobinuria (a strong predictor of mortality, representing a risk of 50%)
- cardiac arrest.

Other complications are outlined in Box 30.8.

Box 30.8 Complications

- Respiratory
  - Secondary infection
  - Aspiration pneumonia
- Cardiovascular
  - Cardiac arrhythmias
  - Pulmonary embolism
- Musculoskeletal
  - Peripheral neuropathy
  - Rhabdomyolysis → myoglobinuria

Table 30.12 Criteria for diagnosis of neuroleptic malignant syndrome

Major criteria	Minor criteria
High fever	Tachycardia
Muscular rigidity	Raised blood pressure
Elevated serum creatine kinase*	Tachypnoea Altered consciousness level Sweating

*No specific laboratory markers exist. Creatine kinase may be mildly or grossly elevated.

Differential diagnosis

Early diagnosis and distinction from other conditions presenting in a similar fashion is crucial in order to prevent fatalities.

Neuroleptic malignant syndrome versus lethal catatonia

Rigidity is intermittent in lethal catatonia. Lethal catatonia demonstrates severe psychotic excitement in the early stages.

Malignant hyperthermia versus neuroleptic malignant syndrome

Compared with MH, NMS demonstrates:

- slow onset
- rigidity of central origin (controversial)
- latency of effect with dantrolene
- uneventful anaesthesia with MH triggering agents
- lack of familial tendency (MH is autosomal dominant).

Drugs of abuse

Ethanol withdrawal, sedative hypnotic withdrawal, cocaine and amphetamine intoxication or monoamine oxidase overdoses must be excluded before NMS is diagnosed. Some of these agents may also release central serotonin, resulting in the central serotonin syndrome.

Neuroleptic heat-stroke

Flaccid muscle tone is the major distinguishing feature.

Management

Non-specific therapy

- Withdrawal of trigger agent.
- Basic resuscitation measures.
- Cooling.

Specific therapy

Dopamine agonists

- Bromocriptine has reduced death rates to below 8%.
- Amantadine has reduced death rates to below 6%.

Dantrolene and bromocriptine

Dantrolene has reduced the death rate to below 9%. It may, however, cause hepatic damage (altered liver enzymes are already present in NMS). The success of dantrolene supports the 'muscle hypothesis', but the time to clinical effect is slow (several days).

Bromocriptine may be the type of choice in patients with NMS associated with hepatic dysfunction.

The relative reduction in death rate holds up at all the levels of syndrome severity in both the dantrolene and bromocriptine groups.

Anticholinergic agents

These drugs are best avoided when rigidity is associated with pyrexia.

Glutamate antagonists

Amantadine and memantine are antagonists at the N-methyl-D-aspartate type of glutamate receptor. They:

- restore the balance between glutaminergic and dopaminergic systems when dopaminergic transmission has been antagonized by neuroleptic drugs
- exhibit hypothermic and central muscle relaxant properties.

These drugs could therefore be effective in the reversal of NMS.

Electroconvulsive therapy

This is controversial, and may only be treating early psychosis following neuroleptic withdrawal rather than NMS.

Re-exposure to trigger agent

Withdrawal of a neuroleptic agent, when treatment is required for severely psychotic patients, is obviously hazardous.

Mortality following reintroduction is variable (17–87%). Mortality may be reduced by:

- low-potency neuroleptic agents
- lowest possible dose of neuroleptic agent
- monitoring of creatine kinase levels.

Anaesthesia

Anaesthetists need to be aware of this syndrome in the context of anaesthesia for ECT. It is important to note that the technique of anaesthesia must not aggravate the muscle disorder or produce the complications of NMS.

It is advisable to avoid succinylcholine in the presence of active muscle disease, as it may release potassium into the circulation and cause rhabdomyolysis. Propofol is best avoided in ECT as it shortens the duration of seizures and increases the frequency of treatment.

Main points

- The pathogenesis of NMS is still not fully understood.
- Early diagnosis is crucial.
- Differential diagnosis remains problematical in the absence of suitable animal models and biological markers for NMS.

- Anaesthesia for NMS patients may continue safely in presence of MH trigger agents.
- The cornerstones of management are withdrawal of the trigger agent and supportive therapy; pharmacological therapy is merely adjunctive.
- Reintroduction of NMS trigger agents is possible, but must be done cautiously.

Bibliography

Adnet P, Lestavel P, Krivosic-Horber R. Neuroleptic malignant syndrome. *Br J Anaesth* 2000; **85**: 129–35.

Anderson WH. Lethal catatonia and the neuroleptic syndrome. *Crit Care Med* 1991; **19**: 1333–4.

Dickey W. The neuroleptic malignant syndrome. *Prog Neurobiol* 1991; **36**: 425–36.

Hard C. Neuroleptic malignant syndrome versus malignant hypothermia. *Am J Med* 1991; **91**: 322–3.

Weller M, Kornhuber J. A rationale for NMDA receptor antagonist therapy of the neuroleptic malignant syndrome. *Med Hypotheses* 1992; **38**: 329–33.

Cross-references

Electroconvulsive therapy, 747
Malignant hyperthermia: clinical presentation, 770

Pacing and anaesthesia

Akbar Vohra

Patient characteristics

Most patients have a history of heart disease:

- ischaemia
- cardiomyopathy
- idiopathic
- congenital
- following cardiac surgery.

There may be other associated conditions:

- peripheral vascular disease
- diabetes
- hypertension.

Preoperative evaluation

History

- Surgical operation, especially site.
- Assessment of cardiac disease.

It is wise to refer the patient to the cardiology department to check the pacemaker function and determine any unusual features of the patient or the pacemaker.

Note that these patients cannot undergo MRI.

Pacemaker function

- Reason for insertion.
- Type of pacemaker:
  - demand (synchronous)
  - fixed (asynchronous)
  - defibrillating.
- When inserted: possibility of electrode displacement if within 4 weeks; possibility of battery failure if a long time ago.
- History of vertigo or syncope (possible battery failure).
- Irregular heart rate (possible competition with intrinsic heart rate).

ECG

- May indicate ischaemia or previous myocardial infarction.
- Confirm pacing capture (if pacing rate > intrinsic rate).
- No intrinsic rhythm (patient is pacemaker dependent).
- Only intrinsic rhythm seen: request cardiology department to test pacemaker function.

Chest X-ray

- Usual assessment of heart size and lung fields.
- Continuity of pacing leads; distal tips within cardiac cavity (especially in patients with chest trauma).

Serum potassium

If high, pacing threshold is increased.

Acid–base balance

Changes may affect pacing threshold.

Additional preparation

A magnet has always been recommended. This is used to convert the pacemaker to a fixed rate if necessary. Modern pacemakers, if checked to be functioning normally, should not need this.

Chronotropic drugs

- Atropine (0.5–3.0 mg): may not be effective.
- Isoprenaline (10–100 μg bolus, or 1–10 μg min^{-1} infusion): note that isoprenaline can decrease SVR.
- Ephedrine (3–30 mg): α and β effects.
- Epinephrine (1:200 000; 0.5–1 mL boluses.)

Diathermy

- Attach plate as far away from the chest as possible.
- Ensure that any current flow does not pass near to the pacemaker.
- No diathermy within 25 cm of the pacing box.
- Bipolar is safer than unipolar mode.
- Transurethral resection of the prostate:
  - cutting mode can interfere, use short bursts
  - coagulation mode should not interfere.
- Request surgeon to use short bursts.
- May need to convert the pacing state to fixed mode if diathermy around chest.
- There is a possibility of phantom reprogramming owing to electromagnetic induction.

Perioperative management

Premedication

Not essential. An opioid or benzodiazepine is suitable.

Monitoring

- Routine minimal monitoring, especially peripheral pulse to confirm cardiac output.

- Invasive monitoring if indicated for operation.
- Caution: possibility of entanglement with pacing wires if inserting central venous or pulmonary artery catheters. These should not be used unless absolutely essential.
- Nerve stimulators can interfere with pacing (caution when using for brachial plexus blocks).

Anaesthetic technique

- Consider local anaesthesia.
- Vasodilatation may be poorly tolerated with fixed heart rates.
- Volatile anaesthetics may increase atrioventricular delay and pacing threshold; avoid halothane.
- Total intravenous anaesthesia may be preferable.
- Caution with succinylcholine:
  - acute release of potassium may increase pacing threshold
  - myopotentials during fasciculation may be abnormally sensed.
- Avoid underhydration.

Postoperative management

- Continue with ECG monitoring.
- Check that the pacemaker programme is correct.

Bibliography

Bloomfield P, Bowler GMR. Anaesthetic management of the patient with a permanent pacemaker. *Anaesthesia* 1989; **44**: 42–6.

Shapiro WA, Roizen MT, Singleton MA, *et al.* Intraoperative pacemaker complications. *Anaesthesiology* 1985; **63**: 319–22.

Zaidan JR. Pacemakers. *Anaesthesiology* 1984; **60**: 319–34.

Cross-references

Cardiomyopathy, 136
Coronary artery disease, 146
Patients with pacemakers and implantable debrillators, 161
Preoperative assessment of cardiovascular risk in non-cardiac surgery, 621

Postoperative oliguria

Brian J Pollard

Definition

Postoperatively the metabolic response to surgery produces sodium retention and decreased free water clearance so that a reduction in urine output is common.

The mean postoperative solute load is 600 mOsmol day^{-1} (range 450–750); this will be increased by intravenous electrolyte solutions. The maximum renal concentrating ability is 1200 mOsmol kg^{-1} H_2O, so the minimum urine volume required is:

$$(600 \text{ mOsmol day}^{-1}/1200 \text{ mOsmol kg}^{-1} \text{ H}_2\text{O}) = 0.5 \text{ kg H}_2\text{O day}^{-1} \approx 20 \text{ mL h}^{-1}$$

Oliguria is conveniently defined as a urine output <20 mL h^{-1} for two consecutive hours.

Pathophysiology

Postoperative oliguria may simply reflect the normal neuroendocrine response to trauma, but often implies one or, more commonly, a number of the factors shown in Table 30.13.

A combination of reduced renal blood flow and prior intrinsic renal damage frequently presents as acute tubular necrosis.

Oliguria is most commonly due to renal hypoperfusion and only rarely from withdrawal of diuretic therapy. Total anuria is usually mechanical in origin but rarely may be due to renal artery occlusion or embolism; beware the patient with a single kidney.

Renal hypoperfusion may not produce oliguria if the ability to concentrate is poor:

- prior renal disease
- diuretic therapy
- the elderly
- sickle cell disease.

Table 30.13 General factors associated with acute renal failure

Reduced renal blood flow	Intrinsic renal damage	Obstruction to flow
Hypovolaemia Poor cardiac output Hypotension (beware diabetes/myeloma) Pre-existing renal damage Renal vascular disease (beware ACE inhibitors) Renal vasoconstriction (beware NSAIDs) Liver failure (hepatorenal syndrome) Sepsis	Hypoxia From prerenal causes Renal vein thrombosis Nephrotoxins Aminoglycosides Amphotericin Chemotherapeutic agents NSAIDs Radiocontrast media (beware diabetes/myeloma/low cardiac output) Tissue injury Pancreatitis Haemoglobinuria Myoglobinuria Tumour lysis (uric acid/xanthine/PO_4) Inflammatory nephritides Glomerulonephritis Interstitial nephritis, including drug-induced Polyarteritis Myeloma Sepsis	Renal or ureteric Calculi Clots Necrotic papillae Pelvic surgery Raised intra-abdominal pressure Prostatic enlargement Bladder neck obstruction Blocked drainage system

ACE, angiotensin-converting enzyme; NSAID, non-steroidal anti-inflammatory drug.

Initial assessment

History

Although a single causative factor which is extremely severe can result in acute renal failure, normally there are a number of predisposing factors (Table 30.14).

Check anaesthetic and other charts for episodes of tachycardia with/without hypotension. From estimates of fluid loss, assess whether adequate volumes of appropriate fluids have been given.

Examination

Physical examination and chest X-ray alone are unreliable in assessing the haemodynamic and volume status in the seriously ill patient in whom cardiac filling pressures often bear little relation to blood volume.

Note any of the following:

- cardiorespiratory
  - tachypnoea
  - tachycardia
  - jugular venous pressure
  - hypotension (check for postural drop)
  - third heart sound
  - absent peripheral pulses/vascular bruits
  - sacral or peripheral oedema
  - cool peripheries
  - reduced skin turgor (assess on forehead or neck)
- abdominal
  - tense abdomen
  - palpable bladder
  - obstructed drainage system
- evidence of infection or systemic disease
  - pyrexia
  - sputum production
  - cloudy urine
  - soft-tissue infection
  - vasculitic or drug rash
  - bruising
  - systemic emboli
  - muscle damage
  - ischaemic tissues
  - compartment syndrome.

Investigations

Consider investigations which will aid diagnosis and monitoring. Exclude obstruction if the cause of oliguria is not immediately obvious.

- Ultrasound to assess:
  - hydronephrosis/thrombosis of renal veins
  - bladder size/catheter location.
- Doppler studies may be helpful in some patients.
- Abdominal X-ray for:
  - calculi in ureter/kidney
  - aortoiliac calcification/nephrocalcinosis.

Sepsis screen

- Chest X-ray.
- Blood cultures.
- Sputum culture.
- Mid-stream sample of urine.

Table 30.14 Patient and perioperative factors associated with acute renal failure

Patient factors	Perioperative factors
Advanced age	Hypotension
Aortic surgery	Arrhythmias
Atherosclerosis (especially aortic)	Hypovolaemia
Cardiac surgery	Diuretic therapy
Chronic renal disease	Preoperative starvation
Cirrhosis	Gastric aspiration/vomiting
Diabetes	Third-space losses, e.g. ileus/obstruction/peritoneal exudate
Heart failure	Diarrhoea/bowel preparation
Hepatobiliary surgery/jaundice	Prolonged tissue exposure/surgical oedema
Hypertension	Blood loss
Myeloma	Hypoxia
Nephrotoxic drugs	Tissue damage/inflammation
Pre-eclampsia/eclampsia	Ischaemia and reperfusion
Sepsis	Major burns
	Multiple fractures/muscle damage
	Pancreatitis
	Haemolysis, e.g. transfusion reactions
	Specific surgical complications, e.g. pericardial tamponade

Blood tests

- Arterial blood gases/lactate.
- Full biochemical profile including electrolytes/urea/creatinine/blood sugar/bicarbonate/calcium/phosphate/liver function tests/C-reactive protein.
- Osmolality.
- Haemoglobin/platelets/white blood count including eosinophils.
- Coagulation studies.
- Amylase.
- Creatinine kinase/myoglobin/uric acid.
- Estimate creatinine clearance since plasma creatinine may not reflect glomerular filtration rate, especially in the elderly with little muscle mass. This can be done on 2 hour urine collection.
- Lactate dehydrogenase/haptoglobin/direct and indirect bilirubin if haemolysis suspected.
- Immunoglobulins and electrophoresis to exclude myeloma.
- Isotope investigations, angiography and renal biopsy may be indicated occasionally.

Urine chemistry

- Sodium, urea and creatinine.
- Osmolality.

Urinalysis

- Blood, protein and myoglobin.
- Microscopy to detect crystals and casts in the urine and to assess red cell morphology:
  - hyaline/granular casts: underperfusion/chronic renal damage
  - tubular casts: acute intrinsic renal injury
  - dysmorphic red cells/casts: glomerulonephritis
  - white cell casts: pyelonephritis/possible interstitial nephritis.

Urinary indices

These are relatively imprecise and become inaccurate after mannitol and loop diuretics. Urinary osmolality and sodium concentration are insensitive discriminators between prerenal azotaemia and acute renal failure.

The fractional excretion of sodium (FE_{Na}) is a more accurate guide to renal integrity:

$$FE_{Na} = (U_{Na}/P_{Na})/(U_{Cr}/P_{Cr})$$

where U_{Na} and U_{Cr} are the urinary concentrations of sodium and creatinine and P_{Na} and P_{Cr} are the respective plasma concentrations.

Table 30.15 shows some common urinary indices.

Management

- Catheterize the bladder when convenient.
- Maintain adequate oxygenation and ventilation.
- Maintain intravascular volume but restrict fluids if oliguric acute renal failure is established and the patient is euvolaemic. Consider invasive monitoring early in high-risk groups.
- Assess fluid deficits and correct accordingly. Postoperative patients have an impaired ability to excrete a water load so avoid excessive dextrose administration.
- Maintain an adequate mean arterial blood pressure (a normal blood pressure of 120/80 mmHg equates to a mean arterial pressure of 93 mmHg).
- Initially, aim for a mean arterial pressure of 60–80 mmHg, *or higher if previously hypertensive or with widespread peripheral vascular disease.*
- Induce a diuresis of at least 30 mL h^{-1}; maintaining urine volume will make fluid management easier:
  - mannitol 20 g (200 mL of 10% solution)
  - furosemide bolus up to 250 mg then infuse at 5–100 mg h^{-1}
  - dopamine 200 mg in 50 mL at 3 mL $h^{-1} \approx 3\ \mu g\ kg^{-1}\ min^{-1}$ in a 70 kg patient (note that dopamine will not prevent acute renal failure.
- In myoglobinuria (also with haemolysis or tumour lysis syndrome), alkalinize the urine (pH > 7) with intravenous sodium bicarbonate and/or acetazolamide (up to 250 mg four times daily, although higher doses may cause confusion).
- For urate nephropathy, add allopurinol (200 mg three times daily).

Table 30.15 Common urinary indices

	Underperfusion	Intrinsic renal failure
U/P osmolality	>1.5	<1.1
U/P creatinine	>40	<20
U/P urea	>20	<10
U_{Na} (mmol L^{-1})	<20	>40
FE_{Na} (%)	<1	>3

FE_{Na}, fractional excretion of sodium; *P*, plasma *U*, urinary.

Bibliography

Baek S-M, Makabali GG, Bryan-Brown CW, *et al.* Plasma expansion in surgical patients with high central venous pressure (CVP); the relationship of blood volume to hematocrit, CVP, pulmonary wedge pressure, and cardiorespiratory changes. *Surgery* 1975; **78**: 304–15.

Bellomo R, Chapman M, Finfer S, *et al.* Low-dose dopamine in patients with early renal dysfunction: a placebo-controlled randomised trial. Australian and New Zealand Intensive Care Society (ANZICS) Clinical Trials Group. *Lancet* 2000; **356**: 2139–43.

Bersten AD, Holt AW. Vasoactive drugs and the importance of renal perfusion pressure. *New Horiz* 1995; **3**: 650–61.

Connors AF, McCaffree DR, Gray B. Evaluation of right-heart catheterization in the critically ill patient without acute myocardial infarction. *N Engl J Med* 1983; **308**: 263–7.

Le Gall JR, Klar J, Lemeshow S, *et al.* The Logistic Organ Dysfunction system. A new way to assess organ dysfunction in the intensive care unit. ICU Scoring Group. *JAMA* 1996; **276**: 802–10.

Sladen RN, Endo E, Harrison T. Two-hour versus 22-hour creatinine clearance in critically ill patients. *Anesthesiology* 1987; **67**: 1013–16.

Star RA. Treatment of acute renal failure. *Kidney Int* 1998; **54**:1817–31.

Cross-reference

Fluid and electrolyte balance, 754

Postoperative pain management

Chandran Jepegnanam

The aim of postoperative pain management should be to provide safe, effective, individualized pain relief to enable quick return to appropriate functional activity.

Effects of uncontrolled pain

Pain after surgery is natural, but it is not an inevitable or harmless consequence of surgery. Uncontrolled pain increases sympathetic activity, increases the stress response to injury and has multisystem consequences. Increased sympathetic activity causes tachycardia, hypertension and increased peripheral vascular resistance, leading to increased oxygen demand. This, coupled with decreased supply because of tachycardia, can precipitate myocardial ischaemia. Pain after abdominal or thoracic surgery can lead to splinting of the diaphragm and chest wall, causing decreased lung volumes, atelectasis, decreased cough, sputum retention, infection and hypoxia. Sympathetic stimulation causes delayed gastric emptying and urinary retention. Pain can also reduce mobility and increase the risk of thromboembolism. The stress response to surgery decreases the humoral immune response and induces a hypercoagulable state. The psychological impact of sustained acute pain, such as after surgery, can alter patients' perception of pain and disability. The very young and very old are at greater risk from the adverse effects of uncontrolled pain after surgery.

Assessment of pain

Assessment is the first step in management of pain after surgery. Assessments in the acute postoperative setting should be at regular, frequent intervals and after every intervention to treat unrelieved pain. The frequency should be determined by the severity of pain and the effectiveness of the analgesic regimen. Pain should be recorded as the fifth vital sign along with blood pressure, heart rate, respiratory rate and temperature.

A thorough assessment of pain should include:

- site of pain, circumstances associated with pain onset (details of surgery)
- character of pain (helpful in identifying visceral and neuropathic components to postoperative pain)
- intensity of pain (both at rest and on movement)
- associated symptoms (e.g. nausea)
- effect of pain on activity and sleep
- relevant medical history (history of pain conditions and treatments, as well as other medical conditions)
- other factors influencing the patient's treatment (belief concerning the causes of pain, expectations of pain relief and reduction required to resume reasonable activity).

Measuring the severity of pain reliably can sometimes be difficult as pain is a subjective, physical and emotional response to potential or actual tissue damage. The main tools available for measuring pain fall into two categories, namely unidimensional scales and multidimensional scales. Unidimensional tools include numeric scales (numeric rating scales, visual analogue scale) and categorical scales (verbal descriptor scale). These can be used as pain relief scales where '0/none' is no relief and '10/complete' is complete pain relief. Unidimensional scales measure one aspect of pain, usually pain intensity. The multidimensional scales such as the Brief Pain Inventory and the McGill Pain Questionnaire are less useful in acute postoperative pain. However, there is a need for a descriptive pain scale to assess acute postoperative neuropathic pain. Pain assessment in special circumstances, such as children and cognitively impaired patients, may need pictorial scales and behavioural scales (Abbey pain scale). In summary, the scale used should be easy to use and one that the patient understands and can be used consistently before and after an intervention.

Basic principles of acute postoperative pain management

Good analgesia should begin before surgery. Planning an analgesic strategy appropriate to the surgical procedure, based on individualized assessment of the patient in terms of previous experience of pain and its treatment, expectations for pain relief and level of pain that would allow reasonable activity, is the first step in good postoperative analgesia.

Using multimodal analgesia, preventive analgesic strategies, providing regular baseline analgesia, making provision for breakthrough/activity-induced pain and prescribing for side-effects of analgesia form the basis of good postoperative analgesia.

The choice of analgesia should be guided by the principles outlined in Table 30.16. Start at the step in the ladder (modification of the World Health Organization's pain ladder) appropriate to the anticipated pain intensity. Use the oral route whenever possible.

If regular analgesia from one section is insufficient:

- exclude a surgical or medical complication
- check that prescribed analgesia has been administered via a viable route
- consider moving to the next step
- increase the dose of the level III agent to regular intervals if pain remains severe.

Paracetamol

- Routes: oral, intravenous.
- Dose: 1 g regularly every 6 hours.
- Side-effects: minimal, danger of liver damage if dose maximum dose exceeded.
- Will provide up to 20% opiate-sparing effect if used regularly with opiates.

Non-steroidal anti-inflammatory drugs

- Routes: oral, intravenous, per rectum.
- Dose: according to drug selected.
- Adjuvant: use of adjuvant therapy with proton pump inhibitors of gastric acid secretion recommended.

Contraindications for the use of NSAIDs

- Impaired renal function.
- Active peptic ulcer disease.
- Dehydrated patients.
- History of asthma induced by aspirin or other NSAIDs.
- Known allergy or intolerance to NSAIDs.
- Bleeding disorders.
- Severe hepatic disease.
- Third trimester of pregnancy.

Use with caution

- Elderly patients.
- Hypertension, heart failure, impaired cardiac function (potential for sodium and water retention, reduction in effect of thiazide diuretics and furosemide).

Opiates

Principles of use in postoperative pain management

- People's perception of pain and response to opiates vary.
- Starting dose of opiates should be tailored to age.
- Maximum dose tolerated is determined by emergence of side-effects.
- Avoid using more than one opiate at a time.
- Avoid using more than one route of administration (except in patients on transdermal opiate administration).
- Breakthrough dose (to bridge the gap) is approximately one-sixth of the total regular dose for 24 hours.
- Patients on long-term opiates for pain or methadone for drug rehabilitation should continue to receive their regular dose (or equivalent if route needs to be changed) perioperatively.

Table 30.16 Pain management strategy

Anticipated pain	Mild	Moderate	Severe
Pain score (rest/ movement)	0–3	4–7	7–10
	Step I	**Step II**	**Step III**
Regular (at timed intervals)	**Simple analgesics** Paracetamol and/or Low-dose weak opiates **Use** Local infiltration or regional blocks whenever possible	**Add** NSAIDs and/or Weak opiates **Use** Local infiltration or regional blocks whenever possible	**Add** Strong opiate **Replace** Weak opiates with strong opiates **Consider** Epidural/PCA
As required	NSAIDs or Weak opiates	Short-acting opiates (e.g. morphine oral/i.v./i.m.)	Short-acting opiates (e.g. morphine oral/i.v./i.m.) PCA/PCEA

i.m., intramuscular; i.v., intravenous; NSAID, non-steroidal anti-inflammatory drug; PCA, patient-controlled analgesia; PCEA, patient-controlled epidural analgesia.

Route of administration of opiate analgesics

- Use oral route whenever possible.
- Intravenous opiate boluses may be required to establish pain control initially.
- If continued use of the parenteral route is required, consider patient-controlled analgesia.
- If patient has had intrathecal opiates, avoid using other opiates or sedative agents.
- Check equianalgesic dose when converting from one route/drug to an other (Table 30.17).
- When converting from oral to transdermal patches or vice versa, consult appropriate conmversion tables (Tables 30.18 and 30.19).

Regional techniques in postoperative pain management

Advantages of regional techniques in postoperative pain

- Better postoperative analgesia.
- Decrease in the use of opiate analgesia leading to a decrease in:
  - postoperative nausea and vomiting
  - itching
  - risk of sedation
  - unplanned admission after ambulatory surgery.

Table 30.17 Approximate equianalgesic doses

Drug	Oral dose (mg)	Parenteral dose (mg)
Morphine	20	10
Hydromorphone	2.6	–
Diamorphine	–	5
Oxycodone	10	10
Buprenorphine	0.8 (sublingual)	0.4
Pethidine	400	100
Tramadol	100	100
Fentanyl	–	0.1
Methadone	10–15	10

Table 30.18 Conversion table for fentanyl patch to morphine

Fentanyl patch (μg h^{-1})	24 hourly oral morphine dose (mg)	Morphine breakthrough dose (mg) (give orally 3–4 hourly as required)
25	<135	20
50	135–224	30
75	225–314	50
100	315–404	60
125	405–494	80
150	495–584	90

Table 30.19 Conversion table for buprenorphine patch to other analgesics

Buprenorphine patch Initial dose	Dihydrocodeine (oral) (mg)	Tramadol (parenteral) (mg)	Tramadol (oral) (mg)	Buprenorphine (sublingual) (mg)	Morphine (oral) (mg)
35 μg h^{-1}	120–240	100–200	150–300	0.4–0.8	30–60
52.5 μg h^{-1}	240–360	200–300	300–450	0.8–1.2	60–90
70 μg h^{-1}		300–400	450–600	1.2–1.6	90–120
2 × 70 μg h^{-1}				1.6–3.2	120–240

- Better patient satisfaction.
- Better dynamic pain relief than opiate analgesia.
- Reduction in length of stay in some cases.

Regional techniques for analgesia fall into three main categories; namely, central neuraxial blocks, peripheral nerve blocks and local infiltration. These can be undertaken as single injections or continuous blocks. Timing of these techniques may have some bearing on the quality of postoperative analgesia. Instituting the blocks before the stimulus prevents central sensitization and also reduces the depth of anaesthesia required. This in turn could improve postoperative analgesia and reduce anaesthetic and analgesic requirements intraoperatively.

Neuraxial blocks are dealt with in other parts of this book. Intrathecal and epidural opiates can be a useful adjuvant to postoperative analgesia. Extended release epidural morphine preparations have been shown to provide analgesia for up to 48 hours after surgery. Issues with neuraxial opiates include delayed respiratory depression with less lipophilic opiates such as morphine and extended release opiate preparations. Care needs to be exercised to avoid other sedating agents when neuraxial opiates are used. Staff in areas caring for these patients should have clear and specific guidelines for monitoring and for management of complications and side-effects.

Peripheral nerve blocks can be used for intraoperative and postoperative analgesia after surgery. Benefits of peripheral nerve blocks need to be balanced against the possibility of motor block and loss of function, which may delay onset of active physiotherapy. Some of the problems can be offset by using low-dose local anaesthetics combined with adjuvants.

In the past few years there has been an accumulation of evidence in favour of wound infiltration techniques and transversus abdominis plane (TAP) blocks. TAP blocks have been shown to improve analgesia, decrease opiate use and improve function in a variety of surgical procedures, including laparoscopic cholecystectomy, total abdominal hysterectomy, caesarean section and laparotomy for bowel surgery. The technique is easy to master and the complication rate is low. TAP blocks can be performed by landmark technique or the use of ultrasound to identify the plane between the internal oblique and transversus abdominis muscles.

Recent meta-analysis showed that continuous wound infiltration leads to decreased pain scores, decreased opiate consumption, less postoperative nausea and vomiting and shorter length of stay in hospital. There was no difference in wound infection rates and patients were generally more satisfied. As in all regional techniques, success depends to a large extent on the skill of the operator. Correct placement of the wound catheter or injection determines the success of the technique.

Pain in special circumstances

Opiate-dependent patients

These patients belong to one of three groups; namely, those who are on long-term opiates for chronic pain, those who are on opiates for cancer pain and those who have been or are currently addicted to opiates. Management of pain after surgery is difficult in this group of patients. It is important to remember that all patients on long-term opiates will be tolerant of opiates but not necessarily addicted. The aim of management should be to manage patient expectations, provide adequate analgesia and prevent or manage withdrawal symptoms. This can be achieved by involving the multidisciplinary team (local drug team, acute pain team, psychologist and pharmacist) early in the process. Management should start with a good preoperative evaluation, setting achievable targets in terms of pain relief with the patient. It is also useful in current abusers of recreational drugs to contact local drug teams to gauge baseline use from street values of drugs. Patients would require a baseline opiate to avoid withdrawal. Regional anaesthesia should be used whenever possible and not contraindicated. In general, a patient will need a higher dose of opiates. It is advisable to avoid immediate release opiates by the parenteral route whenever possible.

In summary:

- 'opioid dependence' does not always mean 'addiction'
- our aim should be to treat the pain not treat the addiction
- these patients are complex and need multidisciplinary management.

Acute neuropathic pain after surgery

Up to two-thirds of patients who have surgery develop chronic postsurgical pain. There are clear examples of early neuropathic pain, such as phantom limb pain after amputation. Mechanisms are poorly understood but believed to be a continuum beginning with the incision; hence, preventive analgesia such as regional techniques before onset of surgery may be useful in prevention. Diagnosis is by maintaining a high index of suspicion in patients who complain of pain inconsistent with the extent of tissue damage, pain in the area of sensory loss or paroxysmal or spontaneous pain, or who on examination exhibit allodynia, hyperalgesia or dysaesthesia. These patients can exhibit a poor response to opiate analgesia.

Most of the evidence for treatment is from chronic pain states such as postherpetic neuralgia and diabetic neuropathy. Current evidence seems to suggest that tricyclic antidepressants and anticonvulsants such as gabapentin are effective in acute neuropathic pain after surgery.

Bibliography

Colvin LA, Wilson JA, Power I. *Acute Neuropathic Pain after Surgery.* Bulletin 15. London: Royal College of Anaesthetists, 2002, pp. 739–43.

Holdcroft A, Power I. Recent developments: management of pain. *Br Med J* 2003; **326**: 635–9.

Liu SS, Richman JM, Thirlby RC, Wu CL. Efficacy of continuous wound catheters delivering local anesthetic for postoperative analgesia: a quantitative and qualitative systematic review of randomized controlled trials. *J Am Coll Surg* 2006; **203**: 914–32.

Macintyre PE, Scott DA, Schug SA (eds) *Acute Pain Management: Scientific Evidence*, 3rd edn. Melbourne: Australian and New Zealand College of Anaesthetists, 2010. See www.anzca.edu.au/resources/books-and-publications.

McDonnell JG, O'Donnell B, Curley G, *et al.* The analgesic efficacy of transversus abdominis plane block after abdominal surgery: a prospective randomised controlled trial. *Anaesth Analg* 2007; 104: 193–7.

Mitra S, Sinatra RS. Perioperative management of acute pain in the opioid dependent patient. *Anaesthesiology* 2004; **101**: 212–27.

Visser EJ. Chronic post-surgical pain: epidemiology and clinical implications for acute pain management. *Acute Pain* 2006; **8**: 73–81.

Cross-references

Epidural and spinal anaesthesia, 707
Regional anaesthetic techniques, 719

Pseudocholinesterase deficiency

Brian J Pollard

Pseudocholinesterase (PChe) is also known as plasma cholinesterase (acylcholine acylhydrolase; E.C.3.1.1.8.). It is a soluble enzyme found in the plasma and manufactured in the liver.

The importance for anaesthesia is that decreased activity may cause a reduction in the rate of hydrolysis and hence a prolonged duration of action of succinylcholine and mivacurium. Note that other agents, e.g. remifentanil, are not broken down by this pathway and are thus unaffected by cholinesterase deficiency. Decreased PChe activity may be inherited or acquired (Tables 30.20 and 30.21).

Determination of PChe activity and phenotype

Biochemical analysis can be undertaken by measuring the rate of hydrolysis of a substrate catalysed by PChe. More commonly, it is described by the percentage inhibition of the hydrolysis in the presence of different inhibitor substances, in particular dibucaine and fluoride. More recently, enzyme assays have been developed and also structural analysis at the molecular level.

Genetically determined changes in PChe activity

More than 50 different mutations are known, and about 25% of subjects in a Caucasian population carry at least one PChe variant. Only a few of these, however, have clinical significance. The cholinesterase activity of the different phenotypes differs qualitatively as well as quantitatively. Because of the above factors, it is not possible to estimate the clinical significance from the PChe activity alone. The phenotype (or genotype) must also be identified (Table 30.22).

Table 30.20 Aetiology of decreased pseudocholinesterase activity

Condition	Change in activity
Physiological variation	
Sex	Males > females
Age	Newborns 50% of adults
Pregnancy	70–80% of pre-pregnancy level until 6–8 weeks after delivery
Disease	
Liver failure	40–70% decrease
Renal failure	10–50% decrease
Malignant tumours	25–50% decrease, depending on the localization
Burned patients	Lowest value 5–6 days after the injury Depending on the degree of injury, the reduction may exceed 80%

Table 30.21 Iatrogenic factors which decrease pseudocholinesterase (PChe) activity

Factor	Decrease in PChe activity (%)
Glucocorticoids, oestrogen	30–50
Cytotoxics	35–70
Neostigmine	5–100
Ecothiopate eye drops	70–100
Bambuterol	30–90
Organophosphates	100
Plasmapheresis (removes PChe)	60–100

● **Table 30.22** Frequency and biochemical characteristics using benzoylcholine as a substrate of the clinically most important pseudocholinesterase (PChe) variants in Caucasian populations

Phenotype	Frequency (%)	PChe activity (U L^{-1})	Dibucaine number
UU	95–97	690–1560	79–87
UA	2–4	320–1150	55–72
AA	0.04	140–730	14–27

Clinical consequences

The clinical implications of decreased PChe activity is principally in relation to succinylcholine. Normally, 90% of an injected dose of succinylcholine is hydrolysed in plasma and only a small amount reaches the neuromuscular receptor. If PChe activity is decreased, more succinylcholine reaches the receptor causing a more profound block with a longer duration of action.

When there is reduced activity in phenotypically normal patients, the duration of action of 1 mg kg^{-1} succinylcholine may be moderately prolonged (20–45 minutes).

In patients who are heterozygous for the normal and the atypical genes (without any other factors which might reduce PChe activity), the duration of action is normal or slightly prolonged (10–15 minutes). More prolonged responses and a phase 2 block may be seen if the PChe activity is further decreased for other reasons (Tables 30.20 and 30.21).

In patients homozygous for two abnormal genes, a very prolonged response (120–180 minutes or even longer) and a phase 2 block are always seen.

Management of prolonged response to succinylcholine

Management depends on the PChe activity and the phenotype. Often the patient's phenotype is unknown. Therefore it is necessary to keep the patient ventilated and anaesthetized and regularly evaluate the response to peripheral nerve stimulation.

In phenotypically normal patients and in heterozygous abnormal patients, a prolonged response can be antagonized with a cholinesterase inhibitor. In homozygous atypical patients, succinylcholine is not hydrolysed in plasma. The effect of a cholinesterase inhibitor is therefore unpredictable and may even potentiate the block. Administration of purified PChe, fresh whole blood or fresh plasma may antagonize the block. However, because of the risks associated with their use, transfusion of blood or plasma cannot be recommended as a routine.

Management of a prolonged response to mivacurium

The rate of hydrolysis of mivacurium is 70–80% of that of succinylcholine *in vitro*.

Low PChe activity in phenotypically normal patients may cause a prolonged block. A prolonged block has been seen in patients with renal and hepatic failure.

In patients heterozygous for the normal and the atypical genes:

- the duration of action may be moderately prolonged (50%)
- the infusion rate is decreased (33%)
- reversal with neostigmine is prompt when two responses to train-of-four (TOF) stimulation are present.

In patients homozygous for two abnormal genes:

- a normal intubating dose causes a very prolonged duration of action (no signs of recovery for 40–180 minutes)
- reversal with neostigmine should not be attempted before two responses to TOF stimulation are present
- purified human PChe can be used, but the exact dose and optimal time are not yet known; FFP or blood should not be given.

Patient follow-up

The patient should be informed about the prolonged block. Enquiries should be made to determine whether there has been any incidence of awareness during the determination of the reason for the prolonged block. If so, the patient might develop severe psychological problems and require counselling. Blood samples should be drawn for determination of PChe activity and phenotype. Warning cards should be issued to the patient and the patient's general practitioner informed.

Bibliography

Belmont MR, Rubin LA, Lien CA, *et al.* Mivacurium. *Anaesth Pharmacol Rev* 1995; **3**: 156–67.

Gätke MR, Østergaard D, Bundgaard JR, *et al.* Response to mivacurium in a patient compound heterozygous for a novel and a known silent mutation in the butyrylcholinesterase gene. *Anesthesiology* 2001; **95**: 600–6.

Head-Rapson AG, Devlin JC, Parker CJR, Hunter JM. Pharmacokinetics and pharmacodynamics of the three isomers of mivacurium in health, in end-stage renal failure and in patients with impaired renal function. *Br J Anaesth* 1995; **75**: 31–6.

Jensen FS, Viby-Mogensen J, Ostergaard D. Significance of plasma cholinesterase for the anaesthetist. *Curr Anaesth Crit Care* 1991; **2**: 232–7.

Jensen FS, Schwartz M, Viby-Mogensen J. Identification of human plasma cholinesterase variants using molecular biological techniques. *Acta Anaesthesiol Scand* 1995; **39**: 142–9.

Jensen FS, Skovgaard LT, Viby-Mogensen J. Identification of human plasma cholinesterase variants in 6.688 individuals using biochemical analysis. *Acta Anaesthesiol Scand* 1995; **39**: 157–62.

Østergaard D, Jensen FS, Skovgaard LT, Viby-Mogensen L. Dose-response relationship for mivacurium in patients with phenotypically abnormal plasma cholinesterase activity. *Acta Anaesthesiol Scand* 1995; **39**: 1016–18.

Østergaard D, Rasmussen SN, Viby-MogensenJ, *et al.* The influence of drug-induced low plasma cholinesterase activity on the pharmacokinetics and pharmacodynamics of mivacurium. *Anesthesiology* 2000; **92**: 1581–7.

Østergaard D, Ibsen M, Skovgaard LT, Viby-Mogensen J. Plasma cholinesterase activity and duration of action of mivacurium in phenotypically normal patients. *Acta Anaesthesiol Scand* 2002; **46**: 679–83.

Østergaard D, Viby-Mogensen J, Pedersen NA, *et al.* Pharmacokinetics and pharmacodynamics of mivacurium in young adult and elderly patients. *Acta Anaesthesiol Scand* 2002; **46**: 684–91.

Viby-Mogensen J. Cholinesterase and succinylcholine. *Dan Med Bull* 1983; **30**: 129–50.

Whittaker M. Cholinesterase. In: Beckman L (ed.) *Monographs in Human Genetics*, vol. 11. Basel: Karger, 1986, pp. 1–125.

Raised intracranial pressure/ cerebral blood flow control

Brian J Pollard

Intracranial pressure

The principal constituents within the skull are the brain, blood and cerebrospinal fluid (CSF). The Monro–Kellie doctrine describes how an increase in the volume of one component must be accompanied by an equal reduction in another to maintain the same pressure (Fig. 30.8).

Initially, the volume increase is compensated for by extrusion of CSF into the spinal sac. When this mechanism is exhausted, further volume increases result in a sudden large increase in intracranial pressure (ICP).

Further brain swelling causes:

- herniation of the temporal lobe through the tentorium and of the cerebellar tonsils through the foramen magnum
- brainstem torsion with reduced cerebral blood flow (CBF) and sudden obstruction of CSF flow with acute hydrocephalus.

Clinical signs of raised ICP

- Nausea and vomiting.
- Frontal headaches on waking.
- Papilloedema.
- Drowsiness.
- Hypertension and bradycardia.

Causes of raised ICP

- Severe head injury.
- Space-occupying lesions (e.g. tumour, subarachnoid haemorrhage).
- Acute hydrocephalus.

Aggravating factors

- Venous obstruction (e.g. from poor neck positioning).
- Raised intrathoracic pressure (e.g. from respiratory obstruction).
- Fibreoptic bronchoscopy increases the ICP significantly in brain-injured patients.

Ameliorating factors

A head up tilt of 30° gives maximal benefit from venous drainage, while minimizing the reduction in cerebral arterial pressure because of the hydrostatic pressure difference between the heart and brain level.

Cerebral blood flow

Normal CBF is 50–65 mL per 100 g min^{-1}.

Regulating factors

- CPP.
- P_ao_2.
- P_aco_2.
- Other (e.g. adenosine, neuropeptides, ions, neurogenic mechanisms).
- CBF doubles as P_ao_2 declines from 50–30 mmHg.

For every 1 mmHg decrease in P_aco_2 between 60 and 20 mmHg, the CBF decreases 1.1 mL per 100 g min^{-1}. The reduction in CBF is maximal when P_aco_2 <25 mmHg. If hypocapnia continues for more than 5 hours the CBF returns to control values.

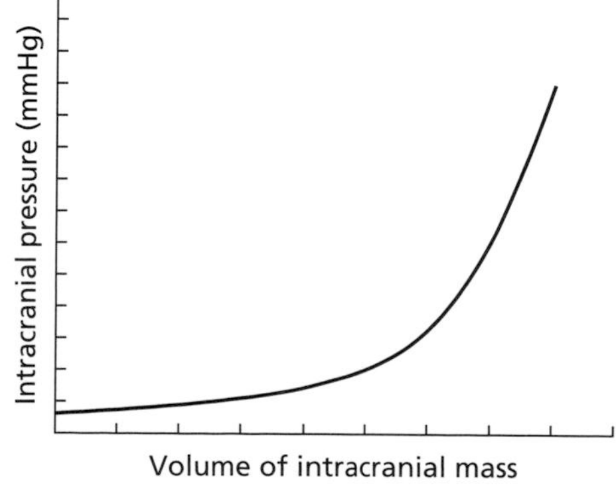

Figure 30.8 Effect of increasing intracranial mass on ICP. Small changes in ICP, initially, become much greater beyond a critical intracranial mass.

Cerebral perfusion pressure

CPP is defined as the difference between the systemic mean arterial pressure and the ICP.

Cerebral vascular resistance

This is proportional to the fourth power of the vessel radius.

Autoregulation

This is the coupling of blood flow to metabolic demand in normal brain by the dynamic interplay of vasoconstriction and vasodilatation in the cerebral vascular bed.

Loss of autoregulation

This occurs:

- at CPP <50 mmHg
- in the traumatized or ischaemic brain
- with vasodilators (e.g. sodium nitroprusside)
- with high doses of volatile agents.

Pharmacological agents that affect CBF

Volatile agents

Halothane and enflurane increase CBF by a direct vasodilating effect on cerebral vasculature. Autoregulation is lost at high concentrations. Hypocapnia prevents the CBF rise.

Isoflurane has an indirect vasoconstricting effect secondary to reducing the metabolic rate and a direct vasodilating effect. Isoflurane provides cerebral protection and ischaemic changes do not develop until the CBF is reduced to 8–10 mL per 100 g min^{-1} (compared with 18–20 mL per 100 g min^{-1} for halothane or when awake). At >1.5 MAC or in damaged brain, the vasodilating effect predominates.

Sevoflurane has similar effects to isoflurane. It is a cerebral vasodilator increasing CBF and decreasing cerebrovascular resistance in a dose-dependent manner. Carbon dioxide reactivity is preserved at 1.5–2.5% inspired sevoflurane concentrations.

Nitrous oxide causes a significant global increase in CBF by direct vasodilatation.

Hypnotics

Propofol causes a reduction in ICP and CPP (not less than 70 mmHg). In patients with intracerebral tumours, there is less tendency to cerebral swelling after opening the dura than when isoflurane or sevoflurane is used. Propofol without narcotic does not prevent the rise in ICP on intubation.

Barbiturates and midazolam produce a dose-dependent reduction in metabolic rate, CBF and cerebral blood volume.

Narcotics

Unless ventilation is supported, narcotics increase ICP secondary to hypercapnia from respiratory depression. Injudicious use can reduce CPP by reducing systemic blood pressure.

Mannitol

The initial effect of a bolus of mannitol is haemodynamic, augmenting intravascular volume and increasing systolic arterial pressure and CPP. With an intact autoregulation reflex, cerebral vasoconstriction and a decreased metabolic rate reduce ICP. With impaired autoregulation ICP falls by 5%, but CBF increases by 17%. The osmotic effect occurring 15 minutes later is less effective in the damaged brain. Mannitol increases flow in the microcirculation, improving oxygen delivery and clearance of vasodilating substances.

Other drugs

- Dexamethasone is used to reduce ICP.
- Dimethylsulphoxide and hypertonic saline have beneficial effects on ICP.
- Succinylcholine raises ICP.
- Calcium channel blockers and magnesium sulphate improve blood flow to ischaemic brain areas.
- In the awake patient, dopamine raises ICP whereas epinephrine and norepinephrine have no effect.
- In the anaesthetized patient, all three inotropes increase ICP. General anaesthesia may alter blood–brain barrier permeability via a central effect.
- Lidocaine reduces ICP in a dose of 1.5 mg kg^{-1}.
- In severe craniocerebral trauma, bitemporal craniotomy has been used to reduce ICP.

Bibliography

Fessler RD, Diaz FG. The management of cerebral perfusion pressure and intracranial pressure after severe head injury. *Ann Emerg Med* 1993; **22**: 998–1003.

Peterson KD, Landsfeldt U, Cold GE, *et al.* ICP is lower during propofol anaesthesia compared to isoflurane and sevoflurane. *Acta Neurochir Suppl* 2002; **81**: 89–91.

Ravussin P, Wilder-Smith O. General anaesthesia for supratentorial neurosurgery. *CNS Drugs* 2001; **15**(7): 527–35.

Walters FJM. Neuroanaesthesia: a review of the basic principles and current practices. *Cent Afr J Med* 1990; **36**: 44–51.

Cross-references

General principles of neuroanaesthesia, 300
Neuromonitoring, 338

Thrombosis and embolism

Niall O'Keeffe

A thrombus is a blood clot which forms within a blood vessel. If a piece breaks off and is carried along in the blood to a distant site, this is an embolus. The effect of the embolus depends on where it ultimately lodges. If on the systemic venous side, it will lodge in a pulmonary vessel. If on the systemic arterial side, it will lodge in a peripheral artery. The symptoms and signs depend on the vessel occluded and the size of the embolus. Thromboembolic disease is a major cause of morbidity and mortality, much of which can be prevented with simple prophylactic measures.

Factors important in the formation of thrombus may still be considered in terms of Virchow's triad:

- abnormality of the endothelium of the blood vessel (e.g. trauma)
- slowing or other disturbances of blood flow
- changes in the composition of the blood, favouring an increase in coagulation potential, e.g. increased platelet aggregation and fibrin formation. Surgery can induce a hypercoagulable state.

Deep vein thrombosis

Deep vein thrombosis (DVT) is a common event in hospital patients. Patients most at risk are listed in Box 30.9. Those with a previous history of DVT or pulmonary embolism, those who are obese and those who have a malignant disease are especially at risk. Prolonged surgery and surgery involving the pelvis, hip and knee are associated with a significant risk of DVT formation.

Diagnosis of DVT

Diagnosis based on clinical features such as leg swelling, pain, warmth and a positive Homan's sign is unreliable. Screening for breakdown products of fibrin is useful in non-surgical patients as a negative result excludes clot formation.

Diagnostic tests for DVT include:

- duplex venous scan: 98% accuracy for proximal thrombi; relatively non-invasive
- venography: the most reliable technique; however, up to 2% of patients may develop a DVT as a result
- impedance plethysmography: sensitive and specific, but not for calf vein thrombi
- radiolabelled fibrinogen scan.

Treatment of deep vein thrombosis

Anticoagulation with unfractionated heparin should be started with a bolus of 100 units kg^{-1} followed

Box 30.9 Risk factors for venous thromboembolism

- Patient factors
  - Age
  - Obesity
  - Varicose veins with phlebitis
  - Immobility (bed rest >3 days)
  - Pregnancy and puerperium
  - Oestrogen therapy (hormone replacement therapy or oral contraceptive pill)
  - Previous DVT or pulmonary embolism in patient or first-degree relative
  - Thrombophilias
- Factors relating to disease or procedure
  - Surgery or trauma, especially to the pelvis, hip or lower limb
  - Long surgical procedures (>90 minutes, or 60 minutes if surgery involves pelvis or lower limb)
  - Malignancy, especially pelvic, abdominal or metastatic
  - Heart failure
  - Recent myocardial infarction
  - Lower limb paralysis
  - Infection
  - Inflammatory conditions
  - Polycythaemia
  - Dehydration
  - Critical care admission

by an infusion of approximately 20 000–30 000 units daily, aiming to keep the activated partial thromboplastin time (APTT) between 1.5 and 2.5 times normal. APTT should be monitored daily. Alternatively low-molecular-weight heparin (LMWH) may be used. Different preparations have different dose schedules and these should be checked before administration. Warfarin is commonly used for longer term treatment. It may be started on the first day, but heparin should be continued until the warfarin becomes effective.

Deep vein thrombosis prophylaxis

Prophylaxis should be related to perceived risk. Low-risk patients may be managed by early mobilization. Patients at increased risk should receive additional prophylaxis. This should include either low-dose subcutaneous heparin (5000 units 8–12 hourly), a LMWH of proven efficacy or fondaparinux 2.5 mg daily. When heparin is contraindicated, consider fondaparinux. Intermittent pneumatic compression or graduated compression stockings should also be used.

Two new oral drugs have recently been licensed for use in patients having hip and knee replacement surgery. Rivaroxaban is a direct inhibitor of factor Xa and dabigatran is a direct inhibitor of thrombin.

Pulmonary embolism

Pulmonary embolism has been reported to account for up to 10% of hospital deaths. Three out of four patients dying from pulmonary embolism have not had recent surgery, emphasizing the importance of prophylaxis in medical patients at risk.

Diagnosis and treatment of pulmonary embolism

Clinical features are often non-specific, making diagnosis difficult. They depend partly on the degree of obstruction and may include tachypnoea, pleuritic or dull central chest pain, tachycardia, cyanosis, raised CVP and gallop rhythm. Massive acute pulmonary embolism usually presents with cardiac arrest. Electrical activity may continue without any cardiac output (electromechanical dissociation or pulseless electrical activity).

Investigations include: ECG (common changes include tachycardia, right bundle branch block, or S1:Q3:T3 in 25% of patients); chest X-ray, which may show pulmonary oligaemia or wedge-shaped opacity; and blood gases, which may show hypoxaemia. Echocardiography often shows an acutely dilated right ventricle with an underfilled left ventricle. Isotope ventilation–perfusion (V/Q) scanning is widely used. It can only be reported as representing a low, moderate or high likelihood of pulmonary embolism. A normal V/Q scan excludes pulmonary embolism. The definitive diagnostic test is a spiral CT pulmonary angiogram.

Initial treatment is supportive with oxygen, fluids and analgesia, depending on the severity of cardiopulmonary disturbance. Specific treatment options include anticoagulation, thrombolysis and pulmonary embolectomy.

Acute minor pulmonary embolism with no haemodynamic disturbance can be treated with heparin as described above, followed by warfarin for a period of 3–6 months.

Acute major pulmonary embolism presenting with haemodynamic disturbance will initially require resuscitation with oxygen and fluids and direct haemodynamic monitoring in a HDU. This should be followed by thrombolysis with streptokinase 250 000–600 000 IU over 20–30 minutes, with or without 100 mg hydrocortisone, followed by 100 000 IU h^{-1} for up to 72 hours. Tissue plasminogen activator produces more rapid resolution of thrombus, but the results are similar after 12–24 hours.

Pulmonary embolectomy is occasionally attempted in major centres but the success rate is not good and it is therefore reserved for massive emboli unlikely to survive without surgery.

Arterial thromboembolism

The source of arterial thromboembolism is often the heart. Over half of all thromboemboli of cardiac origin are the result of atrial fibrillation, particularly when this is associated with mitral stenosis or thyrotoxicosis. Other predisposing conditions include prosthetic valves, recent myocardial infarction with mural thrombus formation and low cardiac output states. Resulting thromboemboli may take the form of peripheral emboli or, more commonly, cerebrovascular events producing a stroke. Studies have demonstrated the benefits of anticoagulation in patients with atrial fibrillation. Although traditionally warfarin has been used, more recently phase 3 trials have shown dabigatran to be superior, although it does not yet have a licence for this indication. It also has the advantages that it does not require routine monitoring and its effects do not last as long.

Bibliography

British Thoracic Society guidelines for the management of suspected acute pulmonary embolism. *Thorax* 2003; **58**: 470–84.

Dunn M, Blackburn T. Anticoagulant treatment of atrial fibrillation in the elderly. *Postgrad Med J* 1992; **68**(Suppl. 1): S57–60.

Goldhaber SZ. Pulmonary embolism. *N Engl J Med* 1998; **339**: 93–104.

Hull RD, Pineo GF. Treatment of venous thromboembolism with low molecular weight heparins. *Hematol Oncol Clin North Am* 1992; **6**: 1095–103.

Mammen EF. Pathogenesis of venous thrombosis. *Chest* 1992; **102**(Suppl. 6): 640S–4S.

National Institute for Health and Clinical Excellence. *Venous Thromboembolism: Reducing the Risk of Venous Thromboembolism (Deep Vein Thrombosis and Pulmonary Embolism) in Patients Admitted to Hospital.* NICE Clinical Guideline 92, 2010. See www.nice.org.uk/guidance/CG92

Proceedings of the Seventh ACCP Conference on Antithrombotic and Thrombolytic Therapy: Evidence Based Guidelines. *Chest* 2004; **126**(3 Suppl.): 163S–696S.

Thromboembolic Risk Factors (THRIFT) Consensus Group. Risk of and prophylaxis for venous thromboembolism in hospital patients. *Br Med J* 1992; **305**: 567–74.

Total spinal anaesthesia

Brian J Pollard

Definition

- Spread of local anaesthetic to block all of the spinal nerves and possibly extending into the brainstem and skull.
- Life-threatening extensive block usually results in severe hypotension, which may progress to cardiovascular collapse, respiratory failure, unconsciousness and cardiac arrest.
- High spinal anaesthesia may produce profound hypotension without respiratory failure.

Physiological effects

See Fig. 30.9.

Cardiovascular collapse

- Total preganglionic efferent sympathetic block.
- Peripheral sympathetic (T1–L2) block leads to loss of vasoconstrictor tone with a profound reduction in SVR and venous return.
- Block of cardiac sympathetic fibres (T1–T4) with unopposed vagal nerve supply results in severe bradycardia.

Respiratory failure

- Progressive intercostal muscles paralysis (rising from T12 to T1).
- Diaphragmatic paralysis (C3–C5).
- Inhibition of respiratory centre owing to a direct effect of local anaesthetic or secondary to cerebral hypoperfusion.

Loss of consciousness

- Direct action of local anaesthetic on the brain.
- Secondary to cerebral hypoperfusion due to severe hypotension.

Aetiology

Intentional

Total spinal anaesthesia (TSA), with respiratory and cardiovascular support, has been used for deliberate hypotension:

- to provide a bloodless operative field, e.g. for ear surgery
- to reduce intraoperative blood loss, e.g. for surgery in a Jehovah's Witness patient.

In chronic pain management, TSA provides transient relief of intractable pain.

Accidental

As a complication of spinal anaesthesia. Most commonly occurs when larger volumes of local anaesthetic are injected accidentally into the subarachnoid space (SAS):

- Central block:
  - extended epidural; increased risk following dural tap
  - caudal block in children
  - false-negative aspiration (no CSF reflux) and test dose

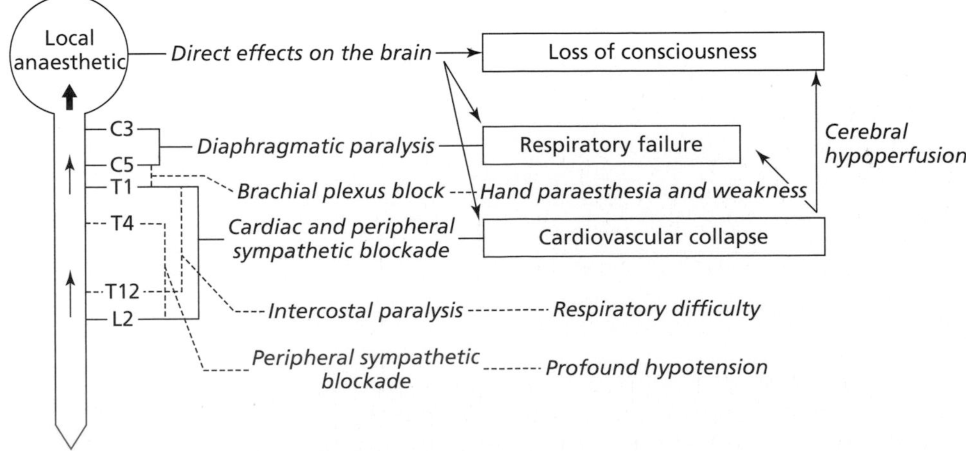

Figure 30.9 Physiological effects of total spinal anaesthesia.

- subdural block
- multicompartment block (epidural, subdural or subarachnoid block with multiholed catheter or Tuohy needle); delayed collapse can develop after previously normal top-ups
- misplaced catheter (initially incorrect place or subsequently migrates into subdural space or SAS).

- Peripheral block. Local anaesthetic spreads to the SAS along the radicular dural cuff or via the perineural space in case of intraneural injection. Cases have been reported after:
  - retrobulbar block
  - stellate ganglion block
  - brachial plexus (interscalene approach)
  - intercostal block
  - paravertebral block
  - lumbar plexus block for total hip replacement.

Diagnosis

One or more of the following (during a potential risk block):

- loss of consciousness
- respiratory collapse
- cardiovascular collapse or cardiac arrest.

Prevention

Pay close attention to details when performing blocks close to the spinal cord.

Factors which may lead to high spinal block are:

- large volume of local anaesthetic for spinal anaesthesia in a short patient
- patient position
- pregnancy (engorgement of epidural veins)
- barbotage
- straining or coughing
- cephalad direction of a small lateral hole spinal needle combined with rapid injection.

Precautions that should be taken when using an epidural catheter are:

- aspirate without a filter and aspirate before each injection (top-ups)
- use a test dose sufficient to produce a reliable subarachnoid block
- test for S1 motor block 10 minutes after epidural injection (10 mL bupivacaine is a reliable test to detect accidental intrathecal injection in an obstetric patient)
- wait sufficient time for the block to occur
- titrate the injected local anaesthetic in incremental doses
- avoid injection during uterine contractions
- it is essential to assess frequently both sensory and motor block.

Precautions to be taken with other blocks are:

- use the shortest practicable needle
- careful aspiration.

Early recognition and treatment of potential total spinal anaesthesia

- Resuscitation equipment and anaesthetic help should be available before any regional block.
- Signs and symptoms:
  - respiratory difficulty (weak voice, inability to cough)
  - upper limb paraesthesia and weakness
  - Horner syndrome (spinal or epidural)
  - cerebral hypoperfusion (restlessness, nausea, vomiting, headache).
- Management directed at restricting spread of local anaesthetic:
  - hyperbaric solution (spinal), anti-Trendelenburg
  - solutions intended for non-subarachnoid use are likely to be isobaric or hypobaric within CSF; the patient should be kept still; a slight head-down tilt will encourage caudal spread of hypobaric local anaesthetic and help to maintain venous return
  - obstetric patients should be managed in a left lateral tilt to avoid aortocaval compression
  - if a dural puncture is not recognized and a volume of local anaesthetic is injected into the CSF, an attempt could be made immediately to withdraw a volume of CSF equal to the local anaesthetic volume through the catheter; some of the drug will theoretically be aspirated and the remainder will be diluted as the CSF is formed.

Treatment

- Support the cardiorespiratory systems until the effects of the high block recede.
- Give 100% oxygen to maximize oxygen supply.
- Cardiovascular support:
  - maintain venous return: elevation of legs; left lateral tilt (obstetric patient); intravenous fluids (colloids or crystalloids)
  - give atropine and vasopressor drugs if required.
- Tracheal intubation and assisted ventilation, which may require general anaesthesia, sedation or muscular relaxation.
- Cardiopulmonary resuscitation if cardiac arrest occurs.

Bibliography

Bonica JJ. *Regional Anaesthesia: Recent Advances and Current Status. High or Total Spinal or Epidural Block.* Oxford: Blackwell Scientific, 1971.

Guterres AP, Newman MJ. Total spinal following labour epidural analgesia managed with noninvasive ventilation. *Anaesth Intensive Care Med* 2010; **38**: 373–5.

Morgan B. Unexpectedly extensive conduction blocks in obstetric epidural analgesia. *Anaesthesia* 1990; **45**: 148–52.

Morton CPJ, Wildsmith JAW. Crises in regional anaesthesia. *Baillieres Clin Anaesthesiol* 1993; **7**: 367–75.

Russell IF. Total spinal anaesthesia: the effect of spinal infusions. In: Reynolds F (ed.) *Epidural and Spinal Blockade in Obstetrics.* London: Baillière Tindall, 1990, pp. 107–20.

Yokoyama M, Itano Y, Kusume Y, *et al.* Total spinal anesthesia provides transient relief of intractable pain. *Can J Anaesth* 2002; **49**: 432–6.

Cross-references

Cardiopulmonary resuscitation, 738
Epidural and spinal anaesthesia, 707
Local anaesthetic toxicity, 767

Transport of the critically ill

Brian J Pollard

Lack of a functioning ITU bed in the patient's parent hospital is statistically the most common reason for transferring critically ill patients. The second is referral for specialist services.

In the UK, as in most developed countries, the demand for critical care services has constantly outstripped the supply. As the demand increases relentlessly, critically ill patients are increasingly being transferred from one hospital to another. This situation is particularly clear in the UK, where there are fewer ITU beds per person than in many other European countries.

It should also be realized that transfers of the critically ill are not benign. When the Canadian Physician Accompanied Transport System was audited, there was a serious morbidity of 7% of transfers and a mortality of 1%.

The public awareness of such problems was heightened by the national media in 1995 in the UK when a victim of a road traffic accident in London was unable to be accommodated in an appropriate local ITU because of a perceived lack of beds. He eventually was flown to Leeds but died during the transfer. The resulting political outcry led to a series of bed bureaux being established to coordinate regional bed availability. These bed services operate systems that are based on daily telephone surveys of critical care beds.

The UK Department of Health document *Comprehensive Critical Care* made the local and regional planning for ITU transfers mandatory. This, in part, has led to the development of critical care networks. Critical care networks are responsible for, among other things, the development of transfer services within defined groups of neighbouring hospitals.

Each network has a lead clinician and manager who are involved in transfer process mapping, protocols and quality assurance programmes. They are also responsible for the availability of appropriate equipment, training and resources to allow the safe and coordinated transfer of the critically ill.

Practical conduct of transfers

Organization within trusts

Transfers for capacity reasons should be kept to a minimum. When a transfer is undertaken it should be to an appropriate local hospital within the designated network.

There must be a consultant in an acute specialty responsible for transfers 24 hours a day. This is usually the ITU consultant. Each patient should be accompanied by two people. One should be medically qualified and have relevant experience and competencies in transport medicine. They should be able to reintubate and resuscitate the patient and be comfortable with the transfer equipment used.

Whether regional retrieval services are utilized depends on local arrangements. If a retrieval team is unavoidably delayed and further delays may lead to a worsened patient outcome, a hospital-based transfer team should be used instead.

Vehicles

Road transport has many advantages. Ambulances with trained paramedic staff are easy and quick to mobilize and are rarely affected by weather. Dedicated retrieval ambulances have many potential advantages, including standardization of gas and power supplies and installation of permanent equipment. However, a substantial workload has to exist to justify such a resource.

There may be situations when air transport may be preferable. The obvious advantage of speed must be balanced against other considerations. Aeromedical transfers by either helicopter or fixed wing aircraft have the following disadvantages:

- organizational delays
- transfer considerations at either end of the journey
- staff involved must have previous aeromedical training
- a fall in atmospheric pressure may lead to an increased F_iO_2 requirement; any gas-containing cavity will tend to expand, e.g. pneumothorax, pneumoperitoneum, intracranial air
- altitude is also accompanied by an increased risk of hypothermia.

Monitoring

Minimal monitoring standards for transfers, as defined by the Intensive Care Society, are:

- continuous ECG
- non-invasive BP (often unreliable in a moving vehicle, and an arterial line should generally be used)
- oxygen saturation (S_aO_2)

- security
- diameter and length.

Do not forget to protect the cervical spine. Anticipate difficult intubation if there is:

- trauma to soft tissues of the face and neck
- midface fractures
- actual or potential injury to the cervical spine
- upper airway burns
- obvious pre-existing conditions (receding mandible, 'buck' teeth).

Consider:

- inhalation induction and direct laryngoscopy
- intubating laryngeal mask airway
- fibreoptic intubation; awake or post induction
- surgical airway, cricothyroidotomy or tracheostomy
- double-lumen tubes if thoracotomy planned.

Ventilation

IPPV in the presence of multiple rib fractures requires a chest drain to prevent a tension pneumothorax developing. In all ventilated patients:

- check air entry bilaterally by listening in midaxillary lines
- monitor $ETco_2$ and O_2 saturation
- measure expired tidal and minute volume, rate and pressure
- adjust F_Io_2, inspired/expired ratio and positive end-expiratory pressure to optimize oxygenation
- consider pressure control ventilation if available.

Difficult ventilation may be due to:

- gastric dilatation (pass a nasogastric or orogastric tube)
- pneumothorax or haemothorax (insert chest drain)
- diaphragmatic hernia.

In patients with chest trauma, over 50% will initially have a normal chest X-ray. Consider CT scan in these patients if time permits or other body areas are being scanned.

A large air leak (e.g. bronchial tear) may require a double-lumen tube.

The final check of the adequacy of ventilation is by analysis of arterial blood gases.

Aim for normocapnia in order not to confuse interpretation of acid–base status (unless there is a head injury).

Circulation

Maintenance of circulating volume is more important than a normal haemoglobin.

- Intravenous access with short, wide cannulae (Poiseuille's law).
- Secure all intravenous lines.
- Whenever possible, avoid intravenous distally to limb fractures.
- Check that the cannula is in the vein before administering drugs/fluids.
- Central venous access can cause pneumothorax or haemothorax.
- Warm all fluids before administration.
- Hartmann's solution is recommended for crystalloid infusions; excessive use of normal saline can lead to acidosis with an associated worse prognosis.
- Use cell savers or autotransfusion when appropriate.
- Aim for urine output 50 mL h^{-1} minimum (excluding diuretics).

Measure blood pressure directly in an upper limb. This is more accurate at low pressures, allows repeat sampling of arterial blood and is less subject to interference (e.g. surgeons).

In patients who present in haemorrhagic shock because of uncontrollable bleeding, do not attempt to resuscitate to normotension – accept systolic BP 70–80 mmHg. Administration of large volumes of fluid simply leads to increased blood loss. Delay aggressive fluid administration until operative control of haemorrhage.

In persistent hypotension:

- ensure monitors are correctly calibrated
- check for occult haemorrhage
- correct profound acidosis (pH <7.2)
- adjust the ventilator to give the lowest mean intrathoracic pressure.

Then consider:

- *Cardiac tamponade*: low BP, pulsus paradoxus, increased CVP. Use fluids and maintain heart rate to preserve cardiac output. Attempt pericardiocentesis if skills available. Maintain spontaneous ventilation as long as possible. Induce anaesthesia using rapid sequence induction with ketamine and succinylcholine.
- *Tension pneumothorax*: low BP, high inflation pressures, hyper-resonant, deviated trachea, increased CVP. Emergency decompression by needle thoracentesis followed by chest drain. Have a high index of suspicion after central line insertion.
- *Neurogenic shock*: low BP, bradycardia, vasodilatation. Use volume expansion initially and institute early measurement of CVP to guide fluid replacement. Atropine and vasopressors may be required when CVP is adequate.
- *Septic shock*: low BP, tachycardia, vasodilatation. Uncommon early after injury and usually associated with abdominal injuries.
- *Myocardial infarction*: low BP, arrhythmias, pulmonary oedema, chest pain (if conscious).

A technique of surgeon-performed ultrasound to assess patients with blunt abdominal trauma is becoming popular in the USA and Europe. Focused assessment with sonography for trauma (FAST) can identify haemoperitoneum. The examination looks at four areas: perisplenic, perihepatic, pelvic and pericardial. However, small fluid collections can be missed and it is recommended that at least two examinations should take place with the second occurring no earlier than 6 hours after the first. Visceral injuries can be missed in the absence of haemoperitoneum.

Disability

Beware when moving or using fractured/injured limbs. Neurovascular injuries may be worsened or caused, especially around joints. Ensure adequate manpower for safe positioning of patients. A head injury is not a contraindication to general anaesthesia. Adequately protect peripheral nerves and pressure areas, particularly the eyes, when prone.

Exposure

Around 66% of trauma patients arrive at hospital hypothermic. This will be worsened by administration of cold fluids and exposure of body cavities (e.g. abdomen, chest) and temperature loss is most severe in the emergency department. Cooling predisposes to arrhythmias; decreases cardiac function, causing an acidosis; adversely affects coagulation; causes left shift of the oxyhaemoglobin curve; and enhances anaesthetic drugs. On recovery, shivering dramatically increases oxygen consumption. Therefore:

- warm all fluids, especially blood
- monitor core and peripheral temperature
- warm and humidify all anaesthetic gases
- cover all exposed parts, including head
- raise theatre temperature when possible
- cover exposed bowel with dry towels or plastic sheet.

Limit initial surgical therapy to life-saving procedures, i.e. 'damage control surgery'. Remember:

- only blood loss kills early
- gastrointestinal injuries cause problems much later
- everything takes longer than you think
- it is easy to miss an injury if you rush
- hypothermia, acidosis and coagulopathy only lead to more of the same
- the best place for a sick patient is in the ITU.

The message regarding hypothermia is mixed. It can be protective by reducing metabolic and oxygen demands, especially in patients with brain injuries and after cardiac arrest. However, it is also part of the triad of death: acidosis, hypothermia and coagulopathy, which lead to worse outcome in trauma.

Monitoring

- ECG
- BP (direct)
- S_po_2
- $ETco_2$
- CVP (or pulmonary artery wedge pressure)
- temperature (core and peripheral)
- urine output
- fluid balance
- ventilatory parameters
- coagulation.

In the elderly trauma patient, early invasive haemodynamic monitoring improves outcome as it facilitates the identification and treatment of cardiovascular instability (low-flow cardiac output syndrome). Occasionally, this may be due to concurrent acute cardiac ischaemia, unrecognized or unreported by the patient.

Postoperative management

On completion of surgery, ensure the following before extubation:

- hypovolaemia corrected
- pH normal
- P_ao_2 acceptable
- temperature >34°C
- reflexes intact
- adequate analgesia.

Any instability requires transfer to an ITU/HDU until problems are resolved, or if there is a risk of the patient developing adult respiratory distress syndrome (Box 30.10).

Beware of problems of transfer, even over short distances.

Remember the secondary survey if not already completed.

Box 30.10 Factors predisposing to adult respiratory distress syndrome

- Aspiration
- Multiple fractures
- Pulmonary contusion
- Blood transfusion >12 units
- Hypotension >30 minutes (<90 mmHg)
- Sepsis
- Risk:
  - 1 factor 18%
  - 2 factors 42%
  - 3 factors 85%

Bibliography

American College of Surgeons Committee on Trauma. *Advanced Trauma Life Support for Doctors*, 6th edn. Chicago: American College of Surgeons, 1997.

Creteur J, Sibbald W, Vincent JL. Hemoglobin solutions: not just red blood cell substitutes. *Crit Care Med* 2000; **28**: 3025–34.

Danks RR. Triangle of death. How hypothermia, acidosis and coagulopathy can adversely impact trauma patients. *J Emerg Med Services* 2002; **27**: 668–70.

Dutton RP, Mackenzie CF, Scalea TM. Hypotensive resuscitation during active hemorrhage: impact on in-hospital mortality. *J Trauma* 2002; **52**: 1141–6.

Ford P, Nolan JP. Cervical spine injury and airway management. *Curr Opin Anaesthesiol* 2002; **15**: 193–201.

Ho MA, Karmaka MK, Contardi LH, *et al.* Excessive use of sodium chloride solution in managing traumatised patients in shock: a preventable contributor to acidosis. *J Trauma* 2001; **51**: 173–7.

Scalea T. What's new in trauma in the past 10 years? *Int Anaesthesiol Clin* 2002; **40**: 1–17.

Shapiro MB, Jenkins DH, Schwab CW, Rotondo MF. Damage control: collective review. *J Trauma* 2000; **49**: 969–78.

Stern SA. Low volume fluid resuscitation for presumed hemorrhagic shock: helpful or harmful? *Curr Opin Crit Care Med* 2001; 7: 422–30.

Cross-reference

Head injury, 16

Transurethral resection of the prostate syndrome

Brian J Pollard

The profound alteration in the functioning of the cardiovascular and nervous systems produced by absorption of large volumes of electrolyte-free irrigation fluid during transurethral resection of the prostate (TURP) is described as the TURP syndrome, although it has also been described in connection with percutaneous ultrasonic lithotripsy, vesical ultrasonic lithotripsy and intrauterine laser endoscopy.

In TURP syndrome, fluid absorption occurs principally through the venous sinuses of the prostatic capsule. Distilled water was the irrigant used originally for TURP, but usage was largely abandoned when it became apparent that the reduction in osmolarity consequent on absorption was responsible for intravascular haemolysis. Water intoxication also occurred and renal failure, due to precipitation of haemoglobin in the renal tubules, was also described. Irrigation by non-electrolyte solutions is necessary in order to reduce dispersion of current through the bladder during electrocautery. Glycine, an amino acid presented as a 1.5% solution, is the most widely used irrigant for TURP and undergoes both renal excretion and metabolism to ammonia by the liver.

Pathophysiology

As fluid absorption becomes significant, a rise in intravascular pressure results in dilution of both proteins and electrolytes. Reduction of oncotic pressure promotes fluid shifts from the vascular compartment into the interstitial compartments, producing oedema in the tissue beds. The syndrome is particularly likely to occur if uptake of fluid exceeds 50 mL h^{-1} during the first 30 minutes of surgery.

Sodium

True water intoxication produces a serum sodium of less than 120 mmol L^{-1}. The low serum sodium seen in the TURP syndrome is not usually associated with a change in serum osmolality. There is often no observable reduction in osmolality in response to the lower serum sodium because irrigating solutions contain osmotically active solutes. It may be the case that a decrease in osmolality, rather than a reduction in serum sodium, distinguishes asymptomatic from symptomatic patients. It has been suggested that the reason for the reduction in serum osmolality seen in some patients is a more rapid diffusion of glycine into the cells. A very low serum sodium is, however, associated with more severe symptoms and a poorer prognosis

Potassium

Transient elevation of the serum potassium has been observed in the absence of haemolysis, and hyperkalaemia may be implicated in the production of cardiac arrest during uptake of irrigating fluid.

Renal function

In severe TURP syndrome renal function may be impaired as a result of acute tubular necrosis, which may be the result of the reduction in renal blood flow produced by hypotension or by renal swelling.

Signs and symptoms

These are related to the volume of irrigant absorbed.

Cardiovascular system

Chest pain may be observed after 20 minutes of absorption and initially reflects hypervolaemia.

Blood pressure may rise initially as a result of hypervolaemia. If plasma sodium is less than 120 mmol L^{-1} a reduction in heart rate is usually observed and profound bradycardia may occur. Reduced myocardial contractility produces wide-ranging ECG abnormalities, including loss of P waves, nodal rhythm, ventricular tachycardia, widened QRS complexes, depression of ST segments and T wave inversion.

Respiratory system

Oedema in the pulmonary vascular bed may result in dyspnoea, cyanosis and pulmonary oedema.

Nervous system

In patients undergoing TURP under spinal or epidural blockade, the first signs of excess absorption have been classically described as mental disorientation and restlessness, often immediately preceded by severe apprehension. Other CNS effects include reduction in level of consciousness and grand mal seizures. Transient blindness has been described and has been attributed to a direct effect of glycine on ocular retinal potentials.

Management

- Early serum sodium measurement should be performed.
- Surgery should be concluded as soon as is feasible and bladder irrigation with warm normal saline should be commenced.
- Ventilation should be appropriately supported.
- Baseline laboratory investigations should include full blood count, electrolytes, arterial blood gases and clotting screen.
- Administration of an intravenous diuretic, usually furosemide in an initial dosage of 20 mg, and concomitant infusion of normal saline may resolve the problem. As a diuresis commences fluid balance should be maintained with normal saline. Further administration of diuretic should be based on assessment of initial diuresis.
- In most centres, administration of hypertonic saline is restricted to the small group of patients demonstrating severe symptoms, e.g. seizures or severe cardiac dysfunction as a result of electrolyte imbalance. Infusion of hypertonic saline must be undertaken with caution, via a central line and with appropriate cardiovascular monitoring, and should not exceed a rate of administration of 100 mL h^{-1} in order to avoid further fluid overload. Measurement of pulmonary capillary wedge pressure is desirable in this situation.
- During the diuresis, the serum potassium should be monitored as hypokalaemia frequently occurs during this phase.

Prevention of TURP syndrome

- The patient requires appropriate preoperative preparation with monitoring of urea and electrolytes. Adequate hydration should be maintained prior to surgery, particularly if elderly or debilitated.
- The main factor in prevention of development of the syndrome is limitation of the duration of the surgical procedure. When possible, resection time should be restricted to less than 1 hour. If fluid is absorbed at a rate in excess of 50 mL min^{-1}, fluid overload of 3 litres may occur within this time frame.
- Haemodynamic stability should be maintained. Significant hypotension reduces the venous pressure in the periprostatic bed and permits excess absorption.
- Caution should be exercised with the height of the bag of irrigation fluid, which, if placed inappropriately high, may increase the hydrostatic pressure generated within the surgical field, thus increasing the risks of absorption.
- Bladder distension should be kept to a minimum and frequent bladder drainage reduces the quantity of irrigant absorbed.
- Techniques now exist for calculation of fluid absorption by addition of trace amounts of ethanol to the irrigation fluid and monitoring of expired ethanol.

Bibliography

Hahn RG. Ethanol monitoring of irrigating fluid absorption in transurethral prostatic surgery. *Anesthesiology* 1988; **65**: 867–73.

Hahn RG. The transurethral resection syndrome. *Acta Anaesthesiol Scand* 1991; **35**: 557–67.

Hawary A, Mukhtar K, Sinclair A, Pearce I. Transurethral resection of the prostate syndrome: almost gone but not forgotten. *J Endourol* 2009; **23**: 2013–20.

Cross-references

Minor gynaecological procedures, 460
Transurethral resection of prostate, 498

Index